SECOND EDITION

Bacterial Pathogenesis

A Molecular Approach

SECOND EDITION

Bacterial Pathogenesis

A Molecular Approach

Abigail A. Salyers and Dixie D. Whitt

Department of Microbiology, University of Illinois, Urbana, Illinois

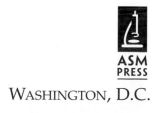

ASM
PRESS

WASHINGTON, D.C.

Address editorial correspondence to ASM Press, 1752 N St., NW, Washington, DC 20036-2904, USA

Send orders to ASM Press, P.O. Box 605, Herndon, VA 20172, USA
Phone: 800-546-2416; 703-661-1593
Fax: 703-661-1501
E-mail: books@asmusa.org
Online: www.asmpress.org

Library of Congress Cataloging-in-Publication Data

Salyers, Abigail A.
Bacterial pathogenesis : a molecular approach / Abigail A. Salyers and Dixie D. Whitt.–2nd ed.
p. ; cm.
Includes bibliographical references and index.
ISBN 1-55581-171-X (softcover)
1. Bacteria diseases—Pathogenesis. 2 Molecular microbiology. I. Whitt, Dixie D. II. Title.
[DNLM: 1. Bacterial–pathogenicity. 2. Bacterial Infections—etiology. 3. Bacterial Infections—prevention & control. 4. Host-Parasite Relations. 5. Virulence. QZ 65 S186b 2002]
QR201.B34 S24 2002
616'.014—dc21

2001045809

10 9 8 7 6 5 4 3 2 1

Cover and interior design: Susan Brown Schmidler
Cover illustration: Terese Winslow

This book is dedicated to Carl Woese, a valued colleague and an inspiring example of a scientist whose creative insights into the evolution and phylogeny of microorganisms have fundamentally transformed the way scientists view microbiology and the evolutionary relationships among all organisms. This book reflects his impact on our thinking about how bacteria can cause disease and how important it is to view the disease process from an evolutionary perspective.

Contents

Preface

The Changing Face of Bacterial Pathogenesis

The first edition of *Bacterial Pathogenesis: a Molecular Approach* was published in 1994 when the field of bacterial pathogenesis research was still in the process of entering the molecular age. At the time, many scientists working in the area advocated focusing on a few well-studied organisms, such as *Escherichia coli* and *Salmonella typhimurium*. They believed that this strategy would furnish basic information about bacterial virulence strategies that would be applicable to most, if not all, bacterial pathogens. This expectation was based on the highly successful use of model organisms to understand such central life processes as DNA replication, transcription, and translation. In retrospect, given what we now know about the mind-boggling diversity of microbes, it seems surprising that *E. coli* and *S. typhimurium* proved to be such good models for the basic metabolic processes that are shared by all free-living cells, including eukaryotes as well as bacteria and archaea.

In the intervening years, several things have happened that have forced scientists to question the model system approach to pathogenesis research. First, although closely related species such as *E. coli, S. typhimurium, Shigella dysenteriae,* and *Yersinia enterocolitica* (which today would have been classified as members of a single species) did prove to have very similar virulence factors, the insights from studies of these species were not necessarily applicable to more distantly related bacteria, such as the gram-positive cocci. Comparisons of genome sequences across genus and phylum lines are revealing that, while there are core functions that are highly conserved—mostly the basic life processes, such as DNA replication, transcription, translation, and the synthesis of amino acids and nucleic acids—there is considerable variety in other genes. This is not surprising given that many of the genes an organism carries are responsible for strategies required to occupy different niches, both inside and outside the human body.

A second realization was that pathogenesis research, far more than basic molecular studies of the past, affects human lives more immediately at the practical level. Given this, does it make sense to focus exclusively on a few paradigm organisms such as *E. coli* and *S. typhi-*

murium when the biggest problem in hospitals today is the gram-positive cocci? The answer, obviously, is to stay with the paradigm organisms but to branch out into areas that have been relatively underdeveloped.

Once one takes the position that pathogenesis research should focus on topics that could become important at the practical level, either for preventing or for treating bacterial diseases, yet another shift in perspective occurs: microbial ecology becomes very important. How many examples do we need of cases in which changes in human practices are accompanied by the emergence of new microbial pathogens before we realize that infectious disease patterns are a reflection of human and microbial ecology? Especially when prevention of disease is the goal of a study, the ecology of the disease-causing microbe and its interactions with potential human hosts become critical considerations. Also, as investigators began to take the concept of host-parasite interactions seriously, more attention had to be given to understanding how microbial interactions with the human body led to the pathology of the disease being studied. The use of cultured mammalian cells as a model for the host side of the host-parasite interaction has been useful, but ultimately the most important features to understand are the mode of entry of a pathogen into the body and why it infects some organs but not others.

All of these influences have combined to produce a field of bacterial pathogenesis that looks very different than it did when the first edition of this text was published. In the second edition, we have tried to capture what we see as the new face of pathogenesis research by paying much more attention to the microbial ecology and pathobiology of different bacterial diseases. When we embarked on this project, we thought that a second edition of an existing book would be easy to write—add a few sections to existing chapters and update the references. This proved to be a serious miscalculation. It soon became clear that we would have to rewrite the book completely to capture not only new research findings but also the new perspective on the host-parasite interaction. In many senses this book is not so much a second edition of the old *Bacterial Pathogenesis* book but the first edition of a book that has the same title.

A major problem we faced as authors was that not only had the feel of pathogenesis research changed, but also the amount of published material had increased manyfold. It was a daunting task for us to keep on top of the material that went into the first edition. The problem of information overload was much worse this time around. We have tried to compensate for the inevitable errors and misunderstandings that we would make if left to our own devices by having each chapter reviewed, often by several reviewers. The reviewers' comments were most helpful, and virtually all of their suggestions have been incorporated into the final text. This is one case in which reviewers can congratulate themselves for having a significant impact on what they spent precious hours reviewing.

Features of the Text

Something that surprised us in the response to the first edition was that so many people liked the simple illustrations. In the first edition, the simplicity of the figures was dictated by our desire to keep the cost of the book as low as possible. We now realize that students appreciate simple figures because they focus attention on critical points and principles. Ever ready to learn from our readers and students, we have kept the same style of illustration in this volume.

Two new features have been added to the chapters in this edition. One appears at the beginning of each chapter that covers a particular bacterium or group of bacteria—a short snapshot of the organism(s) covered in that chapter. The purpose of this feature is to present the organism as an intact entity associated with a particular disease before the student dives into the detailed material presented in the text of the chapter. With so much material available, it is easy for students to get lost in the details and to lose sight of the organism and its niche. This feature was suggested to us by Anne Morris Hooke.

A second new feature is the changed form of the summary section at the end of each chapter. In the first edition, the summary section had a narrative form. We have since concluded that this form of summary is not only of little use to students but even encouraged some of them to think that it can replace the chapter text. In this edition, we have presented the summaries in outline and table form, a summary format that in our experience is much more useful to students and encourages students to process the material covered in the chapter in a slightly different way.

For the most part, the comments of reviewers on the content and organization of the book were positive, but there was one complaint we found a little disturbing—that we had dropped what little bacterial physiology there was in the first edition. This complaint arose from the fact that there was no chapter entitled "bacterial physiology." We strongly disagree with this way of organizing text material. If we have learned anything over the past few decades, it is that bacterial physiology is not an isolated topic that can be summarized neatly in a chapter or two but varies widely depending on the microorganism and its environmental setting. In our view, the physiology of each microorganism should be woven into the chapter that covers that microorganism or presented along with such topics as the action of antibiotics and the characteristics of the host defense systems. Bacterial physiology makes much more sense when it is presented in a real-world context. We also take issue with those who see "bacterial physiology" as synonymous with glycolysis, the tricarboxylic acid (TCA) cycle, and amino acid biosynthetic pathways. In our opinion, toxin production, pilin production, and peptidoglycan synthesis are more appropriate and important aspects of the physiology of bacteria that cause human disease. Also, we have noticed that the minute the subject of glycolysis and the TCA cycle comes up, independent of any relevance to disease, students start to nod off, perhaps never to return to consciousness.

Teamwork

This book has two authors listed on the cover, but as anyone who has gone through the process of book production knows, a book is a group effort that involves not only the authors but also members of the publisher's staff and the reviewers. We are particularly grateful to Jeff Holtmeier and Susan Birch for keeping us on the right path, sometimes with great difficulty, and for always being there to answer our many questions. We also appreciate their patience. It must have been frustrating for them to watch our fits and starts of composition as we came to the daunting realization that it was necessary to completely rewrite this book to bring it up-to-date. We have a new sympathy for publishers who have to fit sometimes-unreliable authors into some sort of rational business plan. We now know why Prozac had to be invented. We also thank Mary McKenney, our copy editor. She has been an all-around good sport and an excellent copy editor. Cathy Balogh deserves thanks for patiently incorporating our many changes into the manuscript.

A major contribution to this text and the original edition was made by the legion of reviewers who patiently read drafts of the chapters and made a number of very useful suggestions. With a few exceptions, we did not know the identity of the reviewers. ASM Press has consented to release this previously confidential list to honor those who selflessly gave their time to make both editions of this book as accurate as possible.

We thank the following reviewers enthusiastically: Alan G. Barbour, University of California, Irvine; Stephen B. Calderwood, Massachusetts General Hospital, Boston; Virginia L. Clark, University of Rochester, Rochester, N.Y.; P. Patrick Cleary, University of Minnesota, Minneapolis; R. John Collier, Harvard Medical School, Boston, Mass.; John Davies, Monash University,

Clayton, Victoria, Australia; Michael P. Doyle, University of Georgia, Griffin; B. Brett Finlay, University of British Columbia, Vancouver; Vincent A. Fischetti, Rockefeller University, New York, N.Y.; Frank C. Gherardini, Rocky Mountain Labs, Hamilton, Mont.; Peter H. Gilligan, University of North Carolina Hospitals, Chapel Hill; Paul A. Gulig, University of Florida, Gainesville; Stuart Hazell, University of Southern Queensland, Toowoomba, Australia; Anne Morris Hooke, Miami University, Oxford, Ohio; Barbara H. Iglewski, University of Rochester Medical Center, Rochester, N.Y.; Ralph R. Isberg, Tufts University School of Medicine, Boston, Mass.; James R. Johnson, University of Minnesota, Minneapolis; David M. Lyerly, Techlab Inc., Blacksburg, Va.; Anthony T. Maurelli, Uniformed Services University of the Health Sciences, Bethesda, Md.; Jeffery F. Miller, University of California, Los Angeles; Virginia L. Miller, Washington University School of Medicine, St. Louis, Mo.; Stephen A. Morse, Centers for Disease Control and Prevention, Atlanta, Ga.; Steve L. Moseley, University of Washington, Seattle; Irving Nachamkin, University of Pennsylvania, Philadelphia; Alison D. O'Brien, Uniformed Services University of the Health Sciences, Bethesda, Md.; Todd Patrick, Mayo Clinic, Rochester, Minn.; David H. Persing, Corixa Corporation, Seattle, Wash.; Daniel A. Portnoy, University of California, Berkeley; Steven J. Projan, Wyeth-Ayerst Research, Pearl River, N.Y.; Thomas M. Shinnick, Centers for Disease Control and Prevention, Atlanta, Ga.; Susan Straley, University of Kentucky, Lexington; Richard A. Strugnell, The University of Melbourne, Parkville, Victoria, Australia; Ronald K. Taylor, Dartmouth Medical School, Hanover, N.H.; Elaine Tuomanen, St. Jude's Children's Research Hospital, Memphis, Tenn.; Janis J. Weis, University of Utah, Salt Lake City; Susan E. H. West, University of Wisconsin, Madison; Tracy D. Wilkins, Virginia Polytechnic Institute and State University, Blacksburg.

We also want to thank two local reviewers, Brenda Wilson and Stanley Maloy, both colleagues at the University of Illinois, who stepped into the breach when we needed specific advice or reviews on an emergency basis. D.W. thanks Greg, whose eyes only occasionally became glazed during what must have seemed at times to be somewhat excessive discussions about "the book."

Finally, we want to thank the many undergraduate and graduate students who have contributed to this edition and the first edition by telling us of their experiences with the text. We have found that, if asked, students are quite willing to express opinions about their textbooks and often make insightful comments.

Foreword

The first edition of Abigail Salyers' and Dixie Whitt's book *Bacterial Pathogenesis: A Molecular Approach* was instantly adopted by most of us who teach bacterial pathogenesis to graduate students and advanced undergraduates. In the foreword of the first edition, I thanked the authors for the extraordinary work they invested in providing such a rich teaching medium. I have now taught a number of classes from this marvelous text, and clearly students like the text and are challenged by the authors' constant urging to consider the implications of the research and ideas that surround the study of bacterial pathogens.

This book is, as the authors state, not so much a second edition as the first edition of a book that has the same title. I agree that the growth of the field called bacterial pathogenesis has undergone a remarkable revolution in the 7 years since the first edition appeared. One revolutionary advance was the study of the cell biology of the interaction between bacterial pathogens and host cells. True, this was mostly the study of bacteria interacting with cultured animal cell models and not the "real world," but the result was the emergence of a new discipline called cellular microbiology, which has spawned two new textbooks and a journal. Moreover, the complete genomes of most of the pathogenic bacteria considered in this book have been sequenced (or, I should say, at least one strain of most of the pathogens mentioned in this book has been sequenced). Already one is inundated by genomic comparisons, bioinformatic analysis, and the use of DNA arrays to study transcription and the host response to interactions between bacteria and their hosts. There is talk of experiments performed "in silico." The authors handle these new technologies and knowledge with aplomb and do a splendid job of explaining the technology and its implications in a way that students will appreciate.

Students and instructors will also appreciate the newer features of this book. The authors now provide a short biography at the beginning of each chapter on a particular pathogen. At the end of each chapter they also provide a summary in a convenient outline form. The illustrations in the book are notable for their simplicity. Better for a student to understand a concept from a simple line drawing than to be hopelessly confused by an artist's multicolored rendition of minutiae.

I noted in the foreword to the first edition my admiration for the personal flavor of the authors' writing and their determination to state their opinions about unsolved ideas. The current version of their book retains this flavor. I'm also pleased to see that the questions for students to consider at the end of each chapter remain an excellent feature of this book.

Salyers and Whitt assert that the discipline of bacterial pathogenesis looks very different to them now than it did when the first edition of the book was published. They pay more attention to microbial ecology and pathobiology of different bacterial diseases as one way to address these changes. They also try to pay more attention to practical aspects of preventing or treating bacterial diseases. Prevention of microbial disease is the ultimate goal of medicine, and it is a goal shared by those of us who study the biology of bacterial pathogenicity. Yet, as one of the oldest practitioners in the field of bacterial pathogenicity, I cannot help but reflect on the fact that my first postdoctoral job in 1960 was with people who had spent most of their lives searching for new vaccines for typhoid, dysentery, cholera, and other infectious diarrheal diseases. With all of the splendid advances in the field, which students will appreciate better after reading this book, it is important to understand that we are still in desperate need of new vaccines against typhoid, dysentery, and cholera and most of the gram-positive cocci and most of the other organisms that are the subject matter of this book. This is humbling and serves to underscore the first chapter, in which the authors warn us, "Never Underestimate the Power of Bacteria." Students need to be aware of this as they read about our unraveling of facts about pathogenic bacteria and how we humans have evolved to resist their onslaught. The study of bacterial pathogenesis still represents a cutting edge of basic and medical research. Understanding bacterial pathogenesis is of inestimable importance for the control of the most important source of human misery. Thus, while this excellent book is a tribute to scientific progress and captures the excitement, enthusiasm, and optimism that the practitioners of bacterial pathogenesis feel, the students who read this book should not come away with the idea that we have gained the upper hand—yet. There is still room for many more editions for generations of students to follow. I hope I'm around to write the foreword(s).

Stanley Falkow
Stanford University School of Medicine
Stanford, California

I

Basic Principles

P HILOSOPHERS AND THEOLOGIANS may glorify humans as the crown of creation, but bacteria view humans more accurately as the proverbial free lunch. By the time humans appeared on the evolutionary scene, bacteria and other microbes had shaped the physicochemical environment of earth and were firmly in charge of the destiny of any subsequent life forms. From the beginning, humans had to come to terms with the microbial world. The fact that there are so many humans on earth today is proof of the fact that humans have successfully adapted to cope with the billions of microbes encountered every day.

Fortunately for us, most microbes seem to be neutral or beneficial to us. There are some, however, that can be injurious to our health. These disease-causing bacteria are the subject of this book. The book is divided in two parts. In part I, we cover the basic principles of infectious disease. Bacterial infections are best viewed as the outcome of a complex set of interactions between bacteria and the defenses of the human body. These interactions include intellectual as well as physical ones; knowledge of the characteristics of disease-causing bacteria and how these bacteria are transmitted is one of the primary protective barriers against infection.

An important part of the infectious disease story is that the pattern of infectious diseases is a dynamic one. This is true both on the personal level and on the larger population level. On the personal level, the outcome of exposure to a disease-causing bacterium is not a foregone conclusion. Depending on the status of a person's defenses and the number of bacteria encountered, a whole gamut of possibilities may ensue, ranging from no disease to symptomatic, even fatal, infection. On a population level, the types of diseases currently circulating can vary with time and place. Epidemics come and go. New types of infections arise. Although microbes have long dominated the Earth, human activities have an impact on the human-microbe interaction. Changing human practices eliminate some diseases and make new ones possible. The chapters in part I are designed to provide an overview of the factors that affect the outcome of human-microbe interactions.

1

The Uneasy Truce: Never Underestimate the Power of Bacteria

Why Bacteria Are Once Again in the Public Health Spotlight

Antibiotics were first introduced into widespread clinical use in the 1950s. The term applied to them at the time, "miracle drugs," gives some indication of the euphoria felt by physicians and the public when this new therapy became available. It was true that prior to this point the medical community had gained greater control over infectious diseases than ever before. In clinics and hospitals, hygienic practices such as hand washing and disinfectant use were reducing the risk of disease transmission. In the community, improved nutrition made people better able to resist infections; less crowded conditions and a clean water supply had reduced disease transmission. Vaccines gave protection against some much-feared diseases. Nonetheless, bacterial infections such as pneumonia, tuberculosis, and syphilis continued to take a heavy toll, and infectious diseases were still a leading cause of death.

Antibiotics appeared as the superweapon that would give humans the final decisive victory over bacteria. In the early euphoria over the success of antibiotics, scientists and policy makers alike concluded that bacterial infections were no longer a threat, and they turned their attention to other problems, such as cancer, heart disease, and viral infections. For the next 3 decades, bacteria were of interest mainly as tractable model systems for studying physiology and genetics and as a source of tools for the new genetic engineering technology that was revolutionizing all of biology. Confidence that bacterial diseases were completely under control was bolstered by the fact that there was a glut of new antibiotics on the market.

Unnoticed by all but a few, the first cracks began to appear in the protective shield against bacterial disease. Antibiotics were no longer the highly profitable products they had once been, especially not compared to heart medications or tranquilizers, which had to be taken daily for long periods of time. Also, antibiotics were becoming harder to find and more expensive to develop. One company after another quietly cut back or dismantled its antibiotic discovery program. For a while, the cracks appeared not to matter. There were still plenty of new antibiotics that still worked on the bacteria that had become

3

resistant to the old standbys like penicillin. Warnings from scientists that bacteria were becoming more resistant to antibiotics were ignored or ridiculed. During the late 1980s, however, scientists began to notice an increase in bacterial infections. By 1995, infectious diseases became one of the top five causes of death in the United States. Even with the AIDS epidemic in full swing, most infectious disease deaths were caused by bacterial diseases such as pneumonia and bacterial bloodstream infections (sepsis). Why was the incidence of bacterial pneumonia and sepsis increasing? For one thing, the population was aging, and older people are more likely to contract these diseases. For another, modern medicine had created an increasingly large population of patients whose immune systems had been temporarily disrupted owing to cancer chemotherapy or immunosuppressive therapy following organ transplants.

Another development that caught many in the medical community by surprise was the appearance of new diseases, dubbed **emerging infectious diseases.** In the past, scientists had assumed that any microorganism capable of causing disease would surely have done so by now, given the millions of years humans had occupied the planet. This view overlooks two important facts. First, bacteria can change their genetic makeup very rapidly to take advantage of new opportunities. Members of some bacterial populations are hypermutable, making it possible for them to try many genetic combinations in seeking the one that is most appropriate for the current environment the bacterium is experiencing. Also, bacteria can acquire genes that confer new virulence traits or resistance to antibiotics from other bacteria. Second, changing human practices, such as the widespread use of air-conditioning and the appearance of crowded intensive care wards in big hospitals, brought susceptible people into contact with microorganisms that had not previously had the opportunity to cause human infections.

Scientists and physicians began to realize that a decisive human victory over bacteria had not occurred and was not going to occur anytime in the future. The best that could be hoped for was a standoff, one that would require constant vigilance to maintain. Something no one liked to contemplate was the specter of the return to the preantibiotic era, at least in the case of some bacterial infections. This prospect is horrific not only from the health standpoint but also from the standpoint of public psychology. The public has been none too happy over the failure of the medical community to cure diseases like AIDS and herpes. To have had a cure and lost it would be a lot more traumatic. This is the kind of thing that brings people down to the town square wielding pitchforks and torches.

This brief account of how bacterial diseases have come back into prominence as a health problem explored the recent past. But to understand fully why bacteria are such formidable opponents, it is desirable to take a longer look at their history, a history that explains their impressive ability to adapt and respond rapidly to whatever humans throw at them.

Ancient History Takes a Toll on Today's Human Health

Bacteria and **archaea,** the two domains of the prokaryotic world, were the first forms of life to appear on ancient Earth, about 3.5 to 4 billion years ago (Figure 1–1). Bacteria and archaea ruled the world undisputed for about a billion years before the first eukaryotes appeared. During this period, they created the global geochemical cycles that made the Earth habitable. Earth is a closed system, and unless compounds that are used are recycled, all life would cease. Bacteria put the first molecular oxygen in the Earth's atmosphere, creating the ozone layer, which protected the Earth's surface from the killing radiation that formerly bombarded it. Life on the surface of the Earth was now possible. By adding molecular oxygen to the atmosphere, bacteria also created conditions that permitted the later evolution of oxygen-utilizing creatures such as us.

In the course of their long history, bacteria developed a variety of other metabolic capabilities that allowed them to survive under an impressive variety of conditions. There are bacteria that can obtain energy by oxidizing sulfide, by reducing sulfate, by oxidizing ammonia, by reducing nitrate, and by oxidizing methane—to name only a few of the vast number of metabolic types represented in the bacterial world. Bacteria also learned how to maximize the plasticity of their genomes, constantly acquiring new DNA and mutating or rearranging existing genes, thereby creating new capabilities that enabled them to colonize the many

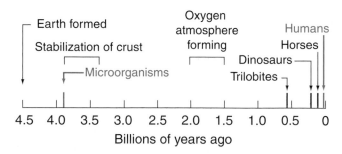

Figure 1–1 Overview of microbial evolution. Microorganisms appeared 3.5 to 4 billion years ago and changed Earth so that higher animals could evolve.

niches the Earth provided. So far, no part of the Earth has been found to be free of bacteria. They live in arctic ice, in the deep subsurface of the land masses, in the surface layer and depths of the oceans, and in boiling hot springs. The genetic plasticity that made the evolution of such metabolically diverse organisms possible stands them in good stead today as they face new challenges and opportunities.

Bacteria became specialists in metabolic diversity, in contrast to eukaryotes, which specialized primarily in morphological diversity. In fact, eukaryotes generally expand their metabolic diversity by acquiring bacteria or archaea as **endosymbionts.** Cells of what later became plants, for example, acquired the ability to photosynthesize by acquiring photosynthetic bacteria as endosymbionts. Some plants also recruited bacterial endosymbionts for their root cells, so that the bacteria could fix atmospheric nitrogen, making the plant self-fertilizing. Animals recruited bacteria and archaea to colonize their intestinal tracts for protective or nutritional reasons. For example, ruminants such as cattle and goats rely on their ruminal bacteria to digest grasses and other forages, producing simple compounds the animal can use.

Bacteria also became experts in how to survive the sort of population crashes that would lead to the extinction of more complex life forms. If the human population were to be reduced from its current level to a few thousand by some catastrophe, could the human race survive, and if so, how long would it take to regain its current population levels? Centuries, millennia? Bacteria routinely experience population crashes even greater in magnitude than this and yet manage to regain their former numbers within weeks or months. No wonder bacteria took antibiotics in stride so easily. After facing voracious protozoa, volcanoes, and ice ages, antibiotics would hardly register as more than a minor annoyance.

About 2.5 billion years ago, the first **eukaryotes** appeared, the single-celled **protozoa.** Although some eukaryotic microbes gain carbon by fixing CO_2 and gain energy from photosynthesis, many protozoa live by feeding on bacteria and archaea. There is an interesting aspect of protozoal grazing that is seldom mentioned. Protozoa have properties similar to human phagocytic cells, which form an important part of the defenses of the human body. Some of these phagocytic cells function mainly to clear bacteria and other invaders from blood and tissue. Others break down bacteria and present segments of their proteins to the cells of the immune system. Some bacteria capable of causing disease have developed strategies for evading phagocytosis or surviving inside phagocytic cells. The evolution of such strategies could well have begun soon after the appearance of the first protozoa. Similarly, some of the toxic proteins that disease-causing bacteria use to kill or alter the functions of human cells could have evolved originally to allow bacteria to return the favor by immobilizing or even feeding on their protozoal adversaries.

If this view of bacterial evolution is correct, then there are likely to be far more bacteria in nature than we thought that are capable of causing disease. Bacteriologists tend to tell anyone who will listen that only a tiny minority of bacteria cause disease. This is true as far as the list of bacteria currently known to cause disease goes, but is this list anywhere near complete? Some people are even questioning whether it is safe to bring samples back from Mars. Is it possible that microbes capable of causing human disease could evolve on a planet without humans? In this case, the low temperature of Mars would seem to preclude the evolution of bacteria that could grow at human body temperature. Yet, there are bacteria (e.g., *Listeria monocytogenes*) that are capable of growing at refrigerator temperatures but can also infect humans. Are there some microorganisms with an even larger range of growth temperatures?

When animals and humans appeared on the evolutionary scene, bacteria immediately took advantage of these new niches for colonization. To a bacterium used to the vagaries of the external environment, where temperature and the availability of water and nutrients can vary widely (and unpredictably), a warm-blooded animal whose temperature is stably maintained and who spends most of its time searching for food and water must be as close as it gets to bacterial heaven. Given this, it should not surprise us that the bodies of humans and animals carry dense bacterial loads, especially in the mouth, intestinal tract, and vaginal tract. Small wonder that the human body is often referred to in the scientific literature on bacterium-human interactions as the "host."

Scientists who study the evolution of insects, animals, and humans have almost completely ignored the selective pressure exerted by the presence of large and diverse populations of bacteria in or on the animal body. As will become evident later in this book, the effects of microbial pressure can be seen clearly in the design of human skin, the intestinal tract, the vaginal tract, and the immune system.

Pressing Current Issues

Having made this digression into ancient history, let us now return to the present and examine some of the public health issues that have brought bacterial infections once again to the forefront. These include emerging infectious diseases, increasing problems with large outbreaks of **food-borne** and **water-borne infections,** **hospital-acquired (nosocomial) infections, bioterror-ism, microbiota shift diseases,** and **antibiotic resistance.**

Emerging and Reemerging Infectious Diseases

The appearance of apparently new bacterial diseases and the reemergence of old diseases that were thought to be under control (at least in developed countries) was an unpleasant shock to the health care community. Emerging and reemerging infectious diseases illustrate an important principle. Disease patterns do change, both because bacteria change and because changing human activities can create new opportunities for bacteria to cause disease. Not all diseases are truly emerging in the sense of being new to the human population. In some cases, the disease has been around for a long time, but the bacterial cause has only recently been identified. These diseases are "emerging" only in the minds of the scientists who study them. Diseases can also wane in importance. The near eradication of syphilis in most developed countries is an example of a waning (submerging?) bacterial disease. Also, old diseases can return if conditions change to favor their reemergence. Since disease patterns can change in different ways and for different reasons, we have invented a new classification system for bacterial diseases that we hope will help to make this important point.

This classification system has four categories: **new-new diseases** (diseases caused by previously unidentified bacteria that have only recently entered the human population), **new-old diseases** (diseases caused by newly recognized pathogens that have been around for a long time), **old-new diseases** (diseases caused by well-known bacterial pathogens that were thought to have been eliminated but have recently reappeared), and **old-old diseases** (diseases caused by long-known bacteria that have remained high in incidence but can be classified as emerging in the sense that the public and the media are only now beginning to notice them). Some examples of bacterial diseases that fall into these different categories are listed in Table 1–1.

NEW-NEW DISEASES. It is difficult to know for sure that a particular disease is really new in the sense that it is appearing for the first time in human history, because collections of clinical specimens go back only 100 years at most. Moreover, because of the great changes that have occurred in medical nomenclature and per-

Table 1–1 Types of emerging, reemerging, or simply ignored bacterial infectious diseases

Category	Definition	Examples
New-new diseases	New diseases caused by newly discovered bacterial species	Lyme disease Legionnaires' disease
New-old diseases	Diseases caused by newly recognized pathogens that have been known for a long time	*Campylobacter* food-borne disease Cat scratch disease Whipple's disease
Old-new diseases	Old diseases with known causes, which were thought to be eliminated but have reappeared	Tuberculosis Cholera Diphtheria (in former Soviet Union)
	Long-known pathogens acquiring traits that make them more dangerous	Antibiotic-resistant bacteria, e.g., *Streptococcus pneumoniae Staphylococcus aureus Enterococcus* spp.
Old-old diseases	Old diseases with known causes that are now being recognized by the public and the media	*Chlamydia trachomatis* Gonorrhea

ceptions of disease, it is difficult to tell from descriptions of diseases written as recently as 100 years ago whether or not the disease is one we see today. (For those who like nothing better than to snuggle down with an impenetrable philosophical text that might just have something important to say, there is a book on the subject of changing human perspectives by Michael Foucault called *The Order of Things*.)

An example of a new-new bacterial disease is **Lyme disease,** which is caused by the spirochete *Borrelia burgdorferi* and transmitted to humans by the deer tick. This disease has probably been around for a long time in the wild rodent population (the white-footed mouse, to be specific). The rise of Lyme disease in the late 20th century was the result of the confluence of three factors. First, the vector of disease, the deer tick, has as its main reservoir the white-tailed deer commonly found in the U.S. Northeast. The bacteria do not infect deer, but deer serve as the major reservoir for the tick, because the blood meal taken from the deer is important for the reproductive cycle of the tick. Second, in the 1980–1990 period, there was a deer population explosion in this area created by reforestation, limitations on hunting deer, disappearance of predators, and climatic factors. Many deer means many ticks. The ticks take a blood meal from the white-footed mice or from humans (as a second choice), and the disease spreads to the human population. Third, because of the increasing tendency of humans to build houses in forested areas or to hike in these areas, contacts between humans and rodents have increased. More deer, more ticks, and more mouse-human proximity lead to an increased likelihood that a deer tick that has taken a blood meal from a mouse infected with *B. burgdorferi* will come in contact with a human and spread that infection to humans (Figure 1–2).

Lyme disease also provides an example of another variable in disease incidence: human gullibility and human greed. Many articles about Lyme disease have appeared in the press, especially in areas where the disease is common. Thus, the public is aware that although the initial symptoms of the disease are transient, long-term neurological damage can occur. There are only about 5,000 reported cases of Lyme disease per year in the United States, so this is not a very common disease. Yet the potentially irreversible long-range consequences experienced by some infected people who were not diagnosed and treated early enough frighten the public.

There is a test for Lyme disease that is not very reliable and can give false-positive results. Some physicians who are unscrupulous—or in a few cases truly believe they are crusaders helping victims of advanced Lyme disease—have opened Lyme disease clinics. These clinics place billboards or radio ads listing the symptoms of advanced Lyme disease, which are so nonspecific that about a third of the people reading the billboard or hearing the ad are sure to have experienced at least one of them. People with one or more of these symptoms are urged to come to the clinic for a free Lyme disease test. Because of the unreliability of the test, which allows a certain latitude in diagnostic interpretation, many of the people who come to the clinic are diagnosed as having Lyme disease and are given expensive multiple-antibiotic therapy, which of course is sold by the clinic itself. A number of these clinics have been shut down, but the fact that they existed in the first place illustrates how fear of an infectious disease that has been overreported in the media can be exploited.

Yet another example of a new-new disease is **Legionnaires' disease,** which is caused by the gram-negative bacterium *Legionella pneumophila. L. pneumophila* has long been ubiquitous in soil and water but until recently was not recognized as a human pathogen. The development that brought *L. pneumophila* into prominence as a human pathogen was the installation of air-conditioning systems in hospitals and hotels. *L. pneumophila* took very quickly to the water-cooling towers of air-conditioning systems, forming bacterial biofilms from which large numbers of the bacteria were shed and entered the water circulating through the air-conditioning system. Through small leaks in the

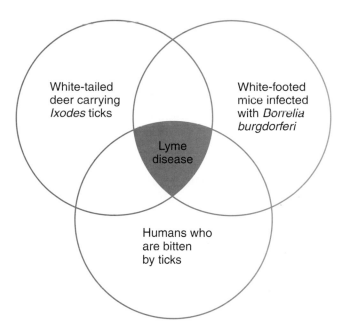

Figure 1–2 Factors leading to the entry of *B. burgdorferi* into the human population. Shaded area represents Lyme disease in humans resulting from the overlap of a large white-tailed deer population carrying *Ixodes* ticks, white-footed mouse populations with *B. burgdorferi* in the bloodstream, and humans who serve as a blood meal for hard-up ticks.

water-bearing coils, *L. pneumophila* entered the air of hotel or hospital rooms in a fine liquid aerosol. The name Legionnaires' disease arose from an outbreak of *L. pneumophila* lung infection that occurred after a Legionnaires' conference in a Philadelphia hotel. The Legionnaires attending the conference were predominantly elderly, and many had a history of smoking and alcohol abuse, two factors that diminish the effectiveness of the lung's defenses against bacteria. Bringing this population of unusually susceptible people into contact with larger numbers of the bacteria than they would normally have encountered created an ideal situation for a new disease to emerge.

Subsequent outbreaks have occurred in hospitals as well as hotels. Many outbreaks have been associated with contamination of air-conditioning water towers by *L. pneumophila,* but some have occurred as a result of nearby construction that puts small particles of contaminated soil into the air to be breathed by hospital patients. More recently, *L. pneumophila* has emerged as a cause of "ventilator pneumonia," a type of pneumonia that occurs in people with tubes introduced deep into the airway to support breathing. The air that flows through the ventilator is humidified, and if the water used to humidify the air becomes contaminated with bacteria, infection can result.

NEW-OLD DISEASES.   An example of a new-old disease is food-borne disease caused by *Campylobacter* species. *Salmonella enterica* serovar Typhimurium has long been known as a prominent cause of food-borne disease, but only recently have *Campylobacter* species been identified as being a common cause. *Campylobacter jejuni, Campylobacter coli,* and other *Campylobacter* species were described many years ago but were thought to be rather uncommon causes of human disease. Advances in the detection of *Campylobacter* species have now revealed that these bacteria are a very common cause of food-borne disease.

Another new-old disease is **cat scratch disease,** which is caused by *Bartonella henselae,* a gram-negative rod. In most medical textbooks, this bacterium is described—if it is mentioned at all—as a rare cause of disease. Another *Bartonella* species, *Bartonella quintana,* was a common cause of disease in World War I. The disease, **trench fever,** was spread by human lice from person to person in crowded military encampments. *B. henselae* was first recognized as a cause of skin nodules and systemic disease in AIDS patients. This species is not spread by lice but rather is acquired from flea-infested cats, which appear to be the natural reservoir. More recently, as methods for diagnosing *B. henselae* infections have improved, the number of known cases has increased and the disease is even being seen in otherwise healthy people.

OLD-NEW DISEASES.   Two of the most troubling recent infectious disease developments were the reappearance of **tuberculosis** in North America and the reappearance of **cholera** in South America. Tuberculosis and cholera are among the most feared bacterial diseases. Approximately one-third of the world's population is infected with the bacterium that causes tuberculosis. Fortunately, most of those who are infected do not develop the fatal form of the disease, but tuberculosis remains one of the leading causes of infectious disease deaths worldwide. Cholera is most commonly seen on the Indian subcontinent, where epidemics of cholera have killed millions of people. In the United States and other developed countries, tuberculosis rates had dropped so low that many people thought the disease had been eradicated. Cholera had become so uncommon in the United States and Latin America after the 1800s that medical textbooks called it an Old World disease.

How did these diseases stage a comeback? During the 1950s and 1960s, aggressive detection and treatment of tuberculosis succeeded in dramatically de-

creasing the incidence of the disease. There is a simple skin test for tuberculosis that is not perfect but is very helpful in identifying people infected with *Mycobacterium tuberculosis,* the bacterium that causes the disease. The treatment of tuberculosis is unusual in that the person being treated must take several antibiotics regularly over a period of 6 months or more. Many people experience unpleasant side effects when taking these drugs. Since the symptoms are brought under control long before the bacterium is eradicated from the body, patient compliance with therapy is usually poor. Thus, a keystone of effective treatment is monitoring of patients by health care workers to make sure they are taking their medications. When the number of tuberculosis cases had dropped precipitously by the early 1970s and remained low, the antituberculosis infrastructure was dismantled and tuberculosis was almost forgotten by the medical community.

During the 1980s, homelessness became a problem as a result of two developments. First, many people who had been incarcerated in mental health facilities were released without adequate support. The intent was good—not to warehouse human beings in inadequate institutions—but the effect was bad in that now the released patients had no regular source of income and shelter. Second, affordable housing disappeared in many urban centers, forcing people who could not afford high rents into the streets. Homeless shelters appeared, places where homeless people were housed in very crowded conditions. Many of the homeless abused alcohol or drugs, and many had human immunodeficiency virus (HIV) infections—all conditions that made them more susceptible to bacterial infections. A similar situation arose in large overcrowded prisons, where many of the prisoners were highly susceptible to diseases like tuberculosis.

These conditions provided a golden opportunity for *M. tuberculosis* to make a big comeback, and epidemics of tuberculosis began to occur. The medical community, caught by surprise and unable to believe that tuberculosis could actually be coming back, was slow to react. Many tuberculosis cases were not detected until the disease was well under way, allowing the infected person to infect many others before therapy was administered. Patients who were given medication were not supervised. Compliance among alcohol and drug abusers proved—not surprisingly—to be very poor, and *M. tuberculosis* had the chance to become resistant to the antituberculosis drugs. **Multidrug-resistant tuberculosis** was born.

Less is known about how the Latin American cholera epidemic originated, but *Vibrio cholerae,* the curved gram-negative rod that causes cholera, was probably introduced into Latin America in the bilge water that was dumped by Asian ships in the harbors of Latin America. Conditions were ripe for an epidemic because water sources throughout much of Latin America are not adequately treated to prevent water-borne spread of disease. Cholera began to spread through Latin America, causing many deaths (Figure 1–3). In contrast to the response of the medical community in the United States to the reemergence of tuberculosis, the Latin American medical community reacted rapidly and aggressively to bring cholera under control. The epidemic was stopped in a surprisingly short period of time, considering that most of the countries involved are poor and lack adequate resources for handling such a medical emergency. The reemergence of tuberculosis and cholera in the Americas illustrates a critically important principle: eternal vigilance is the price of health.

A somewhat different type of infectious disease problem that might be classified as an old-new disease occurs when a long-known bacterial pathogen acquires new traits that make it more dangerous. An example is **antibiotic-resistant bacteria.** Abuse and overuse of antibiotics by physicians and patients have created conditions that foster the appearance of multidrug-resistant pathogens such as *Streptococcus pneumoniae* (the most common cause of pneumonia and a common cause of sepsis), *Staphylococcus aureus* (a cause of pneumonia, sepsis, and wound infections), and *Enterococcus* species (an increasingly common cause of sepsis in hospital patients). Some of these bacteria are now resistant to virtually all known antibiotics. Hospital managers and executives of managed health care companies have become increasingly concerned about antibiotic-resistant bacteria, not only because these bacteria can cause strokes, long-term organ damage, and death, but because the cost to treat patients with antibiotic-resistant infections is 10 to 100 times the cost to treat patients with susceptible infections. Health care administrators are also afraid that if the resistance problem becomes much greater, some types of surgery, such as bypass operations, may become too risky for general use. Antibiotic resistance and its consequences will be discussed in more detail in a later chapter.

Another example of how acquisition of a new trait can turn an old familiar enemy into a new and more frightening one is *Escherichia coli* O157:H7, a strain that causes bloody diarrhea (dysentery) and kidney failure. This strain originally caused ordinary diarrhea, which is seldom fatal except in infants, in whom it can be devastating. Subsequently, O157:H7 acquired genes encoding a protein toxin, and possibly some other as-yet-undetermined traits, that allowed it to cause bloody diarrhea and kidney failure. This example is a

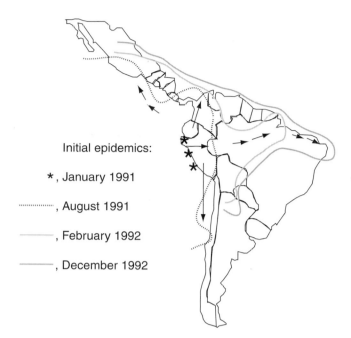

Initial epidemics:

*, January 1991

⋯⋯⋯, August 1991

——, February 1992

——, December 1992

Figure 1–3 Map showing the spread of cholera in the Western Hemisphere, based on surveillance by the Centers for Disease Control and Prevention during 1992. In 1992, 339,561 cholera cases and 2,321 cholera-related deaths were reported from 21 countries in the Western Hemisphere, bringing the total number of reported cases to 731,312 and the total number of deaths to 6,323 deaths since the beginning of the epidemic in January 1991. Map and data obtained from *Morbidity and Mortality Weekly Report.*

bit more problematic than antibiotic-resistant bacteria as an example of old-new disease. It is not clear exactly when *E. coli* O157:H7 acquired its "new" virulence genes; according to biologists who study bacterial evolution, this strain could have arisen thousands of years ago. Either the acquisition of the toxin genes occurred very recently in an old strain of *E. coli,* or there were ecological reasons for the failure of this strain to surface as a cause of human infections until the last decade of the 20th century.

OLD-OLD DISEASES. To complete the symmetry of our classification scheme, we have to include old-old diseases, but we realize that including them under the heading "emerging and reemerging infectious diseases" will strain the credulity of even the least critical reader. Yet there is justification for including them, because the diseases used to exemplify this category have been considered by some to be emerging infectious diseases. As with the new-old diseases, which are emerging in the minds of scientists because of the discovery that a newly described bacterium is an important part of the infectious disease picture, old-old diseases, although not increasing in incidence, are emerging in the sense that the medical community and the public are only now beginning to appreciate their importance.

The resurgence of tuberculosis in the United States received much media attention, yet another epidemic remained almost unrecognized: **bacterial sexually transmitted diseases.** *Chlamydia trachomatis,* currently the most common cause of reportable bacterial infections in the United States, has been virtually ignored by the medical community and the public until very recently. *C. trachomatis* causes a cervical infection that is asymptomatic in about two-thirds of infected women. It also causes urethritis in men that is more likely to be symptomatic, but up to one-fourth of infected men have no noticeable symptoms. People who do not know they are infected are not likely to seek treatment and will continue to spread the disease to others. Although the initial phase of the disease caused by chlamydia is often asymptomatic, untreated cases of disease can have serious consequences for women. Infection of the fallopian tubes can result in closure of the tubes, rendering the woman infertile and creating a risk of ectopic pregnancy (in which the fertilized egg is trapped in the tube, and the embryo develops until it ruptures the tube). Ectopic pregnancy can be fatal.

Similar things can be said about **gonorrhea,** a disease caused by the gram-negative bacterium *Neisseria gonorrhoeae.* Gonorrhea is less common than chlamydial disease in the United States but is still present at levels higher than those in some developing countries. Both gonorrhea and chlamydia may actually be decreasing in incidence, but their incidence remains unacceptably high. Recently, another adverse effect of chlamydia infection has been identified: infection significantly increases a woman's risk of contracting an HIV infection. The level of public awareness of these diseases and of medical concern about them is summed up very well by the title of a 1996 report on bacterial sexually transmitted diseases released by the Institute of Medicine. The title was *The Hidden Epidemic.* These diseases illustrate a very important principle of infectious disease prevention and control: having diagnostic tests and effective treatment is not enough. Until the medical community and the public become aware of and concerned about a disease, it will continue to spread almost unchecked.

Food-Borne and Water-Borne Infections

As is evident from the foregoing section, virtually every type of disease can be, and has been, called an emerging or reemerging infectious disease. This is certainly true of food-borne and water-borne infections. We treat this subject as a separate category because of its unique impact on the public perception of disease risks. Ironically, as the food and water supplies have become cleaner, the public's concern about their safety has become greater rather than less. A review of news articles from the past 2 years makes this quite evident. The integrity of the food and water supplies is a non-negotiable issue as far as the public is concerned, and people who will tolerate the sometimes substantial risks involved in automobile driving, sexual promiscuity, or smoking become far more conservative when the food supply is concerned.

From the 1960s through the 1980s, the public's main concern about the food supply was pesticide residues and other chemical adulterants that might cause cancer. This problem has been largely solved by stringent regulations that limit the amount of pesticide residues and other harmful chemicals that can be in food that is sold for human consumption. More recently, concern has arisen about another hazard that had been around all along but had not been perceived as a threat: food-borne bacterial disease. The catalyst for this abrupt swing in public concern was *E. coli* O157:H7, a strain that can cause kidney failure and death, especially in children. This problem first attracted attention when an outbreak of disease was caused by undercooked, contaminated hamburger dispensed by a fast-food chain. Cases occurred in many western and northwestern states before the source of the outbreak was identified and the contaminated meat was recalled. Since then, numerous cases of *E. coli* O157:H7 infection have been acquired from undercooked meat, radish sprouts, and even apple juice. The apple juice incident, which caused only one death, nearly bankrupted the company that had produced the contaminated juice. The juice had not been pasteurized. The lesson that juice was not exempt from contamination was learned very quickly by the food industry, and it is now uncommon to see unpasteurized juices in supermarkets.

Earlier in the 20th century, outbreaks of food-borne disease tended to be localized. Church socials or business-sponsored employee picnics were the typical sources of such outbreaks. As the food industry became more centralized, however, a different pattern of food-borne disease emerged: the multistate (or even multicountry) outbreak of food-borne disease derived from a single source. In the case of the fast-food outbreak just described, a single processing plant was the source. In 1996 an outbreak of *E. coli* O157:H7 in Japanese schoolchildren was caused by contaminated radish sprouts. The seeds used by Japanese sprouting companies came from a single source in the northwestern United States, where the contamination event probably occurred. The character of food-borne outbreaks had changed considerably from the days of the church social outbreaks. The effect on the public was dramatic. They were reminded not only that contaminated food could kill but that the contaminated product could come from far away and from companies that had formerly had a good reputation for safe food products.

Outbreaks of water-borne bacterial disease continue to be fairly localized. Most of the water-borne outbreaks that have made the news lately have been caused by protozoal parasites such *Cryptosporidium parvum,* but the same conditions that allow protozoal contamination of water—aging pipes and water treatment plants, mammal and bird fecal material in reservoirs—could easily spread bacterial water-borne diseases in the future. The media have picked up on this, as was evident from a cover of *Time* magazine (August 3, 1998) showing *E. coli* cascading out of a kitchen tap. The event that stimulated this amusing bit of media overreaction was an outbreak that occurred among 61 residents of Alpine, Wyoming (total population 470), who drank tap water on one particular weekend. The spring that was the source of the town's tap water had probably been contaminated by a wild animal passing through.

An aspect of water-borne infectious microorganisms that is often overlooked is that contaminated water can produce a contaminated food product if the water is used to wash food. In most cases, water used to wash the dirt off fruits and vegetables prior to shipping is not tap water quality and can be "gray water," which is water processed to remove the worst contamination but not microbiologically clean. At first, vegetarians felt safe because food-borne diseases were so often spread by meat. But people concerned with ensuring food safety privately consider foods that are usually consumed raw, such as fruits and some vegetables, a potentially more serious threat to public health. If meat is properly cooked, the contamination problem is solved, but even careful washing of raw fruits or vegetables may not be sufficient to render contaminated food safe. Salad bars are notorious breeding grounds for bacteria, most of which are innocuous, but their less-than-pure bacteriological status shows a potential route for the spread of disease. In one case, the contamination was not accidental (Box 1–1).

Modern Medicine as a Source of New Diseases

Modern medicine has made impressive breakthroughs in human therapy. Surgeons now routinely transplant new organs into patients whose organs are failing. Cancer chemotherapy is becoming more and more effective. This progress has had a cost, however. Transplant patients and patients receiving cancer chemotherapy have suppressed immune systems. Not surprisingly, these patients can become infected with bacteria never before suspected of being able to cause human disease. These bacteria have been called **opportunists,** because some defense of the body that normally keeps them at bay has to be breached in order for them to have the opportunity to cause infection. Cancer chemotherapy, immune-suppressive therapy given to transplant patients, and perforation of the bowel during surgery are examples of windows of opportunity that open up the human body to such bacteria. For an interesting recent example of an opportunist, see Box 1–2. The term "opportunist" makes such bacteria seem somehow less dangerous than "real" disease-causing bacteria. Do not be fooled by the seemingly innocuous nature of the opportunists. In most developed countries, a person is far more likely to die of an opportunistic infection than of the epidemic diseases that serve as the public's mental image of infectious diseases. Another way in which modern medicine has affected the infectious disease picture is by increasing the human life span. The increasing number of elderly people, whose immune defenses are beginning to decline, provides an expanding population of individuals highly susceptible to infectious disease. Put these elderly people in crowded conditions, such as those experienced in nursing homes, and an even greater opportunity is created for infectious diseases to spread.

Microbiota Shift Diseases

A category of bacterial disease that defies conventional classification consists of diseases that are not caused by a single bacterial pathogen, but rather by a shift in the bacterial population of some part of the human body. Although the natural microbial populations of the human body (microbiota or microflora) are usually protective, shifts in the composition of these populations can have pathological consequences. Diseases of this type do not yet have a name, so we will call them **microbiota shift diseases.** In the chapter on the microbiota of the human body, examples of microbiota shift diseases will be described in detail, but for present purposes one example should suffice: **bacterial vaginosis.**

Bacterial vaginosis is the term used to describe a shift in the vaginal microbiota from a predominantly gram-positive population, dominated by *Lactobacillus* species, to a population of gram-negative anaerobes.

BOX 1–1   Terrorism Hits Oregon Salad Bars

In 1984, a large outbreak of salmonellosis involving at least 750 people occurred in The Dalles, the county seat of Wasco County in Oregon. At the time, a religious commune was at odds with long-term inhabitants over land use restrictions placed on the commune in an attempt by the townspeople to eliminate it. Members of the commune felt that the outcome of an upcoming election was critical to their future ability to grow. In an apparent attempt to disrupt the election, commune members planned to cause an outbreak of salmonellosis that would keep people home from the polls. The 1984 outbreak was a trial run to determine the best way to create the most havoc. At least 10 restaurants were involved, with the salad bar being the main site of intentional contamination. Contamination attempts were also made at local grocery stores, but the most effective source of disease was the restaurant salad bars. Unfortunately for commune members, their trial run was too successful and attracted the attention of the public health department and the police.

Even so, it took nearly a year to trace the epidemic source and to suspect intentional contamination. Such events are fortunately quite rare. Thus, intentional contamination was not even considered at first as a possible explanation for the outbreak. Careful questioning of the victims led investigators to deduce that salad bars had been the source of the outbreak. This in itself was somewhat unusual because large outbreaks of salmonellosis are usually associated with meat, milk, or eggs. Such infections acquired from vegetables, while not unheard of, are relatively uncommon. Meanwhile, interrogation of commune members by police and FBI agents revealed that the commune had been the source of the outbreak. The commune had its own laboratory, where the strain of *S. enterica* serovar Typhimurium was grown and prepared for inoculation of the salad bars. Commune members had apparently gotten the strain by ordering it from the American Type Culture Collection, a widely respected repository of bacterial strains that distributes strains to scientific laboratories for a modest fee. Nearly 2 years after the outbreak, two commune members were sentenced to 1 to 2 years in prison for conspiring to tamper with consumer products. An earlier episode of product tampering involving introduction of cyanide into Tylenol capsules had been responsible for a rash of antitampering legislation. The antitampering laws were used to prosecute the commune members.

Source: T. J. Torok, R. V. Tauxe, R. P. Wise, J. R. Livengood, R. Sokolow, S. Mauvais, K. S. Birkness, M. R. Skeels, J. M. Horan, and L. R. Foster. 1997. A large community outbreak of salmonellosis caused by intentional contamination of restaurant salad bars. *JAMA* **278:**389–395.

For a long time, this condition was not taken seriously by physicians because the only symptoms, if there were symptoms at all, were a sparse discharge and—in some women—a fishy odor. Two papers in a 1995 issue of *The New England Journal of Medicine* changed the status of bacterial vaginosis. One of these papers linked bacterial vaginosis with preterm births. This was an epidemiological association, not proof of a cause-and-effect relationship. The second paper described the result of an intervention study in which antibiotics known to target gram-negative anaerobes were administered to pregnant women with bacterial vaginosis, and the effect on the birth weight of the infant was determined. Antibiotic intervention that returned the vaginal microbiota to normal was associated with normal full-term births, whereas untreated women were significantly more likely to have preterm infants.

More recently, bacterial vaginosis, like chlamydial disease and gonorrhea, has been linked to a higher risk of contracting HIV infections. A major challenge for scientists trained in the analysis of diseases caused by a single species of microorganisms is to learn how to deal intellectually with diseases caused by shifts in bacterial populations consisting of hundreds of species. Undoubtedly, all of the species present are not equal contributors to the disease state, but the situation is far more complex than infections caused by a single species of bacteria.

Genomics

Breakthroughs in DNA sequencing technology now allow scientists to sequence entire bacterial genomes fairly rapidly. Most of the genomes sequenced to date

---

BOX 1–2   Enterprising Bacteria Always on the Alert for New Infection Opportunities

An example of how bacteria can act rapidly to take advantage of new opportunities is provided by an outbreak of pneumonia in an intensive care ward. Many of the patients were very ill and were on respirators to support breathing. The type of respirator being used required that a tube be inserted deep into the airway, an ideal conduit to carry bacteria into the lung. After a number of cases of respirator-associated lung infections, hospital personnel have learned to be very careful not to contaminate the respirator itself or to allow bacterial contaminants to enter the air being forced into the lung.

No one, however, thought about mouthwash. Since patients on respirators are often unable to attend to their own dental hygiene, hospital staff workers use mouthwash to clean and freshen the mouth every day. The cause of the lung infections was identified as *Burkholderia* (formerly *Pseudomonas*) *cepacia*. Although

this species has caused some infections in people with cystic fibrosis, it is generally considered to be a relatively innocuous soil bacterium. In fact, it is used as a biocontrol agent to degrade pesticides such as 2,4,5-trichlorophenoxyacetic acid. *B. cepacia* is ubiquitous in soil and water and apparently managed to contaminate many lots of the mouthwash, which did not contain alcohol and thus contained nothing to discourage bacterial growth. In effect, the hospital workers taking care of the respirator patients were inoculating their teeth and gums daily with a contaminated solution, which placed the bacteria in an ideal location to gain access to the lungs.

Source: Centers for Disease Control and Prevention. 1998. Nosocomial *Burkholderia cepacia* infection and colonization associated with intrinsically contaminated mouthwash—Arizona 1998. *Morb. Mortal. Wkly. Rep.* **47**:926–928.

---

have been those of disease-causing bacteria. There is now a website that keeps track of genomes that have been or are being sequenced. The website is http://www.ornl.gov/microbialgenomes/. Once a **genome sequence** becomes available, scientists examine the open reading frames one by one to try to assess each gene's function. In some cases, this is easy because the gene has already been characterized. In other cases, the tentative identification is made on the basis of similarities to known genes or proteins in the **DNA and protein sequence databases.** Such assignments are useful but should be treated with caution, because many assignments have been based on relatively poor database matches. The best way to approach DNA or protein sequence data is to realize that DNA or protein sequence similarity to known genes is only a hypothesis that needs to be confirmed by more rigorous testing. A sobering fact is that, even in the case of sequences of well-studied bacteria, such as *E. coli* and *Salmonella* species, at least one-third of the genes have no similarity to any known genes. A job for future scientists is to determine the function of these **unidentified reading frames (urfs).**

One example of how DNA sequence information can reveal surprising things about an organism is illustrated by the genome sequence of *B. burgdorferi*, the

spirochete that causes Lyme disease. Scientists noted that there were no genes corresponding to the iron-containing proteins normally found in bacteria. This suggested a radical hypothesis—that *B. burgdorferi* copes with the problem of low iron concentrations in the human body by not using iron at all. Scientists who were trained in an era when every article on iron utilization by bacteria started with words to the effect that "all bacteria require iron" were startled by this suggestion. Biochemical analyses showed, however, that *B. burgdorferi* apparently does live without iron, thus solving one problem most other pathogens have to confront—how to obtain iron in a host whose iron sequestration proteins keep the supply of available iron very low.

Bioterrorism

No discussion of current infectious disease issues would be complete without a mention of **bioterrorism.** Germ warfare—the use of infectious microorganisms as weapons—is an old idea that has, fortunately, never worked very well. This does not mean that it will never be a threat. The nature of germ warfare has been changing in recent years. In the past, the purpose of germ warfare was to kill or incapacitate large numbers of soldiers. This is difficult to do because aerosols of microbes are hard to control, and it is difficult to deliver doses large enough to be effective. Recently, the aim of bioterrorists has changed. Now the goal is to frighten the general population. A small number of deaths is sufficient to achieve this goal. Among bacteria, *Bacillus anthracis,* the cause of anthrax, has been identified as a potentially useful weapon by bioterrorists. *B. anthracis* is a sporeformer and is thus easier to store and more easily "weaponized" than a fragile organism such as *Yersinia pestis,* the cause of bubonic plague. In 1999 the U.S. Army was worried enough about possible anthrax attacks to begin to administer the anthrax vaccine to all soldiers. This caused a great controversy because the efficacy and safety of the anthrax vaccine remain controversial. Another bacterial choice of bioterrorists is *Clostridium botulinum,* the bacterium that produces botulism toxin. Producing botulism toxin in your garage can be hazardous to your health, but botulism toxin is produced commercially for use in a variety of applications, from correcting crossed eyes to eliminating wrinkles. Thus, it is conceivable that commercially produced botulism toxin could be hijacked by terrorists. Whether emptying a load of toxin into a city's water supply would actually result in any deaths is not clear because of dilution of the toxin and breakdown of the toxin in the environment, but it is better to err on the side of caution.

New Solutions, New Hope

New Respect for Prevention

Major changes have been occurring in the approach to controlling infectious diseases, changes that hold great promise for the future. Traditionally, the medical establishments in the developed countries have opted for a treatment-based approach to controlling infectious diseases. Granted, vaccinations were given to prevent some diseases, and doctors used antibiotics prophylactically to prevent others, such as postsurgical infections or infections in cancer chemotherapy patients, but the most common approach to infectious diseases was to wait for an infected person to seek medical help before intervening in the disease process. This approach has been criticized for being expensive and for allowing diseases to gain a foothold in the body before action is taken—a delay that in some cases results in long-term damage to the patient even if the treatment is successful in eliminating the infecting bacterium from the body. Treatment-based approaches have also become much less effective as increasingly resistant bacteria make it more difficult to make the right initial

choices about what antibiotic to use. The physicians' response has been to use more advanced antibiotics to treat infections that might be treatable with less expensive antibiotics and antibiotics that are not so critical for treating diseases caused by resistant bacteria. Physicians have been advised repeatedly to use the front-line antibiotics at first if they must, but to send specimens of tissue or blood to the microbiological laboratory for antibiotic resistance evaluation. The therapy can then be adjusted if laboratory results indicate this is appropriate. Once physicians got used to using the front-line antibiotics, however, they were loath to abandon a strategy that worked for a particular patient. The result has been increased selective pressure for development of bacterial resistance to front-line antibiotics.

A far preferable approach to controlling disease is preventing it in the first place. This approach has been successful in ensuring the safety of food and water. Now, more and more public health officials, hospital managers, and executives of health management organizations are rediscovering that prevention is far more effective—and far less expensive—than treatment. Prevention, once scorned as too low-tech to be fashionable, is suddenly center stage again. For a preventive approach to work, it is first necessary to have information about disease patterns and early warning systems to signal some new disease trend. Led by the Centers for Disease Control and Prevention (CDC), a variety of **surveillance programs** are being implemented to monitor the appearance of new diseases, increased incidence of existing diseases, and occurrence of antibiotic-resistant bacteria. The CDC has been monitoring a subset of infectious diseases for years, but the list of diseases covered was far from exhaustive. Only recently have some major infectious diseases, such as chlamydial infections, been added to the list of reportable diseases. A problem the CDC has had to cope with is that reporting of diseases is voluntary on the part of physicians and state public health departments. Overworked and underfunded state health departments have sometimes (understandably) given reporting of diseases their lowest priority. The CDC and the National Institutes of Health are fighting to alert government agencies to the importance of having consistently funded monitoring programs.

Surveillance—an Early Warning System

An interesting example of a new surveillance program is **Foodnet,** a program that tries to count all cases of salmonellosis and *Campylobacter* food-borne disease in selected states and to estimate from these data the incidence of these diseases nationwide. Prior to the introduction of Foodnet, the CDC had abundant information about large outbreaks of food-borne disease but had no idea how many isolated cases of food-borne disease occurred. Attempts are also being made in several areas to monitor antibiotic-resistant pathogens.

Monitoring disease prevalence is only the first step. Next comes effective action. There are encouraging signs that such programs are beginning to be implemented. A program for prevention of food-borne diseases, **hazard analysis and critical control points (HACCP),** has been implemented by the Food and Drug Administration. Previously, companies waited to test foods for microbiological safety until the final step in food processing. Because it can take days to weeks for microbiology test results to be obtained, and since many products must be shipped immediately for reasons of shelf life and economy, this approach allowed shipments of contaminated food to leave the processing plant and reach many distribution points. HACCP programs monitor the food at control points where contamination is likely to occur. This approach not only lessens the likelihood that contaminated foods will be shipped but identifies contamination problems early so that they can be rectified. At first, the food industry was leery of the HACCP approach, viewing it as a needless and potentially expensive government intrusion. The food industry has now become more enthusiastic about HACCP after seeing how expensive and injurious to the reputation of a company a large recall of contaminated products can be. A good HACCP program not only protects the public from disease but protects the company from recalls and lawsuits. There is still grumbling about specifics, but the HACCP concept seems to be catching on.

Making Hospitals Safe for Patients

Fears concerning increasingly antibiotic-resistant bacteria have led to a number of changes in the way hospitals handle infectious disease problems. Previously, hospitals that had an infection control program often delegated the job of infection control officer to someone of low status who had no authority to confront physicians whose postsurgical infection record was not good or whose prescribing practices were open to criticism. Now this job is being taken much more seriously and is usually held by an infectious disease physician. Communication lines are also being improved. At one time a surgeon could infect numerous patients and never be held accountable, or would not even be informed of such incidents because of a lack of communication between physicians who cared for patients during the postsurgical period and the surgeons who performed the operation.

Managed health care organizations, alarmed at the costs associated with antibiotic-resistant bacterial infections, have started cracking down on physician abuse and overuse of antibiotics. Ironically, cost-cutting measures by the health care plan "bean counters" that earlier pressured physicians to drastically reduce the number of laboratory tests they ordered actually contributed to the resistance problem by encouraging physicians to use the strongest drugs available regardless of need. Thus, although there is still a certain amount of confusion and sending of contradictory signals between managers and physicians, at least a beginning has been made.

A less successful effort—so far—has been the campaign within hospitals to persuade health care workers to wash their hands after each patient and to implement other supposedly standard precautions, such as changing gloves when moving from one patient to another. Because many outbreaks of hospital-acquired infections are thought to be spread by the hands of health care workers, preventing transmission by this route has become an important priority. Unfortunately, health care workers have gotten out of the habit of washing their hands, relying instead on antibiotics to clean up any little messes that result from poor hygiene. The high-stress atmosphere of a modern hospital, in which fewer health care workers are expected to treat more and sicker patients, has made it difficult to perform hygienic procedures by the book. Now that antibiotics are becoming less effective, hygienic practices have become more important than ever.

And Now for the Really Good News— You've Got a Bacterial Infection

Who would have thought that a person could be happy to learn that he or she had a bacterial infection? Yet this is exactly what has happened to people suffering from ulcers and possibly from some other chronic infections. The doctrine has been that infectious diseases are acute diseases that develop rapidly and run their course quickly, whereas chronic diseases—those that last for long periods of time without resolving—are caused by an autoimmune response or a genetic disorder. Examples of chronic diseases are heart disease, Alzheimer's disease, and cancer. But what if these diseases and others like them are caused by microbes? They might be curable by antimicrobial agents or preventable by vaccines or other measures! The discovery that many cases of liver cancer were caused by hepatitis B virus made it possible to prevent

Table 1–2   Some diseases currently suspected of being caused by bacteria

Disease	Suspected microbe
Gastric cancer	*Helicobacter pylori*
Periodontal disease	*Porphyromonas* and other oral bacteria
Atherosclerosis	*Chlamydia pneumoniae*
Low-birth-weight babies (some cases)	Bacterial vaginosis (a shift of the vaginal bacterial population)
Cerebral palsy (some cases)	Placental infection
Rheumatoid arthritis	Unknown
Crohn's disease	*Mycobacterium* spp.

this type of cancer by means of an anti-hepatitis B vaccine. Similarly, the discovery that most gastric and duodenal ulcers were caused by bacteria led to a revolution in the way ulcer patients were treated. Such examples have spawned a revolution that has led to the reinvestigation of virtually every chronic disease, from heart disease to schizophrenia, as being possibly of microbial origin.

Getting the medical community to accept the idea that bacteria cause ulcers took years of acrimonious debate, but once the idea was accepted by clinicians, it took only a short time for them to understand that the implications went far beyond ulcers. Suddenly, clinicians remembered that if a disease is caused by bacteria, it can usually be cured with antibiotics—if diagnosed early enough. What followed was a veritable gold rush to find a bacterial cause for more diseases. A partial list of the diseases currently being reexamined as possibly caused by bacteria is provided in Table 1–2. The scope of this list conveys better than anything else the boundless optimism that surged through the medical community once the implications of *Helicobacter pylori* as a cause of ulcers were fully appreciated. Most of these proposed associations are still controversial as this text goes to press, and many will probably not pan out. Yet if even a few of these diseases become curable because they are found to be caused by bacteria, a treatment revolution will have occurred. More details about some of these associations will be given in subsequent chapters. It is striking how rapidly a too-great skepticism about *H. pylori* as a cause of ulcers metamorphosed into a too-great optimism about the likelihood of making further discoveries of a similar magnitude.

SELECTED READINGS

Alibek, K. W., with S. Handelman. 2000. *Biohazard.* Dell Publishing Co., Inc., New York, N.Y.

Brown, M. R., and J. Barker. 1999. Unexplored reservoirs of pathogenic bacteria: protozoa and biofilms. *Trends Microbiol.* **7:**46–49.

Centers for Disease Control and Prevention. 1998. Preventing emerging infectious diseases: a strategy for the 21st century. *Morb. Mortal. Wkly. Rep.* **47**(RR-15):1–14. (The *Morbidity and Mortality Weekly Report,* despite its rather grim name, is a fascinating up-to-the-minute account of what is happening in the infectious disease world.)

Haffajee, A. D., and S. S. Socransky. 1994. Microbial etiological agents of destructive periodontal diseases. *Periodontology 2000* **5:**78–111.

Hauth, J. C., R. L. Goldenberg, W. M. Andrews, M. B. DuBard, and R. L. Copper. 1995. Reduced incidence of preterm delivery with metronidazole and erythromycin in women with bacterial vaginosis. *N. Engl. J. Med.* **333:**1732–1736.

Hooper, J. 1999. A new germ theory. *Atlantic Monthly* **283**(2):41–53. (An excellent example of "*H. pylori* fever" at work. The scientists interviewed in the article believe that virtually all "big old diseases are infectious.")

Lederberg, J. 1998. Infectious agents, hosts in constant flux. *ASM News* **64:**18–22.

Relman, D. A. 1998. Detection and identification of previously unrecognized microbial pathogens. *Emerg. Infect. Dis.* **4:**382–389.

Van Beneden, C. A., W. E. Keene, R. A. Strang, D. H. Werker, A. S. King, B. Mahon, K. Hedberg, A. Bell, M. T. Kelly, V. K. Balan, W. R. MacKenzie, and D. Fleming. 1999. Multinational outbreak of *Salmonella enterica* serotype Newport infections due to contaminated alfalfa sprouts. *JAMA* **281:**158–162.

Microbial evolution

Microbes appeared 3.5 to 4 billion years ago

Bacteria made Earth habitable for other organisms
> Geochemical cycles
> Atmospheric oxygen
> Ozone layer

Metabolic capabilities allow bacteria to survive under many conditions
> Vast number of metabolic types of bacteria
> Genetic plasticity
> Some bacteria able to grow at temperature extremes

Bacteria have become endosymbionts of eukaryotes

Symbiotic relationships between bacteria and animals
> Protection of animal against infection by pathogens
> Bacteria supply nutrients to animal

Emerging and reemerging infectious diseases

New-new diseases
> Caused by previously unidentified bacteria
> Have recently entered human population
> Take advantage of changes in human lifestyles
> Examples: Lyme disease, Legionnaires' disease

New-old diseases
> Diseases have been known for a long time
> Pathogen causing disease is newly recognized
> Better diagnostic tests have allowed identification of pathogen
> Examples: *Campylobacter* food-borne disease, cat scratch disease

Old-new diseases
> Old disease with known causes
> Once thought to be under control but have reappeared
> Tuberculosis resurgence
>> Treatment infrastructure dismantled
>> Crowded homeless shelters
>> AIDS patients highly susceptible
> Cholera introduced into Latin America, probably in bilge water from Asian ships
> Long-known pathogens acquire new traits
>> Many bacteria become resistant to antibiotics. Examples: *S. pneumoniae*, *S. aureus*, *Enterococcus* species
>> Bacteria acquire genes for virulence factors from other bacteria. Example: *E. coli* O157:H7 acquired toxin genes

Old-old diseases
> Old diseases with known causes
> Recently "discovered" by the media
> Example: bacterial sexually transmitted diseases (*C. trachomatis* infection, gonorrhea)

Food-borne diseases
> *E. coli* O157:H7 increased public concern for food safety
> Centralization of food industry can lead to widespread outbreaks

Water-borne diseases
> Aging water plants and sewage systems allow microbes into water supplies
> Unclean water used to wash produce

(continued)

SUMMARY OUTLINE (*continued*)

Modern medicine as a source of new diseases
- Suppression of immune systems of transplant and chemotherapy patients
- Increased numbers of elderly who are somewhat immunosuppressed
- Infections often caused by opportunists

Microbiota shift diseases
- Infection due to changing proportions of microbes at a particular site in the body
- Example: bacterial vaginosis

Genome sequencing revealing information about virulence factors

Bioterrorism as a potential threat

Controlling disease

Treating diseases successfully does not always prevent damage to patient

Prevention preferable to treating
- Surveillance programs
- Infection control officers in hospitals
- Hand washing and other precautions

Discovery that chronic diseases may be caused by microbes

Has led to search for causative agent for many chronic diseases

Example: gastric ulcers caused by *H. pylori*

QUESTIONS

Answers to the questions can be found in Appendix 2.

1. The number of human deaths is often used as a standard for ranking human diseases in terms of importance. What, if anything, is wrong with this classification scheme?

2. Infectious diseases have obvious deleterious effects on the infected individual. Are there other consequences that reach beyond the infected person to his or her family and to society as a whole?

3. The United States and most developed countries have long had a medical community that focuses on therapy rather than prevention. Why is this the case, and under what conditions might this emphasis be appropriate? Why are scientists arguing for a return to a prevention-based health care system?

4. In our classification of emerging or reemerging infectious diseases, we included antibiotic-resistant bacteria and *E. coli* O157:H7 in the "old-new" disease category. Make the case for and against considering a member of an established disease-causing species that acquires a new trait a new disease entity. What is the significance of such changes in bacterial pathogens?

5. The bacteria that cause cholera and tuberculosis are much more infectious than the so-called opportunists. Why then, are opportunists currently much more of a health concern in developed countries than cholera and tuberculosis?

6. Under what conditions—assuming no new epidemics—could infectious diseases suddenly move to the second or even the first most common cause of deaths in the United States?

7. Do you think humans will ever win the battle against disease-causing bacteria? Why or why not? Is the use of warlike language to describe the relationship between humans and bacteria even accurate?

8. Microbiologists are fond of saying that only a tiny minority of bacteria cause disease. Are there reasons for thinking this might not be true? Could bacteria capable of causing human disease have evolved on Mars?

9. In what sense are bacteria life givers rather than life takers? Is it possible that disease-causing bacteria might have a beneficial role in another context or even in their relationship with the human body?

2

Approaching and Studying Bacterial Diseases

Microbes and Disease

Establishing a Connection—Koch's Postulates

HISTORY AND MODERN RELEVANCE OF KOCH'S POSTULATES. The renewed search for missed infectious diseases, which was sparked by the discovery that the bacterium *Helicobacter pylori* causes most ulcers, brought to the fore an old problem in infectious disease research—how does one prove that a particular microorganism causes a disease? If, for example, you suspect that ulcers or heart disease is caused by a bacterium, how would you test this hypothesis? Keep in mind that scientists involved in this type of research want very much to prove that their hypothesis is correct, because if the disease of interest is caused by a bacterium, this insight could lead to a cure or to improved prevention strategies. Because these scientists have an interest in proving rather than disproving their hypotheses, they have to be especially careful that their hope for a cure does not bias their thinking. Similarly, it may be hard to convince proponents of competing views, such as the scientists who maintained that ulcers were caused by excess stomach acid, not bacteria, that their hypothesis is incorrect, especially if they also have a financial stake in the outcome. The fact that it took over 10 years for the scientific community to accept the idea that ulcers are caused by bacteria shows how long and arduous the process of establishing cause and effect can be.

Proving cause and effect in infectious disease research is not a new problem; it first arose in the 1800s as microbiologists struggled to identify the microorganisms that caused diseases like cholera and tuberculosis. At that time, the idea that disease could be caused by creatures too small to be seen without a microscope was not only new but went against prevailing medical dogma. Naturally, scientists and physicians were even more skeptical than they are today. A German microbiologist, Robert Koch, realized that if the new discipline of infectious diseases was ever to become respectable, it had to have a rigorous scientific basis. To this end, he proposed four criteria for establishing cause and effect that came to be known as **Koch's postulates.**

Koch's first postulate states that the microbe must be associated with the lesions of the disease. That is, the microbe should be found

19

in diseased tissue but not in healthy tissue. The second postulate directs that the microbe must be isolated from the lesions of the disease as a pure culture. The third postulate states that a pure culture of the microbe should cause the symptoms of the disease if it is inoculated into humans or into animals. The fourth postulate states that the microbe must be reisolated in pure culture from the humans or animals used to satisfy the third postulate. Koch's postulates have been invaluable for proving that diseases are caused by microbes. The postulates sound very reasonable and straightforward, but they can be difficult to satisfy in some cases and may not apply universally to all infectious diseases.

THE FIRST POSTULATE: ASSOCIATION OF THE MICROBE WITH THE LESIONS OF THE DISEASE.   Scientists first began to think that bacteria might cause the cardiovascular disease atherosclerosis when they isolated the bacterium *Chlamydia pneumoniae* from atherosclerotic plaques but only occasionally isolated it from healthy blood vessel tissue. Finding *C. pneumoniae* in healthy tissue is not surprising if the characteristics of the bacteria are considered. *C. pneumoniae*, a common cause of mild respiratory infections, invades and lives inside human cells, thus protecting itself from the body's defenses. So, if bacteria from the throat of a person with a respiratory tract infection leaked into the bloodstream, the bacteria might well infect blood vessel cells transiently and thus be found in tissue that looks healthy. The fact that *C. pneumoniae* was occasionally isolated from healthy tissue may be rationalized in this way, but it blurs the clear line implicit in Koch's first postulate. Even worse, although *C. pneumoniae* was isolated from atherosclerotic plaque samples, it was not isolated from all such samples. Thus, *C. pneumoniae* was associated with lesions of the disease most of the time but not all of the time.

Satisfying the first postulate was even more difficult for scientists who were trying to prove that *H. pylori* causes ulcers. Over half the people in developed countries and nearly all of the people in developing countries carry *H. pylori* in their stomachs, but only a small number of these people develop ulcers. As an aside, it is worth pointing out that this same pattern is seen in a number of bacterial diseases; the bacterium colonizes many people, but only those with some predisposing condition develop a symptomatic infection. Koch himself worried about his first postulate, as it became obvious from his studies and those of others that people could be colonized with a disease-causing bacterium but not develop the symptoms of the disease.

Do these examples prove that Koch's first postulate is useless? Not at all. They show that it is very useful for guiding the design of experiments and subsequent discussions about the meaning of experimental results.

What these examples also show, and what Koch himself realized at the time, was that the postulates should not be treated as monolithic requirements.

THE SECOND POSTULATE: ISOLATING THE BACTERIUM IN PURE CULTURE.   The second postulate is also not as easy to satisfy as it sounds. Some bacteria are more difficult to cultivate than others. As was pointed out in chapter 1, bacteria are extraordinarily diverse with respect to their metabolic traits and growth requirements. Although there are some media that can support the growth of many different kinds of bacteria, there is no universal medium on which all bacteria can be cultivated. For example, bacteriologists who work with disease-causing bacteria frequently grow these bacteria by streaking them onto a complex agar medium and incubating the agar plates with ordinary air as the atmosphere. This approach would fail to cultivate *C. pneumoniae*. Because *C. pneumoniae* only grows inside human cells, it must be cultivated using tissue culture cells, not agar medium. Moreover, an atmosphere that has an elevated CO_2 content is required for optimal growth. The fact that *C. pneumoniae* is more difficult to cultivate than many other disease-causing bacteria raises the question of whether the failure to cultivate *C. pneumoniae* from all atherosclerotic lesions could be due to the failure of bacteria present in those lesions to grow in all cases. Although *H. pylori* grows on agar medium, it too requires a special atmosphere.

An extreme example of the difficulty that can arise in attempting to satisfy Koch's second postulate is provided by *Treponema pallidum*, the bacterium that is generally accepted as being the cause of syphilis. *T. pallidum* has a distinctive corkscrew shape and can be seen in the lesions associated with the early stages of syphilis. Yet, *T. pallidum* has never been isolated as a pure culture in laboratory medium, despite many attempts. The closest thing to a laboratory medium for *T. pallidum* is the testicles of a rabbit, which are used as a growth chamber by scientists who work on *T. pallidum*.

A modern alternative to cultivating disease-causing bacteria is to use a molecular biology technique, PCR, to make many copies of a segment of the bacterial chromosome. The DNA sequence of the amplified chromosomal segment can be used to identify the organism. How the process works is described in more detail in chapter 3. This approach has been widely used by scientists who study *C. pneumoniae* because cultivation of the bacteria is so difficult and time-consuming.

THE THIRD POSTULATE: SHOWING THAT THE ISOLATED BACTERIUM CAUSES DISEASE IN HUMANS OR ANIMALS. The third postulate demands that the bacterium isolated in pure culture must produce the disease when inoculated into a human or animal. Of all Koch's postulates, this is often the one that is most difficult to satisfy. Ironically, one of the first critics of this postulate was Koch himself. Less than 2 years after Koch proposed his postulates, he himself ran afoul of it (Box 2–1).

As already mentioned, Koch also had second thoughts about his first postulate once it was discovered that people could carry and shed pathogenic bacteria without having any symptoms (carrier state). It is impressive that Koch himself was far more flexible in his approach to proving cause and effect in infectious disease than some modern-day scientists. Acceptance of the proposal that most ulcers are caused by bacteria was held up for nearly a decade because critics of the idea insisted that Koch's third postulate had to be met.

In recent years, the third postulate has been less of a stumbling block for scientists working on *H. pylori* and *C. pneumoniae*. There are now good animal models for ulcers, but in the early days of *H. pylori* research these models were not available. This led one frustrated scientist to use himself as the guinea pig in an attempt to satisfy Koch's third postulate (see chapter 23). Scientists working on the proposed connection between *C. pneumoniae* and heart disease have used a breed of rabbit that is prone to develop atherosclerosis if fed a high-fat diet to show that infection with *C. pneumoniae* increases the development of atherosclerotic plaques. This demonstration has not convinced some critics, who argue with some justification that the rabbit model is not a perfect replica of the disease in humans. Such objections raise an important issue: how closely should an animal model mimic the disease in humans? One of the early animal models for gastric ulcers was ferrets inoculated with *Helicobacter mustelae*. *H. mustelae* is a close relative of *H. pylori*, but it is not *H. pylori*. Is it acceptable to use a different bacterial species as well as a different animal species to satisfy Koch's third postulate for a human disease?

THE FOURTH POSTULATE: REISOLATING THE BACTERIUM FROM THE INTENTIONALLY INFECTED ANIMAL. Anyone who manages to satisfy the first three postulates will probably be able to satisfy the fourth one with no difficulty. The fourth postulate is important, however. In satisfying the fourth postulate, a scientist shows that the human or animal used to satisfy the third postulate was actually infected and that the lesions of the inoculated human or animal, like those occurring naturally in the disease, contained the microbe. For example, in the case of the rabbit model used to determine whether *C. pneumoniae* would cause atherosclerotic plaques to form, one might object that the reason the plaques formed in the rabbit arteries was not that the arteries were infected by the bacteria but that the bacteria caused a mild respi-

---

BOX 2–1 Koch Backs Off

Scientists sometimes grumble about criticisms of Koch's postulates. After all, they say, Koch's postulates are all we've got. What they may not realize is that the first person to give the old heave-ho to Koch's postulates, at least the third one, was Koch himself. Koch presented his famous postulates in 1882. The ink was barely dry on the paper before, in 1884, Koch was having second thoughts. Koch was passionately interested in cholera and was convinced he had found the causative agent, a curved bacillus ("comma bacillus" to Koch, now known as *V. cholerae*). It turned out that Koch was right, but in 1884 Koch's own postulates were being used against him because there was no animal model for cholera. Here is what Koch had to say to his critics:

> . . . no one ever observes animals with cholera. Therefore, I believe that all the animals available for experimentation and those that often come in contact with people are totally immune. True cholera processes cannot be artificially created in them. Therefore, we must dispense with this part of the proof. This certainly does not mean that there is no proof that comma bacilli are pathogenic. I have already mentioned that even without animal experiments, I can imagine nothing other than that the comma bacilli cause cholera. If a cholera process is finally produced in animals, I will be no more convinced than I am now.

Source: Haffajee and Socransky (1994) quoting from a translation of Koch's essays (K. C. Carter. 1987. *Essays of Robert Koch*, p. xvii–xix, 161. Greenwood Press, Westport, Conn.) in defense of their proposed alternatives to Koch's postulates.

---

ratory illness, which stressed the rabbits enough to increase the rate of plaque formation indirectly. Finding the bacteria in the plaques helped to bolster the contention that the bacteria caused the increase in plaque formation.

IS A FIFTH POSTULATE NEEDED? Technically, scientists working on *C. pneumoniae* have satisfied all four of Koch's postulates if one accepts the rabbit model as a good model for human disease. Nonetheless, there are still skeptics, as there should be, given some of the problems described in the foregoing paragraphs. Similarly, even the use of a human volunteer to show that ingesting *H. pylori* could cause inflammation of the stomach lining did not convince everyone who was skeptical of the *H. pylori*-ulcer connection.

What finally made true believers out of most scientists and physicians in the case of *H. pylori* was the development of an antibiotic therapy that eliminated the bacteria and the symptoms. The proponents of the link between *C. pneumoniae* and heart disease are also taking this route, hoping to find an antibiotic regimen that prevents or cures atherosclerosis. Finding such a regimen may be difficult. Antibiotics that kill a bacterium in the laboratory may not have the same effect in the human body because of the way the antibiotic is distributed and because of local conditions such as the low pH of stomach contents. It took years to find the antibiotic combinations that finally subdued *H. pylori* and caused widespread acceptance of the hypothesis that *H. pylori* causes ulcers. Results to date of clinical trials testing whether antibiotics prevent or cure atherosclerosis have been mixed. Some show an effect and some do not. The tests that do not find an effect have been used to argue that *C. pneumoniae* does not cause atherosclerosis. This argument was also used in the early days of the search for an antibiotic treatment of ulcers.

This type of test was not possible in Koch's time, because antibiotics were not discovered until the 1930s. In a sense, however, a fifth step taken in Koch's time helped convince the skeptics that bacteria caused cholera. Knowing the properties of *Vibrio cholerae*, public health officials were able to prevent the spread of cholera by identifying and shutting off contaminated water sources and, later, by treating water to eliminate *V. cholerae* from the water supply.

The purists can argue about whether a fifth postulate should be added to Koch's original four, a postulate stating that the information about the microbes should enable scientists to design effective therapeutic or preventive measures for eliminating the disease. In practice, however, this phantom fifth postulate will inevitably be invoked and will be seen by many as the ultimate test of a proposed microbe-disease hypothesis.

As should be evident from the foregoing material, it can be very difficult to be absolutely sure that microbe A causes disease X. There is enough room for error in each of Koch's postulates to make absolute certainty a virtual impossibility. The fact that there are still people, some of whom have good scientific credentials, who are not convinced that HIV is the cause of AIDS is an example of this. Moreover, as we have seen in the case of diseases like syphilis, failure to satisfy one or more of Koch's postulates does not necessarily disprove a connection between a microbe and a disease. In the end,

the preponderance of evidence (as the lawyers would say) is what convinces people that there is a cause-and-effect relationship.

THE MICROBIOTA SHIFT DISEASE PROBLEM. If it is difficult to prove a connection between one microbe and a disease, what does one do about diseases such as periodontal disease (associated with gum erosion and tooth loss) and bacterial vaginosis (associated with higher risk for preterm birth), diseases that appear to be caused by shifts in bacterial populations that contain hundreds of species? Scientists working in this area have tried to construct postulates similar to Koch's postulates, in which "pure culture" is replaced by "a shift from one specified population to another." The third postulate presents real problems in this case, because it is difficult to produce specific population shifts in laboratory animals. In the case of periodontal disease and bacterial vaginosis, the phantom fifth postulate may turn out to be of great importance and might become equivalent to Koch's third postulate for single-organism diseases. That is, if the original composition of the bacterial population can be restored, the disease should be cured. This area will be a challenge for future microbiologists, especially if more diseases, such as inflammatory bowel disease, are shown to be microbiota shift diseases.

Concepts of Disease

VARIETIES OF HUMAN-MICROBE INTERACTIONS. The early view of infectious diseases, implicit in Koch's postulates, was that there were microbes capable of causing disease and that exposure to them inevitably caused the disease. Already in Koch's time, however, this simplistic description of infectious diseases was being questioned. Scientists realized that not all people who drank water containing *V. cholerae* developed cholera. Not all people exposed to someone with tuberculosis developed symptomatic disease, even though they could be shown to be infected with the bacterium. Clearly, all humans are not equal in their response to an infectious microbe.

As scientists gained more experience with disease-causing microbes, they further discovered that, just as there are differences in susceptibility from person to person, there are also variations among different strains of the same bacterial species. Sometimes, a bacterium that had been grown too long in laboratory medium lost the ability to infect. Or different isolates of what appeared to be the same bacterium differed in their ability to cause disease. Through the years, a greater appreciation of the complexity of the interaction between microbes and humans has emerged. Today, scientists view the infection process as a multifaceted interaction between the microorganism and the human body. This interaction may result in clearance of the microbe from the body, in asymptomatic carriage of the microbe, or in the development of symptoms. The outcome of a microbe-human encounter depends on the infected person's defenses against disease and on the traits of the infecting strain. Finally, as described in chapter 1, there is an ecology of infectious diseases. Diseases come and go, depending on ecological factors, including changes caused by human activities.

VIEWS OF THE MICROBE-HUMAN INTERACTION. Although everyone agrees that the interactions between microbes and the human body are complex, there are differences of opinion about how these interactions should be understood. Perhaps the most widely held view is that disease-causing bacteria evolved specifically to cause human disease. A second view, which has gained more adherents lately, is that disease-causing bacteria are actually trying to achieve an equilibrium with humans that does not result in disease, and that disease symptoms result when this equilibrium is not achieved. Adherents of this view point to the fact that in many diseases, the number of people who develop serious symptoms is far smaller than the number of people who carry the bacteria without developing any symptoms. A third view is that humans are more often than not accidental hosts of bacteria that may be able to cause human disease but have actually evolved to occupy some other niche. In this view, bacteria entering the human body react by activating stress responses, producing disease symptoms in the process.

Probably each of these views is correct for at least some diseases. For example, a bacterium that causes disease only in humans, has no external reservoir, and causes symptoms in virtually all infected people fits the first view, whereas a bacterium that causes an asymptomatic carrier state in most of the humans it infects fits the second view. A bacterium that spends most of its time outside the human body and only occasionally causes human disease may fit more closely with the third view. The varieties of human-bacterium interactions are so numerous and distinct that there is no one model that fits all diseases.

TERMINOLOGY. The way words are used can reveal a great deal about the philosophy underlying a field. Thus, it is important to scrutinize the language used to describe the host-bacterium interaction, because this language can influence the way we think about such interactions. Accordingly, we introduce here definitions for some terms used frequently in discussions of bacterial pathogenesis. The term "host-parasite" is widely used to describe the human-microbe interac-

tion. This is rather a curious term, when one thinks of it. The host is not in a host-guest situation in the usual sense of the term "guest," where the guest is welcome. Colonization of the body by a bacterium capable of causing disease is called **infection,** and an infection that produces symptoms is called **disease.** Thus, infection does not inevitably result in disease. This use of the term infection is different from its use in the general vernacular, where infection is associated with disease. The word **colonization** means that a bacterium occupies and multiplies in a particular area of the human body. Note that colonization is not synonymous with disease, nor is it necessarily synonymous with infection. Many bacteria that colonize the human body do not cause disease and thus are not considered to be infecting it. The distinction between colonization and infection has been blurred by the realization that some of the supposedly noninfectious bacteria that normally inhabit the human body can cause disease in surgical patients or immunosuppressed people. So, the terms colonization, infection, and disease may vary in their applicability depending on the status of the person colonized.

People who are infected but do not have detectable symptoms are called **asymptomatic carriers.** Asymptomatic carriers form an important group because they are capable of spreading the bacteria they carry to people who may develop disease. Perhaps the most famous example of an asymptomatic carrier is Typhoid Mary. Mary was an asymptomatic carrier of *Salmonella typhi,* the bacterium that causes typhoid fever. Unfortunately, Mary was also a professional cook who managed to transmit typhoid fever to hundreds of people. At one time, she even worked in a hospital. Even after she was tracked down by public health officials and jailed when she refused to give up her profession, she was unable to believe that she was the cause of disease and death that affected so many people who ate her food. Even today among educated people, the concept of asymptomatic carriage is a difficult one to accept, so highly associated are the concepts of infection and disease.

The definition of **symptoms** would seem to be straightforward. Yet this term is also somewhat problematic. Symptoms of a bacterial infection are defined as effects of bacterial infection that are apparent to the infected person. In fact, the term disease (dis-ease) suggests that the infected person feels some discomfort. Yet, infection can result in rather serious damage that is not felt by the infected person at the time. For example, a woman whose cervix is infected with *Chlamydia trachomatis* may feel no pain and experience no vaginal discharge, yet the bacteria are quietly triggering an inflammatory process that fuses her fallopian tubes shut and renders her infertile. Clearly, such women are experiencing disease even though symptoms, as that term is traditionally defined in medicine, are not present, at least in the early stages of the disease.

Virulence (or **pathogenicity**) is defined as the ability of a bacterium to cause infection. **Virulence factor** (or **mechanism of pathogenesis** or **virulence mechanism**) denotes a bacterial product or strategy that contributes to virulence or pathogenicity. Because most of the chapters in this book that deal with individual bacteria contain a section that is titled "virulence factors," it is important to point out that although it is possible to define this term, deciding what counts as a virulence factor is often difficult. In the early days of modern pathogenesis research, things seemed much simpler than they do today. This is probably because the first diseases to be studied in depth at the molecular level were diseases, such as cholera, that were caused by bacteria that produced toxic proteins (toxins), which caused the symptoms of the disease. A toxin is clearly a virulence factor.

As more complex diseases were probed, it became obvious that in some cases, a large number of factors were involved in the ability of a bacterium to cause disease. An experimental definition of virulence factor is that loss of the factor by the bacterium results in a decrease in its ability to cause disease. This seems pretty straightforward, but what does one do about cases in which the loss of two factors reduces the pathogenicity of the bacterium, but loss of each trait separately does not? Or when a trait that is clearly a virulence factor in one type of bacterium is not a virulence factor in another type. Then there are the cases in which loss of the ability to synthesize an amino acid makes the bacterium unable to cause disease. Is biosynthesis of an amino acid, a trait normally considered to be a routine part of the microbe's basic physiology (housekeeping factor), a virulence factor? Even more confusing are the cases in which the loss of a trait makes a bacterium more virulent (see chapter 13, "*Yersinia pestis*, the Cause of Plague"). Throughout this book, you will encounter examples of scientists grappling with the problem of how to define a virulence factor. Either the current definition of virulence factor is inadequate or the entire concept of virulence factor, which implies that a small number of discrete traits make the difference between the ability to cause disease and the inability to cause disease, needs to be rethought.

OPPORTUNISTS. Opportunists are bacteria that normally do not cause disease in healthy people but can cause disease in people whose defenses have been impaired. For example, the bacterium *Pseudomonas aeruginosa* does not infect unless some underlying condition, such as a burn or a wound or cystic fibrosis, makes the person more susceptible to infection. An opportunist might not sound so threatening, but the opportunists are near the head of the list of causes of deaths in hospital patients. Also, the line between the category of opportunist and the category that contains bacteria capable of causing disease in healthy people (primary pathogens) can be difficult to establish. *Streptococcus pneumoniae,* the most common cause of bacterial pneumonia and the most common cause of infectious disease deaths in the United States today, would be considered a primary pathogen by most people. Yet, a person who has had a case of influenza, a viral disease that disrupts an important defense of the lungs, is at much higher risk for developing pneumonia than a healthy person. Similarly, the elderly, whose immune systems are waning in effectiveness, are far more likely to develop pneumonia than younger adults. Does this mean that *S. pneumoniae* should be considered to be an opportunist rather than a primary pathogen?

THE CONTINUUM. The foregoing sections are not intended to debunk the terms commonly used in the field. Scientists have to have terms to describe various aspects of the host-bacterium interaction and the traits of the bacterium that causes disease, and the terms defined here have proved to be very useful. It is important to realize, however, that disease-causing microbes do not always fit into tidy categories with sharp boundaries. There is a continuum of virulence that depends not only on the traits of the microbe but on the traits of the person who encounters it. The language of bacterial pathogenesis is useful only if one understands its limitations. For example, it is not wise to dismiss a bacterium like *P. aeruginosa* as "just an opportunist," as compared to a "true pathogen"; it kills far more people in developed countries than epidemic diseases such as typhoid fever and plague. Also, it is a good idea not to become too rigid in one's use of terms. There are people who would not consider resistance to antibiotics a virulence factor. Yet, resistance is intimately connected with the ability of some bacteria to cause lethal infections.

Measuring Infectivity and Virulence

Animal Models

HUMAN VOLUNTEERS. We start with the best possible model for studying human disease—humans. Human volunteers have been used in many infectious disease studies. Ethical considerations make this approach problematic unless the disease is not life-threatening or is easily treatable. Nonetheless, human volunteers have played an important role in the testing of vaccines against cholera and gonorrhea. Antibiotic intervention trials, such as those to assess the efficacy of antibiotic treatments of ulcers or atherosclerosis, are also ethically defensible, because the treatment presumably either does no harm or may benefit participants.

Some human trials have raised ethical issues. A recent example is provided by the large trials in Thailand and Africa in the 1990s of a short course of zidovudine (AZT) therapy to prevent mother-to-infant transmission of HIV. Developing countries cannot afford the long-term AZT regimen used in developed countries to prevent maternal transmission of HIV, a regimen that starts early in pregnancy and continues for months after childbirth. Physicians had begun to suspect that a much shorter course of AZT would protect newborns nearly as well and a lot more cheaply. The controversy over ethics arose because the control group received a placebo, whereas the trial group received the short-term course of AZT. Although this seems at first glance to be a rational design, it would not be approved in any developed country. The ethically acceptable test design in developed countries would be to compare women treated with the long course of AZT, a treatment known to be effective, with those treated with the shorter course. Scientists in the United States and Europe questioned the ethics of the short-course trial on the basis that the trial applied a different ethical standard to people in developing countries than the one applied to people in developed countries. Why were scientists in developed countries, especially the United States, so upset over the ethical issues raised by this test? One reason is a human trial called the Tuskegee experiment, which was conducted in the United States under the auspices of the precursor of today's National Institutes of Health (Box 2–2). Although most scientists practicing today were not around when that infamous example of unethical science was perpetrated, its chilling implications are still very real to older scientists, who are determined that such an experiment or anything remotely like it will never be repeated.

There is another type of human trial, which might be called "involunteer studies," in which infectious disease outbreaks are studied in retrospect to obtain information about disease transmission in humans. One example is the case of a school bus driver who unintentionally infected a number of schoolchildren with tuberculosis before his disease was diagnosed. A retrospective study of various aspects of this case provided information about the factors affecting tuberculosis transmission. For example, the likelihood of infection was directly linked to the amount of time a child spent on the bus. The fact that 40 minutes a day versus 10 minutes a day made a discernible difference in the infection rate gave scientists a new appreciation of how infectious tuberculosis actually is. Similarly, retrospective studies of food-borne disease outbreaks have helped to determine what types of people are most likely to develop a life-threatening form of the disease. Such information helps to identify victims of future outbreaks early enough for effective treatment.

NONHUMAN ANIMAL MODELS. For most studies of infectious diseases, nonhuman animals are the models of choice. Laboratory rodents are the most widely used models for infectious disease research because they are small and more easily (and cheaply) housed and cared for than larger animals such as pigs and baboons. Although rodents are very closely related to humans on the evolutionary scale, there are a number of important differences. Anatomically they are similar to humans except that they have fur and tails, a more prominent cecum where humans have a vestigial appendix, and a very different microbiota. Rats do not have a gallbladder. A fact that is frequently overlooked but could be a factor in the use of rodents to study intestinal disease is that rodents practice coprophagy (routine ingestion of one's own feces), whereas humans do not (except unintentionally via unwashed hands). There are undoubtedly many other differences, as is evident from the very different course some human diseases have in rodents. For example, *Salmonella enterica* serovar Typhimurium, which causes diarrhea in humans, causes a systemic disease in mice that most closely resembles the human disease typhoid fever (caused by *S. typhi*). Yet *S. typhi*, which can be deadly in humans, does not infect mice. There are a number of examples of this type.

Although rodents have been the models of choice, there are more exotic models. These include ferrets (as a model for ulcers) and guinea pigs. Recently, the nematode *Caenorhabditis elegans* has been proposed as an animal model for bacteria, such as *P. aeruginosa*, that infect many different hosts. In fact, some scientists have been looking into plants as a model for infectious disease studies. For the most exotic animal model yet, however, see Box 2–3.

Ideally, an **animal model** for a human infection would develop a disease whose symptoms and distribution of bacteria in the body mimicked the human form of the infection. Similarly, the disease should be acquired by the same route as in humans. How far to trust a model that does not satisfy these criteria is a matter of judgment. Rather than establishing rigid criteria for whether an animal model is good or bad, a variety of factors need to be considered. Have studies using the animal model produced insights that are consistent with observations of the disease in humans? Has research on the animal model led to effective interventions in human disease? More recently, another criterion has surfaced, the ease with which the animal model can be manipulated genetically. One of the primary rea-

BOX 2–2   The "Tuskegee Experiment"—a Shameful Chapter in Infectious Disease History and a Warning to Young Scientists

Syphilis, a bacterial disease, was widespread in the southeastern United States in the 1930s. The first treatment for syphilis—arsphenamine (an arsenical) and bismuth—was introduced in the early 1930s. At that time, a decision was made by the U.S. Public Health Service in Alabama to withhold treatment from 400 black men for the purpose of learning more about the development and pathology of the disease. The men, most of whom were sharecroppers and could not afford medical care, were offered free "health care," something unknown in their experience. This care consisted of regular visits to a clinic, where they were treated for any ailments other than syphilis and where detailed records could be kept of the progression of the disease.

The first decision to withhold therapy has been defended on the basis that arsphenamine treatment had some serious side effects and was not a foolproof cure, although it cured many treated individuals. But when penicillin became available in the 1940s and proved to be an effective and nontoxic cure for syphilis, the decision to continue to withhold therapy was criminal. This study continued until 1972. The study was dubbed the "Tuskegee experiment" because some of the laboratory facilities at Tuskegee University were used, but the study was designed and carried out by people working for public health agencies.

When this study was discovered and made public in 1973, it provoked extensive congressional hearings, which formed the basis for current ethical rules governing the use of human volunteers. The U.S. government, after a long delay, offered free medical care to the men involved but not to their infected wives or children who were infected because of being born to syphilitic mothers. Grudgingly, health care was later extended to family members, but it took a lawsuit on behalf of the men to prod the government to offer a cash settlement, small by today's standards. To the end, the Public Health Service officials refused to acknowledge any wrongdoing and continued to defend the study on the basis that the men would not have had treatment anyway because of the lack of knowledge of medical services and their poverty—an argument that infuriated rather than convinced critics of the study.

This painful chapter in U.S. medicine had almost been forgotten—a fact that itself raises some serious questions about how well we are training students in bioethics—when it resurfaced in connection with the controversial AZT trial design. Critics of the AZT study invoked the Tuskegee precedent in their outrage over the fact that different standards of medicine were being applied to people in the developing world than to people in the developed world. Defenders of the AZT study pointed out that the women involved in the AZT trials would not, under normal conditions, have received any therapy, but that defense was unacceptable to critics of the study design and recalled the use of the same argument to defend the syphilis study.

Source: J. H. Jones. 1993. *Bad Blood. The Tuskegee Syphilis Experiment.* Simon & Schuster, New York, N.Y.

---

sons for putting forth the nematode *C. elegans* as an animal model is that there are many mutant strains of *C. elegans,* thus making it possible to investigate the effect of host traits in the development of a disease. There are few scientists who would not agree that an imperfect animal model is better than no animal model at all.

A good reason for remaining flexible on the laboratory-rodent-as-model issue is the increasing number of available mouse strains with specific genetic alterations. These include not only the so-called **knockout mice,** which have disruptions in specific genes, but also what we might call "knockin mice," which have had human genes introduced into their genome. One such mouse is the Le^b mouse, which carries the human Lewis b antigen (one of the blood group antigens [carbohydrates on the surface of human cells]). This mouse model has been used to study *H. pylori* infections because the Lewis antigen appears to be a receptor for attachment of *H. pylori* to gastric cells and gastric mucin. Such mutant animals offer vast new possibilities for research on infectious diseases, possibilities that are only beginning to be explored. The availability of these ani-

BOX 2–3   A Bloodcurdling Animal Model

Despite repeated assurances from scientists that vampires do not exist, a segment of the public seems to place more credence in novels and movies than in the opinion of scientists; they persist in holding onto a belief in vampires. Accordingly, a group of Scandinavian scientists decided to do the superstitious a public service (or leg pulling?) by testing the old hypothesis that vampires can be repelled with garlic. Unfortunately for the scientists wanting to conduct the studies, vampires are not easily come by, so they had to resort—as scientists often do—to an animal model. They chose the medicinal leech, *Hirudo medicinalis*. Leeches are readily available because the medicinal leech has recently become respectable once again in medical circles for its ability to prevent the formation of clots and internal accumulations of blood (hematomas). Hematomas and clots interfere with the healing of surgically reattached fingertips or ear segments because they block the circulation of blood to the reattached area. A person with a reattached fingertip or other body segment has only to place a medicinal leech on that appendage for a short time every few days to eliminate clotting and hematoma formation. End result? Happy patient, happy leech.

The Scandinavian scientists borrowed a few leeches and set up an experiment in which leeches were given the opportunity to choose a garlic-smeared hand or a garlic-free hand for their next meal. The results of this experiment demonstrated that leeches actually preferred the garlic-smeared hand to a clean one. The difference was statistically significant. The scientists conducting this study modestly declined to extrapolate their results too recklessly, but their findings definitely raise questions about the efficacy of garlic as a vampire repellant. Does anyone else think these scientists have a little too much time on their hands? At least this study shows that, contrary to the usual portrayal of scientists in movies, scientists do know how to have fun.

Source: H. Sandvik and A. Baerheim. 1994. Does garlic protect against vampires? An experimental study. *Tidsskr. Nor. Laegeforen* 114:3583–3586.

mals is particularly important given the slowly accumulating examples of specific genetic defects that make people more resistant to certain types of infectious diseases. Heterozygous carriage of the sickle-cell trait confers partial immunity to malaria. Homozygous carriage of a defective chemokine receptor gene confers resistance to HIV. As studies of human genetic variation (some fortunate rather than deleterious) expand in scope, we will gain a better understanding of how human genetic variation affects patterns of susceptibility to bacterial infections.

ID_{50} AND LD_{50}. Because virulence factors are defined as factors that allow a bacterium to infect and cause symptoms, measuring properties such as infectivity is an important part of virulence studies. Two common measures widely used to define virulence in animal models are **ID_{50}** and **LD_{50}**. The ID_{50} is the number of bacteria necessary to infect 50% of the animals exposed to the bacterium (Figure 2–1). The LD_{50} is the number of bacteria needed to kill 50% of the animals. Plots of number of animals infected or killed versus number of bacteria in the inoculum are sigmoidal, not linear. To locate the 50% point precisely, one uses statistical methods such as the procedure of Reed and Muench or probit analysis. These methods not only determine the 50% point mathematically but also provide a measure of experimental error that is important for deciding whether two ID_{50} or LD_{50} values differ from each other by a statistically significant amount. The reason the 50% value is determined rather than the 100% value is that it is much easier to determine the 50% value accurately because it is in a region of the curve where maximum change occurs. Students who have trouble with the concept that the lower the LD_{50} or ID_{50}, the more lethal or infectious the bacterium is, might make use of the following dictum: when it comes to LD_{50} or ID_{50}, less is worse.

ID_{50} and LD_{50} have proved to be useful measures of infectivity and lethality, but they have some important limitations. First, they are very crude measures, which reflect the cumulative effect of the many steps involved in colonization and production of symptoms. Their lack of sensitivity means that the failure of a mutation to lower the ID_{50} or LD_{50} does not necessarily mean that the mutation did not affect an important virulence de-

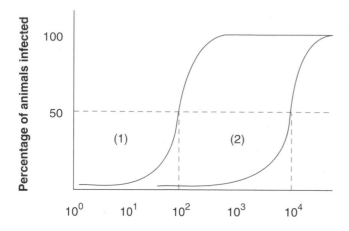

Log (number of bacteria/animal)

Figure 2–1 Typical curves obtained when determining ID_{50} values for bacteria with different levels of infectivity. For bacterium (1), it requires only 10^2 organisms per animal to cause disease in 50% of the animals ($ID_{50} = 10^2$). In comparison, for bacterium (2), it requires 10^4 microbes per animal to cause disease in 50% of the animals ($ID_{50} = 10^4$). Therefore, bacterium (1) is more infectious than bacterium (2), because it requires fewer cells to cause disease.

terminant; rather, it could mean that the effect was not gross enough to be detected by these assays. In this connection, it is important to remember that animal models are generally designed to give the bacteria as much of an edge as possible, so that infection can be obtained reproducibly in most or all of the animals. A trait that might be critical to establishing an infection in the more challenging environment of the body of an immune-competent human might not be as critical in an animal model when the animal was chosen for its high susceptibility.

Another limitation is that ID_{50} and LD_{50} at best provide relative measures of virulence when comparing different strains of a species or different mutants of the same strain. They are misleading when used to compare two different diseases. For example, the bacterium that causes cholera has an ID_{50} of about 10,000 bacteria when ingested by humans, whereas the bacterium that causes bacterial dysentery has an ID_{50} of 10 to 20. At first glance, this might appear to indicate that the bacterium that causes dysentery is more virulent than the bacterium that causes cholera, but this is not the case. In fact, cholera is often a fatal disease whereas bacterial dysentery seldom causes death in adults. The difference in ID_{50} is due to the relative ability of the two species of bacteria to survive passage through the acid environment of the stomach, the first step in infection by an ingested pathogen. Thus, comparisons of ID_{50} or LD_{50}

values must be made with care and are best applied to assessing the relative infectivity or lethality of closely related strains of bacteria.

COMPETITION ASSAYS. A way to make infection experiments more sensitive than the ID_{50} and LD_{50} assays is to use a competition assay. In this assay, the animal is infected with a mixture of mutant and wild-type bacteria. After giving the bacteria time to establish themselves, samples are taken from various parts of the animal, and the ratio of mutant to wild type is determined. If the ratio of mutant to wild type is the same as in the infecting dose, the mutation had no detectable effect on virulence, but if the wild type outcompetes the mutant, the mutation clearly had a negative effect. One reason this type of assay is more sensitive than the ID_{50} or LD_{50} assays is that the mutant and wild type are competing for the same turf. A second reason is that the ratio of mutant to wild type can be quantified more accurately than the ID_{50} or LD_{50}. Also, this assay may enable the investigator to use fewer animals.

Tissue Culture and Organ Culture Models

TISSUE CULTURE. Although animal models are the "gold standard" of research on bacterial virulence, animals present a complex system in which many variables cannot be controlled. Cultured mammalian cells are commonly used to provide a more easily controlled system for investigating the host-bacterium interaction. Tissue culture cells can be grown in defined media under reproducible conditions, and only one cell type is represented. With tissue culture cells, it is easier to do experiments involving radioactive compounds and to introduce foreign DNA. Tissue culture cells also cost less per day to house than laboratory rodents, do not fight with each other, and have seldom been known to escape from their cages. As useful as cultured cells are for studying the bacterium-host interaction, they have some important limitations that must be kept in mind when interpreting results of experiments. Because of the critical role tissue culture cells have played in molecular investigations of the bacterium-host cell interaction, it is important to understand these limitations.

A major limitation of cultured mammalian cells is that they are often derived from a tumor, whose cells have lost growth control and may have changed in other ways. A second way to immortalize cells is to plate them in tissue culture medium and select for those few cells that are capable of unregulated growth. This process stresses the cells to such an extent that their chromosomes undergo numerous mutations, gene rearrangements, and gene duplications. These mutations are not only uncharacterized (because they are so numerous and so complex), but they are not easily reproducible. Two separate sets of primary cells from the same source, which are treated in exactly the same way to produce immortalized cell lines, will have different combinations of mutations and rearrangements. Thus, not only are cultured cells far from being genetically identical to cells in the organ from which they were derived, but different lines developed from the same type of cell are not necessarily identical. Cell lines that are passed repeatedly in culture will continue to develop new mutations. Thus, the fact that two different investigators are using a cell line with the same name does not mean that they are using genetically identical cell lines.

Tissue culture cell lines lose many traits of the original tissue from which they were derived. To make the transition from a differentiated, nondividing cell to a rapidly dividing cell, cultured cells must be stripped of many of the properties that made them the type of cell they were in the first place. A consequence of this is that bacterial and viral pathogens that are highly specific for a particular tissue when causing an infection in an intact animal are frequently able to invade cultured cells derived from tissue they do not normally infect. Probably this is due to loss of a receptor that was present on cells in the original tissue and that was responsible for the tissue specificity of the pathogen. Loss of the primary receptor uncovers secondary receptors that are present on many types of cells.

Cells in culture are no longer in the same environment as cells in the organ of origin, and many genes that were expressed by cells in an intact organ are not detected in cultured cells. This gene expression problem can be corrected to some extent by addition of hormones to the culture medium and by providing an artificial **extracellular matrix** for the cells to grow on, but no one has yet managed to make an immortalized cell line into a completely faithful replica of the same cells in the body. A related problem is that most cultured cells lose their normal shape and distribution of surface antigens. Cells in an intact animal are usually **polarized.** That is, different parts of the cell are exposed to different environments, e.g., lumen, adjacent cells, and underlying blood and tissue. Membranes on different sides of polarized cells contain different sets of proteins, a feature that is presumably important for their function.

This is illustrated in Figure 2–2 for a layer of mucosal cells, but the same considerations apply to cells in other parts of the body. In a layer of normal mucosal cells, the **apical surface** is exposed to the external environment (e.g., the lumen contents in the gastrointestinal tract), whereas the **basal** and **lateral surfaces** are in contact with the extracellular matrix (a combination of proteins and polysaccharides that "glue" the cells together). Mucosal cells in the gastrointestinal tract and some other tissues are also connected to each other by **tight junctions,** proteins that make a tight impermeable connection between the adjacent cells. By contrast, tissue culture cells grown as nonconfluent monolayers do not have differentiated surfaces, and proteins that are found only on the apical or basal-lateral surface of cells in vivo may be distributed over the entire surface of such cells, assuming they are produced at all. Allowing the cells to grow to confluence does not necessarily solve this problem. It is usually necessary to provide an extracellular matrix substitute and to provide hormones to obtain a polarized monolayer in culture. Production of a polarized monolayer in culture has been achieved for some types of cell lines, but the expression and distribution of relevant surface molecules should still be checked before concluding that a polarized cell monolayer in culture is the same as tissue in the intact animal. In practice, this is seldom done.

Still another problem with cultured cells as representatives of human mucosal surfaces is that real mucosal surfaces are covered with mucus and bathed in solutions that are difficult to mimic in an in vitro system. For example, the fluid bathing the small intestinal and colonic mucosal cells is anaerobic and contains bile salts. The fluid bathing the vaginal mucosal cells and the bladder mucosal cells also has a low oxygen concentration and high concentrations of compounds such as urea or lactic acid that could have an effect on mucosal cell physiology. Finally, real tissues usually consist of multiple cell types, not of a single cell type.

The fact that there are problems with existing cell lines does not mean that such cell lines are not extremely useful. If their limitations are kept in mind, cultured cells can be a marvelous tool for discovery. Once a new phenomenon has been discovered in cultured cells (e.g., attachment of bacteria to a mammalian cell receptor or reorganization of host cell cytoskeleton), experiments can be designed that use organ cultures or animals to test the importance of the phenomenon in vivo. It is not uncommon to find that a mutation that affects the ability of a bacterium to infect a tissue culture cell has no effect when tested in animals, so taking the study from tissue culture cells to the animal is an important step. Tissue culture cells can be important for generating hypotheses, which can then be tested in the intact animal. It is a mistake, however, to take the results obtained from studies of tissue culture cells and extrapolate directly from them to the disease in humans.

The development of many new reagents for probing the interior of a mammalian cell or changing its chemical environment has generated opportunities for sophisticated new approaches to studying the bacterium-

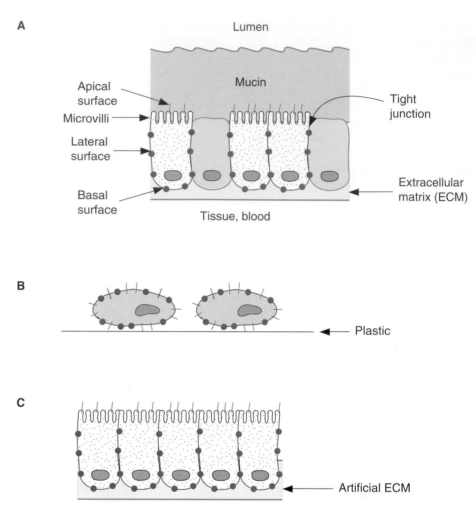

Figure 2–2 Differences between cells of an actual mucosal membrane and tissue culture cells. (**A**) Actual membrane in vivo. (**B**) Nonconfluent, nonpolarized tissue culture cells. (**C**) Polarized monolayer of tissue culture cells.

│ , apical antigens; ● , basolateral antigens

host cell interaction. For example, dyes or monoclonal antibodies that bind specifically to host cell cytoskeletal components have been used to follow cytoskeletal rearrangements caused by bacteria attaching to and invading mammalian cells. Calcium has proved to be both a signal for bacterial regulatory systems and an activator of bacterial toxins inside host cells. A number of reagents are available that either detect calcium levels inside tissue culture cells or alter those levels. In the case of organ cultures, techniques for in situ detection of proteins and mRNA make it possible to detect the elevated expression of bacterial genes in a particular tissue. These are only a few of many examples of reagents and approaches that are currently being generated by scientists interested primarily in the activities of mammalian cells but that could prove equally applicable to studies of the bacterium-host cell interaction. It is likely that future work on bacterium-host cell inter-

actions will be influenced profoundly by studies taking place today in cell biology laboratories.

ORGAN CULTURES. Organs or portions of them can be kept viable for short periods of time. Such tissues are called organ cultures. Organ cultures provide a better model of what transpires in an animal or human host than tissue culture cells, but they may be more difficult to obtain. Scientists who study adherence of bacteria to skin cells have benefited enormously from the popularity of cosmetic surgery, which generates large amounts of skin tissue. Similarly, hysterectomies make fallopian tube and uterine tissues available. But the number of people lining up to donate portions of their liver or heart is rather limited. We will return to the issue of organ cultures in the context of specific diseases in later chapters.

Good Information about the Pathology of a Disease

A topic that is very important but is seldom discussed is the quality and quantity of information about how a disease progresses in humans and—perhaps even more important—the extent to which basic scientists in the field are aware of this information. There are some fields, such as tuberculosis research, in which scientists are fortunate to have a vast store of information about how the disease progresses in the human body. Also, scientists working in the field are almost all conversant with this body of knowledge and refer to it on a regular basis to assess whether their experimental findings make sense in the context of the real world. Unfortunately, this is not the case in all areas of pathogenesis research. It is important for young scientists (and old ones too) to acquire some knowledge of human physiology, or the physiology of whatever animal they are using as a model, and to know as much as possible about where the bacteria are in the body, how the disease progresses, and what types of damage are done. Against this background, results of experiments on tissue culture cells and other ex vivo model systems are more likely to be interpreted correctly and to be productive of new insights than the results of experiments done in vacuo. Therefore, we have tried to introduce this type of material wherever possible, although a really complete treatment is clearly beyond the scope of this book.

SELECTED READINGS

Falkow, S. 1998. What is a pathogen? *ASM News* **63:**359–366.

Groisman, E. A., and H. Ochman. 1994. How to become a pathogen. *Trends Microbiol.* **2:**289–294.

Haffajee, A. D., and S. S. Socransky. 1994. Microbial etiological agents of destructive periodontal diseases. *Periodontology 2000* **5:**78–111. (This paper discusses Koch's postulates in an interesting new way. See Box 2–1.)

McFall-Ngai, M. J. 1998. The development of cooperative associations between animals and bacteria: establishing detente among domains. *Am. Zoologist* **38:**593–608. (This is another interesting paper that questions whether "virulence factors" might actually be better described as "colonization factors.")

Tyler, K. D., G. Wang, S. D. Tyler, and W. M. Johnson. 1997. Factors affecting reliability and reproducibility of amplification-based DNA fingerprinting of representative bacterial pathogens. *J. Clin. Microbiol.* **35:**339–346.

SUMMARY OUTLINE

Koch's postulates

First postulate
- Bacteria must be associated with the lesion
- Problem: some bacteria colonize without causing symptomatic disease

Second postulate
- Bacteria must be isolated in pure culture
- Problem: some bacteria cannot be cultivated

Third postulate
- Isolated bacterium must produce disease when inoculated into human or animal
- Most difficult postulate to satisfy
  - Disease too serious to use in human volunteers
  - No animal model exists

Fourth postulate
- Bacteria must be reisolated from intentionally infected animal or human

Proposed fifth postulate
- Information about the microbe should enable scientists to design effective therapeutic or preventive measures

Microbiota shift diseases
- Many microbes involved in infection
- Difficult to satisfy Koch's postulates

(continued)

Concepts of disease

Varieties of human-microbe interactions

Not all people are equal in their response to a pathogen

Not all strains of a bacterial species have equal ability to cause disease

Views of human-microbe interactions

Disease-causing bacteria evolved specifically to cause human disease

Disease symptoms result when equilibrium does not develop between disease-causing bacteria and humans

Humans are accidental hosts of bacteria that normally occupy another niche

Terms used in bacterial pathogenesis

Infection: colonization of the body by a bacterium capable of causing disease

Disease: infection that produces symptoms

Colonization: bacterium occupies and multiplies in a particular area of the body

Asymptomatic carrier: an infected person who does not have symptoms

Symptoms: effects of bacterial infection apparent to infected person

Virulence (pathogenicity): ability of a bacterium to cause disease

Virulence factor: bacterial product or strategy that contributes to virulence or pathogenicity

Opportunists: bacteria that normally do not cause disease in healthy people but can cause disease in people with impaired defenses

Measuring infectivity and virulence

Human volunteers

Best model systems

Ethical issues

Retrospective studies of outbreaks

Nonhuman animal models

Do not always respond in same way as humans

Rodents most common models

Many strains available

Some carry human genes

ID_{50} and LD_{50}

ID_{50}: number of bacteria necessary to cause infection in 50% of animals exposed to bacterium

LD_{50}: number of bacteria needed to kill 50% of animals exposed

Somewhat crude measures

Provide relative measures when comparing different strains of a species or mutants

Misleading when comparing different diseases

Competition assays

Animals infected with mutant and wild-type bacteria

Change in ratios measured after period of time

More accurate than ID_{50} and LD_{50}

Tissue culture models

Cultured mammalian cell lines used

More easily controlled than whole animals

Limitations

Often derived from tumors

Selected for ability to grow in unregulated manner

Mutations, gene rearrangements

Separate sets of cells not identical

(continued)

SUMMARY OUTLINE (continued)

      Lose many traits of original tissue and respond differently to microbes

      Lose normal shape and distribution of surface antigens, e.g., polarity

      Not covered by mucus or bathed in solutions found in intact animal

    Important as first step in determining virulence factors; can then be tested in intact animals

Organ culture models

    Better models than tissue culture

    More difficult to obtain than isolated cells

QUESTIONS

Answers to the questions can be found in Appendix 2.

1. Three views of bacterial pathogens were presented. In one view, disease-causing bacteria evolved specifically to cause disease in humans. (They're out to get you!) In the second view, bacteria evolved to colonize certain sites in a certain animal and cause disease when they do not establish an equilibrium with their host. (They're out to dine at your expense!) In the third view, humans were often accidental hosts for bacteria whose traits were not designed for colonizing or infecting humans. (They're lost and not happy about it!) What sort of traits in a bacterial pathogen would convince you that one of these views is the best explanation for a particular disease?

2. Why are scientists so reluctant to let go of Koch's postulates even though scientists often chafe—as Koch himself did—under their restrictions? Why are Koch's postulates, with all their problems, still as relevant today as they were when Koch first proposed them?

3. Using leeches as models for vampires is a humorous example of an animal model, yet it illustrates some of the problems encountered when choosing an animal model and then deciding how much credence to give the results of animal model experiments. What problems and what advantages of animal models does this rather silly example illustrate?

4. What should the criteria be for a nonhuman animal model to be acceptable as a stand-in for humans? Under what conditions would you favor allowing human volunteers to be used as guinea pigs?

5. Describe the type of disease that would have a low ID_{50} but a high LD_{50}. Is it possible to have a disease for which LD_{50} is an appropriate measure but not ID_{50}? Is there a combination of high or low ID_{50} and high or low LD_{50} that should not be possible?

6. What limitations do organ cultures have as model systems?

7. What is the nutritional version of Koch's postulates?

Molecular Approaches to the Diagnosis and Characterization of Bacterial Infections

Seeking Insights into Virulence

Molecular Koch's Postulates

Just as microbiologists in the second half of the 19th century struggled with the question of how to prove that a particular bacterium caused a particular disease, microbiologists in the second half of the 20th century struggled with the question of how to prove that a particular gene or genes contributed to virulence. If Koch were alive today, he would no doubt be flattered by the fact that the initial attempts to answer this question used his postulates as a guide, but he would not be surprised to see the new postulates debated just as hotly as the postulates he put forward. There have been several versions of molecular Koch's postulates, but most of them read as follows: First, the gene (or its product) should be found only in strains of bacteria that cause the disease and not in bacteria that are avirulent. Second, the gene should be "isolated" by cloning. Third, disrupting the gene in a virulent strain should reduce the virulence of the bacterium. Alternatively, introducing the cloned gene into an avirulent strain should render the strain virulent. Finally, it should be demonstrated that the gene is expressed by the bacterium when it is in an animal or human volunteer at some point during the infectious process.

Today, this view of virulence genes seems overly simplistic, but at the time, attempts to establish a set of criteria for what would be called a "virulence gene" was instrumental in getting the field off to a running start. This version of molecular Koch's postulates also did a service because almost immediately it generated dissatisfaction with this simple view of virulence factors and fueled discussions that have led to a more sophisticated (but probably still not entirely correct) view of virulence.

Virulence as a Complex Phenomenon

Rather than critique the early versions of molecular Koch's postulates, it makes more sense to consider how molecular methods have provided new ways to investigate how bacteria cause disease. In retrospect, a critical experiment done on *Salmonella enterica* serovar

Typhimurium presaged what is now being learned from genomics and other ultramodern approaches. The investigators introduced transposons into a virulent strain of serovar Typhimurium. Transposons are DNA segments that integrate nearly randomly in DNA. Since most transposon insertions disrupt a gene, introducing a transposon into a population of bacterial cells and isolating members of that population that have received a transposon creates a large set of mutants, each of which has a different transposon insertion and thus potentially a different phenotype. For purposes of this study, the investigators defined "virulence" as the ability of serovar Typhimurium to grow inside macrophages. They screened thousands of transposon-generated mutants for the ability to survive and grow inside macrophages. Their results led them to conclude that at least 200 genes (over 5% of the chromosome) were involved in the ability of serovar Typhimurium to survive in macrophages, and these genes were scattered all over the bacterial chromosome.

Today, comparisons of the genome sequences of, say, Salmonella serovar Typhimurium and Escherichia coli K12 (an avirulent E. coli strain) or of serovar Typhimurium and Salmonella typhi (the cause of typhoid fever) show that the differences are many and are scattered throughout the chromosome. Clearly, virulence is multifactorial. Also, it has become clear that genes important for virulence in one strain may also be found in a nonvirulent strain of the same species. Thus, the assumption implicit in the first postulate, that only virulent organisms contain virulence genes, is flawed in much the same way as the assumption underlying Koch's first postulate, that all people harboring a pathogen would have symptomatic disease. These limitations of the simple view of virulence that underlies the early versions of molecular Koch's postulates are not applicable in all situations. The cloning and disruption of virulence genes remain a fundamental and important part of pathogenesis research today.

A number of attempts have been made to cope with the multifactorial nature of virulence by designing methods, such as the transposon mutagenesis approach just described, that do not focus on one or a few genes but seek mutations that affect some general feature of pathogenic bacteria, such as the ability to survive inside a phagocyte, or expression of the gene when the bacteria are in an animal, or survival of the bacteria in the animal. Two of the best-known recent examples of this approach are the in vivo expression technology (IVET), which seeks genes that are expressed only in the animal, and signature-tagged mutagenesis, which seeks transposon insertions that eliminate the ability of a bacterium to survive in the animal. These approaches will be described in more detail later in this chapter. Both of them have identified numerous genes as being important in the animal. More often than not, the genes identified by these approaches have proved to be genes that would be considered housekeeping genes or stress response genes. Perhaps what this is telling us is that it is the entire physiology of the bacterium, not just a few genes, that is important.

The Importance of Bacterial Physiology

DECIPHERING THE GENOME SEQUENCES. The era of genome sequencing filled scientists working in the area of bacterial pathogenesis with the heady notion that the availability of genome sequences would magically unlock the secrets of bacterial pathogens. Very quickly, however, they began to understand that there would be a small problem. How does one translate strings of A's, T's, G's, and C's into phenotypic traits such as production of toxins or ability to evade phagocytosis? At first, it appeared that this question had a simple answer: have a computer translate the DNA sequence into an amino acid sequence and search the protein databases for proteins of known function that had a similar sequence.

This strategy has been very powerful in cases where it has suggested testable hypotheses about gene function, but there is a problem. About one-third of all genes are not recognizable in this way; their deduced amino acid sequences have no significant matches in the databases. (How "significant" is defined varies somewhat from one scientist to another, but usually this means that the percentage of amino acid identities should be at least 20%.) In addition to the sequences that are not recognized at all, there are sequences for which the tentative identification is questionable. For example, a deduced amino acid sequence that contains a consensus ATP binding site may be identified as an ATPase, when it actually has a completely different function. As many as one-fifth of the supposedly identified genes may fall into this misidentified category. Whoops.

People who have taken a biochemistry course sometimes have a hard time believing such figures. They invoke the large number of pathways and enzymes described in biochemistry texts. This brings us to another problem with the sequence databases. Many of the enzymes and other proteins described in biochemistry texts were characterized before the days of protein sequencing. Determining the N-terminal amino acid sequence of a purified protein provides an amino acid sequence that can be converted to a DNA sequence and thus can be matched with a gene in the genome sequence. In many cases, the genes for familiar proteins are not recognizable in the genome sequence databases because there is no partial amino acid sequence to link them to the DNA sequence. Whoops again.

PARTIAL SOLUTIONS.   One strategy for moving from a genome sequence to function is **microarrays.** Microarrays are chips that contain DNA segments representing all the genes in a genome. These chips are used to identify genes that are expressed under certain conditions by hybridizing the array with mRNA from the organism grown under different conditions. An example is shown in Figure 3–1. In this example, iron-regulated genes are being sought. RNA from a bacterium grown in low-iron medium and RNA from bacteria grown in high-iron medium are obtained, labeled, and hybridized separately with two chips containing the DNA from that bacterium's genome.

If expression of a gene is stimulated by low-iron conditions, the RNA that hybridizes to it should be more abundant when bacteria are grown under low-iron conditions than when the same bacteria are grown under high-iron conditions. A comparison of the hybridization patterns of the two chips identifies such genes. Going back to a master list of the genes represented on the chip allows scientists to tentatively identify those genes whose expression is stimulated when iron levels are low.

Such an iron-regulated gene may not be involved in acquisition of iron, however. Production of some virulence factors, such as protein toxins, may be linked to iron levels only insofar as the bacteria are using low iron levels to sense that they are in a mammalian host. Still, the microarray strategy (or chip technology, as this approach is also known) does help to narrow the possibilities of how a gene might function.

DEFINING THE "LIFE" OF THE MICROBIAL PARTY. Ultimately, flashy technological fixes such as microarrays are not going to solve the problem of putting flesh on the skeleton provided by genome sequences. It is going to take a new initiative to advance our knowledge of bacterial physiology to the point that the sequence information becomes truly decipherable. More than that, interactions between different pathways remain to be elucidated. As subsequent chapters on individual microbes will show, the expression of different virulence genes is coordinated, and the proteins they encode are highly interactive. How are we to understand this second layer of complexity, to move beyond the function of gene products to the interaction of these products with those of other genes? In other words, it's time to return to studies of bacterial physiology.

Unfortunately, the way bacterial physiology is normally presented to students only serves to convince them that bacterial physiology is a more powerful soporific than any prescription medication. This is a problem, because a better understanding of bacterial physiology is the most likely way to get at the essence of what it means to be a living organism. The genome sequence of a tiny bacterium called *Mycoplasma genitalium,* which contains about 300 genes, currently stands as the simplest genome of a free-living organism. Sad to say, over 111 of these genes were not recognizable as having a known function. What is exciting about this small genome is that it raises the hope that if scientists could understand the function and interactions of this small number of gene products, they would finally have a grip on what "life" means. Scientists who define their function will be pushing into an intellectual frontier that has never been entered before.

Molecular Microbe Hunting

Role of Molecular Methods in Diagnosis

An important factor in the initial association of a bacterium with a disease is the ability to identify the bacterial species. Once the cause of a disease is established, it is often important to be able to follow individual strains of a bacterial species in outbreaks. If an outbreak is caused by a particular strain that is being spread from a central focus, the strategy for stopping the outbreak will be different from the strategy dictated by isolated cases of disease popping up independently. For example, a tuberculosis outbreak in a prison or homeless shelter could be due to a single individual who served as the focus of infection. In that case, identifying and treating that individual and then following up on contacts is the approach that makes the most sense. If different individuals with tuberculosis are entering the facility, giving rise to disease caused by many different strains, screening arrivals for disease status is likely to make the greatest impact.

Molecular methods are helping to meet the challenge of responding to a rapidly changing disease picture. Although classical cultivation-based identification and monitoring methods have dominated clinical microbiology in the past, the new molecular methods are slowly but inexorably displacing the traditional cultivation-based methods, not only in research laboratories but also in clinical laboratories. The reasons for this switch are evident from a tour of the typical clinical laboratory. Stacks of petri dishes and microtiter dishes fill benchtops and incubators. Many different types of media and different atmospheric conditions have to be used to cultivate the variety of microorganisms that are known to cause human disease. One advantage of molecular methods is that they tend to use the same reagents (e.g., PCR primers) for identifying different bacteria. In a sense, these reagents serve as a universal "molecular medium," supplanting the plethora of different media types used in cultivation-based approaches.

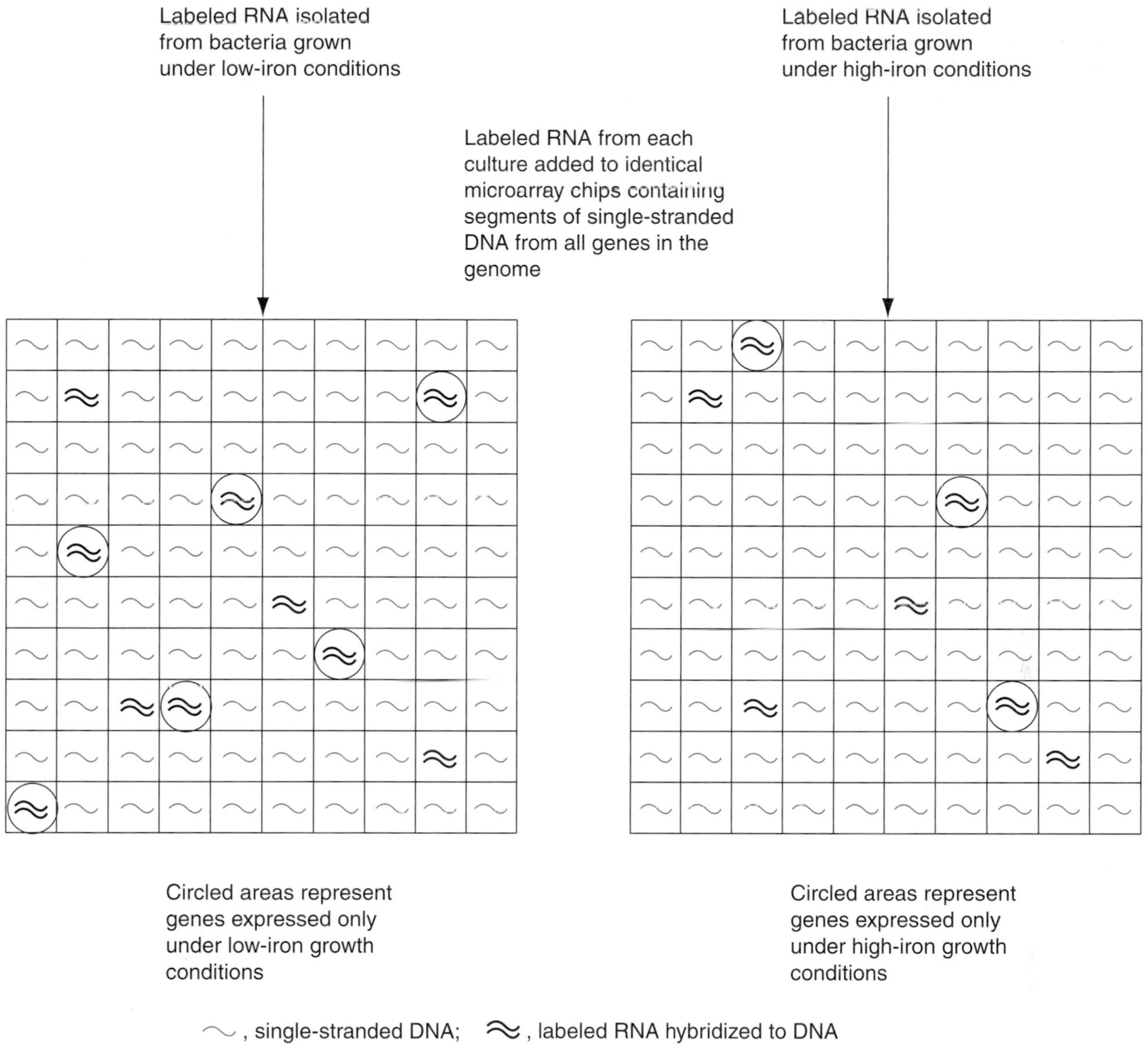

Figure 3-1 Microarrays. Microarrays are chips that contain DNA segments representing all the genes in a genome. Each square contains a segment of single-stranded DNA from a particular gene. In this figure, genes regulated by iron are being sought. mRNA from bacteria grown under low-iron conditions and mRNA from a different set of bacteria grown under high-iron conditions are isolated and labeled and incubated with two separate, identical chips. The mRNA binds to DNA of the gene from which it was transcribed. The label on the chips is detected, and from this it is possible to determine which gene was expressed under one, both, or neither of the growth conditions.

Molecular tests are usually quicker to perform than cultivation-based tests. It is true that *E. coli* can still be identified by cultivation-based methods almost as rapidly as with molecular methods, but not many other pathogenic bacteria grow as rapidly and are as easily cultivated as *E. coli*. Some bacteria, such as the bacterium that causes gonorrhea (*Neisseria gonorrhoeae*), require special atmospheric conditions and are difficult to keep alive in the laboratory. Others, such as the bacterium that causes tuberculosis, take weeks to form colonies on agar media. For such bacterial pathogens, molecular methods are an attractive option.

Nonetheless, cultivation-based methods still dominate clinical microbiology laboratory practice for two reasons. First, molecular methods were introduced, with an abundance of hype, before the technology was reproducible and robust enough to meet the high standards of clinical laboratories, where lives (and lawsuits) hang on the accuracy of test results. Second, clinical laboratory technologists are familiar with the cultivation-based technologies. Many of the older technologists had no training in molecular biology techniques and felt uncomfortable with them. The objection voiced most often, however, is that, although molecular methods can identify the species of the bacterium, one needs the cultivated organism to ascertain susceptibility to antibiotics. Some scientists think that this barrier could be overcome by putting to use the information that has been gathered about types of resistance genes found in various groups of bacteria, but this has not been done in a systematic way.

The force that is most likely to propel molecular strategies to the fore is cost. Cultivation-based microbiological analysis is expensive in terms of personnel, reagents, and space. Molecular methods, which are often more amenable to automation than cultivation-based methods, should be cost-effective as well as rapid. Also, to be blunt, molecular methods are usually "no-brainer" procedures, in which the technician uses a kit and follows a simple set of instructions. Cultivation-based identification procedures require both active intellectual involvement and wisdom on the part of the technologist, not to mention an instinct based on years of experience. This type of experience is not only expensive for hospitals and clinics but is rapidly disappearing.

There are already a bewildering variety of molecular tests on the market. Rather than trying to include all of these here, we will introduce some of the most commonly used types of tests and introduce other types of tests, where appropriate, in chapters on specific bacteria. There are two types of molecular surveys: those designed to identify the cause of a patient's disease or follow particular strains in an outbreak and those designed to identify genes responsible for the ability of a bacterium to cause disease. In this chapter, we will survey examples of both types of tests.

PCR

The realization that bacteria can be identified rapidly and accurately by obtaining the sequence of their rRNA genes has introduced a new era in bacterial identification. The revolution first hit in environmental microbiology, where nothing equivalent to the detailed identification algorithms of clinical microbiology existed. The procedure was simple: use primers that recognize

the conserved regions of 16S rRNA genes to amplify the gene (Figure 3–2), obtain a partial sequence, and then compare it with the growing sequence databases. It is now possible to identify an unknown bacterial isolate within 24 h by this approach; once this process is automated, the time will shrink still further. This method uses the same reagents for all bacterial species, because primers recognize conserved regions of 16S rRNA, which are almost universal in bacteria. Even better, this approach has now been used to identify bacteria that are not amenable to cultivation.

The first success of this approach in clinical microbiology was the identification of the bacterium that causes a rare form of intestinal disease called Whipple's disease. A bacteriumlike form could be seen in tissues of infected people, but attempts at cultivation had been unsuccessful. Finally, with the use of this technique, the bacterium associated with Whipple's disease was given a name: *Tropheryma whippelii*.

If the specimen of interest contains a mixture of microbial species, for example, the microbiotas of the human body, things get a little more complicated, but the approach still works. After using PCR to amplify rRNA genes from bulk DNA, the amplified regions (amplicons) are cloned to separate different rRNA genes from different bacterial species, and the clones are sequenced. This approach is currently being used to characterize the main members of complex bacterial populations, such as those found in the human colon. Although sequencing through hundreds of clones is no longer the scientific tour de force it once was, it is still beyond the power of many laboratories, and this limits widespread application of this approach.

Checkerboard Hybridization

Still another recent innovation that can be used to sort rapidly through many samples and many bacterial species is a technology called **checkerboard hybridization** (Figure 3–3A). The probes are applied to a membrane filter, which has been placed on a screen over an empty chamber that is connected to a vacuum line. The probes are applied in lines, using a special template that makes a waterproof seal with the filter so that cross-

Figure 3–2 Using PCR to detect microbes in a clinical specimen. PCR primers (solid dark bars) recognize segments of DNA on either side of the region to be amplified. The amplified segment can be detected by DNA hybridization or by fluorescently labeled bases incorporated during amplification.

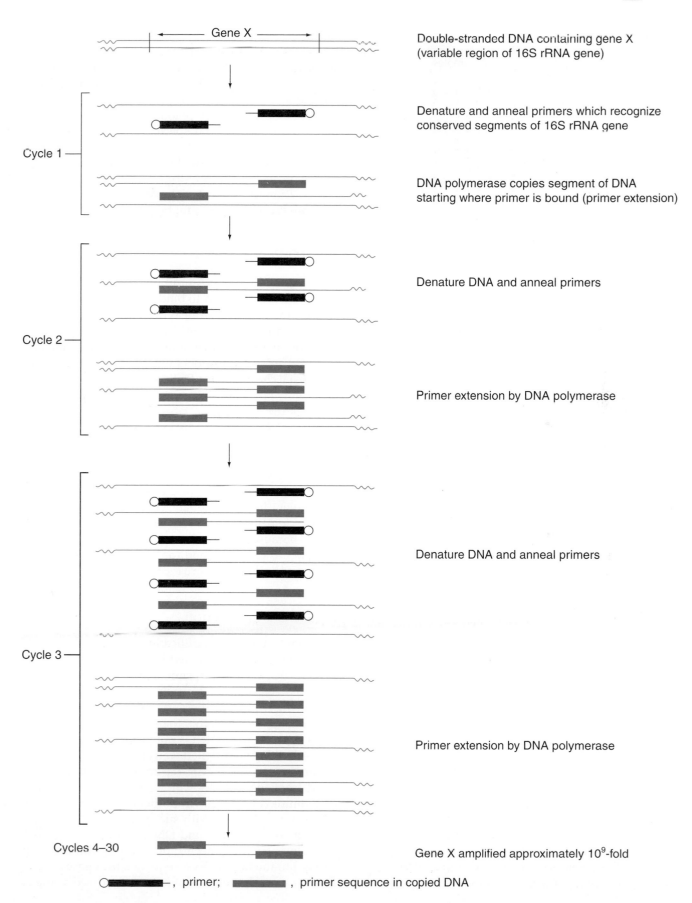

Double-stranded DNA containing gene X
(variable region of 16S rRNA gene)

Cycle 1

Denature and anneal primers which recognize
conserved segments of 16S rRNA gene

DNA polymerase copies segment of DNA
starting where primer is bound (primer extension)

Cycle 2

Denature DNA and anneal primers

Primer extension by DNA polymerase

Cycle 3

Denature DNA and anneal primers

Primer extension by DNA polymerase

Cycles 4–30

Gene X amplified approximately 10^9-fold

⊙▬▬▬ , primer; ▬▬▬ , primer sequence in copied DNA

A

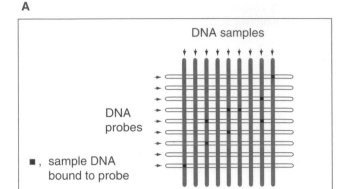

DNA samples

DNA probes

■ , sample DNA bound to probe

B

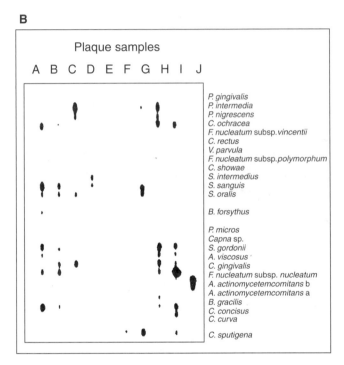

Plaque samples

A B C D E F G H I J

P. gingivalis
P. intermedia
P. nigrescens
C. ochracea
F. nucleatum subsp. vincentii
C. rectus
V. parvula
F. nucleatum subsp. polymorphum
C. showae
S. intermedius
S. sanguis
S. oralis

B. forsythus

P. micros
Capna sp.
S. gordonii
A. viscosus
C. gingivalis
F. nucleatum subsp. nucleatum
A. actinomycetemcomitans b
A. actinomycetemcomitans a
B. gracilis
C. concisus
C. curva

C. sputigena

Figure 3–3 Checkerboard hybridization. (**A**) Probes are first applied in lines on a membrane filter. Labeled amplicons of rRNA genes are applied in lines perpendicular to the probe lines. DNA bound to the probes is seen as a dark spot. (**B**) Results of a checkerboard hybridization experiment used to identify bacteria in a sample from a patient with periodontal disease. (Adapted from S. S. Socransky et al., *BioTechniques* **17:**788–792, 1994.)

contamination is prevented. A vacuum applied to the lower chamber draws the fluid (which contains the probe) onto the filter. rRNA genes in the same sample are amplified using PCR with fluorescently labeled nucleotides. The labeled amplicons are applied to the filter, which contains the probe, in lines that run perpendicular to the probe lines. After an incubation period to allow DNA sequences similar to the probe DNA to hybridize to the probe, the labeled DNA is removed, and

the filter is washed with buffer to remove unhybridized DNA. Bound fluorescent DNA is visualized as dark spots. In Figure 3–3B, checkerboard hybridization is being used to identify the bacteria in a sample taken from the gums of someone with periodontal disease. Periodontal disease is a microbiota shift disease involving many different bacterial species. Using checkerboard hybridization, scientists at the Forsythe Dental Institute in Boston, Mass., are trying to learn how much person-to-person and lesion-to-lesion variability there is in the composition of the bacterial population found below the gum line in the periodontal pocket.

RAPID-PCR

In the case of 16S rRNA amplification using PCR, the primers were designed to bind specifically to one type of gene and to produce one type of amplicon. A variant of PCR, called **random-primed (RAPID)-PCR,** uses a random mixture of nucleotide hexamers as primers in PCR. Because the hexamers will bind to many sites on a bacterial chromosome, PCR will produce a mixture of differently sized amplicons, which appear as multiple bands after electrophoretic separation and staining. RAPID-PCR can easily distinguish between different strains of a bacterial species and has been used to determine the source of an outbreak. A limitation of this procedure is that the banding pattern can vary from laboratory to laboratory and even from experiment to experiment in the same lab. This problem should not cause scientists to dismiss RAPID-PCR in its various forms, because there are many ways in which this simple and attractive method for tracing strains could be improved and made more reproducible.

Ligase Chain Reaction

A different type of amplification, called **ligase chain reaction (LCR),** is illustrated in Figure 3–4. In contrast to PCR, the two specific primers hybridize to sequences immediately adjacent to each other. If the sequence alignment is perfect, the ends of the primers will be close enough to each other to be covalently attached by DNA ligase. If the match is not perfect, the ends of the primers will not be aligned well enough for DNA ligase to join them. As with PCR, the bound primers are separated from the test DNA in a denaturation step, and then unused primers have another chance to bind to the DNA and be linked. With successive rounds of denaturation, renaturation, and DNA ligase action, primer pairs increase in concentration if they bind tightly enough to the target DNA sequence for ligase joining. Finally, a wash step removes unhybridized primers, and then a denaturation step removes the bound primers and primer pairs from the test DNA one final time.

Usually, one primer is labeled and the other is not. The unlabeled primer binds to beads coated with single-stranded DNA segments that hybridize to single-stranded DNA from the unlabeled primer. If the primers were linked by DNA ligase, the label will bind to the beads and be retained. Unlinked labeled primer is washed away. Fluorescent label attached to the beads indicates that the bacterial species recognized by the primers is present in the sample.

An important recent application of LCR is a test to detect chlamydial disease. *Chlamydia trachomatis*, a major cause of bacterial sexually transmitted disease, grows inside cells of the female cervix and the male urethra. The bacteria are too tiny to see with an ordinary microscope and must be grown in tissue culture cells or detected with fluorescent antibodies. To get enough cells containing chlamydia for either of these tests to give a detectable reaction, clinicians used to have to swab the cervix through a speculum or, in males, scrape cells off the urethra—an uncomfortable and painful process. LCR is far more sensitive than serological tests and much cheaper than growing cells in tissue culture. LCR is sensitive enough to detect *C. trachomatis* in a urine sample, eliminating the need for invasive sample collection methods.

Ribotyping or Insertion Sequence Typing Using Restriction Fragment Length Polymorphisms (RFLP)

Perhaps the simplest molecular typing system for tracking bacterial strains is ribotyping and related methods. The drawback to these approaches is that much more DNA is needed than in the amplification-based systems. DNA from a bacterial strain is digested with restriction enzyme. The fragments are separated by electrophoresis and are transferred to a membrane filter. The filter is incubated with a probe that hybridizes to rRNA genes. Most bacteria have more than one rRNA gene, so the resulting pattern will have more than one band. Depending on the restriction enzymes chosen, the pattern of hybridizing bands can be species specific or strain specific. For greater confidence in cases where strains are being tracked, it is customary to use several different restriction enzymes in separate digestions to generate different patterns from the same strain. For example, if two strains have the same *Hin*dIII pattern, they may not have the same *Eco*RI pattern.

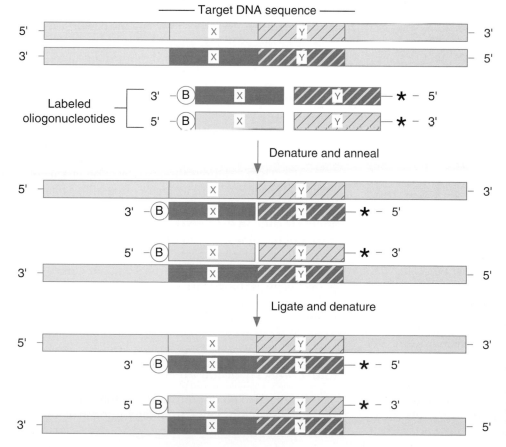

Figure 3–4 LCR amplification. Streptavidin linked to beads is used to capture biotin-labeled DNA, and then the amount of label attached to beads is measured. B, biotin. Asterisks indicate label. (Reprinted with permission from N. C. Engleberg, *ASM News* **57:**183–186, 1991.)

A similar method, but with a different hybridization probe, is widely used to track *Mycobacterium tuberculosis* strains. This approach takes into account the fact that virtually all *M. tuberculosis* strains carry multiple copies of an insertion sequence, IS*6110*. DNA from each strain is treated with one or more restriction enzymes, the fragments are separated electrophoretically and transferred to a membrane filter, and the filter is treated with a probe that hybridizes with IS*6110*. An example is provided in Figure 3–5.

PFGE

Another conceptually simple approach to strain typing is **pulsed-field electrophoresis (PFGE)**. DNA is extracted from the bacterial cell in a way that does not shear it. It is then incubated with restriction enzymes that cut in only a few places on the bacterial chromosome. The resulting fragments are too large to migrate far in an ordinary agarose gel placed in an electric field. The DNA molecules soon stop moving as they become physically trapped in the gel. If, however, the electric field switches direction (pulses) frequently, the DNA can snake its way further into the gel and be separated on the basis of size. PFGE has been used in outbreaks of *Salmonella javiana* to trace the strain back to the contaminated food and food handlers responsible for the outbreak (Figure 3–6). PFGE has the advantage of sim-

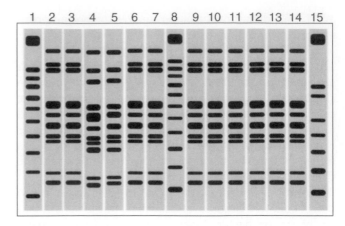

Figure 3–6 PFGE fingerprints of *S. javiana* isolates from a suspected food-borne outbreak. Digestion of the DNA with *Xba*I generated several large fragments of DNA. Lanes 1, 8, and 15, standard DNA markers; lanes 4 and 5, *S. javiana* unrelated to the outbreak; lane 2, isolate from leftover chicken sandwich; lanes 3, 11, 12, 13, and 14, samples from patients; lanes 6, 7, 9, and 10, isolates from food handlers. (Reprinted with permission from R. Lee, J. Peppe, and H. George, *J. Clin. Microbiol.* **36:**284–285, 1998.)

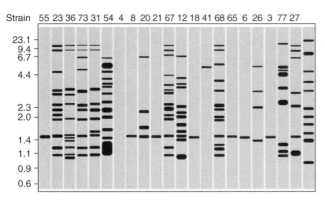

Figure 3–5 RFLP Southern blot of *M. tuberculosis* DNA using IS*6110* as a probe. Chromosomal DNA was digested with the restriction enzyme *Pvu*II. Numbers on the left indicate sizes of standard DNA fragments (in kilobase pairs). As you can see, different strains of *M. tuberculosis* give different banding patterns, so in an outbreak, if most strains have the same banding pattern, you could conclude that a single strain was causing the outbreak. (Reprinted with permission from D. Van Soolingen, P. E. W. de Haas, P. W. M. Hermans, P. M. A. Groenen, and J. D. A. van Embden, *J. Clin. Microbiol.* **31:**1987–1995, 1993.)

plicity. It uses ordinary ethidium bromide staining and does not require special fluorescent dyes and fluorescence detectors or time-consuming hybridization steps. It does require special care in lysing the bacteria so that very large pieces of DNA remain intact, and a pulsed-field gel apparatus costs several thousand dollars.

Identifying Virulence Factors Experimentally

The first virulence factors to be characterized at the molecular level were bacterial toxins, proteins that damage host cells. The activity of these proteins on eukaryotic cells clearly marks them as factors that allow bacteria to cause disease. Other factors, such as the ability to adhere to human tissues via adhesins and the ability to force uptake of a bacterium by a normally nonphagocytic cell via adhesins, also seem likely to contribute to disease. But what about the factors that our current imperfect view of the disease process might have missed? Several approaches have been developed to find such factors.

Cloning, Transposon Mutagenesis, and Transcriptional Fusions

One approach to identifying the traits that contribute to virulence is to clone genes from the pathogen of interest

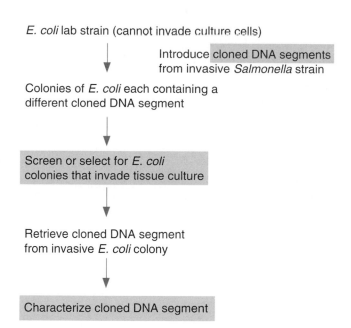

E. coli lab strain (cannot invade culture cells)

Introduce cloned DNA segments from invasive Salmonella strain

Colonies of E. coli each containing a different cloned DNA segment

Screen or select for E. coli colonies that invade tissue culture

Retrieve cloned DNA segment from invasive E. coli colony

Characterize cloned DNA segment

Figure 3–7 Identifying virulence genes by cloning them in *E. coli*. Example: cloning a gene(s) from a *Salmonella* strain that allows *E. coli* to invade tissue culture cells.

(organism X) into a strain of *E. coli* that is avirulent and look for genes that make *E. coli* virulent (Figure 3–7). For example, ordinary laboratory strains of *E. coli* do not adhere to or invade tissue culture monolayers. Thus, potential adhesins and invasins can be identified by selecting for clones that contain DNA segments that enable *E. coli* to adhere to or invade these monolayers. This type of strategy has worked in some cases to identify candidate virulence genes, but it has some important limitations. Because standard cloning procedures isolate only small portions of the total bacterial genome, usually less than 30 kbp, this approach works best if only one or a few linked genes are sufficient to give the desired phenotype. Also, this approach requires that the gene(s) of interest be expressed in *E. coli* (or whatever avirulent host is being used). Not surprisingly, this approach has been most successful when applied to bacterial species closely related to *E. coli*.

A second approach (Figure 3–8), which is one of the more widely used strategies for identifying virulence genes, is to make random mutations in the genome of pathogen X by using a transposon and then screen the transposon-generated mutants for loss of virulence. **Transposons** are DNA segments that integrate almost randomly. The ones commonly used as genetic tools carry a selectable marker, such as an antibiotic resistance gene. By introducing a transposon into X and selecting for colonies expressing the selectable marker,

the investigator generates a collection of mutants, each of which contains a single transposon insertion. This approach has the advantage that every selected colony carries some type of mutation, and virtually all of these mutations disrupt a gene. Another advantage of transposon mutagenesis is that the transposon serves as a marker to locate the gene of interest and can be used to clone the gene later. This is an important trait in bacterial species in which the sophisticated genetic mapping tools needed to locate and clone point mutations are not available. Still another advantage of **transposon mutagenesis** is that it can be used to identify virulence genes that are not expressed in *E. coli* or are not closely linked to other virulence genes on the chromosome. These advantages explain why transposon mutagenesis is so widely used in bacterial pathogenesis research.

Two limitations of the transposon mutagenesis approach should be kept in mind. First, transposons often carry transcriptional terminators. If a transposon lands in the first gene in an operon, it will eliminate expression not only of that gene but also of downstream genes as well; i.e., transposon insertions are polar. The avirulent phenotype of the mutant could thus be due either to loss of expression of the gene interrupted by the transposon or to loss of expression of downstream genes in the operon. A second limitation is that transposon insertion mutations can only be obtained in genes that are not essential for growth on the selective medium. A transposon insertion in a gene essential for growth will not be isolated, because the bacteria will not survive to form a colony. This could be considered an advantage if one assumes that the most interesting virulence genes are the ones that are not expressed by bacteria growing in laboratory medium but that are induced specifically in an animal host. For a description of an animal model that can be used for screening transposon-generated mutants, see Box 3–1.

A third approach to identifying virulence genes is based on their regulation. Virulence genes are frequently organized in regulons, different genes in different locations that are controlled by the same regulatory proteins. Thus, if one virulence gene has been identified in the organism and shown to be regulated in a particular way, other genes can be sought that are regulated in the same way. These genes might be members of the same regulon as the known virulence genes and, if so, might be virulence genes themselves. Identification of potential virulence genes by their regulatory properties is done by using **transcriptional fusions** (also called **operon fusions**). In a transcriptional fusion, a hybrid is created which contains the promoter-operator of a virulence gene fused to a structural gene encoding some easily assayable enzyme (**reporter**

Transposon (▬ Q^R ▬) introduced into invasive bacterial cells

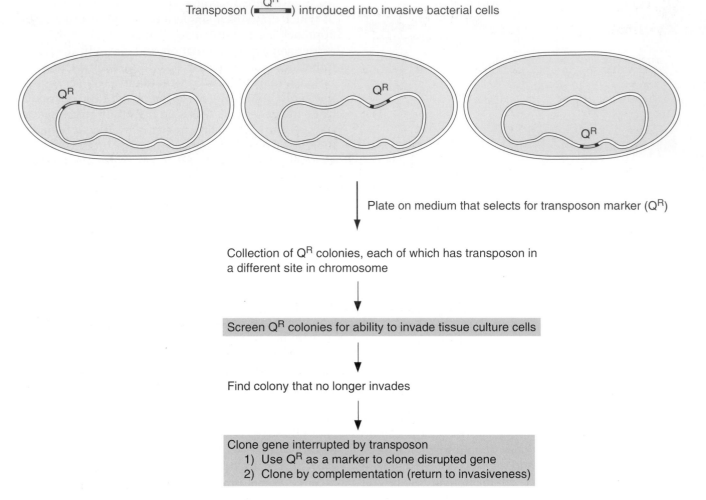

Plate on medium that selects for transposon marker (Q^R)

Collection of Q^R colonies, each of which has transposon in a different site in chromosome

Screen Q^R colonies for ability to invade tissue culture cells

Find colony that no longer invades

Clone gene interrupted by transposon
  1) Use Q^R as a marker to clone disrupted gene
  2) Clone by complementation (return to invasiveness)

Figure 3–8   Identifying virulence genes by transposon mutagenesis. Example: identifying a gene(s) needed for invasion of tissue culture cells by a *Salmonella* strain.

gene). The most popular reporter gene is *lacZ,* the gene that encodes **β-galactosidase.** Other commonly used reporter genes are *uidA,* the gene encoding *E. coli* **β-glucuronidase (GUS),** and *cat,* the gene encoding **chloramphenicol acetyltransferase (CAT).** In the hybrid construct (Figure 3–9), the ribosome binding site is provided by *lacZ.* Thus, although RNA polymerase starts transcription from the regulated promoter-operator region of the virulence gene, only β-galactosidase is translated from the transcript. Thus, β-galactosidase is expressed under conditions in which the virulence gene would normally have been produced. Thus, for example, if the original virulence gene were expressed at higher levels at 37°C than at 25°C, β-galactosidase activity of the fusion strain would be produced at higher levels at 37°C than at 25°C. β-Galactosidase activity is readily detected on plates or in liquid assay systems by using **chromogenic substrates.** A popular chromogenic substrate is an **indolyl-galactoside** called **X-Gal,** which turns blue when the galactosyl bond is cleaved by the enzyme. Thus, in the example mentioned above, colonies containing a fusion of the temperature-regulated virulence gene to *lacZ* would be blue at 37°C and white or light blue at 25°C. Not only is it easier to assay β-galactosidase activity than it is to assay most virulence proteins, but β-galactosidase poses none of the hazards associated with, for example, an exotoxin.

A transcriptional fusion can be created by cloning *lacZ* in the correct orientation downstream of the virulence gene promoter-operator region. This is feasible when the virulence gene has already been cloned. In cases where the investigator wants to locate genes regulated in a particular way, a transposon-based strategy

BOX 3–1   Worms as Animal Models Revisited

Those of you who sneered at our use of the medicinal leech study (where the leeches were a stand-in for vampires) as an example of animal models carried a bit too far, prepare to receive your comeuppance. Researchers interested in identifying virulence factors of *Pseudomonas aeruginosa*, a gram-negative pathogen that is a common cause of infection in burn patients and people with cystic fibrosis, have turned to the worm *Caenorhabditis elegans* as a stand-in for mice and humans. Screening random transposon-generated mutants of *P. aeruginosa* in mice would be expensive and time-consuming, but *C. elegans* is smaller and much easier to work with. Also, there are no government regulations regarding the proper care and housing of worms. It turns out that *P. aeruginosa* kills *C. elegans* and that inactivation of some of the same virulence genes important for infection of mice is also important for infection in *C. elegans*. Accordingly, *C. elegans*, which has heretofore served mainly as a model for development of complex eukaryotic animals, has now been proposed as a model for *P. aeruginosa* infections in humans. *C. elegans* is being used as an initial screening tool for identifying mutants that are less virulent, as indicated by their inability to kill *C. elegans*.

Source: M. W. Tan, L. G. Rahme, J. A. Sternberg, R. G. Tompkins, and F. M. Ausubel. 1999. *Pseudomonas aeruginosa* killing of *Caenorhabditis elegans* used to identify *P. aeruginosa* virulence factors. *Proc. Natl. Acad. Sci. USA* 96:2408–2413.

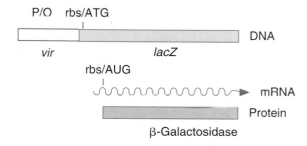

Figure 3–9   Transcriptional fusion of a virulence gene promoter/operator (P/O *vir*) to the promoterless reporter gene for β-galactosidase (*lacZ*). Although the *lacZ* DNA segment lacks the original promoter of the gene, it still has its ribosome binding site (rbs) and start codon (ATG). Thus, β-galactosidase will be regulated the same as the virulence gene.

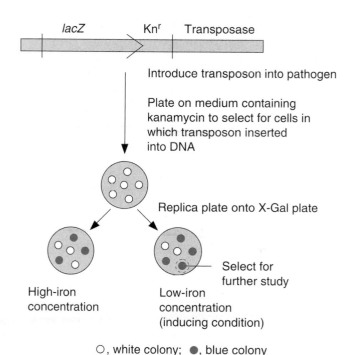

Figure 3–10   Use of a transposon carrying *lacZ* to generate *lacZ* fusions. Transposase allows the DNA carrying promoterless *lacZ* to integrate in the genome.

is used. The transposon carries the promoterless *lacZ* gene and a selectable antibiotic resistance marker (Figure 3–10). Selection for antibiotic resistance generates a set of random insertions of the transposon into the bacterial chromosome. Colonies carrying transposon insertions are then screened for regulated expression of *lacZ*. Only a portion of the transposon insertions will fuse *lacZ* to promoters, and only a fraction of these fusions will be regulated in the desired manner. Suppose the genes being sought are expressed at a high level only under low-iron conditions. In this case, colonies carrying transposon insertions would be replica plated

onto high-iron medium and low-iron medium, both containing X-Gal. Colonies containing the desired fusions will be blue on the low-iron plates but white or light blue on the high-iron plates.

Once a fusion to a regulated virulence gene is obtained, either by cloning or by transposon insertions, the strain containing the virulence gene-*lacZ* fusion can be used to find regulatory genes that control expression of the virulence gene. This is illustrated in Figure 3–11. The strain containing the virulence gene-*lacZ* fusion is mutagenized (by chemical mutagenesis or by using another transposon), and the resulting colonies are screened either for colonies exhibiting aberrant regulation, i.e., colonies that do not turn blue under inducing conditions (possible loss of an activator) or colonies that turn blue under both inducing and noninducing conditions (possible loss of a repressor).

When a gene has been tagged by a *lacZ* fusion or by a transposon insertion, it can be cloned. The transposon antibiotic resistance gene can be used as a selective marker to obtain a clone carrying the transposon and a segment of the DNA into which it had inserted. The DNA adjacent to the transposon insertion point can then be used as a hybridization probe to clone the wild-type locus. Alternatively, the gene can be cloned by **complementation.** A collection of cloned DNA segments can be introduced into this mutant background, and clones that complement the mutant to give a wild-type phenotype can be found by screening or selection. Once a clone is obtained, even a partial DNA sequence of the cloned DNA can provide considerable information. In species such as *E. coli* or *Salmonella* serovar Typhimurium, for which complete genome sequences are available, a few hundred base pairs of DNA sequence from a gene may identify the gene if it has already been sequenced. Alternatively, by looking for highly conserved amino acid sequence motifs, it is sometimes possible to guess the identity of a cloned gene.

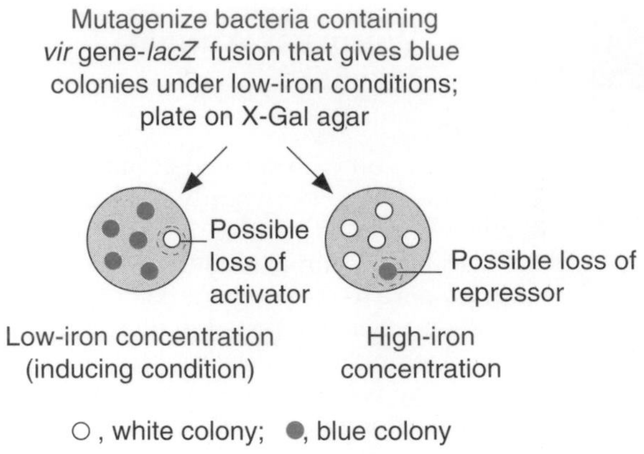

Finding Genes That Are Expressed In Vivo

A major limitation of the above approaches to locating virulence genes is that the selections involve growth and screening on bacteriological medium. Because no bacteriological medium or in vitro system is a perfect mimic of the environment inside the animal body, the best way to select or screen for interesting mutations would be to do it in an animal. A method for identifying genes that are expressed by bacteria infecting an animal has now been developed: **IVET (in vivo expression technology).** IVET is being used to search for genes that permit *Salmonella* serovar Typhimurium to cause a typhoidlike disease in mice. The approach is based on the observation that purine auxotrophs of serovar Typhimurium are unable to infect mice. To find promoters that are expressed in the animal, a promoterless version of the purine biosynthetic gene (*purA*) is introduced at random into the chromosome of a strain in which *purA* has been deleted, the collection of fusions is inoculated into an animal, and surviving clones are isolated. Presumably, the bacteria that were able to survive in the

Mutagenize bacteria containing *vir* gene-*lacZ* fusion that gives blue colonies under low-iron conditions; plate on X-Gal agar

Possible loss of activator

Possible loss of repressor

Low-iron concentration (inducing condition)

High-iron concentration

○ , white colony; ●, blue colony

Figure 3–11 Screening mutants of a *lacZ* fusion strain for mutants with aberrant regulatory properties.

animal contained a fusion of *purA* to some gene that is expressed in vivo.

To generate the pool of fusion clones, serovar Typhimurium chromosomal DNA is digested with restriction enzymes into 4- to 6-kbp fragments, and these fragments are cloned upstream of an artificial operon consisting of a promoterless *purA* gene fused to a promoterless *lacZY* incorporated into a plasmid (Figure 3–12). Cloning is done in *E. coli.* A pool of these plasmids is introduced into a strain of serovar Typhimurium that contains a deletion in its *purA* gene. The plasmid used for cloning does not replicate in serovar Typhimurium because it requires a replication gene, *pir*, for autonomous replication, a gene that is not provided in the serovar Typhimurium strain. Thus, in serovar Typhimurium the plasmids integrate into the chromosome. Selection for antibiotic-resistant colonies of serovar Typhimurium produces a collection of bacteria in which the plasmid has integrated into different places in the serovar Typhimurium chromosome by homologous recombination. Some of these integrated plasmids will place the *purA* gene downstream of a promoter that is expressed in vivo, and these are the clones that will survive when the mixture is inoculated into a mouse.

The reason homologous recombination via cloned fragments of serovar Typhimurium DNA is used to generate fusions instead of the transposon method described earlier is that the transposon insertion disrupts the gene it enters, whereas many of the homologous recombination events will leave a copy of the wild-type gene intact. This is important, because the investigators are after genes that are essential for survival in the animal and thus do not want to disrupt the genes to which fusions are made. A pool of integrated *purA-lacZY* fusions is injected into mice. The bacteria that survive in the mouse are then plated on medium on which the

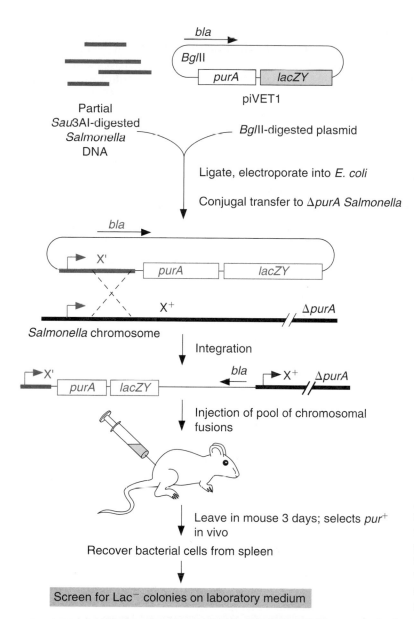

Figure 3–12 IVET for detecting genes that must be expressed for the bacteria to survive in the mouse. *bla*, gene for ampicillin resistance; *purA*, promoterless gene necessary for purine utilization; *lacZY*, indicator gene; *X*, gene into which construct was integrated; *X'*, partial copy of *X*. (Adapted from M. J. Mahan, J. M. Slauch, and J. J. Mekalanos, *Science* **259:**686–688, 1993.)

expression of the *lacZ* can be detected. The rationale for this step is that promoters that are expressed constitutively will be LacZ$^+$ on indicator plates. The investigators are particularly interested in genes that are *not* expressed during growth on laboratory medium but were specifically expressed in the animal. Thus, the desired colonies are those which are *not* Lac$^+$ on the indicator plates. Interestingly, the genes so far identified by IVET have turned out to be housekeeping genes (see chapter 2).

The IVET approach is a crude one, and its discovery record so far has been disappointing. At best, it will identify a set of genes that are expressed at some point in the infection process. A detailed analysis of the genes and gene products by in situ hybridization is necessary to determine where and when during the course of infection the gene was expressed. A more serious problem with this approach is that it only detects genes that are transcribed at elevated levels in the host. Gene products that may be activated posttranscriptionally in response to host signals will be missed. Nonetheless, the IVET approach provides one way to identify genes that may be necessary for survival in the animal. These shortcomings, however, have not deterred scientists from using this or similar approaches in the hope of identifying important new virulence genes.

The type of medium used to determine whether the gene is expressed during growth on laboratory medium also can cause problems. Many scientists use

Lactose-MacConkey agar to differentiate Lac⁺ from Lac⁻ colonies. This medium contains bile salts, which may be an important signal in vivo for gastrointestinal pathogens. Thus, some insertions identifying new virulence genes may be discarded as Lac⁺ in vitro when in fact the decision is based on an artifact of medium composition. Also, body temperature is the inducer of at least some important virulence genes. Insertions in such genes could be missed because the plates are incubated at 37°C and thus induce gene expression on laboratory media. More careful attention should be given to the means used to determine which insertions to study further and which to discard.

Signature-Tagged Mutagenesis

An in vivo form of transposon mutagenesis is **signature-tagged mutagenesis** (Figure 3–13). Instead of a single transposon, this method uses a mixture of variants generated from a single transposon. The mixture is obtained by cloning a collection of random oligomers into a transposon. Thus, each transposon has its own individual "tag," the oligomer it carries. (A library containing a mixture of transposons, each with its individual tag, is available from the original inventors of this technique.) The transposon library is transformed or electroporated into the target bacterial strain, and transformants (electroporants) that received a transposon insertion somewhere in their chromosome are detected by selecting for the antibiotic resistance gene carried on the transposon. Individual colonies, each representing a different random mutation, are saved on master plates or in wells of a microtiter dish. The mixture of transposon-containing isolates is then used to inoculate an animal. After the infection develops, the organ of choice is removed. PCR primers that recognize the portions of the transposon that flank the oligomer are used to amplify the mixture of tags. Restriction enzyme digestion then removes the primer region, leaving only a mixture of tags.

PCR is done with radiolabeled nucleotides or with nucleotides labeled with other indicators (e.g., biotinylated nucleotides) so that the mixture of tags can be used to probe the original collection of transposon-generated mutants. Any of these original mutants that does not hybridize with the mixture of probe tags represents a mutant that was lost during the infection process, presumably because it had a mutation that made it less virulent. These "lost" mutants are recovered from the original master plate and examined further to determine why they are less virulent. Since the

transposon insertion marks the site of mutation and since the sequence of the transposon is known, the transposon can be used as a marker to clone out the chromosomal DNA that was interrupted by the transposon. The chromosomal DNA is sequenced to determine whether it is a known gene or something new.

Molecular Mania—a Boon or a Boondoggle?

There is some good news and some bad news about the plethora of new molecular approaches to diagnosing disease and seeking answers to the question of how bacteria cause disease. The good news is that novel and imaginative new methods continue to appear at a breathtaking rate. The old view of the animal or the tissue culture cell as a black box that would never be opened is being challenged, and the challenges are forcing scientists to think in new ways about how bacteria cause disease. The fact that methods like IVET and signature-tagged mutagenesis, which were devised to identify virulence genes, continue to turn up housekeeping genes or genes of unknown function has made it necessary to ask to what extent the concept of "virulence factor"—a small collection of genes that distinguish a pathogen from a nonpathogen—is correct. Information coming out of studies that employ these methods is forcing scientists to rethink virtually all the dogma about what makes a bacterium a pathogen.

The good news—that novel and imaginative new methods continue to appear at a breathtaking rate—is also the bad news. In such an atmosphere, old and young scientists alike can be distracted from substantive questions by flashy new technologies. Hardly anyone working on bacterial pathogenesis has escaped the experience of finding that new technologies can be a distraction as well as an aid.

Still, on balance, the new molecular revolution that has transformed the study of bacterial diseases has had a positive influence, as long as there is a bit of skepticism in the mix. The most dangerous mistake that can be made in the rush to be on the cutting edge of new technologies is that access to the pre-molecular biology body of knowledge is lost. It is interesting that some of the top scientists in various fields of bacterial pathogenesis have begun to dip into the old literature again, even as their laboratories follow up the latest technologies. Just as the molecular revolution has opened many new vistas on infectious diseases, a synthesis of the past insights of such giants as Koch, Pasteur, and the microbiologists of the early 1900s with the new insights that technology makes possible may well be the wave of the future.

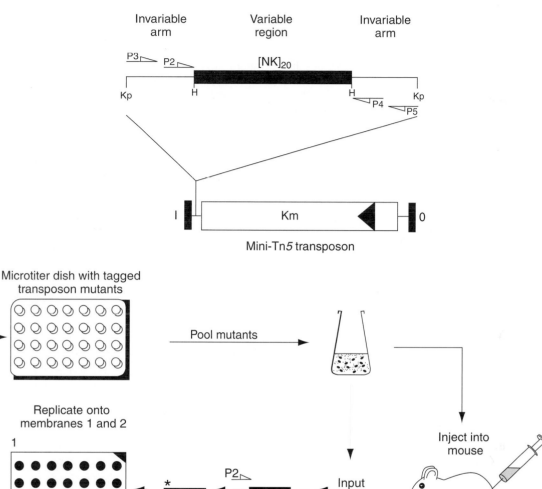

Figure 3–13 Signature-tagged mutagenesis used for simultaneous identification of *Salmonella* serovar Typhimurium virulence genes based on transposon mutagenesis and negative selection. P, primers; Kp, *Kpn*I; H, *Hind*III; I and O, ends of mini-Tn5; Km, kanamycin resistance gene. Asterisk indicates labeled tag. (Adapted from M. Handfield and R. C. Levesque, *FEMS Microbiol. Rev.* **23:**69–91, 1999.)

SELECTED READINGS

Bender, J. B., C. W. Hedberg, J. M. Besser, D. J. Boxrud, K. L. MacDonald, and M. T. Osterholm. 1997. Surveillance for *Escherichia coli* O157:H7 infections in Minnesota by molecular subtyping. *N. Engl. J. Med.* **337:**388–394.

Eisenstein, B. I. 1990. New molecular techniques for microbial epidemiology and the diagnosis of infectious diseases. *J. Infect. Dis.* **461:**595–602.

Fredricks, D. N., and D. A. Relman. 1996. Sequence-based identification of microbial pathogens: a reconsideration of Koch's postulates. *Clin. Microbiol. Rev.* **9:**18–33.

Handfield, M., and R. C. Levesque. 1999. Strategies for isolation of in vivo expressed genes from bacteria. *FEMS Microbiol. Rev.* **23:**69–91.

Heithoff, D. M., C. P. Conner, and M. J. Mahan. 1997. Dissecting the biology of a pathogen during infection. *Trends Microbiol.* **5:**509–513.

Leboux, D. E., F. Sanschagrin, and R. C. Levesque. 1999. Defined oligonucleotide tag pools and PCR screening in signature-tagged mutagenesis of essential genes from bacteria. *BioTechniques* **26:**473–478.

Mahan, M. J., J. W. Thomas, J. M. Slauch, P. C. Hanna, R. J. Collier, and J. J. Mekalanos. 1995. Antibiotic-based selection for bacterial genes that are specifically induced during infection of a host. *Proc. Natl. Acad. Sci. USA* **92:**669–673.

Socransky, S. S., C. Smith, L. Martin, B. J. Paster, F. E. Dewhirst, and A. E. Levin. 1994. "Checkerboard" DNA-DNA hybridization. *BioTechniques* **17:**788–792.

Tyler, K. D., G. Wang, S. D. Tyler, and W. M. Johnson. 1997. Factors affecting reliability and reproducibility of amplification-based DNA fingerprinting of representative bacterial pathogens. *J. Clin. Microbiol.* **35:**339–346.

Van Soolinger, D., P. E. W. de Haas, P. W. M. Hermans, P. M. A. Groenen, and J. D. A. van Embden. 1993. Comparison of various repetitive DNA elements as genetic markers for strain differentiation and epidemiology of *Mycobacterium tuberculosis. J. Clin. Microbiol.* **31:**1987–1995.

SUMMARY OUTLINE

Molecular Koch's postulates

Address how a particular gene contributes to virulence

First postulate: gene (or its product) should be found only in strains of bacteria that cause the disease

Second postulate: gene should be "isolated" by cloning

Third postulate: disruption of genes in virulent strain should reduce virulence

Fourth postulate: gene is expressed by bacterium during infectious process in animal or human

Now clear that virulence is multifactorial

Importance of bacterial physiology

Genome sequencing coupled with database searches
　　One-third of genes not recognized
　　Tentative identification may be questionable
　　Gene for known proteins may not be recognizable in databases

Microarrays
　　Consist of chips that contain DNA segments from all genes in the genome
　　mRNA from bacteria growing under specific conditions isolated and added to chip
　　Used to identify genes expressed under certain conditions

Microbial physiology will be essential to understand interaction of many gene products

Molecular methods in diagnosis

Quicker and less expensive than cultivation-based tests

PCR
　　Sequence of 16S rRNA amplified and sequenced
　　Used to identify bacteria that cannot be cultivated

(continued)

Checkerboard hybridization—can be used to identify bacterial species contained in a sample with many species

RAPID-PCR—yields mixture of amplicons of different sizes
  Can distinguish between different strains of a bacterial species
  Used to determine source of outbreaks
  Somewhat variable

LCR
  Amplification technique involving one labeled and one unlabeled primer
  Example: used to detect C. trachomatis in urine

Ribotyping using RFLP
  DNA digested with restriction enzymes
  Fragments separated by electrophoresis
  16S rRNA genes detected with labeled probes

PFGE
  Large segments of DNA separated by switching direction of electric fields
  Does not require special fluorescent dyes

Identifying virulence factors experimentally

Cloning—clone genes from pathogen into avirulent strain of E. coli and look for genes that make E. coli virulent

Transposon mutagenesis
  Introduce transposon with selectable marker into pathogen to generate collection of mutants
  Several advantages
    Every selected colony has a mutation
    Transposon is marker for gene of interest
    Used to identify virulence genes not expressed in E. coli
  Limitations
    Transposons carry transcription terminations—insertions are polar
    Mutations can only be obtained in genes not required for growth on selective medium

Transcriptional fusions—used to identify potential virulence genes by their regulatory properties
  Promoter-operator of virulence genes fused to reporter gene (e.g., lacZ) to form hybrid
  Reporter protein synthesized only under conditions in which virulence gene would normally be expressed

IVET
  Used to detect genes essential for bacterial survival in animal
  Look for genes that are not expressed in vitro
  Genes detected so far are housekeeping genes

Signature-tagged mutagenesis
  In vivo form of transposon mutagenesis
  Mixture of isolates containing transposons with oligomer tag used to inoculate animal
  After infection develops, organ or tissue of interest removed
  Tags amplified, digested, and labeled
  Mixture of labeled tags used to probe original mutants
  Any mutant not hybridizing with probe is examined to determine why it is less virulent

QUESTIONS

Answers to the questions can be found in Appendix 2.

1. Scientists have proposed a molecular version of Koch's postulates for associating a bacterium with a disease (see chapter 2). In view of the new methodologies described in this chapter, can you suggest modifications of these postulates?

2. The genomes of a number of bacterial pathogens have now been completely sequenced. How might the availability of this information affect the definition of virulence factors?

3. Critique the statement: if you compare the genomes of a pathogen and a closely related nonpathogen (e.g., *Salmonella* serovar Typhimurium and *E. coli* K12), the differences will be the virulence genes.

4. PCR amplification of rRNA genes, combined with sequencing, can provide a quick identification of bacteria. What are the limitations of this approach?

5. How could PCR be used to determine whether a strain of bacterium is resistant to an antibiotic? Keep in mind that there are hundreds of resistance genes for which sequences are available. How would you go about limiting the genes you have to PCR amplify to a manageable number?

6. Techniques such as PFGE and ribotyping can be adjusted to discriminate between different strains or between different species (or subspecies). What adjusts the specificity?

7. Why are techniques such as IVET and signature-tagged mutagenesis continuing to turn up housekeeping genes rather than the "virulence genes" the inventors of these methods envisioned? (If you have a good explanation for this, publish it right away. A lot of us are waiting for the answer.)

8. How is a gene fusion like a microarray, and how is it different?

9. If you have the genome sequence of a bacterial pathogen, would you still need to clone genes, or does cloning become obsolete?

4

The First Line of Defense against Infection: Prevention and the Phagocytic Cell Response

An Ounce of Prevention

The Human Brain—the First Line of Defense against Infection

Much that has been written about the first-line defenses of the human body has focused on the nonspecific defenses that protect the body against invading bacteria in a way that is not bacterium specific. Although the nonspecific defenses are an early response to infection, they are the first-line defenses only if one considers that the bacteria have already entered the body. In fact, the true first line of defense against infection is an effective strategy for preventing disease-causing bacteria from entering the body in the first place.

The germ theory of disease developed by Pasteur and Koch and other early microbiologists led to a medical revolution not just because it stated that tiny bacteria could sicken and kill people, but because it gave public health officials a means of telling good water from bad and good food from bad. Perfectly clear water is not necessarily safe. Ask someone who has gotten giardiasis, a particularly debilitating form of diarrhea caused by a protozoan, *Giardia intestinalis,* by drinking water from clear mountain streams. Similarly, dirty-looking, murky water may nonetheless be safe. Being able to tell good water from bad and having a criterion for when treatment of the water had made it safe allowed scientists for the first time to formulate principles of water treatment and food safety that actually worked to protect people.

The germ theory of disease also allowed public health officials to intervene more effectively to stop the spread of epidemics. Consider plague during the Middle Ages as a case in point. The officials responsible for preventing the spread of plague to their cities correctly deduced that people with plague could spread the disease. In some cities, sailors were quarantined aboard incoming ships for a month or more to see if they developed the disease. This strategy did not work, however, because the city officials missed the rat connection. Rats were running to and fro between the quarantined vessels and the city, carrying the disease into people's homes. If public officials had had some way to identify this route of disease transmission, their attempts to intervene might have been effective. Also, knowing the cause of an infection has helped to identify asymptomatic carriers such as Typhoid Mary. Because of the existence of asymptomatic carriers, prevention measures that focused only on the sick would also have been ineffective in preventing the spread of typhoid fever. A little knowledge can sometimes be a lifesaving thing.

The medical establishments of the developed world have become so focused on intervention that the notion of prevention has become distinctly unfashionable. But prevention is by far the preferable option. Once bacteria or other pathogens enter the human body, there will be collateral damage to human tissues as a result of the body's attempts to control the incursion—just as firefighters sometimes cause as much damage as the fire they are trying to control.

Two good examples of the power of prevention are provided by the recent outbreaks of West Nile virus encephalitis in the New York area and earlier Ebola virus outbreaks in Africa. Once it was established that West Nile virus was spread by mosquitoes, the solution to preventing more deaths became obvious—spray to eliminate the mosquitoes. In the case of Ebola virus, health workers were almost helpless in the face of the outbreaks until it was established that the virus was spread not by insects and not by aerosols, but by direct contact. Once this was understood, effective strategies for preventing the spread of the disease could be implemented. This is the reason that Ebola virus and West Nile virus did not spark a global epidemic, as they might have done in earlier times.

Similarly, have you ever wondered how hundreds, possibly thousands, of scientists have worked day in and day out with large quantities of infectious HIV without being infected? The answer is that if you know what you are dealing with, you can contain the risks and work with something as potentially deadly as HIV or drug-resistant tuberculosis without contracting the disease. The human brain is by far the most effective deterrent of disease available. Having said this, it is important to point out that the human brain can be a cantankerous cuss and people can behave in counterproductive ways despite knowing better. A case in point is hand washing—or lack thereof—by health care workers caring for hospital patients. Patients would be better protected if all the hand-wringing over hospital-acquired infections caused by bacteria that have become impervious to most antibiotics were to be replaced by more hand washing and more effective use of gloves to prevent transmission of such infections (Box 4–1).

Nonspecific and Specific Defenses

Definitions

Humans and other animals were born into a world that was and still is dominated by bacteria. Given this, it is not surprising that the body evolved sets of overlapping defenses that keep blood and tissue free of bacteria. One set of defenses targets bacteria in general by recognizing such general bacterial signals as lipopolysaccharide (LPS) and lipoteichoic acid (LTA). These defenses are called nonspecific defenses. This term is not quite accurate because the response involves recognition of bacterial LPS and LTA by specific receptors. Nonetheless, the term is useful because it emphasizes the fact that this defense system is multipurpose. The **nonspecific defense system** is also the first defense on the scene when an infection begins because it is always present. Examples of nonspecific defenses are skin, epithelial cells, mucin, phagocytic cells, and complement.

A second set of defenses is specific for a particular type of bacterium and is thus called the **specific defense system** or the **immune system.** When a bacterium is first encountered, the specific defenses are not immediately available and will take days to weeks to rise to full strength. In subsequent encounters with the same bacterium, however, the specific defenses appear almost immediately. Examples of specific defenses are antibodies and cytotoxic T cells. This chapter and chapter 5 will focus on the nonspecific defenses of the body. The specific defenses will be covered in chapter 6.

Connections between Nonspecific and Specific Defense Systems

Although the distinction between nonspecific and specific defenses is useful for emphasizing the differences between these defenses, it is somewhat artificial because the nonspecific and specific defenses interact with each other in a number of ways. The two systems are controlled and organized by a complex set of proteins called **cytokines** and **chemokines.** These proteins are produced by cells of both the nonspecific and specific defense systems and by nondefense cell types such as the endothelial cells that form the walls of blood vessels.

Another connection between the two systems is that antibodies (a specific defense) help phagocytes (a nonspecific defense) to ingest and kill bacteria. Antibodies can also activate the nonspecific defense **complement,** a set of blood proteins that have bactericidal activities. The defense systems are well designed to play a protective role and are remarkably effective in fulfilling that role, but both the nonspecific and the specific defense systems have a dark side. In the case of the nonspecific defenses, the dark side is a life-threatening condition called **septic shock,** which can occur if bacteria infect and persist in the bloodstream (**sepsis** or **septicemia**). Septic shock will be discussed in chapter 5. The dark side of the specific defenses is **autoimmune disease,** a condition that occurs if the immune system

BOX 4–1 Hand Washing Past and Present—a Lesson in Learning and Forgetting

The idea that physicians and nurses should wash their hands before treating a new patient is a relatively recent innovation. Ignaz Semmelweis, the man credited with making hand washing a standard part of medical practice, lived and practiced medicine in the mid-1800s. Although he was not the first physician to make the connection between contaminated hands and the spread of disease by physicians to their patients, he was the first to prove that proper disinfection of hands could dramatically reduce hospital-acquired infections. Semmelweis had noted that two maternity wards in the Vienna Lying-in Hospital had very different mortality rates. In one, the death rate due to childbed fever (a common cause of death in women of the period) was about 3%, whereas in the second ward it was over 10%. This fact was well known to women entering the hospital, who considered assignment to the second ward to be a virtual death sentence. Both wards were equally crowded, with three patients sharing each bed, the sick mixed indiscriminately with the well, and both wards contained women of similar socioeconomic status. The only difference was that women in the first ward were attended by student midwives, and the women in the second ward were attended by male medical students. Semmelweis noted that the medical students frequently went to the ward to make vaginal examinations after dissecting cadavers, some of whom had died of childbed fever.

The student midwives in the first ward were not only not dissecting cadavers but were expected to pay more attention to physical cleanliness than the medical students. Semmelweis deduced that the medical students were transmitting childbed fever (which we now know is caused most frequently by the bacterium *Streptococcus pyogenes*) to their patients because they failed to cleanse their hands properly. In 1846, he began to require that all midwives and medical students wash their hands with a chlorine solution before examining patients. The death rate in both wards promptly dropped to 1%, something the women who came to the ward appreciated but Semmelweis's male detractors did not. Semmelweis's discovery remained controversial for many years and it was

only in the early 1900s that hand washing was universally accepted as an essential medical practice.

Today, proper disinfection of hands is one of the most basic and firmly entrenched of clinical procedures, especially for surgeons. Nonetheless, the advent of antibiotics and the consequent decrease in deaths due to hospital-acquired infections has led some surgeons to neglect this important practice.

A particularly dramatic example of this was provided by a surgeon in a large northeastern U.S. hospital who started bypassing the rigorous surgical scrub procedure because he was troubled by dermatitis on his hands. He trusted to the two pairs of surgical gloves, which were commonly worn during operations. But tiny holes in gloves can be made by contact with sharp objects or bone fragments. Also, the surgeon was using mineral oil to ease the irritation to his hands, and mineral oil undermines the integrity of surgical gloves. This physician managed to contaminate heart valve implants in a number of patients with *Staphylococcus epidermidis* before he was identified as the source of the outbreak. *S. epidermidis* is commonly found as part of the resident microbiota of the skin, where it is not normally pathogenic, but it can cause infections if introduced into the body through wounds. Infections of heart valve implants usually cannot be treated effectively with a simple course of antibiotics, not only because of the high resistance level of *S. epidermidis* strains but also because of the formation of bacterial biofilms that are more resistant to antibiotics than individual bacteria. Thus, the patients with the infected valves had to endure a second operation to remove and replace the infected valve, not to mention additional damage to the heart due to the infection.

As is evident from the date on the reference cited at the end of this box, this case occurred in the 1980s. Does this mean that such cases have ceased to occur? Not at all. This case was used because it is a classic example of the hand-washing problem, but there have been many other cases since. The difference between the 1980s and the first decade in the 21st century is that today the surgeon in this case

(continued)

BOX 4–1   Hand Washing Past and Present (*continued*)

would probably have been discovered before he infected so many people, because infectious disease surveillance systems in hospitals have improved. But the attitude and behavior that sparked this sorry episode were still rampant in many hospitals in the 1980s.

The silver lining in this particularly black cloud is that the accountants for the insurance agencies have finally figured out how much the lack of hand washing and improper use of gloves is costing them, and they are mounting increasingly vigorous campaigns in favor of

hand washing and against health care workers who ignore these simple but effective precautions. In fact, relatives of hospital patients are being urged to question unhygienic practices they witness. The lawyers are circling. Who knows? It might even become safe to enter a hospital in the coming years.

Source: J. M. Boyce, G. Potter-Bynoe, S. M. Opal, L. Dziobek, and A. A. Medeiros. 1990. Tracing the source of a *Staphylococcus epidermidis* "outbreak" in a hospital. *J. Infect. Dis.* **161**:493–499.

---

attacks the body itself rather than a bacterial invader (see chapter 6).

Septic shock and autoimmune diseases are extreme examples of an important principle: the nonspecific and specific defenses of the human body are potentially destructive forces, for humans as well as for bacteria. Their protection comes at a price. Just as calling in the SWAT team can result in harm to bystanders once the bullets start flying, the nonspecific and specific defenses do a certain amount of collateral damage to tissues near the site where the invader is being attacked. In fact, many of the symptoms of bacterial infections, such as fever, tissue damage, pus, and pain, are caused not so much by direct action of the invaders themselves as by the cells of the defense systems harming human tissue as an accidental by-product of their effort to eliminate the bacterial invader.

This understanding of the origin of symptoms of bacterial infections, septic shock, and autoimmune disease suggests an obvious therapeutic maneuver: intervene to dampen the nonspecific or specific defense systems when they spin out of control. Because cytokines and chemokines are the orchestrators of these defense responses, they should be good targets for therapeutic compounds to counter an out-of-control defense response. Yet, one of the biggest medical disappointments of the past 2 decades has been the failure of one cytokine inhibitor after another to have any demonstrably beneficial effect in human trials. Ironically, just as the cytokine system can go out of control and wreak havoc with the human body, the failure of cytokine antagonists to perform well enough to justify their use in human medicine has put a number of biotech start-up companies out of business. On the bright side, however, there is one success story. Patients receiving cancer che-

motherapy, which impairs the phagocytic cell component of the nonspecific defense system, are now being given a protein, granulocyte colony-stimulating factor, which stimulates bone marrow to replenish the phagocytic cells killed by the chemotherapeutic drugs. Also, some new antisepsis drugs look promising. Results of attempts to treat autoimmune disease have been promising, but here too, progress has been disappointingly slow.

Fashion Statement

Scientists like to think that their decisions are made on objective grounds, and they usually are. Yet, there is no question that scientists are influenced by fashion. For many years, the immune system (specific defense system) was considered to be a "hot" area of investigation. The nonspecific defenses, by contrast, were considered rather dull and uninteresting. Worse, many scientists assumed that everything about the nonspecific defenses that was worth knowing had already been discovered. This lack of research interest in the nonspecific defenses made it easy to ignore them at all levels and to forget that, as the body's first line of defense against bacteria trying to invade the body, they are arguably the most important line of defense. Fortunately, this view has shifted dramatically during the past decade. Starting with an explosion of interest in the cytokine/chemokine regulatory network, which not only organizes the immune response but also controls some of the nonspecific defenses, interest has spread to the nonspecific defenses such as neutrophils. There has always been an interest in septic shock, but new technologies and new insights have pushed work on that problem to a new level. The nonspecific defenses are no longer ho-hum.

Epithelia

Epithelia, the layers of cells that cover the external and internal surfaces of the body, are an important initial defense against pathogenic bacteria. The epithelial cells found in different body sites differ considerably in their properties, but they have some features in common. The epithelia that line the respiratory, intestinal, and urogenital tracts consist of tightly packed cells, which are attached to each other by protein structures called **tight junctions** and **desmosomes** (Figure 4–1). The tight binding of epithelial cells to one another prevents bacteria from transiting an epithelial layer. To get through epithelia, bacteria must either take advantage of breaches caused by wounds or be capable of invading epithelial cells, passing between them or passing through them to get to underlying tissue. By contrast, the cells that line blood vessels or lymphatic vessels (**endothelium**) are not tightly bound to one another, because the cells of the defense systems must be able to move freely from blood to tissues. Unfortunately, this feature also allows bacteria to move into and out of blood and lymphatic vessels and into tissue.

A second feature of epithelial cells is that they are attached to a basement membrane (**basal lamina**), which consists of a matrix of glycoproteins. The surfaces of an epithelial cell that are attached to other cells or to the basal lamina (**basolateral surfaces**) have a different protein composition from the surface that faces outward (**apical surface**). Cells with this property are said to be polarized. Epithelial layers that cover surfaces where absorption or secretion is taking place, e.g., in the intestinal tract, usually consist of a single layer of epithelial cells (**simple epithelium**). Other surfaces, such as the female cervix or the skin, are composed of many layers of epithelial cells (**stratified epithelium;** Figure 4–2). Epithelial cells in different sites vary in shape. Some have a flattened shape (**squamous** cells), some are cube shaped (**cuboidal** cells), and some are tall and thin (**columnar** cells; Figure 4–2).

Simple epithelia are more vulnerable to bacterial invasion than stratified epithelia because invading bacteria only have to pass through one layer of cells to gain access to underlying tissue. Most of the surfaces that are exposed directly to the environment (e.g., skin and mouth) are covered by stratified epithelia, whereas simple epithelia are found in internal areas, such as the intestinal tract. We will use the term mucosal layer or mucosal cells to denote the simple epithelia of these internal areas. Epithelia are protected by an array of nonspecific and specific defenses. Some of these defenses are listed in Tables 4–1 and 4–2. Other defenses are more specific for certain areas of the body, such as the eyes or the respiratory tract. For example, tears contain ly-

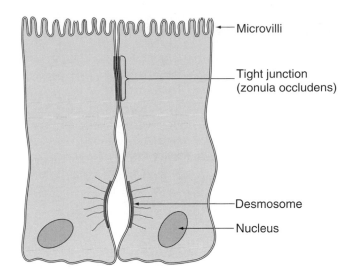

Figure 4–1 Intestinal epithelial cells showing tight junctions and desmosomes.

sozyme, an enzyme that degrades the peptidoglycan wall of bacteria. Such site-specific defenses will be described in later chapters that deal with infections of particular body sites. For the present, we will focus on defenses that are found in many areas of the body.

Defenses of Skin

Chemical and Physical Barriers to Bacterial Colonization

Bacteria are unable to penetrate intact skin unaided. This is why skin infections are usually associated with breaches of skin caused by wounds, burns, or insect bites. Why is intact skin such an effective barrier to bacterial invasion? A number of characteristics combine to make skin inhospitable to bacterial growth, as well as difficult to penetrate. Skin is composed of two layers, the epidermis (outer layer) and the dermis (inner layer). The epidermis consists of stratified squamous cells, most of which are keratinocytes. Keratinocytes produce the protein keratin, which is not readily degraded by most microorganisms. As cells from the dermis are pushed outward into the epidermal region, they produce copious amounts of keratin and die. This layer of dead keratinized cells forms the surface of skin. The dead cells of the epidermis are continuously shed. Thus, bacteria that manage to bind to epidermal cells are constantly being removed from the body.

Skin is dry and has an acidic pH (pH 5), two features that inhibit the growth of many pathogenic bacteria, which prefer a wet environment with a neutral pH. Also, the temperature of skin (34 to 35°C) is lower than

A Simple squamous epithelium

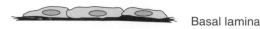

Basal lamina

B Simple cuboidal epithelium

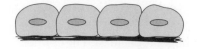

Basal lamina

C Stratified squamous epithelium

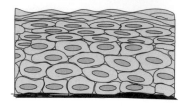

Basal lamina

D Simple columnar epithelium

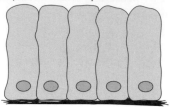

Basal lamina

E Ciliated columnar epithelium

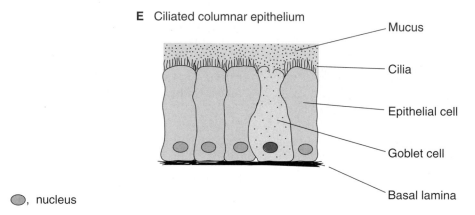

Mucus

Cilia

Epithelial cell

Goblet cell

Basal lamina

, nucleus

Figure 4–2 Different types of epithelial cells. (**A**) Simple squamous epithelium. (**B**) Simple cuboidal epithelium. (**C**) Stratified squamous epithelium (upper layers of cells are dead; typical of skin). (**D**) Simple columnar epithelium. (**E**) Ciliated columnar epithelium showing goblet cells, which secrete mucus.

that of the body interior (37°C). Accordingly, bacteria that succeed in colonizing skin must be able to adapt to the very different internal environment of the body if they manage to reach underlying tissue. Hair follicles, sebaceous glands, and sweat glands offer natural breaches in the skin that can be used by some bacteria to move past the skin surface. These natural breaches are protected by lipids that are toxic to many bacteria and by the enzyme lysozyme, which degrades the peptidoglycan cell wall of bacteria. Some pathogenic bacteria are capable of infecting hair follicles or sweat glands. This is why skin infections such as boils or furuncles are commonly centered around hair follicles.

Normal Microbiota

The defenses of the skin do not completely prevent bacterial growth, as is evident from the fact that there are bacteria capable of colonizing skin. Normally, these are innocuous gram-positive bacteria, a mixture of cocci and rods. A bacterial population that is found continuously in some body site without causing disease is called the resident microbiota of that site. The skin microbiota helps to protect against pathogenic bacteria by occupying sites that might be colonized by pathogenic bacteria. It also competes with incoming pathogens for essential nutrients. The microbiota does not completely prevent colonization of skin by potential pathogens, but colonization by pathogenic bacteria is usually transient.

Since transient colonization with pathogens can occur, and since even normally harmless skin bacteria can cause infections under certain conditions, hand washing and disinfection of hands provide a barrier to infection of oneself and other people. In hospitals, latex gloves provide yet another barrier.

Table 4–1 Defenses of skin

Defense	Function
Dry, acidic environment	Prevents growth of many bacteria
Dead, keratinized cells	Keratin is hard to degrade, and dead cells discourage colonization
Sloughing of surface cells	Removes bacteria that adhere
Toxic lipids, lysozyme	Protect hair follicles, sweat glands, and sebaceous glands
Normal microbiota	Competes with pathogens for nutrients, colonization sites
Underlying immune cells (Langerhans and other cells)	Combat bacteria that manage to reach the dermis and tissue below it

Defenses of the Dermis

Bacteria that manage to get past the epidermis through cuts or burns encounter another defense of skin: Langerhans cells. Langerhans cells belong to a class of cells called **dendritic cells** that process invading bacteria and activate the specific defenses (antigen-presenting cells; see chapter 6). The skin has its own specific defense system, called the skin-associated lymphoid tissue (SALT). This defense system has become the focus of those interested in using patches coated with tiny needle points to deliver vaccines as well as those interested in arthropod-transmitted infections.

When Skin Is Breached

Members of the skin microbiota normally do not cause human infections, unless they are introduced into the body by catheters or surgery. *Staphylococcus epidermidis,* a common skin bacterium that is normally innocuous, has been implicated in postsurgical and catheter-

related infections. (*S. epidermidis* was the bacterial villain in the surgeon-transmitted infections described in Box 4–1.) Relatively nonpathogenic bacteria like *S. epidermidis* would be killed rapidly by the defenses of the bloodstream unless they can reach an area that is somewhat protected from host defenses, such as the plastic surface of a heart valve implant. In that case, they can multiply and produce quite serious infections. **Catheters** inserted into veins can provide skin-associated bacteria with a conduit into the bloodstream, thus bypassing the defenses of the epidermis and dermis. Catheter-associated infections have become a serious enough problem in hospitals that companies manufacturing catheters are developing catheters that are impregnated with antibacterial compounds.

Surgical wound infections and catheter-associated infections caused by skin bacteria, especially *S. epidermidis,* have become an ever more serious problem because of the fact that *S. epidermidis* has become resistant to most available antibiotics. It is now clear that at least some antibiotics are exuded in sweat. Also, ointments containing antibiotics are widely used in the treatment of such skin conditions as acne and rosacea (unnaturally red skin). These treatments can last for months or years. Thus, it is not surprising that *S. epidermidis* has become resistant to a variety of antibiotics.

Common Themes

Before moving from the skin to mucosal surfaces, let us summarize some of the features of the skin defense system that will be echoed in subsequent discussions of the defenses of other areas of the body. First, surfaces are usually protected by both chemical and physical barriers. Second, bacteria that breach these nonspecific defenses encounter a specific defense system analogous to the SALT, which backs up the nonspecific defenses. Third, many body surfaces, interior as well as exterior, are protected by a complex population of bacteria specific to that area (normal microbiota). These bacterial

Table 4–2 Defenses of mucosal surfaces, both nonspecific and specific

Defense	Characteristic	Protectants	Function
Mucus	Glycoprotein matrix	Lysozyme	Digests peptidoglycan
		Lactoferrin	Sequesters iron, prevents growth of bacteria
Cryptdins and other defensins	Antibacterial peptides produced by the host		Toxic for many bacteria
Antibodies (sIgA)	Protein complexes		Specifically bind certain bacteria
Cells of immune system underlying the mucosal surface or extruded between epithelial cells			Engulf and kill bacteria or kill bacteria by bombarding them with toxins

populations are predominantly composed of gram-positive bacteria, although there are sometimes significant gram-negative members of the population. Finally, although the microbiota of a site is usually protective, members of this population can cause disease if the conditions are right.

Defenses of Mucosal Surfaces

The respiratory tract, the gastrointestinal tract, and the urogenital tract are topologically "inside" the body, but they are exposed constantly to the outer environment and foreign materials. These areas have a temperature of around 37°C and a pH of 7.0 to 7.4, and most are bathed in fluids, ideal conditions for the growth of bacteria. These vulnerable epithelia are protected from bacterial colonization by a formidable array of chemical and physical barriers (Table 4–2).

An important protection of many internal epithelia is mucus. Mucus is a mixture of glycoproteins produced by goblet cells, a specialized cell type incorporated into the epithelial layer. Mucus has a viscous, slimy consistency, which allows it to act as a lubricant. It also plays a protective role because it traps bacteria and prevents them from reaching the surface of the epithelial cells. Mucus is constantly being produced, and excess mucus is shed in blobs that are expelled. Bacteria trapped in mucus are thus eliminated from the site. In the gastrointestinal and urinary tracts, the flow of liquids through the area removes the mucus blobs. In the respiratory tract and fallopian tubes, there are specialized cells, **ciliated cells,** whose cilia are constantly waving in the same direction. The waving action of the cilia propels mucus blobs out of the area.

Another protective role of mucus is to hold proteins that have antibacterial activity (Table 4–2). Lysozyme is one such protein. It is most effective against the cell walls of gram-positive bacteria but can digest the gram-negative cell wall if breaches in the outer membrane are made by membrane-disrupting substances, such as the bile salts found in the intestine. Lactoferrin, an iron-binding protein in mucus, sequesters iron and deprives bacteria of this essential nutrient. Lactoferrin has long been appreciated as a defensive protein but has recently taken on new importance as a regulatory protein (Box 4–2).

Toxic peptides, called defensins, kill bacteria by forming channels in their membranes, collapsing the proton motive force that is essential for bacterial survival. Defensins have been found in the mouth, on the tongue, and in the crypts of the small and large intestine. Defensins in the mouth may be the reason why infections of the tongue are so uncommon and why animals lick wounds. In the crypts of the intestinal mucosa,

defensins are presumably protecting the intestinal stem cells, which divide constantly to replenish the intestinal mucosa.

A member of the specific defense system, the antibody secretory immunoglobulin A (sIgA), is found in mucin. Antibodies are proteins that bind to specific sites on bacteria or other pathogens. sIgA is thought to increase the stickiness of mucin by attaching to mucin sugars by one end, leaving its bacteria-binding ends free to trap bacteria trying to reach the mucosal layer.

Mucosal cells are constantly being replaced, and old cells are ejected into the lumen. In fact, mucosal cells are one of the fastest dividing populations of cells in the body. Thus, bacteria that manage to reach and colonize a mucosal surface are constantly being eliminated from the mucosal surface and can only remain in the area if they can divide rapidly enough to colonize newly produced cells. Defenses such as lactoferrin help to reduce the growth rates of bacteria sufficiently to allow ejection of mucus blobs and sloughing of mucosal cells to clear bacteria from the area.

Most mucosal surfaces are protected by a normal microbiota. Exceptions are the uterus and upper female genital tract and the urinary tract. The species composition of the microbiota of different parts of the body varies appreciably from one site to another. Nonetheless, all have in common the fact that gram-positive bacteria predominate. Shifts in these populations can be pathological, as is seen from diseases such as periodontal disease and bacterial vaginosis (see chapter 1).

As was the case with skin, mucosal surfaces generally have an underlying population of immune cells. This mucosal defense system (which is distinct from the defense system that defends blood, lymph nodes, and other organs) is called the **mucosa-associated lymphoid tissue (MALT)** or the **gastrointestinal-associated lymphoid tissue (GALT).** These specific defense systems are composed of macrophages, T cells, and B cells, and their principal purpose is to produce a type of antibody that is secreted into mucus, sIgA. We will return to the MALT (or GALT, if you prefer) in chapter 6.

Phagocytes and Nonspecific Cytotoxic Cells: Defenders of Blood and Tissue

A Versatile Defense Force

The defenses of epithelial surfaces are highly effective in preventing pathogenic bacteria from entering tissue and blood, but from time to time bacteria succeed in breaching these surfaces. Bacteria that get into tissue and blood encounter a formidable defense force, the phagocytic cells. **Phagocytes** are cells that ingest and

BOX 4-2   Lactoferrin—New Roles, New Importance

For decades, lactoferrin has been considered to be just one of the many foot soldiers of the nonspecific defense system. Lactoferrin is found mainly in breast milk and other secretions. It binds iron, and its role as a defense was thought to be similar to that of other iron-binding proteins: to reduce levels of available iron during an infection, thus depriving invading bacteria of the iron they need for growth. Although there is still controversy about the roles of lactoferrin, it seems likely that lactoferrin does a lot more for the human body than just deprive bacteria of iron. The iron-binding role of lactoferrin is not in question, and lactoferrin in mother's milk may be an important defense of infants against diarrheal disease—a common killer of infants in places where the water supply and the food supply are not clean.

Lactoferrin also helps neutrophils, the cells that ingest and kill bacteria, to do their destructive job (see later section of this chapter). Lactoferrin has a very basic N-terminal region. Proteolytic cleavage during a neutrophil attack releases N-terminal peptides (lactoferricins), which are very effective in binding bacterial LPS and permeabilizing gram-negative bacteria. So far, most of the evidence for a bactericidal role for lactoferrin peptides comes from in vitro studies. Yet feeding lactoferricins to mice prevented enteric bacteria from transiting the intestinal wall, so proof of an in vivo bactericidal activity may soon be available.

Many cells of the nonspecific and specific defense systems have receptors for lactoferrin. As you will learn in chapter 5, this is also true for two other families of proteins, cytokines and chemokines, which regulate the nonspecific and specific defense responses. A number of reports have already begun to appear that claim activities for lactoferrin that are similar to those associated with cytokines and chemokines. That is, lactoferrin elicits various responses by binding to different cells of the defense systems. Lactoferrin may be regulatory in another sense, by functioning as a regulator of transcriptional expression of some other regulatory genes.

Finally, lactoferrin could play a protective role. When neutrophils attack invading bacteria, they spew reactive forms of oxygen into the environment. These reactive forms of oxygen are just as toxic to human cells as to bacteria. They are especially dangerous when they interact with iron released by dying cells. Lactoferrin, by sequestering iron in an area where a neutrophil attack is occurring, may help protect human cells in the area from toxic reactions that occur owing to iron-catalyzed reactions involving reactive forms of oxygen. Apparently, lactoferrin is about to be elevated from lowly foot soldier to a leadership role in the specific and nonspecific defenses. Lactoferrin provides a good example of the numerous ways in which the response to infecting bacteria is coordinated and controlled. More such examples of this complex coordination and control will be seen with cytokines and chemokines.

Sources: J. Brock. 1995. Lactoferrin: a multifunctional immunoregulatory protein. *Immunol. Today* **16**:417–419; P. P. Ward, C. S. Piddington, G. A. Cunningham, X. Zhou, R. D. Wyatt, and O. M. Conneely. 1995. A system for production of commercial quantities of human lactoferrin: a broad spectrum antibiotic. *Biotechnology* **13**:498–503.

---

kill bacteria. Another type of nonspecific defense cell is the **natural killer (NK) cell.** NK cells attack infected human cells. Once thought to be a defense mainly against viral infections, these cells are now known to serve also as an important defense against bacteria that invade and grow inside human cells. The characteristics of different nonspecific phagocytic and NK cells and their relationships to cells of the specific immune defense system are illustrated in Figure 4–3. The phagocytes include **polymorphonuclear leukocytes** (also called **PMNs** or polys or neutrophils), **monocytes,** and **macrophages.**

Monocytes are the precursors of macrophages. Macrophages are included here as members of the nonspecific defense system, but they will appear again as important members of the specific defense system. This is due to the fact that although some macrophages act to ingest and kill bacteria in a nonspecific way, others present antigens to cells of the immune system. A cell type that is closely related to macrophages is the dendritic

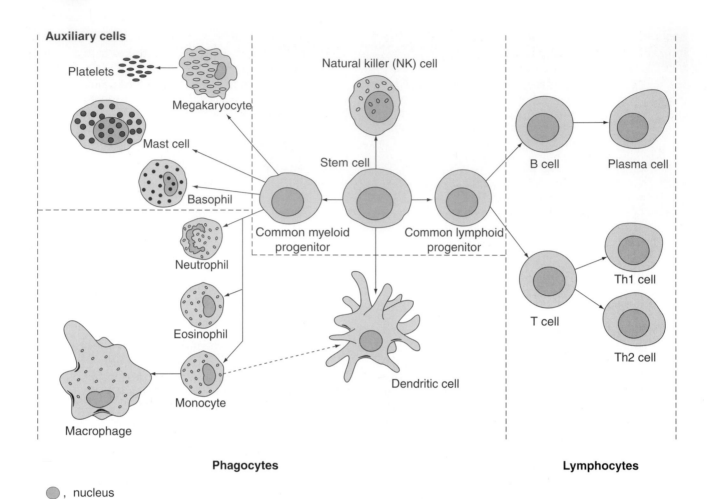

Figure 4–3   Characteristics and differentiation of the various types of leukocytes of the human body. Leukocytes can be divided into three groups: auxiliary cells (platelets, megakaryocytes, mast cells, and basophils), phagocytes (neutrophils, eosinophils, monocytes, macrophages, and dendritic cells), and lymphocytes (T and B cells and plasma cells). Arrows indicate the order of development of different cell types. A dashed arrow indicates uncertainty.

cell. Dendritic cells, whose name comes from the fact that they are covered with spiny projections that look like the dendrites of neurons, are instrumental in initiating and stimulating the immune response. They form a link between the nonspecific and immune responses because they are activated by microbial products such as LPS. The activities of these cells will be described in more detail in chapter 6.

Another type of cell that participates in the defense against bacterial infections is the **mast cell.** Mast cells congregate around blood vessels. If any foreign material is detected, the mast cells release granules that contain histamine, a compound that makes blood vessels leakier (**vasodilation**). This helps the PMNs and NK cells, which are normally circulating in blood, to leave the bloodstream and move to the site of infection. Monocytes also circulate in blood and then differentiate

into macrophages as they leave the bloodstream and migrate into tissue.

Distribution of Phagocytic and Cytotoxic Cells

BLOOD.   PMNs, monocytes, and NK cells are produced in the bone marrow and then released into the bloodstream. PMNs are the most abundant and the most short-lived of these cells. All of these cell types are capable of doing a significant amount of damage to tissue. It is not easy to kill bacteria, which are tough little critters, and considerable firepower has to be brought to bear to destroy them. If this firepower is released into surrounding tissue, human cells become vulnerable targets. The body protects itself from these potentially toxic cells by keeping them in a quiescent state in the bloodstream unless danger threatens. Only when infection triggers various signaling pathways (e.g., cytokine production) that alert these cells to prepare for battle do the PMNs and NK cells pass through the blood vessel walls and enter tissues by a process called **transmigration.** In the process, they become activated to have greater killing power. Monocytes are longer-lived and less numerous than PMNs. Monocytes start out in the blood but later leave the bloodstream to migrate into tissues. As they do this, they develop into macrophages, a more actively phagocytic cell with greater destructive power.

Although PMNs and NK cells are normally found mainly in blood, monocytes leave the bloodstream and differentiate into macrophages as a normal part of regenerating the specific and nonspecific defenses of tissues. During an infection, this process is accelerated. When bacteria enter tissue, cytokines stimulate PMNs to become more actively phagocytic as they leave the bloodstream and migrate to an infected area, but they do not develop into a different type of cell, as monocytes do. There are two types of macrophage: free and fixed macrophages. Free macrophages are found in most types of tissue and migrate through them in search of invaders to ingest and destroy. Fixed macrophages are stationary and are found in organs that filter blood or lymph. The dendritic cells play an important part in triggering the specific immune response in many parts of the body. Some examples of dendritic cells are the **Langerhans cells** of the skin, the **Kupffer cells** of the liver, **alveolar macrophages** of the lung, **spleen macrophages,** and **dendritic cells** of the lymph nodes.

During an infection, the release of circulating phagocytic and cytotoxic cells from bone marrow into the bloodstream is markedly increased. Passage of these cells from the bloodstream into tissue also increases, but the net effect is an increased concentration of nonspecific defense cells in blood. A high number of PMNs in blood is a useful **diagnostic indicator of infection.** During an infection, PMNs are being produced so rapidly in bone marrow and dumped so quickly into the bloodstream that the immature form of PMNs (called **bands** because their nuclei look like bands) are seen in blood. The presence of bands is another sign of infection.

How do PMNs know when to leave the blood vessels and where to go? Two groups of proteins alert PMNs to leave the bloodstream and guide them to their destination. One is the **complement** system, which consists of proteins that are activated by contact with invading bacteria or by interaction with antibodies bound to foreign material. The second group of proteins is the **cytokine/chemokine** system. Cytokines are proteins that mediate the inflammatory response to microbial

antigens and other types of tissue damage. They also participate in activating cells of the immune system. Chemokines are small cytokines that guide phagocytes to where an infection is occurring. They may also play a role in orchestrating the immune response to an infection. Cytokines and chemokines are produced by a number of human cell types, including monocytes, macrophages, endothelial cells, lymphocytes, and fibroblasts. How complement and cytokines work together to direct the phagocytes and cytotoxic cells to an infected area and activate them in the process is described in detail in chapter 5.

Recently, chemokines have been in the news because of their relationship to HIV infection. Chemokines and cytokines can act as messengers because the cells whose activities they direct have receptors that bind them and cause the cell to respond to their presence. The T cells (T-helper cells) and macrophages that are the targets of HIV have a chemokine receptor, which cooperates with the main HIV receptor, CD4, to allow the virus to bind to these cells in such a way as to invade them so that it can replicate. People whose cells lack the chemokine receptor CCR5 are immune to HIV or develop AIDS a lot more slowly than people with this receptor.

LYMPH. Another fluid that is monitored and sterilized by phagocytes is lymph, the fluid that moves through the lymphatic system. Lymphatic vessels are tubes composed of overlapping endothelial cells. These tubes are organized into a complex network similar in complexity to the circulatory system that carries blood to all parts of the body. The role of lymphatics is to prevent excess buildup of fluid in tissue and to recycle blood proteins. Normally, blood fluids and proteins leak from blood vessels of capillary beds to feed cells, donate oxygen, and remove carbon dioxide. Blood fluids also provide protective blood proteins such as complement, cytokines, and chemokines. Fluids that leak from blood vessels are not readily reabsorbed, however, by the blood vessels.

Lymphatic endothelial cells are tethered to the muscle bed. Thus, when the level of fluids in an area becomes high enough, the pressure causes muscle cells to separate, pulling the overlapping endothelial cells of the lymphatic vessels apart. This creates openings that allow fluid from the surrounding area to enter the lymphatic vessels. This fluid is then returned to central holding areas, such as the thoracic duct, where it is dumped back into the bloodstream.

The inflammatory response to bacterial infection creates a buildup of fluid in tissue, leading to opening of the lymphatic vessels. We experience the accumulation of blood fluids as swelling and redness that appears around infected wounds. In such situations, bacteria can enter lymphatic vessels. Because the fluid in lymphatic vessels is returned to the bloodstream, the lymph must be cleansed before it reenters the bloodstream. This task is accomplished by lymph nodes located along the lymphatic vessels.

Lymph nodes contain macrophages and the cells of the immune system (dendritic cells, T cells, and B cells). Bacteria that enter a lymph node are usually killed by the macrophages, but there are bacteria that are able to evade this fate. Some of the most dangerous pathogens are the ones that can survive and multiply in the lymph nodes. An example of such a pathogen is *Yersinia pestis,* the cause of bubonic plague. *Y. pestis* growing in lymph nodes creates an inflammatory response so intense that it causes the lymph nodes to become grossly distended, producing the buboes that give bubonic plague its name. A less pronounced, but still detectable, swelling of lymph nodes occurs during many types of bacterial infections and serves as a diagnostic sign of infection.

In chapter 6, you will learn that macrophages and dendritic cells of the lymph nodes also act as antigen-presenting cells and stimulatory cells that potentiate the specific defense response against bacteria. Thus, the lymph nodes not only sterilize lymph but also act as sites where the specific defense system is alerted that an infection is under way.

How Phagocytes Kill Bacteria

The steps in phagocytic killing of a bacterium are shown in Figure 4–4. The phagocyte first forms pseudopods that engulf the bacterium. After engulfment, the bacterium is encased in an endocytic vesicle called the **phagosome.** The phagosomal membrane contains ATPases that pump protons into the phagosome interior, reducing the internal pH to about 5. Phagocytes also carry antibacterial proteins that are as toxic to the phagocytes and surrounding tissue cells as they are to their bacterial targets. Accordingly, they are stored in an inactive form in **lysosomal granules.**

Fusion of a lysosomal granule with the phagosome to form the **phagolysosome** releases the lysosomal proteins into the phagolysosome interior. The low pH of the phagolysosome generated by the ATPases of the phagosome membrane activates lysosomal proteins. Lysosomal proteins have three main types of killing activity. Some lysosomal proteins are **degradative enzymes,** such as proteases and lysozyme, which destroy surface components of bacteria. Other lysosomal proteins, such as **defensins,** insert themselves into membranes, creating pores that cause the bacterium's cytoplasmic components to leak into the surrounding environment. A third type of lysosomal protein, **myeloperoxidase,** produces reactive forms of oxygen that are toxic to many bacteria. Myeloperoxidase is only ac-

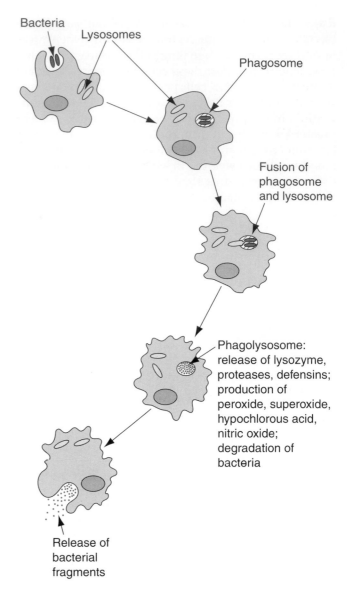

Figure 4–4 Steps in ingestion and killing of bacteria by phagocytes. Bacteria are first engulfed by endocytosis into a phagosome. Fusion of phagosomes and lysosomes releases toxic enzymes and proteins that kill most bacteria. Debris from dead bacteria is then released by exocytosis.

tivated when it is brought into contact with an **NADPH oxidase,** which is located in the phagosome membrane, and when the resulting complex is exposed to the low pH of the phagolysosome interior. The reaction catalyzed by the myeloperoxidase complex is $NADPH + 2O_2 \rightarrow 2O_2^-$ (superoxide radical) $+ NADP^+$.

Superoxide radical is highly reactive. Its toxicity is due to the fact that it oxidizes disulfide linkages and thus inactivates essential bacterial surface proteins. It can also damage nucleic acids, because iron plus superoxide can disrupt bonds that hold the DNA bases together (Fenton reaction) to create breaks in the DNA.

Superoxide is so reactive, however, that most of it does not react directly with bacterial proteins but converts spontaneously to H_2O_2 (peroxide) or reacts with chlorine to form hypochlorous acid (the active ingredient in bleach). Both peroxide and hypochlorous acid are toxic to bacteria for the same reason superoxide is toxic: they oxidize and inactivate essential bacterial proteins. The generation of toxic forms of oxygen by phagocytes is called the **oxidative** (or **respiratory**) **burst.** During an infection, cytokines stimulate increased production of lysosomal enzymes, thus increasing the killing potential of the oxidative burst.

Just Say NO

Human monocytes and macrophages produce nitric oxide (NO). NO is toxic in its own right, attacking bacterial metalloenzymes, proteins, and DNA. In addition, it can combine with superoxide to form peroxynitrite ($OONO^-$), a very reactive molecule that oxidizes amino acids and is toxic both for bacteria and for human cells. Synergistic reactions between NO and superoxides during the oxidative burst may help make the burst more toxic for bacteria. NO may also regulate the functions of phagocytic cells as well as other cells of the specific defense response. NO has been implicated in so many areas of human and animal physiology that the journal *Science* chose it as the "molecule of the year" in 1992.

During an infection, cytokines trigger human cells to produce NO. In blood, the stable end products of NO oxidation, nitrite and nitrate, increase, thus indicating that NO is being produced. NO may contribute to some of the symptoms of disease, including vascular collapse and tissue injury. Mice lacking NO synthetase, an enzyme necessary for NO production, tolerate bacterial endotoxin with fewer toxic side effects than normal mice. A decade ago, one controversy over NO was whether it was produced by human cells and had any role in human response to infection. Today, the question has changed to: is there anything NO is not involved in? The answer appears to be NO, but the jury is still out.

Collateral Damage

Although phagocytic cells are effective killers of bacteria and are essential for clearing invading bacteria from an infected area, the body can pay a high price for this service. During active killing of a bacterium, lysosomal enzymes are released into the surrounding area as well as into the phagolysosome. Released lysosomal enzymes damage adjacent tissues and can be the main cause of tissue damage that results from a bacterial infection. Also, PMNs kill themselves as a result of their killing activities, and lysosomal granules released by

dying PMNs contribute further to tissue destruction. Pus, a common sign of infection, is composed mainly of DNA from dead PMNs and tissue cells. Because phagocytes cause collateral damage to tissue cells when they combat an invader, it is important for the body to tightly regulate their numbers, location, and activation state. This is why the body has a complex set of signals (e.g., complement, cytokines) that stimulate phagocytes to leave the bloodstream and enter tissues only in sections of the body where the invading bacteria are located. This same set of signals upregulates the phagocytes' killing ability, making sure that activation occurs only as they approach the site of the infection (see chapter 5).

Killing by Nonspecific Cytotoxic Cells

Although nonspecific cytotoxic cells, such as NK cells, do not ingest their target, their mode of killing resembles that of phagocytes in most other respects. Like phagocytic cells, they store their toxic substances in granules. When they bind to a target, such as an infected human cell, binding stimulates release of these granules. Thus, instead of ingesting a bacterium or infected cell, the nonspecific cytotoxic cells bombard infected cells. The granule proteins of cytotoxic cells are not the same as those of the lysosomal granules of macrophages and PMNs, but they have some similar functions. For example, cytotoxic cell granules contain a protein called **perforin** that enters the membrane of a target cell and causes channels to form. These channels allow other granule proteins, a set of proteases called **granzymes,** to enter the target cell. One effect of this assault appears to be to force the target cell to initiate apoptosis, a process by which the cell kills itself (discussed in chapter 6).

SELECTED READINGS

Brock, J. 1995. Lactoferrin: a multifunctional immunoregulatory protein? *Immunol. Today* **16:**417–419.

Fang, F. C. 1997. NO contest: nitric oxide plays complex roles in infection. *ASM News* **63:**668–673.

Janeway, C. A., P. Travers, M. Walport, and J. D. Capra. 1999. *Immunobiology. The Immune System in Health and Disease,* 4th ed. Garland Publishing, Inc., New York, N.Y.

Kaufmann, S. H. E. 1999. Killing vs. suicide in antibacterial defence. *Trends Microbiol.* **7:**59–61.

Medzhitov, R., and C. Janeway. 2000. Innate immunity. *N. Engl. J. Med.* **343:**338–344.

Tannock, G. W. 1994. *Normal Microflora,* p. 1–47. Chapman & Hall, Ltd., London, England.

Veenstra, D. L., S. Saint, S. Saha, T. Lumley, and S. D. Sullivan. 1999. Efficacy of antiseptic-impregnated central venous catheters in preventing catheter-related bloodstream infection. *JAMA* **281:**261–267.

SUMMARY OUTLINE

Nonspecific defenses

   Communicate with specific defenses via cytokines and chemokines

   Always present

   May cause septic shock

   Responsible for some of the symptoms of bacterial infections

Epithelia

   Layers of cells covering skin and mucosal surfaces

   Tightly bound together; prevent bacterial transit

   Cells attached to basement membrane

   Cells are polarized—different proteins on basolateral and apical surfaces

   Simple epithelium—one layer of cells

   Stratified epithelium—many layers of cells

Defenses of skin

   Chemical and physical defenses

   Epidermis

      Outer layer consists of stratified squamous epithelial cells

      Most cells are keratinocytes

         Produce keratin and then die

         Layer of dead cells at surface of skin continuously shed

         Maintain acidic pH of skin

      Natural breaches in skin

         Hair follicles, sebaceous and sweat glands

         Protected by toxic lipids and lysozyme

      Normal microbiota

         Occupies sites that might be colonized by pathogens

         Competes with pathogens for nutrients

         May cause infection if introduced into body

            Enter through wounds, catheters

            Often resistant to antibiotics

   Dermis is lower layer of skin

      Langerhans cells (dendritic cells)

      Process invaders and stimulate specific defense system

      SALT

Defenses of mucosal surfaces

   Mucus often covers surface

      Mixture of glycoproteins

      Produced by goblet cells

      Traps bacteria

      Contains antibacterial proteins

         Lysozyme degrades peptidoglycan

         Iron-binding proteins deprive bacteria of iron

         Defensins

            Form channels in bacterial membranes

            Found in mouth and small and large intestine

      sIgA (part of specific defenses) found in mucus

(continued)

Mucosal cells divide rapidly and are sloughed regularly; carry attached bacteria along

Normal microbiota protects most mucosal surfaces

MALT—part of specific defense system

Phagocytes

Ingest and kill bacteria

Monocytes
  Produced in bone marrow
  Precursors of macrophages
  Circulate in bloodstream

Macrophages
  Important in both specific and nonspecific defense systems
  Closely related to dendritic cells
  May be free or fixed
    Langerhans cells of skin
    Kupffer cells of liver
    Alveolar macrophages
    Spleen macrophages
    Dendritic cells of lymph nodes

Mast cells
  Congregate around blood vessels
  Produce histamine
    Causes vasodilation
    Helps phagocytes and natural killer cells to leave bloodstream

PMNs
  Produced in bone marrow; released into bloodstream
  Most abundant, shortest-lived phagocytes
  Leave blood and enter tissue (transmigration) to attack bacteria
  Become more active in response to cytokines
  Numbers in bloodstream increased during infection—used diagnostically to indicate infection
  Respond to proteins of complement system and cytokine/chemokine system
  Monitor lymphatic system
  May cause collateral damage by releasing toxic compounds

Mechanisms for killing bacteria
  Bacteria engulfed by pseudopods, taken up in endocytic vesicle (phagosome)
    Interior of phagosome acidified
    Phagosome fuses with lysosomal granules (contain toxic proteins)
      Low pH of phagosome activates three types of lysosomal proteins
        Degradative enzymes destroy surface components of bacteria
        Defensins create pores in bacterial membranes
        Myeloperoxidase produces reactive forms of oxygen (oxidative burst) that oxidize and
          inactivate bacterial proteins
  NO
    Produced by monocytes and macrophages as well as many other cell types
    Attacks bacterial proteins and DNA
    Can combine with superoxide
    May regulate phagocytes and cells of specific defense system

(*continued*)

SUMMARY OUTLINE (*continued*)

NK cells

Important defense against intracellular pathogens

Circulate in bloodstream but move to tissues in response to invaders

Do not ingest bacteria

Attach to infected human cells

Release granules that bombard infected cell with toxic proteins

Perforin—creates channels in membrane of target cell

Granzymes—proteases that stimulate apoptosis in target cell

Lymphatic system

Complex network similar to blood circulatory system

Removes fluids from tissues and recycles blood proteins—returns them to bloodstream

Lymph monitored and sterilized by phagocytes

Lymphatic vessels composed of endothelial cells

Lymph nodes located along lymphatic vessels

Contain macrophages, dendritic cells, and lymphocytes

Site where specific defense system alerted

QUESTIONS

Answers to the questions can be found in Appendix 2.

1. If, for some reason, you decided that you had to figure out whether the ability to prevent infectious diseases was a nonspecific or specific defense, how would you categorize it? There are links between the nonspecific and specific defenses. Are there links between preventive strategies and the nonspecific and specific defenses?

2. In what sense are *S. epidermidis* infections an example of how changing human practices can provide new opportunities for bacterial pathogens? *S. epidermidis* is classified as an opportunist. Why is this the case?

3. Explain why infections of the skin occur more often in folds of the skin or under bandages than in regions of skin exposed to the air.

4. If lysozyme is present in saliva and mucus and is most effective against gram-positive bacteria, why are gram-positive bacteria such prominent members of the microbiota?

5. How and why do the defenses of mucosal surfaces differ from those of the skin? How do they resemble each other?

6. What kinds of evasive action could a bacterium take to prevent itself from being killed by a phagocyte? (Hint: consider the steps in the killing process.)

7. Why do neutrophils circulate in blood? Why don't they migrate permanently into tissue, as the macrophages do?

8. Inflammation near the skin is characterized by redness and swelling. What causes these symptoms?

5

The First Line of Defense, Continued: Complement, Chemokines, and Cytokines

The barriers of skin and mucosa, together with the phagocyte defense system, are a powerful deterrent to invading bacteria. There is another arm of the nonspecific defenses that is highly complex but equally important—the blood proteins that direct the phagocyte defense system and, in the case of chemokines and cytokines, the specific immune response as well. Because complement, chemokines, and cytokines form links between the nonspecific phagocyte defense system and the specific defenses, it is appropriate to treat them as a separate topic. The inspection of these critically important proteins and their functions also leads naturally to a dark side of the nonspecific defenses—septic shock. Septic shock is a major killer of patients who acquire infections while in the hospital.

Characteristics and Roles of Complement

Complement is a set of proteins produced by the liver. These proteins circulate in blood and enter tissues all over the body. Complement proteins are inactive until a proteolytic cleavage event converts them to their active form. The cascade of proteolytic cleavages of complement components that occurs during an infection is called complement activation. Complement components, some of which are multiprotein complexes, are usually designated by a "C." There are nine of these components, C1 to C9. Activated proteolytic cleavage products are indicated by an "a" or "b," where "a" designates the smaller and "b" designates the larger of the two proteolytic products. Thus, for example, complement component C3 is proteolytically cleaved into a large fragment (C3b) and a smaller fragment (C3a) during complement activation.

Complement activation can be initiated in three ways. A newly discovered initiation method involves protein trimers called **mannose-binding lectins,** a type of **collectin.** Collectins are calcium binding lectins (proteins that bind very specifically to sugar residues). The mannose-binding lectins bind the mannose residues that are commonly found on the surfaces of bacteria but not on human cells. Collectins are produced by the liver and are part of what is called the **acute-phase response** to an infection, the initial onslaught by a variety of proteins, including iron-binding proteins, that makes it difficult for bacteria to multiply. Collectins bound to the surface of bacteria not only sequester the bacteria into clumps that are eliminated from the body by phagocytic cells but can also activate the complement cascade (Figure 5–1).

Certain molecules found on the surfaces of bacteria trigger the complement cascade directly without the intervention of collectins. This has been called the **alternative pathway.** The best-characterized complement-triggering bacterial surface molecule is lipopolysaccharide (LPS) found in the outer membrane of gram-negative bacteria. Complement-activating molecules of gram-positive bacteria, fungi, protozoans, and metazoans are not as well characterized, but they also appear to be lipid-carbohydrate complexes.

Finally, antibodies of the specific defense system can activate complement similarly to collectins by binding to the surface of bacteria and interacting with complement proteins. Antibodies are blood proteins but differ from collectins in that they are produced by B cells, not the liver, and they bind to very specific sites on the bacterial surface, not nonspecifically to a ubiquitous bac-

terial molecule such as mannose or LPS. Thus, both the nonspecific and specific defense systems can trigger the complement cascade. This is yet another example of a link between the nonspecific and specific defenses.

Before examining the pathways for complement activation in detail, it is helpful to understand the roles of the activated proteins they produce. Regardless of how the complement pathway is activated, the same key activated components, **C3a, C3b, C5a,** and **C5b,** are produced (Figure 5–1).

C3a and C5a stimulate mast cells to release their granules, which contain vasoactive substances that increase the permeability of blood vessels and thus facilitate the movement of phagocytes from blood vessels into tissue. C5a also acts together with cytokines to signal phagocytes to leave the bloodstream and guides them to the infection site. Once PMNs or monocytes have left the bloodstream, they move along a gradient of C5a to find the locus of infection. At the site of infection, C3b binds to the surface of the invading bacterium

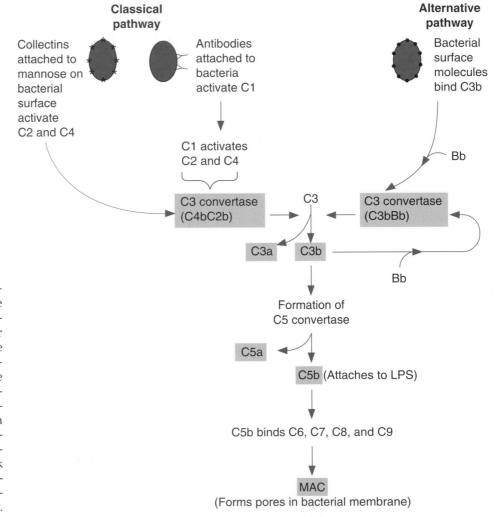

Figure 5–1 Main steps in activation of complement by the classical and alternative pathways. These pathways differ only in the steps that initiate formation of C3 convertase. Important activated products are C3b (which opsonizes bacteria), C3a (which acts as a vasodilator), C5a (which acts as a vasodilator and attracts phagocytes to the area), and C5b-C9 (MAC [membrane attack complex], which inactivates enveloped viruses and kills bacteria). LPS, lipopolysaccharide.

and makes it easier for phagocytes to ingest the bacterium. This activity is called **opsonization.**

Without opsonization, phagocytes have difficulty ingesting a bacterium unless the bacterium is trapped in a small space. The reason is that most bacteria do not stick to the phagocyte surface, so the action of pseudopod encirclement can actually propel the bacterium away from the phagocytes, much as a fish slips from your hands as you try to grab it. Phagocytes have surface receptors that bind C3b (Figure 5–2). Thus, complement component C3b allows the phagocyte to immobilize the bacterium so that it can be engulfed more efficiently. Antibodies, like C3b, can also act as opsonins because a portion of the antibody, the Fc portion, is recognized by phagocyte receptors. But antibodies bind to specific molecules on the surface of one type of bacterium, whereas C3b binds nonspecifically to any surfaces not coated, as human cells are, by sialic acid. The combined effect of C3b and antibodies is synergistic in stimulating uptake of bacteria by phagocytes.

Another role of activated complement components is direct killing of bacteria. Activated component C5b recruits C6, C7, C8, and C9 to form a membrane-damaging complex in the membranes of some types of microorganisms (e.g., enveloped viruses, gram-negative bacteria, some gram-positive bacteria). This complex is called the **membrane attack complex (MAC).** Formation of the MAC inactivates enveloped viruses and kills bacteria by punching holes in their membranes.

Steps in Complement Activation

The steps in complement activation by the classical and the alternative pathways are shown in more detail in Figure 5–3. The **classical pathway** (so named because it was the first to be discovered) is initiated when the Fc regions of two immunoglobulin G (IgG) molecules or one IgM molecule bound to the surface of a bacterium are cross-linked by C1, a multiprotein complex (Figure 5–3A). Binding of C1 to the antibodies causes C1 to release one of its components, producing a form of C1 that cleaves C4 to C4a and C4b. C4b binds to the bacterium's surface at a site near C1. C1 also cleaves C2 to C2a and C2b. Collectins also stimulate cleavage of C2 and C4. C2b binds to C4b to complete the **C3 convertase** complex. C3 convertase cleaves C3 to C3a, which diffuses away from the site and C3b, which binds to the bacterium's surface. Bound C3b has two functions. Some C3b acts as an opsonin to enhance uptake by phagocytes, and some C3b binds to the C3 convertase complex to form the **C5 convertase** complex, which cleaves C5 to C5a and C5b. C5a diffuses away from the site, whereas

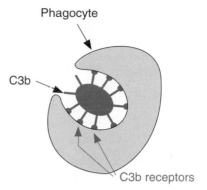

Opsonization by C3b

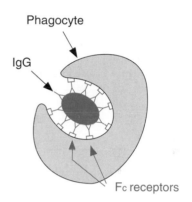

Opsonization by IgG

Figure 5–2 Opsonization of a bacterium by activated complement component C3b and antibodies. Combined opsonization by both C3b and antibodies considerably enhances the uptake of the bacterium by phagocytes. IgG, immunoglobulin G.

C5b binds the bacterium's surface. C5b recruits C6, C7, C8, and C9 to form the MAC.

Activation via the **alternative pathway** (so named because it was discovered after the classical pathway) bypasses C1, C2, and C4 and relies on C3 as the initiating component (Figure 5–3B). As C3 circulates in blood and tissue, it is occasionally activated to produce a form that interacts with water to assume a conformation similar to that of C3b. This activated form (C3-H₂O) binds to nearby surfaces. Tissues of the body are coated with sialic acid residues, which preferentially bind a serum protein, H. C3-H₂O can interact with H to form a complex that produces C3b, but the C3b remains bound to H. This binding changes the conformation of C3b and targets it for proteolytic cleavage and destruction by serum protein I.

If C3-H₂O instead binds a bacterium's surface, it is more likely to encounter serum protein B, which binds to the bacterium's surface better than protein H. Once

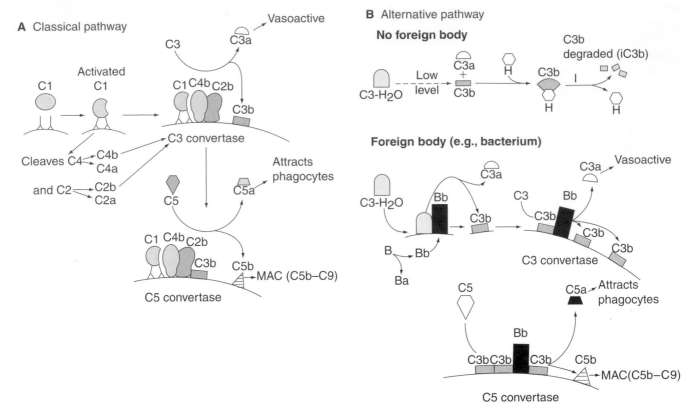

Figure 5–3 Activation of complement. (**A**) Classical pathway. Two IgG molecules or one IgM molecule attached to the surface of a bacterium bind complement component C1, causing an autoproteolytic event that activates it. C1, C4b, and C2b bind to one another and to the bacterium's surface to form C3 convertase. Addition of C3b produces C5 convertase, which triggers assembly of the membrane attack complex (MAC). The mannose-binding lectins or collectins activate the classical pathway similarly to antibodies, except that they interact with C4 and C2 rather than C1. After that point, both are the same. (**B**) Alternative pathway. C3-H$_2$O, an activated form of C3 that resembles C3b in conformation, is normally produced at low levels. If it binds a host cell surface, which preferentially binds serum factor H, H binds to C3b produced by the C3-H$_2$O complex and targets it for destruction by serum protein I. If C3-H$_2$O binds to the surface of a bacterium, it can form a complex with Bb (C3 convertase). Addition of more C3b produces C5 convertase, which triggers assembly of the membrane attack complex (MAC).

C3-H$_2$O binds to B on the bacterium's surface, another serum protein, D, cleaves B to Ba and Bb. The resulting C3-H$_2$O/Bb complex produces C3b, which can then bind Bb to form a C3/C5 convertase. The initial C3bBb complex is the C3 convertase, which cleaves C3 to form more C3a and C3b. The newly generated C3b binds to the same bacterial surface, and when this bound C3b comes in contact with the C3bBb complex already on the surface, this new complex becomes the C5 convertase. Some bacteria produce a polysaccharide surface coating, called a **capsule,** which preferentially binds serum protein H, rather than B. The effect of this is to eliminate C3b as it is deposited on the surface and to prevent effective opsonization of the bacterial surface.

In both the classical and alternative pathways, it is important to keep the accelerated production of C3a, C3b, C5a, and C5b under control. To this end, most C3b molecules on the bacterium's surface are proteolytically cleaved to produce iC3b. iC3b is an effective opsonin but cannot help to form a C3 or C5 convertase complex.

Role of Cytokines and Chemokines in Directing the Phagocyte Response

Cytokines are glycoproteins produced by a variety of cells, including monocytes, macrophages, NK cells, endothelial cells, lymphocytes, and fibroblasts. Chemokines are small peptides that have many of the same functions, especially attracting phagocytes and activating them, much as complement components C5a and C3a do. Cytokines are larger than chemokines and play a central role in regulating the activities of the cells of the nonspecific and specific defense systems. Figure 5–4 gives an overview of the nonspecific responses to infection and shows how many of these responses rely on cytokines. Just as complement is activated by bacterial surfaces, cytokine release is triggered by interaction between cytokine-producing cells and molecules on the surfaces of the invading bacterium. In the case of gram-negative bacteria, the outer membrane LPS that activates complement is also the molecule that stimulates cytokine production. Although the surface molecules of other types of bacteria that activate complement and stimulate cytokine release have not been nearly as well studied, it appears likely that the same

surface molecules on these bacteria both activate complement and stimulate cytokine production.

The process by which bacterial surface molecules trigger cytokine release is best understood in the case of LPS. LPS is released from the bacterial surface by the lysis of bacteria. LPS binds to **CD14,** a protein receptor on macrophages and other cytokine-producing cells (Figure 5–5). Binding of LPS to CD14 triggers a signal transduction pathway that culminates in cytokine production and release by the stimulated cell. CD14 is a somewhat unusual signal transducer because it is anchored in the macrophage membrane by **glycosylphosphatidylinositol (GPI)** rather than being part of a membrane-anchored protein complex, as most better-known signal-transducing receptors are. Usually, signal-transducing proteins have a membrane-spanning tail that is exposed in the cytoplasm and interacts with various signal-transducing enzymes to

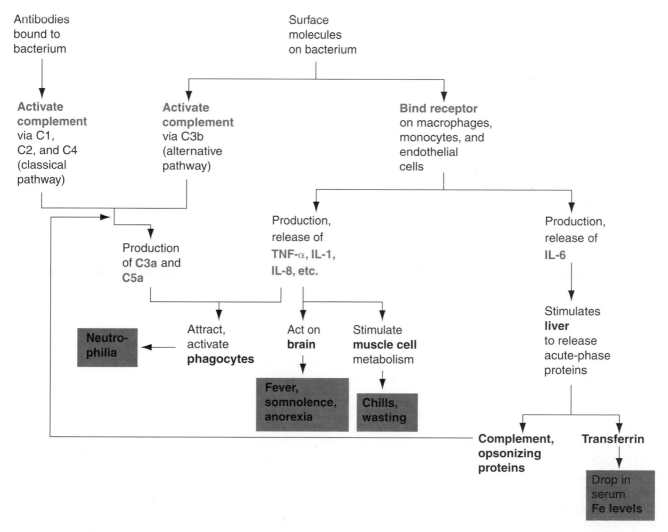

Figure 5–4   Overview of nonspecific responses to infection and the effects of cytokines on these responses. Cytokines include TNF-α, IL-1, and IL-6.

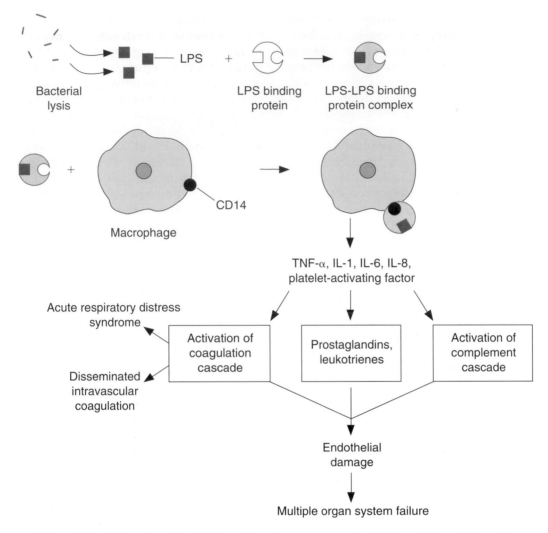

Figure 5–5 Triggering of cytokine release by gram-negative LPS and the role in septic shock. TNF-α, tumor necrosis factor alpha, and IL, interleukin, are cytokines.

trigger the phosphorylation cascade that transmits the signal. How CD14 transmits its signals is just beginning to be understood, and the answer seems to be that it interacts with other cell surface proteins that actually mediate the signal transduction.

Before proceeding to the proteins that might serve the signal transduction function, let us first consider a protein that is involved in the interaction between CD14 and LPS, **LPS binding protein.** LPS bound to LPS binding protein interacts more effectively with CD14 than does unbound LPS. Presumably, the complex formed by LPS, LPS binding protein, and CD14 is more effective at initiating a signal than is LPS binding to CD14. A long-standing mystery is how cells such as endothelial cells and fibroblasts, which do not normally have CD14 on their surfaces, nonetheless respond to LPS by producing cytokines. The answer may lie in the fact that

macrophages cleave the GPI-CD14 bond to release CD14 in a soluble form. This soluble form of CD14 appears to enable other cell types, which do not normally produce CD14, to respond to LPS. How CD14, aided by LPS binding protein, allows endothelial cells, for example, to react to LPS is unknown. Until recently, little was known about how lipoteichoic acid (LTA), a surface lipid-carbohydrate molecule found in gram-positive bacteria, and peptidoglycan fragments from both gram-positive and gram-negative bacteria caused cytokine release. Apparently, LTA and peptidoglycan fragments also bind to CD14 and through this interaction elicit cytokine production. It is not yet clear whether there are specialized LTA binding proteins, analogous to LPS binding protein.

Still another class of receptors for LPS and possibly for other bacterial molecules such as LTA and peptidoglycan fragments has been discovered—in a rather unusual way. Scientists working on the fruit fly *Drosophila melanogaster* identified a transmembrane receptor called Toll that was required for resistance to fungal infections. Activation of Toll leads to activation of gene expression via a signal transduction pathway. A search for a human equivalent of Toll revealed a group of proteins called **Toll-like receptors (TLRs).** At least some of the TLRs seem to be able to interact with LPS and peptidoglycan fragments, and TLRs may be the missing link in the signal transduction cascade that transduces a signal to the interior of the cell being activated. This discovery has led to the solution of one mystery. Certain inbred strains of mice do not respond to LPS. One such strain is C3H/HeJ. It turns out that these mice have a mutation in a TLR that prevents the interaction between LPS and TLR. TLRs probably interact with CD14 and carry out the actual signal transduction process initiated by binding of CD14 to LPS, because TLRs are proteins that span the cytoplasmic membrane.

During an infection, macrophages and other cells, such as endothelial cells, release a variety of cytokines. Some of these appear early in the infection and are responsible for upregulating host defenses. Others appear late in the infection and help to downregulate the defense response. Among the earliest cytokines to appear are **granulocyte-macrophage colony-stimulating factor (GM-CSF)** and **interleukin 3 (IL-3).** These cytokines trigger the release of monocytes and granulocytes (especially PMNs) from the bone marrow into the circulation (Figure 5–6). Other early-appearing cytokines, such as **tumor necrosis factor alpha (TNF-α), IL-1, gamma interferon (IFN-γ),** and **IL-8,** stimulate the monocytes and granulocytes to leave the bloodstream and migrate to the site of infection. The steps in this process are illustrated for PMNs in Figure 5–6.

Normally, PMNs move rapidly through the blood vessels with a rolling motion, occasionally colliding with one of the vessel walls. TNF-α, IL-1, and IFN-γ stimulate endothelial cells to produce a set of surface proteins called **selectins.** These selectins bind to proteins on the surface of PMNs and other blood cells, causing them to bind loosely to the endothelium. This loose binding slows the movement of the PMNs. Other selectins appear on the endothelial cells, and IL-8 stimulates PMNs to produce proteins called **integrins** on their surfaces. The integrins bind another set of cytokine-stimulated proteins on the endothelial cell surface, the **intercellular adhesion molecules (ICAMs),** to generate a tighter attachment between PMNs and endothelial cells. This stops the movement of the PMNs and causes them to flatten against the blood vessel wall. The slowing and stopping of the PMNs is called **margination.** The PMNs then force themselves between endothelial

cells, a process that is assisted by a protein called **platelet-endothelial cell adhesion molecule (PECAM).** The process of moving from the bloodstream into tissue is called **transmigration** or extravasation. Complement components C3a and C5a assist in transmigration by causing mast cells to release vasoactive amines, which dilate blood vessels and make them leakier. Dilation of blood vessels is also assisted by the cytokine **platelet-activating factor (PAF).** PAF triggers mast cells to produce a number of vasoactive compounds from the membrane lipid, arachidonic acid. These compounds include the leukotrienes and prostaglandins.

Once the PMN has moved out of the blood vessel and into surrounding tissue, it follows the gradient of C5a to the infection site (chemotaxis). Some bacterial peptides also attract PMNs. As PMNs move through tissue, cytokines TNF-α, IL-1, IL-8, and PAF activate the PMNs' oxidative burst response so that the PMNs arrive at the infection site with their full killing capacity in force. A similar activation occurs in the case of monocytes and the macrophages into which they develop as they move to the infected area. IFN-γ further stimulates the killing ability of macrophages, producing activated macrophages. Note that using cytokines and activated complement components, which are in highest concentrations near the infected area, as signals to control the activities of PMNs ensures that the PMNs will exit the blood vessel near where the infection is occurring and not in other areas of the body. Also, the fact that activation of the phagocytes occurs only as they are moving into the infected area reduces the chance that they will inadvertently damage tissues outside the infected area.

The result of the process just described is that PMNs and other phagocytic cells leave the blood vessels near the infection site in high numbers. Some underlying conditions reduce the effectiveness of this signaling system and reduce the transmigration of PMNs. These include steroid use, stress, hypoxia, and alcohol abuse. Their inhibitory effect on transmigration may explain why these underlying conditions are frequently associated with increased susceptibility to infection.

The combination of complement activation, cytokine release, phagocyte transmigration/activation, and production of prostaglandins and leukotrienes is called the inflammatory response or **inflammation.** Cytokines that aid in this process are called proinflammatory cytokines. Common symptoms of localized inflammation are redness, swelling, heat, and pain. The redness and swelling are caused by blood fluids leaking out of the vessels as phagocytes marginate. The increased temperature of the area also results from the increased blood flow through the area. The source of the pain is still not clearly understood but is probably due to the combined effects of cytokines, prostaglandins, and co-

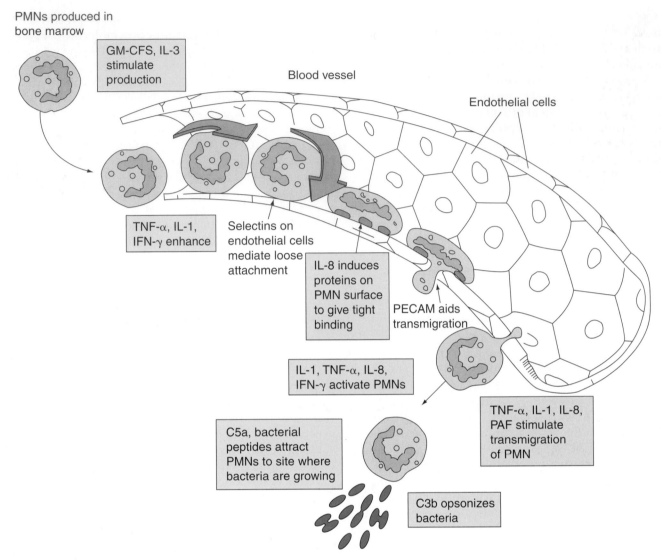

PMNs produced in bone marrow

GM-CFS, IL-3 stimulate production

Blood vessel

Endothelial cells

TNF-α, IL-1, IFN-γ enhance

Selectins on endothelial cells mediate loose attachment

IL-8 induces proteins on PMN surface to give tight binding

PECAM aids transmigration

IL-1, TNF-α, IL-8, IFN-γ activate PMNs

TNF-α, IL-1, IL-8, PAF stimulate transmigration of PMN

C5a, bacterial peptides attract PMNs to site where bacteria are growing

C3b opsonizes bacteria

Figure 5–6 Roles of various cytokines in directing the exit of PMNs from the bloodstream at particular sites. Initially, new proteins are expressed on the surfaces of PMNs and endothelial cells, permitting a loose reversible binding. This gives PMNs a rolling motility as they flow through the blood vessel. Other cytokines cause changes in the cell surfaces that result in tighter binding. The PMNs stop moving, flatten against the vessel wall, force themselves across the endothelial wall, and then move chemotactically along a C5a gradient. PAF, platelet-activating factor; PECAM, platelet-endothelial cell adhesion molecule.

agulation cascade components on nerve endings in the inflamed region.

If the phagocytes are successful in eliminating the invading bacterium, a second set of cytokines begins to predominate. These cytokines (e.g., IL-4, IL-10, and IL-13) downregulate production of TNF-α and reduce the killing activities of phagocytes, thus allowing the phagocyte defense system to return to its normal, relatively inactive, level.

Other Activities of Cytokines

Some of the other roles of the proinflammatory cytokines are also illustrated in Figure 5–4 and explain common symptoms of infectious diseases other than localized infection: fever, somnolence, malaise, anorexia, chills, decrease in blood iron levels, and weight loss. Cytokines IL-1 and TNF-α interact with the hypothalamus and adrenal gland to produce fever and somnolence. Somnolence is interpreted by the patient as a feeling of malaise. Indifference to food, which can also characterize this state, explains the anorexia. TNF-α and other cytokines stimulate muscle cells to increase their metabolic rate and catabolize proteins to provide fuel for the mobilization of host defenses. Increased metabolism of muscle cells may be the cause of chills seen in some types of systemic infections. If the infection persists, the combination of anorexia and muscle cell breakdown of protein results in weight loss and visible loss of muscle tissue (wasting).

The cytokine IL-6 stimulates the liver to increase the production of a set of proteins called acute-phase proteins. These include complement components (to regenerate complement components used up during complement activation), LPS binding proteins (to continue stimulation of cytokine production as long as bacteria are detected in the body), two general opsonins (mannose binding protein and C-reactive protein), and transferrin. Transferrin is an iron binding protein that sequesters iron. Transferrin-iron complexes are taken up by macrophages, which remove the iron and recycle the transferrin to scavenge more iron. In this way, the levels of iron in blood drop to an even lower level than normal, which severely limits the multiplication of most bacteria.

Stress and Resistance to Disease: Connections between the Nervous System and the Immune System

For many years, researchers and clinicians have noted an association between stress and susceptibility to infectious diseases. Two well-studied examples are the increased susceptibility to tuberculosis and the reactivation of latent herpes simplex virus infections in people exposed to various forms of stress. Does the fact that stress is often associated with increased incidence of infection prove there is a cause-and-effect relationship, and if so, what is the mechanism by which stress affects the immune system? As the result of recent studies, some insights into relations between the nervous system and the immune system are beginning to come into focus. A diagram of some of the interactions between the nervous system and the immune system that might explain how stress can cause reduced efficacy of immune responses is shown in Figure 5–7.

The two parts of the nervous system that appear to be most important in influencing the immune system are the **sympathetic neurons** and the **hypothalamic-adrenal cortex-pituitary axis.** Stress stimulates the hypothalamus to release **corticotropin-releasing factor (CRF),** which in turn stimulates production of **adrenocorticotropic hormone (ACTH)** by the pituitary gland.

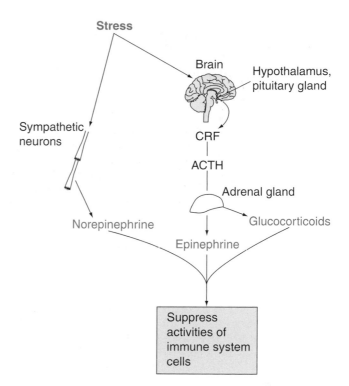

Figure 5–7   Proposed model for the effect of stress on the defense systems of the human body. Stress causes the sympathetic neurons to produce norepinephrine and the hypothalamus to produce corticotropin-releasing factor (CRF). CRF stimulates production of adrenocorticotropic hormone (ACTH), which stimulates the adrenal gland to produce glucocorticoids. The adrenal gland also produces epinephrine. Glucocorticoids, epinephrine, and norepinephrine reduce the activities of cells of the nonspecific and specific defense systems.

ACTH stimulates production of **glucocorticoids** by adrenal cells. Monocytes, macrophages, and the B and T cells of the specific defense system have glucocorticoid receptors. This may explain why the activities of these cells, such as cytokine production and development of specific immunity, are downregulated in a stressed individual (Box 5–1). **Norepinephrine** produced by sympathetic neurons and **epinephrine** produced by the adrenal gland also suppress immune cell activities. Normally, these hormones serve as part of the protective feedback loop that stops the inflammatory process when it is no longer needed. Apparently, stress inappropriately activates this feedback loop to a point where it becomes detrimental to host defense systems.

The Dark Side of the Nonspecific Defenses: Septic Shock

An example of how inappropriate functioning of host defenses can lead to disastrous consequences is pro-

BOX 5–1   Proof at Last! Examinations Are Bad for Your Health!

Many of the studies looking into a possible connection between stress and the immune system have focused on people experiencing long-term stress as a result of divorce, family discord, or caring for a family member with Alzheimer's disease. Some studies, however, have examined the effects of short-term stress caused by examinations. In one such study (Glaser et al., 1992), second-year medical students taking a 3-day examination were the subject of study. The students were inoculated with hepatitis B vaccine. The initial injection was given on the third day of the semester's first 3-day test. Booster shots were given on the third day of later examinations that took place at least a month apart. Before each vaccine injection, blood samples were taken and tested to determine the level of antibodies against hepatitis B virus in the blood. At the time of each injection, the students were also questioned to ascertain their level of anxiety about the examinations that they were taking. All of the students developed high levels of serum antibodies to the virus, but those who reported the highest levels of anxiety tended to develop an antibody response more slowly than those who were less stressed. Loneliness was also correlated with a slower antibody response.

The conclusion is obvious: instead of making students take examinations, we should make them go out on dates. Needless to say, this was not one of the conclusions stated in the paper describing the study.

Unfortunately for medical students, an earlier study examining the effect of examinations on the ability of medical students to mount an antibody response to hepatitis B vaccine concluded that the most stressed students actually developed *higher* antibody levels than less stressed students (Petry et al., 1991). Of course, since the level of antibody in this study was measured much later in the vaccination schedule than in the other study, the investigators could not determine whether development of the antibody response was slower in the most stressed students. So there is still room for hope.

Sources: L. J. Petry, L. B. Weems, and J. N. Livingstone. 1991. Relationship of stress, distress, and the immunologic response to a recombinant hepatitis B vaccine. *J. Family Pract.* **32**:481–486; R. Glaser, J. K. Kiecolt-Glaser, R. H. Bonneau, W. Malarkey, S. Kennedy, and J. Hughes. 1992. Stress-induced modulation of the immune response to recombinant hepatitis B vaccine. *Psychosomatic Med.* **54**:22–29.

vided by septic shock. Septic shock is a form of shock caused by bacterial infection. Other causes of shock include massive crush injuries and burns. In people with septic shock, vascular resistance and blood pressure drop despite normal to high cardiac output. The heart rate increases as the body tries to compensate for decreasing blood pressure. Another sign that is frequently associated with septic shock is **disseminated intravascular coagulation (DIC),** which can be seen as blackish or reddish skin lesions (petechiae).

Septic shock is a serious condition because severely reduced levels of blood flow deprive essential organs of oxygen and nutrients. The consequent failure of organs such as kidneys, heart, brain, and lungs is the cause of death from septic shock. **Septicemia** (bacteria multiplying in the bloodstream) occurs in more than 500,000 patients per year in the United States alone. A quarter of the patients with septicemia die in the hos-

pital. Even those who survive may have long-term aftereffects, such as stroke or permanent damage to the lungs or other organs. Moreover, those who survive an episode of septic shock have a significantly greater risk of dying during the next 5-year period than people with the same underlying conditions but no episode of shock. Septic shock is serious business—serious expensive business, as hospital administrators and insurance executives are quick to point out.

The all-inclusive term "sepsis" has now been defined more precisely in an effort to aid diagnosis of the various stages of disease. Septic shock occurs in four stages. The first stage of shock, **systemic inflammatory response syndrome (SIRS),** is characterized by temperature over 38°C or under 36°C, a higher than normal heart rate, a higher than normal respiratory rate, and an unnaturally high or unnaturally low neutrophil count. The second stage, **sepsis,** is SIRS with a culture-documented infection, i.e., laboratory results proving the presence of bacteria in the bloodstream. The third stage, **severe sepsis,** is characterized by organ dysfunction and very low blood pressure. The fourth stage, **septic shock,** is characterized by low blood pressure despite fluid administration.

How does a bacterial infection of the bloodstream produce such serious consequences? From previous sections of this chapter, it is evident that the body goes to great lengths to confine the inflammatory response to certain areas of the body. Septic shock is an example of what happens when an inflammatory response is triggered throughout the body. Shock occurs when bacteria or their products reach high enough levels in the bloodstream to trigger complement activation, cytokine release, and the coagulation cascade in many parts of the body. The effects of this are illustrated in Figure 5–8. High levels of cytokines, especially TNF-α, IL-1, IL-6, IL-8, and IFN-γ, cause increased levels of PMNs in the blood and encourage these PMNs to leave the blood vessels throughout the body. This leads to massive leakage of fluids into surrounding tissue. PMNs and macrophages activated by IFN-γ also damage blood vessels directly, resulting in loss of fluid from blood vessels. Activation of complement throughout the body further increases the transmigration of phagocytes. The vasodilating action of C3a, C5a, leukotrienes, and prostaglandins contributes to leakage of fluids from blood vessels and further reduces the ability of blood vessels to maintain blood pressure. Some cytokines cause inappropriate constriction and relaxation of blood vessels, an activity that undermines the ability of the circulatory system to maintain normal blood flow and normal blood pressure. Widespread triggering of the coagulation system produces the clots that can plug capillaries (DIC). More seriously, it depletes the blood of essential clotting factors, so that damage to endothelial cells caused by phagocytes and cytokines leads to small hemorrhages in many parts of the body. Hemorrhages not only contribute to hypotension but also damage vital organs.

Once septic shock enters the phase in which organs start to fail, it is virtually impossible to treat successfully, and the death rate exceeds 70%. Treatment is most likely to be effective if it is begun early in the infection. Diagnosis of septic shock in its early stages is not straightforward, however, because the early symptoms of shock (fever, hypotension, tachycardia) are so nonspecific. Also, the transition from the early stages to multiple organ failure can occur with frightening rapidity. Hundreds of thousands of cases of septic shock occur in the United States each year. Many of these cases occur in patients hospitalized for some condition other than infectious disease. Accordingly, a massive effort

has been made to develop new techniques for treating septic shock more successfully, especially in cases where the disease has reached the point that treatment with antibacterial agents is no longer sufficient to avert disaster. Early efforts to combat septic shock centered on administration of glucocorticoids, which downregulate cytokine production, but there is now general agreement that glucocorticoid treatment is not effective in treating most types of shock. More recently, attention has focused on the cytokines, such as TNF-α, which seem to play such a central role in the pathology of shock. Antibodies or other compounds that bind and inactivate cytokines have been tested for efficacy in clinical trials. The outcome of early clinical trials has been disappointing, but newer anticytokine agents now being tested appear to be more promising. Nonetheless, it is clear that this type of therapy will never be as effective as catching septic shock in its very early stages.

Antibiotic therapy administered early enough can stop the shock process, but the right antibiotic must be chosen. This means more laboratory tests, once more bringing physicians into conflict with health management organizations that want to save money by minimizing tests. Microbiological testing tends to be expensive because it requires skilled technicians and is less automated than other types of clinical tests. Although it is true that tests for bacterial identification and antibiotic susceptibility cost money, septic shock costs even more. If the causative bacteria are resistant to most antibiotics, the cost of treatment can rise by as much as 100-fold. Moreover, patients who have developed shock and survived may experience strokes and permanent damage to vital organs. The effect of shock, in terms of future risk of untimely death, can last years beyond the actual shock experience.

And then there are the lawsuits. Patients who, through neglect and misdiagnosis, develop strokes or other long-term damage are starting to sue hospitals. Consumer advocates are also suing to obtain information about infection rates in hospitals, particularly those infections leading to serious conditions like septic shock. The rate of postsurgical infections is higher than most people realize, especially in crowded urban hospitals with large intensive care wards. Increasing antibiotic resistance is only making things worse. Not surprisingly, hospitals guard their figures on the incidence of hospital-acquired infection, keeping them in strict secrecy. In spring 1998, an article appeared in the *New York Times* about a unique arrangement among several New York City hospitals that would allow them to share information about antibiotic resistance patterns in their hospitals. This deal had taken months to broker because hospital officials were worried that another hospital would leak their infection statistics to the press

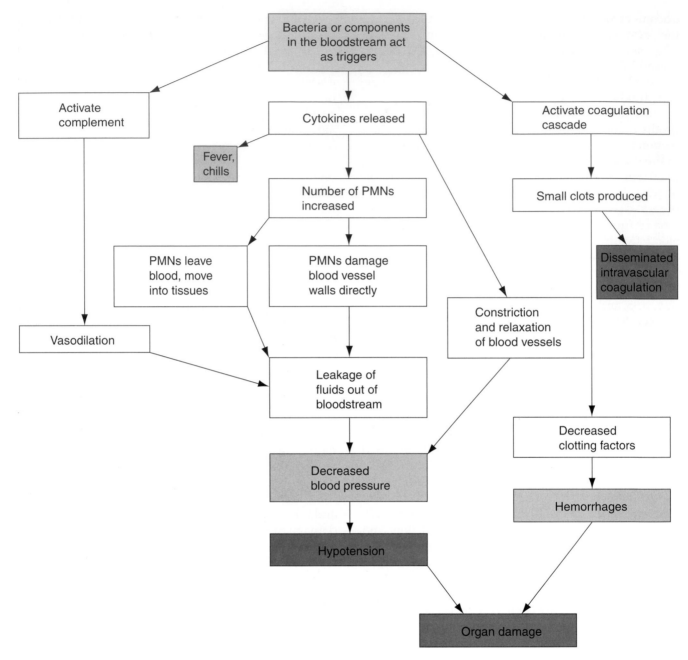

Figure 5–8 Sources of hypotension, disseminated intravascular coagulation, and internal hemorrhages seen in cases of septic shock.

in a move to attract more business to the hospital with the lowest infection rate.

One impediment to early diagnosis of shock has already been mentioned: the nonspecific nature of the signs and symptoms of shock. Another impediment to early diagnosis is that so many different types of bacteria can cause septic shock. Bacteria are the microorganisms most frequently implicated in septic shock, but many different species of gram-positive and gram-negative bacteria can cause shock. Because no single

antibiotic is effective against all of these bacterial pathogens, it is important to determine the species of the bacterium causing the infection as well as its susceptibility to antibiotics. Doing this more rapidly is a challenge for future research and is the key to timely and effective intervention strategies. Preventive strategies will also play a role. These include hand washing and other hygienic measures, as well as reduction in the length of time patients are immunocompromised (e.g., by cancer chemotherapy) or are exposed to conditions such as catheterization that increase their chance of being infected.

SELECTED READINGS

Baggiolini, M. 1998. Chemokines and leukocyte traffic. *Nature* **392:**565–568.

Chaudhary, P. M., C. Ferguson, V. Nguyen, O. Nguyen, H. F. Massa, M. Eby, A. Jasmin, L. Hood, and P. S. Nelson. 1998. Cloning and characterization of two Toll/Interleukin-1 receptor-like genes TL3 and TL4: evidence for a multi-gene receptor family in humans. *Blood* **91:**4020–4027.

Dinarello, C. A. 1996. Thermoregulation and the pathogenesis of fever. *Infect. Dis. Clin. N. Am.* **10:**433–449.

Hoffman, J. A., F. C. Kafatos, C. A. Janeway, Jr., and R. A. B. Ezekowitz. 1999. Phylogenetic perspectives in innate immunity. *Science* **284:**1313–1318.

Medzhitov, R., and C. Janeway. 2000. Innate immunity. *N. Engl. J. Med.* **343:**338–344.

Parham, P. 2000. *The Immune System.* Elsevier Science Ltd., London, England.

Quartin, A. A., R. M. H. Schein, D. H. Kett, and P. N. Peduzzi. 1997. Magnitude and duration of the effect of sepsis on survival. *JAMA* **277:**1058–1063.

Sheridan, J. F., C. Dobbs, D. Brown, and B. Zwillig. 1994. Psychoneuroimmunology: stress effects on pathogenesis and immunity during infection. *Clin. Microbiol. Rev.* **7:**200–212.

Warren, H. S. 1997. Strategies for the treatment of sepsis. *N. Engl. J. Med.* **336:**952–953.

Wenzel, R. P., M. R. Pinsky, R. H. Ulevitch, and L. Young. 1996. Current understanding of sepsis. *Clin. Infect. Dis.* **22:**407–413.

Wheeler, A. P., and G. R. Bernard. 1999. Treating patients with severe sepsis. *N. Engl. J. Med.* **340:**207–214.

SUMMARY OUTLINE

Characteristics and roles of complement

Consists of nine inactive proteins produced by liver (C1 to C9)

Activated by proteolytic cleavage of components

Classical pathway activated in one of two ways
  Mannose-binding lectins (collectins) bind mannose residues on bacteria
  Antibodies bind to bacterial surface

Alternative pathway activated by binding of bacterial surface molecules (e.g., LPS) to complement components

Key activated components
  C3a—stimulates mast cells to release histamine
  C5a—stimulates mast cells to release histamine; acts as chemoattractant for phagocytes
  C3b—nonspecifically binds to bacteria; enhances engulfment by phagocytes (opsonization)
  C5b plus C6, C7, C8, and C9 form MAC, which directly kills some bacteria

Classical pathway
  Activation by mannose-binding lectin
    Mannose-binding lectin binds to mannose on surface of bacteria
    Binding stimulates cleavage of C2 (C2a + C2b) and C4 (C4a + C4b)
    C2b + C4b bound close to C1 = C3 convertase
    C3 convertase cleaves C3 to C3a, C3b
    C3 convertase + C3b forms C5 convertase (forms C5a, C5b)
  Activation by antibodies binding to bacterial surface
    Initiated when C1 cross-links Fc portions of antibodies
    Activated C1 cleaves C2 (C2a + C2b) and C4 (C4a + C4b)
    C3 convertase cleaves C3 to C3a, C3b
    C3 convertase + C3b forms C5 convertase (forms C5a, C5b)

(continued)

Alternative pathway
  Initiated by C3 which has been activated by H$_2$O
  Activated C3 binds surface of bacterium next to protein B
    B converted to Bb by protein D
    C3-H$_2$O/Bb produces C3b
    C3b + Bb forms C3/C5 convertase
In both pathways, most C3b molecules on the bacterium's surface are cleaved to iC3b, preventing
  excess production of C3a, C3b, C5a, C5b

Chemokines

Small peptides produced by many cell types

Attract and activate phagocytes

Activities similar to cytokines

Cytokines

Glycoproteins produced by numerous cell types

Release triggered by interaction between cell producing the cytokine and invading bacteria
  LPS on gram-negative bacteria released when bacteria lyse
  LPS binds CD14 on macrophages or other cytokine-producing cells
  Binding triggers signal transduction leading to cytokine release
  LPS bound to LPS binding protein interacts with CD14—more effective trigger of signal trans-
    duction
  LTA and peptidoglycan fragments bind CD14 to elicit cytokine release
TLRs
  Transmembrane receptors in human cells
  Interact with LPS and peptidoglycan fragments
  May interact with CD14 and carry out the signal transduction process initiated by binding of
    LPS to CD14
Early cytokines upregulate defenses
  GM-CSF, IL-3 trigger release of monocytes and granulocytes from bone marrow into blood-
    stream
  TNF-α, IL-1, IFN-γ, IL-8 stimulate monocytes and granulocytes to leave bloodstream and mi-
    grate to site of infection
    Stimulate endothelial cells to produce selectins
    Selectins bind PMNs, slow movement (rolling motility)
    IL-8 stimulates PMNs to produce integrins, which bind ICAMs on endothelial cells—stops
      PMN movement, flattens PMNs (margination)
    PECAM on endothelial cells assists PMNs to move out of bloodstream into tissue (transmi-
      gration)
      Transmigration assisted by vasoactive amines produced by mast cells
      Blood vessels dilate in response to PAF (triggers production of leukotrienes, prostaglandins)
    PMNs follow gradient of C5a to infection site (chemotaxis)
    Cytokines activate oxidative burst of phagocytes only as they leave bloodstream
  IL-4, IL-10, IL-13 downregulate production of TNF-α, reduce killing activities of phagocytes
Inflammation
  Combination of complement activation, cytokine release, PMN transmigration/activation, and
    production of prostaglandins and leukotrienes
  Redness and swelling—due to blood fluids leaking out of blood vessels

(*continued*)

SUMMARY OUTLINE (*continued*)

Increased temperature—due to increased blood flow in area

Pain—due to action of cytokines, prostaglandins, and coagulation cascade products on nerve endings

Stages of septic shock

Due to inflammatory response throughout the body

SIRS—first stage

Temperature either above or below normal

Increased heart rate

Increased respiratory rate

Neutrophil count abnormally high or low

Sepsis—SIRS plus culture-documented infection

Severe sepsis

Multiple organ system failure

Very low blood pressure

Death rate 70%

Septic shock—low blood pressure despite fluid replacement

No effective treatment once organs start to fail but early diagnosis difficult

QUESTIONS

Answers to the questions can be found in Appendix 2.

1. How do the functions of various activated complement components resemble the functions of cytokines and chemokines?

2. Why does the body have such a complex system (complement plus cytokines) for directing the activities of the phagocytes? What is this system trying to achieve?

3. Why are there two pathways for activating complement?

4. What is the point of using proteolytic cleavage to activate complement? Why aren't the molecules simply made in their active form?

5. In septic shock, why does blood pressure fall?

6. Why are antibiotics (chemicals that kill bacteria) ineffective after a certain point in the course of septic shock, even though the causative bacterium is susceptible to them? Make an educated guess as to why so many of the anticytokine therapeutic agents have failed.

7. How would you attract the attentions of a good-looking phagocyte?

6

The Second Line of Defense: Antibodies and Cytotoxic T Cells

Effective as they are, the nonspecific defenses do not protect the body against all invading microbes. In fact, the ability to evade one or more of the nonspecific defenses is a characteristic of most disease-causing microbes. To cope with such microbes, the body has evolved a second defense system, the **specific defense system,** which includes **antibodies** and **cytotoxic T cells.** The specific defenses do not appear immediately when a microbe is first encountered. Several days or weeks may pass before the specific defense response begins to develop. Only upon subsequent encounters with the same microbe do the specific defenses appear rapidly and at full strength. Vaccination is a strategy for eliciting the specific defenses without actually having to endure the first episode of the disease.

Understanding how the specific defenses are induced and how they protect the body from infection is important for understanding how vaccines work, how they are designed, and what is the best administration route. Although vaccines have been important in preventing disease, the yield of successful vaccines has been disappointingly small. New technologies and new insights into how the specific defense response develops may help to break down some of the barriers that have prevented development of vaccines against diseases such as AIDS, gonorrhea, chlamydial disease, tuberculosis, and malaria, which are serious causes of morbidity and mortality throughout the world.

In this chapter, we start with a description of two of the main players in the specific defense system, antibodies and cytotoxic T cells. We will then delve into the complex series of steps that produce these defenses. Also important is the body's strategy for remembering past infectious experiences so that if the infectious microbe is encountered again, as it almost certainly will be, the specific defenses are prepared to respond rapidly to the invader.

Antibodies

Characteristics of Antibodies and Their Diverse Roles in Preventing Infection

Antibodies are protein complexes produced by **B lymphocytes** (B cells). This rather bland description is accurate as far as it goes but fails to convey the amazing variety of tasks performed by these relatively simple molecules. To understand how they perform so many diverse tasks, it is first necessary to understand how an antibody is put together. The structure of an antibody monomer is shown in Figure 6–1. The monomer consists of two heavy chains and two light chains. (The words "heavy" and "light" refer to the size of the protein, with the heavy chain being the larger of the two.) The heavy and light chains are held together by a combination of disulfide bonds and noncovalent interactions. Antibodies have two important domains: the variable region (Fv), which contains the antigen-binding end of the antibody, and the other end, the constant portion (Fc), which interacts with complement or phagocytic cells via a glycosylated region of the protein. An **antigen** is defined as any material the body recognizes as foreign. For the purposes of this chapter, "antigen" will mean an infectious microbe or some component of it. Examples of other types of antigens are nonhuman animal proteins, macromolecules on organs from a noncompatible donor, and the pollens of some plants.

An antibody monomer has two **antigen-binding sites,** each of which recognizes and binds to the same specific segment of an antigen. The antigen-binding sites are grooves in the antibody ends that bind tightly only to a molecule having one particular structure, an **epitope.** An epitope on a protein antigen can vary in size from 4 to 16 amino acids, although most are 5 to 8 amino acids in length. Complex antigens, such as microbes, contain many possible epitopes. In practice, however, a subset of the epitopes on an antigen dominates the specific response to that antigen. Why some epitopes are highly **immunogenic** (eliciting a robust antibody or T-cell response) whereas others are only weakly immunogenic is still not well understood. Differences in immunogenicity have important practical consequences. For example, it is now possible to produce epitope-sized peptides synthetically. Peptides are not only much cheaper to produce than proteins, which must be purified by time-consuming biochemical procedures, but they also make it possible to target an antibody or cytotoxic T-cell response toward one or more specific regions of an antigen.

Directing the specific defenses toward particular epitopes is important because not all immunogenic epitopes elicit a **protective** response. Some immunogenic epitopes, for example, are buried within a folded protein on a microbe's surface. Eliciting an antibody response to such an epitope is useless because the antibody will not be able to bind it. Some microbial proteins have regions that vary considerably from one strain to another. Antibodies or cytotoxic cells that recognize highly variable regions of microbial proteins will be

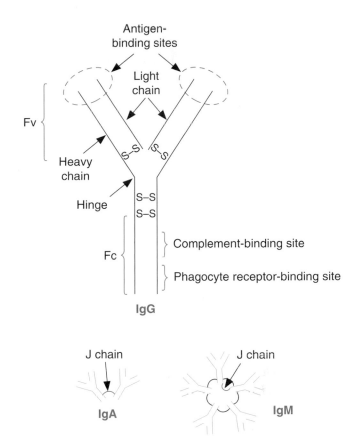

Figure 6–1   Structures of IgG, IgA, and IgM. The antigen-binding sites are the regions of the antibody molecule that recognize the target epitope. The Fc region of the molecule is responsible for complement activation and mediates binding to phagocyte receptors during opsonization.

useful only against a limited number of strains. A better strategy is to target regions of microbial proteins that are highly conserved, i.e., that are found on all strains of the microbe. Using peptide epitopes as vaccines makes it possible to program a specific defense response directed toward exposed, conserved epitopes.

Serum Antibodies

IgG, THE MOST COMMON ANTIBODY TYPE.   There are several types of antibodies, which have somewhat different roles (Table 6–1). IgG, a monomer, is the most prevalent type of antibody in blood and extravascular fluid spaces (Figure 6–1). There are four subtypes of human IgG (**IgG1** to **IgG4**). These subtypes differ in the amino acid sequence and disulfide cross-linking of their heavy chains (primarily in the Fc portion) and also in their function. IgG1 is the most abundant of the IgG subtypes. IgG1 and IgG3 are called **opsonizing antibodies** because these two subtypes are the most effective in opsonizing microbes (Table 6–1). IgG2 and IgG4

Table 6–1 Protective roles of serum antibodies IgG and IgM

Role	IgG1	IgG2	IgG3	IgG4	IgM
Neutralize toxins	+	+	+	+	+
Neutralize microbes (prevents binding to a target host cell)	+	+	+	+	+
Opsonization Fc portion binds					
PMN receptors	+	−	+	−	−
Macrophage receptors	+	−	+	+	+
Complement activation	+	+	+	−	+
Cross placenta	+	+	+	+	−

opsonize poorly, if at all. Opsonization of an antigen by IgG facilitates ingestion of the opsonized antigen by phagocytic cells. In the case of infected tissues, which are too large to ingest, IgG mediates attachment of a cytotoxic cell to the tissue, and the cytotoxic cell employs a bombardment strategy to kill the infected cell. This is called **antibody-dependent cell-mediated cytotoxicity (ADCC).** It is commonly associated with NK cells, but phagocytes can also be involved. ADCC serves as a defense against intracellular pathogens.

IgG1, IgG2, and IgG3, but not IgG4, also activate complement, but it takes at least two IgG monomers bound close together so that C1 can bind to the Fc regions of both IgG monomers. Binding to two monomers is necessary to activate C1 to initiate the complement cascade. IgG is the only antibody type that crosses the placenta and is responsible for protecting an infant during the first 6 months of life until the specific defenses are fully developed. (Warning: as indicated in Box 6–1, the nomenclature used to describe human IgG is not the same as that used to describe murine IgG. So IgG1 of mice does not necessarily have the same features as IgG1 of humans. We mention this now because later we will see that this explains why different papers on the development of the immune response may seem at first to contradict each other but actually do not. We will return to this nomenclatural problem in the section on the Th1/Th2 responses to infection.)

IgM, THE EARLIEST APPEARING ANTIBODY. IgM consists of five monomers, which are connected to each other and to a peptide called the **J chain** (Figure 6–1). IgM predominates in the initial antibody response against a pathogenic microbe, whereas IgG predominates in the response to sustained or subsequent infections by the same microbe. This feature of the immune response is useful for diagnostic purposes. Diagnostic tests that detect IgM are used to determine whether a

BOX 6–1 Are You a Man or a Mouse?

This archaic challenge, issued to someone showing classic symptoms of cowardice, in the hopes of getting him or her to act decisively and courageously, actually applies as well to antibodies. Although humans and mice are much more closely related than many of us would like to admit, there are subtle but real differences between some antibody classes found in humans and mice. Accordingly, there is also a somewhat different nomenclature used to designate these antibody classes. These different designations can be confusing, especially in the case of the IgG subtypes. A guide to the different antibody designations in humans and mice is provided below:

Human	Mouse
IgG1	IgG2a
IgG2	IgG2b
IgG3	None
IgG4	IgG1
IgM1 IgM2	IgM
IgE	IgE

Why such differences occur between closely related species remains a fascinating but unanswered question.

patient is experiencing a first infection with a particular microbe. Because IgG can circulate in serum for long periods, detectable IgG levels can either signal the presence of a current infection that is well under way or can simply be the residue of a previous infection. IgM is the most effective activator of complement. A single molecule of IgM is sufficient to activate complement via the classical pathway because it has five Fc regions that can be easily cross-linked.

Both IgG and IgM bind to the surfaces of bacteria and viruses and prevent them from attaching to and invading target host cells (**neutralization of the microbe**). Antibodies do this very effectively because they are bulky molecules that block interactions between microbial surface proteins and the receptors they recognize on host cells. Antibodies can also neutralize toxic proteins produced by bacteria (**exotoxins**) because exotoxins must first bind to a specific host cell receptor before they can exert their toxic effect. Antibodies bound to the exotoxin prevent the exotoxin binding portion from binding to the receptor (**toxin neutralization**).

IgE, THE ALLERGY-ASSOCIATED ANTIBODY. A serum antibody with a different function from that of IgG and IgM is **IgE**. IgE is an antibody monomer and is thought to play a protective role against metazoal pathogens, although this idea has become somewhat controversial. IgE levels rise during metazoal infections, but increased levels associated with infection do not necessarily mean that the response is protective. IgE binds to **mast cells,** and if two IgE molecules are cross-linked by a polyvalent antigen, the mast cell releases granules containing **histamine** and other **vasoactive compounds.** Release of mast cell granules in the vicinity of the intestinal wall may provoke an allergic response that ejects parasitic metazoans from the intestine. Many of the symptoms of metazoal infections are traceable to the effects of increased levels of IgE.

In developed countries, where metazoal infections are relatively uncommon, IgE is most often associated with noninfectious diseases, such as allergies or asthma. The most serious complication of the massive release of mast cell granules is anaphylaxis, which can rapidly kill a person. An interesting point to ponder is that the human body evolved over millions of years to cope with worm infestations. IgE seems to be part of that response. In recent times, in developed countries, we have eliminated worms from our intestinal landscape. Is the rise in allergies and asthma seen in all developed countries due to an immunological imbalance caused by elimination of a former enemy, leaving the worm-oriented part of the specific and nonspecific defenses with nothing to do except get into fights with allergens and human tissue? Rest assured that this is not the start of a "bring back the worms" initiative, but it is interesting to think about the possibly negative consequences of an abrupt change (in evolutionary terms) in our exposure to invaders that have been with us from antiquity.

Secretory Antibodies—Antibodies That Protect Mucosal Surfaces

IgA is an antibody type found in low concentrations in serum in its monomeric form. The role of IgA in blood and tissue is to aid in the clearance of antigen-antibody complexes from the body. By far the most important form of IgA, however, is **secretory IgA (sIgA),** which plays a key role in the defense of mucosal surfaces. sIgA

consists of two IgA antibody monomers joined by a peptide J chain to which another peptide, called **secretory piece,** has been attached. The secretory piece is acquired when IgA is transported through the mucosal layer into the mucin layer (see later section). The main role of sIgA is to attach to incoming microbes or microbial toxins and trap them in the mucin layer, thus preventing them from reaching the mucosa. sIgA can trap microbes in mucus because the Fc portion of sIgA binds to glycoprotein constituents of the mucin layer. sIgA binding to the surface of a microbe or toxin also prevents the microbe or toxin from binding to receptors on mucosal cells. sIgA does not activate complement. sIgA is secreted into mother's milk, as well as into the mucous layer. Thus, sIgA, like IgG, serves as an important protection against infection for young infants who have not yet developed their own set of immune responses.

Affinity and Avidity

A characteristic of antibody binding to antigens, which is of critical importance in determining the effectiveness of the antibody, is the **avidity** of the antigen-binding site for the epitope it binds. Avidity is a combination of **affinity** (the strength of the interaction between an antigen-binding site and an epitope) and **valence** (the number of antigen-binding sites available for binding epitopes on an antigen). A single epitope can elicit a mixture of antibodies that vary considerably in affinity. The reason for this variation may be that since the body cannot "know" in advance what epitopes it will encounter, it responds to one by producing a variety of antibodies with slightly different antigen-binding sites, among which will be some binding sites that have a high affinity for the antigen. In fact, as the antibody response to an epitope develops, the antibodies with the highest affinity eventually predominate.

High affinity is important, but it is not sufficient to ensure that an antibody bound to an epitope retains its hold on the epitope. Since the binding between antigen-binding sites and epitopes is noncovalent, the interaction is reversible. Thus, there is an "off rate" as well as an "on rate" associated with antibody binding to an epitope. The importance of valence is that an antibody with a higher valence will be significantly less likely to detach from the antigen to which it is bound than an antibody with a lower valence. If two antigen-binding sites of an antibody monomer bind to two adjacent epitopes on an antigen, the probability that both of them will detach at the same time is much lower than the probability that a single antigen-binding site will detach from its epitope. Thus, higher valence can improve the strength of binding of an antibody to an epitope by orders of magnitude. Some types of antibodies, such as IgM and sIgA, have a higher valence number than IgG because they are composed of more than one monomer and can thus bind to four (sIgA) or 10 (IgM) epitopes. These antibodies thus have a greater avidity for antigens than does IgG, which is a monomer.

High avidity for an antigen is important for neutralizing microbes and toxins, opsonizing microbes, and activating complement. Moreover, phagocytic cells more rapidly clear antibodies that bind to their antigens with high avidity from the body. This is a desirable feature because the longer antibody-antigen complexes remain in circulation, the more likely they are to deposit in the kidneys or other blood-filtering organs, where they can activate complement and cause an inflammatory response that damages the organ.

Cytotoxic T Cells

Cytotoxic T cells have a role in killing infected host cells similar to that of NK cells. The difference between cytotoxic T cells and NK cells (which are very like T cells in many respects) is that cytotoxic T cells have receptors that are specific for a particular epitope on a microbial antigen. Thus, whereas NK cells will kill host cells infected with a variety of intracellular pathogens, cytotoxic T cells kill only cells infected with one particular type of microbe. ADCC, like cytotoxic T-cell killing, is also specific for a particular microbe because the normally nonspecific PMNs are directed by antibodies to attack target infected host cells. Cytotoxic T cells, ADCC, and NK cells are an important part of the defense response against intracellular pathogens because killing infected cells may be the only way to attack these pathogens, which are protected by their intracellular location from antibodies and complement.

Cytotoxic T cells are related to T-helper cells but differ from them in that cytotoxic T cells have a protein called **CD8** on their surfaces, whereas T-helper cells have a different protein, **CD4,** on their surfaces. As you will see later in this chapter, these different proteins help make sure that T-helper cells and cytotoxic T cells interact with the right cell types. T-helper cells interact primarily with the professional antigen-presenting cells of the specific defense system, such as macrophages and dendritic cells, and with B cells (the antibody-producing cells), whereas cytotoxic T cells can attack most of the cell types in the body if they are infected. It would hardly do for cytotoxic T cells to start attacking uninfected cells nonspecifically.

How do cytotoxic T cells attack and kill intracellular bacteria? The answer to this question has long been controversial. In particular, it was unclear whether cytotoxic T cells simply killed infected human cells or

also killed microorganisms directly. Recent studies have shown that the cytotoxic T cells do both. Cytotoxic T cells have two mechanisms for killing infected human cells. Cytotoxic T cells bind to infected cells using a T-cell receptor on their surface that recognizes microbial antigens being displayed on the surface of the infected cell. The cytotoxic T cell then produces proteolytic enzymes (granzymes) that trigger **programmed cell death (apoptosis)** in the infected cell. This type of attack kills the infected cell but not the microbes. Released microbes, however, can then be taken up by activated macrophages that are better able to kill them. Alternatively, the cytotoxic T cell can use granules that contain two proteins, **perforin** and **granulysin,** to attack the microbes (Figure 6–2). Perforin enters the host cell membrane and forms holes in it, killing the cell. Perforin also helps a second T-cell granule protein, granulysin, to enter the infected cell. Granulysin is not very effective in lysing host cells, but it is very effective in killing bacteria. Presumably, granulysin kills bacteria the way perforin kills eukaryotic cells—by creating holes in their membranes. Holes in the bacterial membrane collapse the proton motive force that the bacteria use to gain energy. Perforin may also help to deliver other antibacterial lysins, which remain to be discovered, into intracellular compartments of host cells.

Production of Activated Cytotoxic T Cells and Antibodies

Processing of Protein Antigens by APCs

When microbes or their products first enter the body, professional **antigen-presenting cells (APCs)** ingest them or their proteins. There are three types of APCs—macrophages, dendritic cells, and B cells. The APC degrades protein antigens and displays the resulting peptides on its surface on a protein complex called the **major histocompatibility complex (MHC)** (Figure 6–3). Two types of MHC complexes, **MHC-I** and **MHC-II,** have been known for some time. Recently, a third antigen-presenting molecule has been added: **CD1 molecules.** CD1 molecules present lipid or glycolipid antigens rather than peptide antigens. In the past, immunologists have focused almost exclusively on peptide antigens because proteins and peptides are easier to characterize than carbohydrate or lipid-containing molecules. Also, peptide antigens elicit a strong immune response. Finally, peptides are relatively simple molecules. They consist of amino acids linked by a single type of bond, the peptide bond. Carbohydrate oligomers, by contrast, can be linked by any of 12 glycosidic linkages. Lipids also contain more than a single type of linkage.

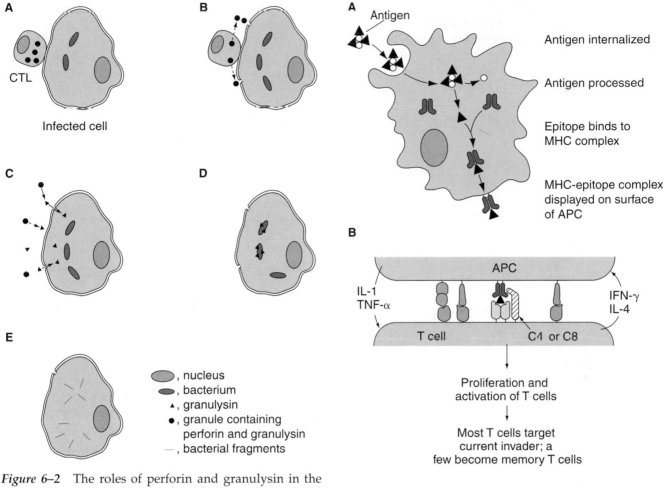

A CTL

Infected cell

B

C

D

E

, nucleus
, bacterium
, granulysin
, granule containing perforin and granulysin
—, bacterial fragments

Figure 6–2 The roles of perforin and granulysin in the killing of bacteria that have infected a host cell. (**A**) Cytotoxic T cell (CTL) recognizes the infected cell. (**B**) CTL releases granules containing perforin and granulysin; perforin creates pores in the infected cell membrane. (**C**) Granulysin enters subcellular compartments through the pores created by perforin. (**D**) Granulysin attaches to and kills bacteria. (**E**) Host cell with degraded bacteria.

A Antigen

Antigen internalized

Antigen processed

Epitope binds to MHC complex

MHC-epitope complex displayed on surface of APC

B

IL-1 TNF-α   APC   IFN-γ IL-4

T cell   C4 or C8

Proliferation and activation of T cells

Most T cells target current invader; a few become memory T cells

, epitope-MHC complex;   , T-cell receptor

Figure 6–3 Antigen processing by APCs (exemplified by a macrophage) leads to activation and increased proliferation of T cells. (**A**) The macrophage binds a cognate T cell, making multiple contacts. (**B**) Formation of a tight complex stimulates the APC to produce cytokines that stimulate T-cell activation and proliferation.

Unfortunately, many of the bacterial antigens recognized by the immune system are lipid, carbohydrate, or lipid-carbohydrate antigens. Gram-negative LPS and gram-positive LTA are excellent examples. *Mycobacterium tuberculosis,* the cause of tuberculosis, provides a cornucopia of lipid-saccharide antigens not found in most other bacteria. Examples of this type continue to be discovered. Accordingly, some immunologists have begun to study the processing of lipid-carbohydrate antigens. Their first big find was CD1, a protein complex that presents *M. tuberculosis* lipid antigens, and probably lipid antigens from other sources as well. So far, four forms of human CD1 have been found, CD1a to CD1d. The steps in processing and displaying lipid antigens

appear to be similar to those shown in Figure 6–3 for peptide antigens, with CD1 taking the place of the MHC molecule. CD1 is related at the amino acid sequence level to MHC-I and MHC-II but has obviously diverged from them during evolution. In what follows, we will concentrate our attention on MHC-I and MHC-II for the simple reason that relatively little is known about CD1. But brace yourself for new literature on CD1 in the future, as intrepid immunologists begin to enter the quagmire of bacterial lipid and lipid-carbohydrate antigens.

The type of MHC used to display the peptide epitope determines whether the APC will stimulate production of cytotoxic T cells or activate T-helper cells, which in turn will stimulate production of antibodies or activation of macrophages. Display on MHC-I allows the APC to activate and stimulate the proliferation of cytotoxic T cells. Display of an epitope on MHC-II leads to activation and proliferation of T-helper cells, which aid in the production of antibodies or produce IFN-γ, which activates macrophages and cytotoxic T cells.

How the APC decides whether to display an epitope on MHC-I or MHC-II has received a lot of attention, because an understanding of the properties that lead to each type of presentation is critical for the design of vaccines. Although this area is still quite controversial, some basic rules are beginning to emerge. Pathogens, such as viruses and bacteria that can enter the cytoplasm or nucleus of an APC (intracellular pathogens), are most likely to elicit an MHC-I display of their antigens (Figure 6–4). Even particulate antigens that do not escape the phagocytic vesicle can elicit an MHC-I-linked display. By contrast, soluble antigens, such as peptides or proteins from lysed bacteria, are displayed mainly on MHC-II. Thus, to use peptides to elicit a cytotoxic T-cell response, it is desirable to present the peptides in particulate form, e.g., bound up in a complex consisting of inert materials which will encourage their processing via the MHC-I pathway.

Interaction between APCs and T Cells: the T-Cell-Dependent Response

T cells have specialized protein complexes on their surfaces called **T-cell receptors.** The genes encoding T-cell receptor proteins undergo extensive rearrangements during development of the T cells. The result is a pool of T cells with surface receptors that recognize a variety of epitopes. When an APC displays a particular MHC-I-peptide or MHC-II-peptide complex on its surface, only a few of the vast pool of available T cells will have a T-cell receptor capable of recognizing that MHC-peptide combination. These T cells bind the MHC-peptide complex via their T-cell receptors. Cytotoxic T cells have a protein on their surfaces, CD8, which helps the T-cell receptor respond to peptides displayed on MHC-I. CD8 binds to MHC-I and stabilizes the interaction between the MHC-I-peptide complex and the T-cell receptor. T-helper cells have a different surface protein, CD4, which helps their T-cell receptors respond to peptides displayed on MHC-II; CD4 stabilizes the interaction between the MHC-II-peptide complex and T-cell receptor. Other proteins on the surface of the APC and the T cell, called costimulatory molecules (e.g., CD54, CD11a/CD18, CD58, CD2), must also interact to make the binding between APC and T cell tight enough to stimulate the APC to release cytokines (e.g., IL-1, TNF-α). The cytokines stimulate the T cell to proliferate and become activated. The contacts between different surface proteins of the APC and the T cell help ensure that specific binding of the correct T-cell receptor to an MHC-peptide complex will result in T-cell activation. Once activated, T cells begin to proliferate. Most of the resulting T cells are involved in combating the invading microbes. A few of the T cells, however, become **mem-**

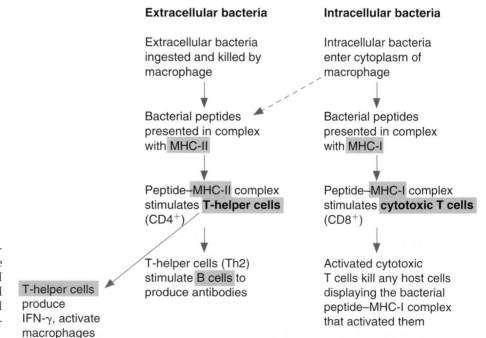

Figure 6–4 Characteristics of antigen (Ag) determine whether the antigen is presented on MHC-I (to trigger the cytotoxic T-cell [TC] response) or on MHC-II (to trigger the T-helper cell response).

Extracellular bacteria

Extracellular bacteria ingested and killed by macrophage

Bacterial peptides presented in complex with MHC-II

Peptide–MHC-II complex stimulates **T-helper cells** (CD4⁺)

T-helper cells (Th2) stimulate B cells to produce antibodies

T-helper cells produce IFN-γ, activate macrophages

Intracellular bacteria

Intracellular bacteria enter cytoplasm of macrophage

Bacterial peptides presented in complex with MHC-I

Peptide–MHC-I complex stimulates **cytotoxic T cells** (CD8⁺)

Activated cytotoxic T cells kill any host cells displaying the bacterial peptide–MHC-I complex that activated them

ory cells. Memory T cells are T cells that persist for long periods in the body and constantly monitor blood and tissue for the epitope they recognize. Upon subsequent contacts with the epitope, e.g., during an infection, these memory cells are stimulated to proliferate. Memory cells allow the body to respond to a second encounter with a microbial invader much more swiftly than it did after the initial encounter.

Some bacteria and viruses produce proteins, called **superantigens,** that interfere with the natural progression of T-cell activation. Superantigens force a close association between APCs and T cells that would not normally occur because the receptors on the macrophages and T cells are not a good match. Whereas normally only a fraction of a percent of T cells would interact specifically with a particular macrophage presenting an antigen on its cell surface, superantigens can cause up to 20% of T cells to participate in such interactions. As the cytokine signaling begins, cytokines are produced at higher levels than normal, and this overreaction can trigger septic shock. As described in chapter 5, septic shock is usually initiated by LPS or other bacterial surface components.

The role of activated cytotoxic T cells is to recognize infected cells, because virtually all cells of the body produce MHC-I. If a cell is infected, it displays epitopes from the invading microbe on MHC-I. The T-cell receptor, usually composed of alpha and beta subunits, recognizes this MHC-I-peptide complex in much the same way it recognized the MHC-I-peptide complex on the surface of the APC. Binding of a cytotoxic T cell to the surface of an infected cell causes the cytotoxic T cell to release cytolytic or apoptotic proteins that can kill the infected cell. The role of activated T-helper cells is to stimulate antibody production by B cells. Activated T cells can also use IFN-γ to activate macrophages to give them a greater killing capacity.

The Th1/Th2 View of Immunity Development

A new theory of how T-helper cells influence the development of different types of immune response has emerged. In recent years, the theory has become more controversial rather than less but is still widely accepted. According to this theory, there are two subtypes of T-helper cells, Th1 and Th2 (Figure 6–5). Both are descended from the same cell type, Th0. The decision to produce Th1 cells is triggered when PMNs produce IL-12, which stimulates NK cells to produce IFN-γ, which in turn stimulates Th0 cells to differentiate into the Th1 form (Figure 6–5). IL-4 is thought to stimulate Th0 cells to develop into Th2 cells. Whether Th0 cells differentiate into Th1 or Th2 cells is very important. Th1

cells produce IFN-γ, which helps to activate macrophages and cytotoxic T cells. Th1 cells also stimulate B cells to produce some subclasses of antibodies, but these are antibodies that do not opsonize very well. Thus, Th1 cells influence the immune system to produce a type of response that is effective mainly against intracellular pathogens.

Th2 cells activate eosinophils and stimulate B cells to produce antibodies of the IgG1 class. IgG1 is the most effective of the opsonizing antibodies. Th2 cells also stimulate production of antibodies of the IgE class, the class associated with the allergic or antimetazoan response. Th2 cells produce IL-10 and IL-13, cytokines that downregulate some cells of the immune system. Thus, the Th2 response produces effective opsonizing antibodies, which are important for helping phagocytes clear extracellular bacterial pathogens. The Th2 response is important for the control of metazoal infections because IgE and eosinophils are critical factors in this control.

A fact that has long puzzled and frustrated scientists trying to develop vaccines is that a vaccine may elicit high titers of antibody and still not be protective. The difference in effectiveness of the Th1- and Th2-type responses, both of which result in stimulation of antibody production, may help to explain at least some cases in which this has happened.

Production of Antibodies by B Cells

Once T-helper cells are activated, they seek and bind to **B cells** that are displaying the appropriate MHC-II-peptide complex. Only a few cell types, such as B cells, produce MHC-II, so the use of MHC-II helps T-helper cells bind specifically to B cells. Binding of a T-helper cell to a B cell involves a set of multiprotein contacts similar to that which occurs between the initial APC cells and T cells (Figure 6–6). Tight binding of the T-helper cell to the B cell stimulates the T-helper cell to produce cytokines, which in turn stimulate the B cell to proliferate and differentiate into the form that secretes antibodies. A fraction of activated B cells become **memory B cells.** In subsequent encounters with the same antigen, antibodies on the surfaces of the memory B cells bind the antigen and stimulate the B cell directly to proliferate and secrete antibodies. This is a much more rapid response than the APC-initiated process. During an infection, both the APC-initiated response and direct B cell stimulation by antigen binding can occur, but the APC-initiated process is more important in the initial reaction to the microbe, whereas direct B-cell stimulation by antigens is more important for antibody production in subsequent encounters.

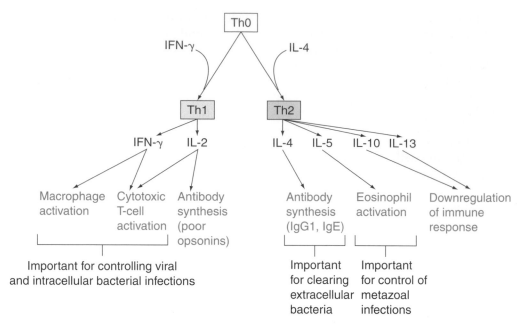

Figure 6–5 Model for development and roles of Th1 and Th2 cells in humans. Antibody nomenclature for mice is somewhat different.

Links to Nonspecific Defenses

For the human body to have the nonspecific defenses acting independently of the specific defenses would be inefficient, especially since the two types of defense can act synergistically. Not surprisingly, there are a lot of links between the two systems. One set of links is **cytokines** and **chemokines.** PMNs contribute to the Th1/ Th2 decision-making process through cytokine production. Complement comes up in connection with both C3b-mediated opsonization and interaction with antibodies to kill bacteria directly. Macrophages can act as APCs or phagocytic cells. Th1 cells activate macrophages to greater killing power.

T-Independent Antigens

The APC-T-cell pathway responds to protein antigens but not necessarily to nonprotein antigens, such as polysaccharides and lipids. Because T cells are not involved in responding to antigens of this type, such antigens are called **T-independent antigens.** Polysaccharides and lipids can elicit an immune response in children and adults, but not in infants under the age of 2 years. Thus, the ability to respond to T-independent antigens develops after birth. This is an important consideration, because it means that vaccines consisting of T-independent antigens are not effective until an infant has become old enough to respond to these antigens.

T-independent antigens provoke an antibody response but not a cell-mediated response because they interact directly with B cells. Unactivated B cells display the antibody they produce on their surfaces. Polysaccharides and lipids are characterized by repetitive epitopes. If these epitopes bind to antibodies exposed on the surface of a B cell, they cause cross-linking of the antibodies. Cross-linking of surface antibodies stimulates the B cell to increase production of more antibodies and to release them (Figure 6–7). The T-independent response is particularly important for protection against bacterial pathogens that can avoid phagocytosis by covering themselves with a polysaccharide layer (capsule). Such bacteria are not effectively opsonized by C3b. They are ingested and killed by phagocytes only if antibodies that bind to capsular antigens are elicited and act as opsonins.

Although the T-independent response provides protection against capsule-producing bacteria, it has some important drawbacks. First, the antibody response elicited by T-independent antigens is not as strong as the T-cell-dependent response. Nor is it as long lasting, because no memory cells are developed. Second, the main antibodies elicited by T-independent antigens are IgM and IgG2. IgG2 does not opsonize, and IgM does so less effectively than IgG1 and IgG3. Third, as already mentioned, young infants do not mount a T-independent response. Unfortunately, infants are one of the highest risk groups for contracting serious infections due to capsule-producing bacteria (e.g., pneumonia and meningitis). A strategy for improving the immune response

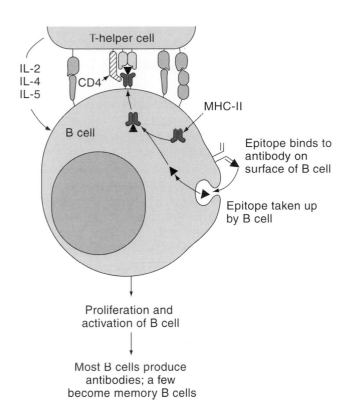

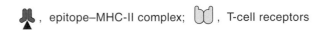

, epitope–MHC-II complex; , T-cell receptors

Figure 6–6 Th cells find and activate B cells presenting the same epitope on their MHC-II. For simplicity, only some of the accessory proteins involved in binding and activating the B cell are shown.

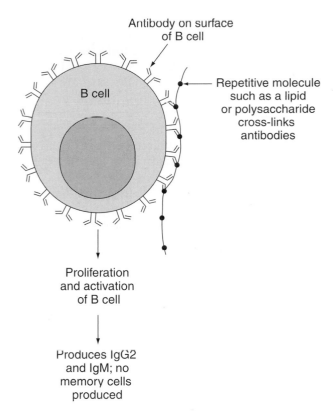

Figure 6–7 T-independent production of antibodies.

to T-independent antigens and extending this response to infants is to covalently link a portion of the polysaccharide capsule to a protein. Such a vaccine is called a **conjugate vaccine.** APCs, noted more for their muscle than for their high intelligence, process conjugate vaccines as if they were proteins and elicit a T-dependent response that ultimately results in production of antibodies that recognize the polysaccharide antigen. This immune response is long-lived and produces opsonizing antibodies IgG1, IgG3, and IgG4.

The account just given of the T-independent response to polysaccharides is the one currently favored by immunologists. Questions about the accuracy of this account can be raised, however, when one considers the protection record of the vaccine against *Streptococcus pneumoniae*, which consists of capsular polysaccharides. According to the currently accepted version of the T-independent response, this vaccine should confer only short-term immunity. In fact, in young adults this vaccine confers immunity that lasts for many years. Does

this indicate that there may be some sort of memory response to polysaccharide antigens? Stay tuned for future developments. One aspect of this account of the T-independent response remains, unfortunately, correct. Infants are not protected at all by polysaccharide vaccines. A conjugate vaccine that protects against *S. pneumoniae*, a major cause of earache, pneumonia, and meningitis, has now reached the market. Unfortunately, this vaccine covers only 7 of the nearly 100 serotypes of *S. pneumoniae*.

Mucosal Immunity

A very important immune response to infectious diseases, but one that is less well understood than the humoral or cell-mediated responses, is the response that produces sIgA. The first step in many microbial infections is colonization and invasion of a mucosal surface. sIgA can prevent such infections by blocking colonization. Thus, whereas the cell-mediated or humoral antibody responses may cause damage to tissues in the area where infection is occurring, the sIgA-mediated defense is completely innocuous to the host, because it occurs in the mucin layer. Skin and mucosal surfaces all have associated lymphoid tissues. The best studied of these systems is the gastrointestinal-associated lymphoid tissue (GALT) found in the **follicles** and **Peyer's patches,** which are most highly concentrated in the ileum and rectum. Similar lymphoid tissues are found in the respiratory and vaginal tracts. This group of mucosal immune systems is called mucosa-associated lymphoid tissue (MALT). Skin also has a similar system, called the skin-associated lymphoid tissue (SALT). The Langerhans cells of the epidermis are the APCs of this system.

The cells of the GALT are illustrated in Figure 6–8. The **M (microfold) cell** takes up antigens from the lumen of the intestinal tract and passes them to GALT macrophages, which presumably act as the APCs. The process by which GALT macrophages process antigens and elicit production of cytotoxic T cells or antibodies is the same as that described in earlier sections, except that the macrophages, B cells, and T cells of the GALT home specifically to mucosal membranes and appear not to be part of the humoral immune system. Memory T and B cells stimulated by antigen processing at the GALT can migrate to other mucosal sites and vice versa. Thus, stimulation of one of the MALT sites results in general mucosal immunity. This characteristic of the MALT system is what makes **oral vaccines** feasible. Initially, oral vaccines stimulate the GALT, but sIgA against vaccine antigens is later detectable in other sites. Thus, an oral vaccine can be used to elicit immunity to respiratory and, presumably, genital pathogens.

Currently, efforts are being made to develop vaccines administered by inhalation, so that stimulation of the bronchial MALT would produce an sIgA response at other MALT sites. These vaccines would have the advantage that they need not pass through the stomach. Vaccines that target the GALT have to be capable of surviving the low-pH and protease-rich stomach environment, a barrier that has proved problematical in some cases. Administering vaccines by rectal or vaginal suppositories is theoretically possible, but this strategy has not been actively pursued to date.

When the GALT is stimulated, one outcome is production of IgA (Figure 6–8). IgA binds to the **poly-Ig receptor** on the basal surface of mucosal cells and is then taken up and carried in vesicles to the apical surface, where it is released. Release involves proteolytic cleavage of the receptor, and a portion of the receptor remains attached to the IgA, making it sIgA. Activation of the GALT can also lead to production of cytotoxic T cells. These cells probably remain on the basal side of the mucosa, although it is possible that during an infection some of them migrate to the apical surface, especially in areas where damage to the mucosa has occurred. GALT cytotoxic T cells are important for

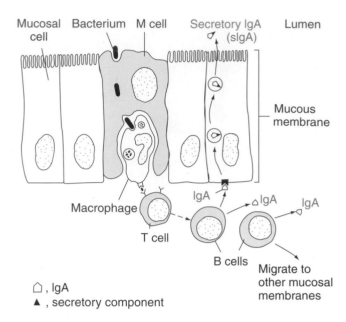

Figure 6–8　Cells of the GALT. M cells and their associated lymphoid cells (T and B cells) are sometimes called follicles. Collections of follicles are called Peyer's patches.

protection against viral infections of the gastrointestinal tract and some bacterial infections in which the bacteria multiply inside mucosal cells.

One of the many mysteries associated with the intestinal immune mucosa is the role of a type of mucosal cell called **gamma-delta T cells.** The majority of gamma-delta T cells are CD8$^+$ T cells and would thus be grouped with cytotoxic T cells. However, whereas cytotoxic T cells of the humoral immune system have T-cell receptors composed of alpha and beta protein subunits, the **intestinal epithelial lymphocytes (IELs)** have a T-cell receptor composed of related but somewhat different protein subunits called gamma and delta. Gamma-delta T cells account for fewer than 4% of circulating CD8 cells, but they account for as many as 10 to 15% of the mucosal cells in the gastrointestinal tract; in some parts, such as the colon, the level may be as high as 40%. Recently, some light has been shed on their role. In fact, gamma-delta T cells have gone very rapidly from being cells in search of a function to cells to which too many functions are now attributed.

A particularly intriguing feature of gamma-delta T cells has been that these cells have a very limited repertoire of antigen recognition. Whereas there are thousands, perhaps millions, of types of cytotoxic and T-helper cells, each of which recognizes a different antigen, the gamma-delta T cells seem to recognize only a limited number of antigens. Also, gamma-delta T cells appear to bypass the macrophage antigen presentation step and recognize nonpeptide antigens that have not been processed. This is T-cell heresy at its best. T cells were named to indicate that these are cells that *must* first pass through the thymus, an organ that contains APCs, which give the T cells their marching orders. Gamma-delta T cells are not thymus derived and are relatively nonspecific. How could they play any role in the response to infection? Yet there are certainly a lot of them populating the mucosal membranes of the body. As the old saying goes, if there are this many ants, the picnic must be a success.

The mystery surrounding the function of the gamma-delta T cells has been cleared to some extent by the discovery that gamma-delta T cells respond primarily to two human protein complexes related to MHC-I, **MICA** and **MICB.** These proteins are displayed on the surface of cells that are stressed by being infected. Does this relative lack of specificity mean that they should be classified as members of the nonspecific defense system? No, but it illustrates our previously stated caveat that, although drawing a line between the so-called specific and nonspecific defenses may be useful from a pedagogical point of view, it obscures the many linkages that exist between the two systems. Alternatively, the gamma-delta T cells may have specificity that has not yet been determined.

Another role attributed to gamma-delta T cells is production of factors that help turn off the inflammatory response. Gamma-delta T cells also produce cytokines that stimulate alpha-beta cytotoxic T cells to migrate to the area and eliminate damaged cells. Finally, gamma-delta T cells produce growth factors that may aid in repair of damaged epithelia. Perhaps the best way to describe the role of gamma-delta T cells is as a busboy who doubles as a bouncer. The gamma-delta T cells not only take part in the battle against invaders but help with the cleanup and repair process that returns the body to normal and reestablishes the mucosal membrane after an attack by invaders. As if that were not enough to keep a T cell busy, gamma-delta T cells appear not only to stimulate T-helper-cell activities but also to secrete chemokines to help orchestrate the activities of the neutrophils and monocytes.

The GALT is not an unmixed blessing. Normally, bacteria that pass through M cells are killed by the GALT macrophages. Some bacterial pathogens, however, have acquired the ability to avoid this fate and use the GALT as an entryway into the body. Because the M cell is an antigen sampling cell, it usually does not take up substantial amounts of an antigen because only a few bacteria or other antigens are sufficient to stimulate a GALT-mediated immune response. The bacteria that use the GALT as an entryway into the body stimulate M cells to transport them in higher than usual numbers.

Such bacteria must also be able to survive an attack by the GALT macrophages.

Development of the Specific Response System from Infancy to Adulthood

Human infants do not develop fully effective specific and nonspecific defenses until they are 1 to 2 years of age. For a period up to 1 year of age, maternal antibodies that were transferred through the placenta during gestation or secreted in breast milk during infancy protect them at least partially. Circulating maternal antibodies can actually interfere with an infant's immune response to some antigens because high levels of antibody to a particular epitope discourage the development of an antibody response to that epitope. This is a consequence of immune regulation that normally protects the body from overreacting to a particular epitope. The dampening effect of circulating maternal IgG is the reason that some vaccines are not given to infants less than 1 year of age. The transition between the protection conferred by maternal antibodies and the development of the infant's own immune system provides pathogenic microbes with a window of opportunity and is one of the reasons that children under the age of 2 are particularly vulnerable to infectious diseases. The nonspecific defenses of infants are also underdeveloped before age 2. Infants have very low levels of NK cells and are deficient in mannose-binding protein, one of the acute-phase proteins produced by the liver that help to opsonize some types of microbes.

The Dark Side of the Specific Defenses— Autoimmune Disease

The interactions between cells of the specific defense system are highly complex, as is evident from Figures 6–3 and 6–6. These interactions are important because they help to ascertain that the contacts between immune cells are occurring in response to foreign antigen presentation events and are not accidental associations between cells of the immune system and human cells. They are the insurance that the immune system will not go out of control and attack human cells. This safeguard is sometimes breached when bacterial antigens mimic human antigens. In such cases, the specific defenses can mount an attack that targets human tissues. If the tissue is heart tissue or tissues of other vital organs, the misguided attack (autoimmune response) can be lethal. In later chapters, we will encounter examples of such misguided attacks by the specific immune defenses, a set of conditions called autoimmune diseases. Bacteria that elicit an autoimmune response are particularly difficult targets for vaccines, because the vaccine may induce an autoimmune response that causes damage to the body. Thus, one of the concerns of vaccine producers is to make sure that their vaccine does not elicit an auto-immune response. If a vaccine elicits such a response, it can make the disease worse rather than preventing it when the vaccinated person is exposed to the bacterium.

SELECTED READINGS

Del Prete, G., and S. Romagnani. 1994. The role of Th1 and Th2 subsets in human infectious diseases. *Trends Microbiol.* **2:**4–6.

Delves, P. J., and I. M. Roitt. 2000. The immune system. The first of two parts. *N. Engl. J. Med.* **343:**37–49.

Delves, P. J., and I. M. Roitt. 2000. The immune system. The second of two parts. *N. Engl. J. Med.* **343:**108–117.

Kagnoff, M. F. 1996. Mucosal immunology: new frontiers. *Immunol. Today* **17:**57–59.

Mak, T. W., and D. A. Ferrick. 1998. The gamma-delta T-cell bridge: linking innate and acquired immunity. *Nat. Med.* **4:**764–765.

Murray, J. S. 1998. How the MHC selects Th1/Th2 immunity. *Trends Immunol.* **4:**157–163.

Prigozy, T. I., and M. Kornenberg. 1998. Presentation of bacterial lipid antigens by CD1 molecules. *Trends Microbiol.* **6:**454–459.

Stenger, S., D. A. Hanson, R. Teitelbaum, P. Dewan, K. R. Niazi, C. J. Froelich, T. Ganz, S. Thoma-Uszynski, A. Melian, C. Bogdan, S. A. Porcelli, B. R. Bloom, A. M. Krensky, and R. L. Modlin. 1998. An antimicrobial activity of cytolytic T cells mediated by granulysin. *Science* **282:**121–125.

Yuan, D., C. Y. Koh, and J. A. Wilder. 1994. Interactions between B lymphocytes and NK cells. *FASEB J.* **8:**1012–1018.

SUMMARY OUTLINE

Antibodies

Characteristics
    Protein complexes produced by B cells
    Monomer consists of two heavy chains, two light chains
    Have two antigen-binding sites that bind to epitope region of antigen
    Fc portion binds complement or receptor on phagocytes

Classes of antibodies
    IgG
        Most prevalent type in serum
        Four subtypes (IgG1 to IgG4)
            IgG1 most abundant
            IgG1 and IgG3 are opsonizing antibodies
        ADCC
            IgG mediates attachment of NK or PMN to host tissue
            Cytotoxic cell kills infected cell
        IgG1, IgG2, and IgG3 activate complement
        IgG can cross placenta
    IgM
        Occurs as pentamer
        Contains a J chain
        Predominates in early antibody response
        Most effective activator of complement
    IgG and IgM can neutralize microbes or toxins and prevent binding to host cell
    IgE
        Monomeric
        May protect against metazoal pathogens by interacting with eosinophils
        If two IgE molecules bound to mast cell are cross-linked, mast cell releases vasoactive compounds

(*continued*)

IgA
    Occurs as a monomer in serum
    Secretory IgA (sIgA) found in mucus
        Two monomers joined by J chain
        Secretory piece added as IgA transported through mucosal membrane
        Traps microbes in mucus
    Aids clearance of antigen-antibody complexes from body
    Secreted in milk, protects infants

Characteristics of antibody binding to antigen
    Affinity—strength of interaction between antigen-binding site and epitope; binding reversible
    Valence—number of antigen-binding sites for binding to epitopes; the higher the valence, the
        less likely antigen will detach from antibody
    Avidity—combination of affinity and valence

Cytotoxic T cells

Have CD8 on surface

Kill infected host cells

T-cell receptor on surface composed of alpha and beta protein subunits
    Recognizes microbial antigens being displayed on surface of infected cell
    One subtype triggers apoptosis
        Kills host cell, not bacteria
        Released bacteria may be taken up by activated macrophages
    Second subtype uses granules containing two proteins
        Perforin forms holes in host cell membrane; helps granulysin enter cell
        Granulysin kills intracellular bacteria by collapsing their proton motive force

Important in protecting against intracellular pathogens

Production of activated cytotoxic T cells and antibodies

Processing of protein antigens by APCs
    APC degrades protein antigens of ingested microbe
    Peptides displayed on surface on MHC
        Display on MHC-I stimulates proliferation of cytotoxic T cells
        Display on MHC-II stimulates proliferation of T-helper cells
            May lead to production of antibodies
            May aid in production of IFN-γ (activates macrophages and cytotoxic T cells)
    Lipids and glycolipids displayed on CD1 molecules
    Properties that determine whether epitope is displayed on MHC-I or MHC-II
        Intracellular pathogens and particulate antigens displayed on MHC-I
        Soluble antigens displayed on MHC-II

Interaction between APCs and T cells—T-cell-independent response
    Body contains pool of T cells with receptors that recognize many different epitopes
        Only a few will recognize a particular MHC-epitope complex on an APC
        T-cell receptor binds MHC-peptide complex
    CD8 on cytotoxic T cells helps T cell respond to MHC-I-epitope complexes
    CD4 on T-helper cells helps T cell respond to MHC-II-epitope complexes
    Other surface proteins (costimulatory molecules) of APC and T cell interact—APC releases cy-
        tokines; ensures specificity of binding and T-cell activation

(*continued*)

Activated T cells proliferate
  Most involved in controlling invading microbes
  A few become memory cells
Superantigens force nonspecific interaction between APCs and T cells

Cytotoxic T cells
  Recognize infected cells because almost all cells of body produce MHC-I
  Bind to infected cell, release cytokines that can kill infected cell

T-helper cells
  Recognize cells infected with specific microbe
  Two types: Th1 and Th2
  Th1
    IL-12 produced by PMNs stimulates NK cells to produce IFN-γ
    IFN-γ stimulates Th0 to become Th1
    Th1 produces IFN-γ
      Activates macrophages and cytotoxic T cells
      Stimulates B cells to produce antibodies (poor opsonizers)
    Most important for viral and intracellular bacterial infections
  Th2
    IL-4 stimulates Th0 to become Th2
    Activate eosinophils
    Stimulate B cells to produce IgG1 (good opsonizer) and IgE
    Produce IL-10 and IL-13—downregulate immune response
    Most important in controlling extracellular bacterial and metazoal infections

Production of antibodies by B cells
  Activated Th cells bind to B cells displaying MHC-II-peptide
  Binding stimulates Th cell to produce cytokines
  Cytokines stimulate B cell to proliferate and differentiate
    Most will produce antibodies
    Some will become memory B cells
      Respond more rapidly than APC-initiated process
      Most important in subsequent encounters with microbe

Links to nonspecific defenses
  Cytokines and chemokines
  Complement
  Macrophages
  B cells and NK cells interact

T-cell-independent antigens
  Commonly polysaccharides or lipids
  Elicit immune response in children, adults (not infants)
  Provoke antibody, not cell-mediated response
  Repetitive epitopes cross-link antibodies on B cell
    B cell increases production of antibodies
    No memory cells develop
  Important defense against pathogens with polysaccharide capsules
  Drawbacks
    T-cell-independent response is not as strong as T-cell-dependent response; less long lasting
    Fewer opsonizing antibodies produced

(*continued*)

        Infants do not mount such a response
            Some important pathogens that infect infants have capsules
            Conjugate vaccines (polysaccharide linked to protein) may induce response to polysaccharide in infants

Mucosal immunity

Skin and mucosal surfaces have associated lymphoid tissue

GALT
    Part of MALT
    Found in follicles and Peyer's patches (concentrated in ileum and rectum)
    Components of GALT
        M (microfold) cell—takes up antigens from lumen, passes them to macrophages (act as APCs)
        Macrophages, B cells, and T cells of GALT home to mucosal membranes
        Memory B and T cells produced in any MALT site can migrate to other MALT sites—makes oral vaccines feasible
    Stimulation of GALT results in production of IgA
        IgA binds poly-Ig receptor on basal surface
        Carried in vesicle to apical surface; released
        Portion of receptor (secretory component) remains attached; makes it sIgA
    Stimulation of GALT can lead to production of cytotoxic T cells
    IELs—another type of cytotoxic T cell
        T-cell receptor on these cells made up of gamma and delta subunits instead of alpha and beta
        Account for less than 10% of circulating CD8 cells
        Make up as much as 40% of intestinal mucosal cells
        Respond to MICA and MICB
            Similar to MHC-I
            Displayed on surface of infected cells
    Produce factors that turn off inflammation
    Produce growth factors—aid repair of epithelial cells
    GALT may serve as entryway for some pathogens (stimulate M cells to take them up)

Development of specific responses

Requires 1 to 2 years for immune system to develop in infants

Initial protection acquired from maternal antibodies

Autoimmune disease

Occurs when bacterial antigens resemble human antigens; antibodies attack host antigens

Antibacterial defenses attack host cells

QUESTIONS

Answers to the questions can be found in Appendix 2.

1. Does the fact that sIgA does not activate complement make it less effective than IgG in preventing infection?

2. Explain how the structure of an antibody is designed to facilitate the functions of antibodies, e.g., why an antibody has at least two antigen-binding sites and why it has an Fc portion.

3. Why is a Th cell needed to mediate APC-initiated antibody production? Why don't the B cells bind directly to APCs?

4. Explain why direct antigen activation of cytotoxic T cells and B cells is more important than APC-initiated activation in subsequent encounters with a microbe. Why is the APC-initiated pathway needed at all?

5. There are many interactions between the nonspecific and specific defense systems. List as many of them as you can and explain how they work. Why are these interactions important? Are all of them beneficial?

7

Vaccination—
an Underappreciated
Component of the Modern
Medical Armamentarium

Vaccines—a Major Health Care Bargain

The Current Vaccine Situation

Vaccines are nontoxic antigens that are injected, ingested, or inhaled to induce a specific defense response without having to go through the disease process. A good vaccine can provide lifelong immunity to an infectious disease. Vaccines are not only much cheaper than diagnosis and treatment of infections after they have started, but they also reduce human suffering because they prevent disease from occurring in the first place. Finally, in cases where there is no effective therapy for an infection, vaccines are the only way to protect patients who are exposed to the causative agent. Vaccines are clearly a major health care bargain.

If vaccines are so important, why aren't there more of them? Many of the barriers to vaccine development are financial, legal, and political rather than scientific. In the market economies of the developed countries, there are few financial incentives to develop and produce vaccines, especially vaccines that would have their greatest impact in the developing world. Vaccines are not nearly as profitable as mind-altering drugs or heart medications, which have to be taken daily for long periods. In recent years, development and testing of vaccines have focused on diseases that are widespread and usually not serious, such as otitis media in children. Such vaccines are the ones most likely to be profitable. Of course, these vaccines may have wider effects. For example, the vaccine against otitis media, which is usually caused by *Streptococcus pneumoniae,* may also protect against bacterial pneumonia or meningitis caused by this same species. There is no point in lambasting the pharmaceutical industry for putting profit ahead of human health; they are for-profit companies that need to have a healthy bottom line to survive. Rather, the solution to the problem of stimulating vaccine development, especially vaccines that would be important mainly in the developing world, is to acknowledge that there are financial disincentives that limit enthusiasm for vaccine development in the private sector and to find ways of countering these disincentives.

There are also legal reasons for industry's lack of enthusiasm for vaccine development. There have been numerous lawsuits based on

101

alleged, rare side effects of vaccines. Such lawsuits can be quite expensive for companies, especially when they involve children. And juries may not appreciate the fact that many of the alleged side effects of vaccines are not supported by scientific studies. In 2000, a U.S. congressman became convinced that his grandchild was autistic because of a vaccine the child had received. It took over a year and a blue ribbon commission to prove there was no basis for the accusation. Such public allegations encourage parents of children with neurological problems to contemplate lawsuits.

There is no question that each new vaccine carries a risk that rare, serious side effects may occur. In an era when most people in developed countries have not experienced the horrors of an outbreak of smallpox, polio, whooping cough, or diphtheria, have not watched a child die of bacterial meningitis, or have not witnessed the anguish of a mother who gives birth to a malformed child because she contracted rubella during pregnancy, it is not surprising that most people do not appreciate the tremendous benefit vaccines confer. It is easy to take these benefits for granted and to focus instead on the rare side effects that are the inevitable cost of such benefits.

There is, however, a growing subset of the world's population that is rediscovering the enormous benefits vaccines can confer—those who suffer greatly from the absence of an effective vaccine. People whose relatives die of bacterial pneumonia or endocarditis, people whose children are dying of malaria or diarrheal disease, people infected with HIV, and people at risk from drug-resistant tuberculosis are examples of groups who look longingly at the miracles performed by such successful vaccines as the polio vaccine and the smallpox vaccine. If a vaccine became available tomorrow that prevented any of these current disease problems, even if it had common and sometimes serious side effects, people who are at risk would line up to be vaccinated because they have done the risk-benefit analysis and seen that the risk-benefit ratio is definitely in their favor. In the case of diseases that progress slowly, such as tuberculosis and HIV (in at least some people), a vaccine might even effect a cure by eliciting a protective immune response and giving the body new powers to repel the microbial invader.

A continuing public relations problem is making people aware of past dangers so that they are willing to accept the tiny risk of preventing the return of those terrible times. During the 1990s, the CDC produced a series of advertisements that attempted to do just this. In one, a child is shown riding a tricycle along the shoulder of a major superhighway with trucks and cars whizzing by. A voice in the background likens this situation to failing to vaccinate a child in a timely manner. In another ad, a baby is shown lying perilously close to the edge of a steep cliff, with large waves crashing against the rocks below and no protecting adult in sight. Apparently, this campaign was terminated early because of a negative response on the part of viewers, but anyone who has seen the photographs from the 1940s and 1950s of hundreds of children confined to iron lungs or of children with deformed legs moving haltingly on crutches—all victims of polio, a disease that is now being eradicated thanks to an effective vaccine—will appreciate that the media images were not too far from reality.

One of the authors of this book remembers seeing in a Paris museum a small but poignant sculpture of a woman with her hands raised in prayer over an infant in a crib. The title was "Woman praying for the life of a child stricken with cholera." In the developing world today, many infants still die of diarrheal diseases caused by a variety of bacteria and viruses, diseases that might be prevented by vaccines. The economists would be quick to point out that cleaning up the water and food supply would be an even more effective preventive measure. This is true, if governments could be convinced to invest in these important public health measures rather than investing in expensive arms procurement programs.

But even if a country decided to invest in sanitation programs, the safety net would take long enough to develop that children would be at risk for many years to come; it takes time for an entire country to be brought into compliance with rigorous sanitation standards. Even in rich countries such as the United States, which has a state-of–the-art water and food supply protection system, there have been large failures of sanitation. So vaccines have an important role to play as countries struggle to protect their populations against waterborne and food-borne infections. Vaccines play an even bigger role in countries whose leaders seem not to be interested in improving the quality of food and water for the majority of citizens.

Perhaps the greatest moral failure of the 20th century is not widespread drug abuse or the hundreds of civil wars that have reduced countries to penury, but the abandonment of the developing countries by the developed countries that have the money to invest in vaccine development. In developing countries, acute respiratory disease, diarrheal disease, tuberculosis, malaria, and HIV loom as the major causes of death. Of these, only HIV, and more recently tuberculosis, have received much funding for vaccine development. Oddly enough, a vaccine to prevent HIV infection, a relatively new disease, is farther along the development path than an effective vaccine against tuberculosis, a much older danger to human health.

There are also formidable technical barriers to development of vaccines against some of the diseases considered most important today: AIDS, malaria, gonorrhea, tuberculosis, and pneumonia. To understand some of the technical problems that have frustrated development of vaccines against these infectious diseases, it is first useful to understand how successful vaccines work, because the successful vaccines illustrate traits of infectious microorganisms that make them amenable to development of a vaccine. Microorganisms that do not have these traits pose a much greater vaccine challenge. It is also encouraging to recall that, despite the poor showing in recent years, there have been some highly effective vaccines developed in the past.

A New Form of Child Abuse (as if We Needed One)

Not everyone is equally enthusiastic about vaccines, and there is a small but vocal group of individuals who are refusing to have their children vaccinated. Moreover, antivaccination activists are now working to make refusal of vaccinations possible for people who cannot claim religious grounds for their objections. Why would parents willingly expose their children to such horrible diseases as diphtheria and whooping cough, which used to kill many thousands of children? Not because these diseases have disappeared. If you need to be convinced that these diseases are still around, consider the "involunteer experiment" done in the United Kingdom during the 1980s. In response to sensational and highly inaccurate news accounts of alleged serious side effects of the vaccine against whooping cough, parents of young children began to refuse to have them vaccinated. This vaccine is the "P" (for pertussis) part of the DTP vaccine routinely administered to infants and toddlers. Parents demanded—and their children received—a DT formulation that lacked the pertussis vaccine. The effects of this miscalculation were tragic but unfortunately entirely predictable. An epidemic of whooping cough occurred in the United Kingdom, in which 100,000 children were infected and 36 died. Those children who survived went through a horrible experience. The disease produces a cough so violent and repetitive that the child has a sense of suffocating. Permanent brain damage occurred in some of those who survived.

Given this, why would any parent refuse to have a child vaccinated? Most of these parents are well intentioned and believe allegations that vaccines cause all manner of evils, in particular, neurological damage. The reason for this association is easy to understand. Most neurological problems in children appear in the first few years of life, the time when virtually all children in developed countries are receiving their vaccinations. But, as we stressed *ad tedium* in chapter 2, association is not proof of cause and effect. In particular, in cases where over 80% of the population receives a particular treatment, that treatment will be associated with everything. As for the argument that there are fewer cases of neurological disorders in developing countries where vaccinations are not available, the sad fact is that most children in such countries who develop neurological problems do not live long enough to be counted.

The degree of misinformation that has characterized arguments advanced by the antivaccination activists is best illustrated by the actions of the 1994 Miss America, the first Miss America to have a disability—deafness. Miss America told reporters that she was deaf because she received the DTP vaccine as a child and suffered neurological damage in the form of hearing loss as a consequence. Finally, her pediatrician came forward to explain that her deafness was actually the result of a case of meningitis caused by the bacterium *Haemophilus influenzae* type b, which used to be a common cause of childhood meningitis. Those children who survive childhood meningitis frequently suffer such disabilities as deafness and blindness. Why is childhood meningitis much less common today, especially cases caused by *H. influenzae* b? You guessed it—the introduction of a successful new anti-*H. influenzae* b vaccine! So the 1994 Miss America, under the impression that she was saving children from what she had suffered, was actually putting more children at risk for developing her disability.

In an attempt to introduce some medical rationality into the debate over vaccine safety, the Institute of Medicine, an independent research agency sponsored by the National Academy of Sciences, undertook a painstaking review of the alleged side effects of vaccines in 1994. Their conclusions, which are summarized in Table 7–1, were that there is little or no evidence for most of the alleged side effects of vaccines and, where there might be a connection, the side effects are rare and mostly not of the most serious type. The benefit figures, which are almost never included in sensational press articles about vaccines, are impressive. For vaccines administered in the United States, the reduction in incidence of the targeted disease has been at least 96%, and in most cases 99% or higher. Reductions of nearly 100% in the case of diseases such as polio have made it possible to attempt to eradicate the disease. This has already been accomplished with smallpox, and if it were not for the bioterrorists eyeing the few remaining stocks of smallpox virus in scientists' freezers, we could safely forget smallpox, a disease that killed millions of people in

Table 7–1   Summary of conclusions based on evidence regarding the possible association between specific adverse effects and receipt of childhood vaccines, by determination of causality—Institute of Medicine, 1994[a]

DT/Td/tetanus toxoid[b]	Measles vaccine[c]	Mumps vaccine[c]	OPV/IPV[d]	Hepatitis B vaccine	*Haemophilus influenzae* type b (Hib) vaccine
1. No evidence was available to establish a causal relationship					
None	None	Neuropathy Residual seizure disorder	Transverse myelitis (IPV) Thrombocytopenia (IPV) Anaphylaxis (IPV)	None	None
2. Inadequate evidence to accept or reject a causal relationship					
Residual seizure disorder other than infantile spasms Demyelinating diseases of the central nervous system Mononeuropathy Arthritis Erythema multiforme	Encephalopathy Subacute sclerosing panencephalitis Residual seizure disorder Sensorineural deafness (MMR) Optic neuritis Transverse myelitis Guillain-Barré syndrome Thrombocytopenia Insulin-dependent diabetes mellitus	Encephalopathy Aseptic meningitis Sensorineural deafness (MMR) Insulin-dependent diabetes mellitus Sterility Thrombocytopenia Anaphylaxis[e]	Transverse myelitis (OPV) Guillain-Barré syndrome (IPV) Death from SIDS[f]	Guillain-Barré syndrome Demyelinating diseases of the central nervous system Arthritis Death from SIDS[f]	Guillain-Barré syndrome Transverse myelitis Thrombocytopenia Anaphylaxis Death from SIDS[f]
3. Evidence favored rejection of a causal relationship					
Encephalopathy[g] Infantile spasms (DT only)[h] Death from SIDS (DT only)[h,i]	None	None	None	None	Early-onset Hib disease (conjugate vaccines)
4. Evidence favored acceptance of a causal relationship					
Guillain-Barré syndrome[j,k] Brachial neuritis[j]	Anaphylaxis[e]	None	Guillain-Barré syndrome (OPV)[k]	None	Early-onset Hib disease in children ages ≥ 18 mos whose first Hib vaccination was with unconjugated vaccine

(continued)

Europe and wiped out whole populations of Native Americans.

Those who refuse to have their children vaccinated are—quite consciously, in some cases—taking advantage of a phenomenon known as the **herd effect.** The herd effect arises from the fact that an unvaccinated person in a population that is mostly vaccinated will be protected from disease because there are not enough susceptible people in this population to allow an infectious disease outbreak to materialize. There is a serious defect in this reasoning, however, given the increase in international travel due to the globalization of the economy. Children who have not been immunized against viral diseases such as measles and mumps, for example, and who have been protected from measles and mumps during childhood years because of the herd effect, would be ill advised to travel during their adult years to areas of the world where measles or mumps is endemic. For reasons that are still not well understood, these diseases have a much more serious effect if they

Table 7–1 Summary of conclusions based on evidence regarding the possible association between specific adverse effects and receipt of childhood vaccines, by determination of causality—Institute of Medicine, 1994[a] (*continued*)

DT/Td/tetanus toxoid[b]	Measles vaccine[c]	Mumps vaccine[c]	OPV/IPV[d]	Hepatitis B vaccine	*Haemophilus influenzae* type b (Hib) vaccine
5. Evidence established a causal relationship					
Anaphylaxis[j]	Thrombocytopenia (MMR)	None	Poliomyelitis in recipient or contact (OPV)	Anaphylaxis	None
	Anaphylaxis (MMR)[e]				
	Death from measles-vaccine–strain viral infection[f,l]		Death from polio-vaccine–strain viral infection[f,l]		

[a] Reprinted from CDC. 1996. Update: vaccine side effects, adverse reactions, contraindications, and precautions—recommendations of the Advisory Committee on Immunization Practices (ACIP). *Morb. Mortal. Wkly. Rep.* **45**(RR-12):1–35. This table is an adaptation of a table published previously by the Institute of Medicine (IOM) (K.R. Stratton, C.J. Howe, and R.B. Johnston [ed.]. 1994. *Adverse Events Associated with Childhood Vaccines: Evidence Bearing on Causality*. Institute of Medicine, National Academy Press, Washington, D.C.). IOM is an independent research organization chartered by the National Academy of Sciences. The National Childhood Vaccine Injury Act of 1986 mandated that IOM review scientific and other evidence (e.g., epidemiologic studies, case series, individual case reports, and testimonials) regarding the possible adverse consequences of vaccines administered to children. IOM constituted an expert committee to review and summarize all available information; this committee created five categories of causality to describe the relationships between vaccines and specific adverse events.

[b] DT, diphtheria and tetanus toxids for pediatric use; Td, diphtheria and tetanus toxoids for adult use.

[c] If the data derived from studies of a monovalent preparation, then the causal relationship also extended to multivalent preparations. If the data derived exclusively from studies of the measles-mumps-rubella (MMR) vaccine, the vaccine is specified parenthetically. In the absence of data concerning the monovalent preparation, the causal relationship determined for the multivalent preparations did not extend to the monovalent components.

[d] For some adverse events, the IOM committee was charged with assessing the causal relationship between the adverse event and only oral poliovirus vaccine (OPV) (i.e., for poliomyelitis) or only inactivated poliovirus vaccine (IPV) (i.e., for anaphylaxis and thrombocytopenia). If the conclusions for the two vaccines differed for the other adverse events, the vaccine to which the adverse event applied is specified parenthetically.

[e] The evidence used to establish a causal relationship for anaphylaxis applies to MMR vaccine. The evidence regarding monovalent measles vaccine favored acceptance of a causal relationship, but this evidence was less convincing than that for MMR vaccine because of either incomplete documentation of symptoms or the possible attenuation of symptoms by medical intervention.

[f] This table lists weight-of-evidence determinations only for deaths that were classified as sudden infant death syndrome (SIDS) and deaths that were a consequence of vaccine-strain viral infection. However, if the evidence favored the acceptance of (or established) a casual relationship between the vaccine and a possibly fatal adverse event, then the evidence also favored the acceptance of (or established) a causal relationship between the vaccine and death from the adverse event. Direct evidence regarding death in association with a vaccine-associated adverse event was limited to (a) Td and Guillain-Barré syndrome, (b) tetanus toxoid and anaphylaxis, and (c) OPV and poliomyelitis.

[g] The evidence derived from studies of DT. If the evidence favored rejection of a causal relationship between DT and encephalopathy, then the evidence also favored rejection of a causal relationship between Td and tetanus toxoid and encephalopathy.

[h] Infantile spasms and SIDS occur only in an age group that is administered DT but not Td or tetanus toxoid.

[i] The evidence derived primarily from studies of DTP, although the evidence also favored rejection of a causal relationship between DT and SIDS.

[j] The evidence derived from studies of tetanus toxoid. If the evidence favored acceptance of (or established) a causal relationship between tetanus toxoid and an adverse event, then the evidence also favored acceptance of (or established) a causal relationship between DT and Td and the adverse event.

[k] This conclusion differs from the information contained in the Advisory Committee on Immunization Practices recommendations because of new information that became available after IOM published this table.

[l] Deaths occurred primarily among persons known to be immunocompromised.

strike teens or young adults than if they occur in children. Parents who refuse to have their children vaccinated are setting them up for a dangerous future.

The Success Stories

Some of the vaccine success stories are summarized in Tables 7–2 and 7–3. For a very different but heartening example of a vaccine success story, see Box 7–1.

The successful antibacterial vaccines listed in Table 7–3 are administered routinely to all children in the population in developed countries. A vaccine that illustrates some features associated with vaccines that are highly effective and have few side effects is the trivalent vaccine **DTaP.** The "D" and "T" in DTaP are detoxified

forms of bacterial toxins (**toxoids**). Vaccines like D and T, which consist of one or a few purified proteins, are called **subunit vaccines.** Because they are soluble, they elicit an antibody response rather than a cell-mediated response. This is effective in the case of diphtheria and tetanus because toxins circulating in the bloodstream, not invasive infection, cause the symptoms of these diseases. In both diseases, bacteria grow in a localized site of the body (throat in the case of diphtheria, wound in the case of tetanus). The protein toxin released by the bacteria enters the bloodstream and damages essential organs. Vaccination with DT elicits an antibody response that neutralizes diphtheria and tetanus toxins. Thus, even if the bacteria that cause diphtheria and tetanus repeatedly colonize a person, no symptoms will develop because an immediate antibody response neu-

Table 7–2 Baseline 20th century annual morbidity (cases of disease) before the vaccine became available and 1998 morbidity from nine diseases with vaccines recommended before 1990 for universal use in children[a]

Disease	Baseline 20th century annual morbidity	1998 morbidity	% Decrease
Smallpox	48,164[b]	0	100
Diphtheria	175,885[c]	1	100[d]
Pertussis	147,271[e]	6,279	95.7
Tetanus	1,314[f]	34	97.4
Poliomyelitis (paralytic)	16,316[g]	0[h]	100
Measles	503,282[i]	89	100
Mumps	152,209[j]	606	99.6
Rubella	47,745[k]	345	99.3
Congenital rubella syndrome	823[l]	5	99.4
Haemophilus influenzae type b	20,000[m]	54[n]	99.7

[a] Reprinted from *Morb. Mortal. Wkly. Rep.* **48:**243–247, 1999.

[b] Average annual number of cases during 1900–1904.

[c] Average annual number of reported cases during 1920–1922, 3 years before vaccine development.

[d] Rounded to nearest tenth.

[e] Average annual number of reported cases during 1922–1925, 4 years before vaccine development.

[f] Estimated number of cases based on reported number of deaths during 1922–1926, assuming a case-fatality rate of 90%.

[g] Average annual number of reported cases during 1951–1954, 4 years before vaccine licensure.

[h] Excludes one case of vaccine-associated polio reported in 1998.

[i] Average annual number of reported cases during 1958–1962, 5 years before vaccine licensure.

[j] Number of reported cases in 1968, the first year reporting began and the first year after vaccine licensure.

[k] Average annual number of reported cases during 1966–1968, 3 years before vaccine licensure.

[l] Estimated number of cases based on seroprevalence date in the population and on the risk that women infected during a childbearing year would have a fetus with congenital rubella syndrome.

[m] Estimated number of cases from population-based surveillance studies before vaccine licensure in 1985.

[n] Excludes 71 cases of *Haemophilus influenzae* disease of unknown serotype.

tralizes circulating toxin. Although the vaccine regimen produces long-term immunity to diphtheria and tetanus, a tetanus booster is usually administered to persons with the sort of wounds that are associated with tetanus, to make sure that antibody levels are high enough to be protective. Bacteria that produce toxins, which circulate in blood and are responsible for causing the symptoms of the disease, are among the easiest vaccine targets.

The DTaP vaccine has to be administered in five separate injections. This example illustrates a common problem with subunit vaccines. Prolonged exposure to antigens is needed to generate a good memory T and B cell response. Since subunit vaccine components do not replicate in the body, they must be administered repeatedly to elicit a maximally effective memory response. A solution to this problem, which is currently under study, is to have the vaccine proteins produced by a microbe that is cleared from the body after a few rounds of division or to encapsulate vaccine proteins so that they are released slowly over a period of time (see later section).

Diphtheria and tetanus toxoids have virtually no side effects. This was not true of the "P" part of the old DTP vaccine. The old form of the P vaccine consisted of whole killed *Bordetella pertussis* cells. The pertussis vaccine has been very successful in preventing whooping cough, a disease that was once a common killer of children, but it has some troublesome side effects. In about 20% of infants given the old form of P, side effects range from generalized discomfort, which makes the infant fussy for a couple of days, to convulsions. The pertussis vaccine may also cause hearing loss or irreversible brain damage in some children, although this side effect is extremely rare. The reason the pertussis vaccine has so many side effects compared to diphtheria and tetanus toxoids is that it consists of whole killed bacteria and is thus a complex mixture of components, some of which (e.g., LPS) are toxic.

There are now some new, more defined versions of the pertussis vaccine. These vaccines usually consist of a toxoid form of a toxin produced by *B. pertussis*, **pertussis toxin,** plus a **surface adhesin** of *B. pertussis*. The new subunit vaccines are called **acellular pertussis vaccines (aPs)** to distinguish them from the old whole-cell vaccine. The aP vaccines have fewer side effects than the P vaccine, although they still have more side effects than diphtheria and tetanus toxoids. The pertussis vaccine story illustrates the general principle that the simplest vaccines, which consist of only one or a few well-defined antigens, are the ones least likely to cause side effects. Also, at least in theory, the simple vaccines should make it easier to target the desirable type of immune response. As already mentioned in the case of DT, subunit vaccines, being soluble antigens, elicit an antibody response rather than a cell-mediated response. Whooping cough is a more invasive disease than tetanus or diphtheria because the bacteria invade and replicate in the airway. Since *B. pertussis* replicates extracellularly, at least in the early stages of the infection, antibodies that neutralize the toxin and opsonize the bacteria are sufficient to control the infection. A cell-

Table 7–3   Antibacterial vaccines administered to all children in the United States

Component name	Composition	Disease prevented	Administration
D	Diphtheria toxoid	Diphtheria	Injected as part of DTP or DTaP
T	Tetanus toxoid	Tetanus	Trivalent vaccine
P	Whole killed bacteria (*Bordetella pertussis*)	Whooping cough	
aP	Pertussis toxoid, adhesin proteins (acellular vaccine)	Whooping cough	
Hib	Polysaccharide-protein (conjugated vaccine) (*Haemophilus influenzae* type b)	Infant and childhood meningitis	Injected
PCV	Conjugated vaccine containing polysaccharide capsules from seven types of *Streptococcus pneumoniae* linked to protein	Otitis media (perhaps meningitis, pneumonia)	Injected

mediated response is not essential in this case, as it would be if the bacteria multiplied intracellularly.

From the foregoing description, it might appear that subunit vaccines like D, T, and aP consist solely of the purified protein antigens. Although proteins given alone can produce an immune response, they work much better if they are given in conjunction with an adjuvant. **Adjuvants** are compounds that aid antigens to stimulate the immune response. They appear to work by trapping the antigens in complexes, from which the antigen is released fairly slowly, thus prolonging exposure to the antigen. In the case of peptide vaccines, adjuvants are essential to elicit an immune response because peptides given alone not only do not elicit an immune response but can actually cause the body to ignore the epitope (**anergy**). The only adjuvant currently licensed for use in the United States is **alum,** an aluminum salt. Other adjuvants are currently under development. A particularly interesting type of adjuvant, which may solve the problem of having to administer DTaP so many times, is **microspheres** made of resorbable suture material or some other inert substance that gradually breaks down in the body. The proteins are encapsulated in the adjuvant material and are thus released slowly over a period of time. By administering a mixture of microspheres of differing sizes, it is hoped that the vaccine will be released over a long enough period that a memory response will be elicited with only one or two injections. Another strategy is to use molecular techniques to make a live, avirulent bacterial vaccine strain that produces the protein antigen (or portions of it) on its surface.

Another powerful adjuvant comes from an unexpected source: the bacterium that causes cholera (*Vibrio cholerae*). As you will see in a later chapter, *V. cholerae* causes a massive dehydrating watery diarrhea because

it produces a toxic protein complex called cholera toxin. For reasons that are still not completely apparent, cholera toxin is a very effective stimulator of the antibody-specific immune response. Don't worry, we are not asking you to ingest large doses of cholera toxin. Instead, cholera toxin is being used experimentally to stimulate immune responses to vaccines administered through the skin. There is currently a lot of interest in how to create vaccines that do not require needle injections but can be administered intranasally or by skin patches (via tiny prongs that do not penetrate far enough to cause pain). Cholera toxin appears to stimulate immune responses to various antigens by the skin-associated lymphoid system. This response is often accompanied by a general mucosal immune response, a very desirable feature. And since your skin cannot develop cholera, cholera toxin used in this way as an adjuvant should be completely safe.

Another successful antibacterial vaccine is the one that protects against childhood meningitis caused by the gram-negative bacterium *H. influenzae* b (hence the vaccine name, **Hib**). *H. influenzae* b used to be the most common cause of meningitis in children and also caused epiglottitis, a rare but rapidly progressing disease that can close the airway and lead to suffocation. *H. influenzae* b also causes pneumonia, particularly in the elderly. Unlike the bacteria that cause diphtheria, tetanus, and whooping cough, *H. influenzae* does not produce a protein toxin. Instead, *H. influenzae* coats its surface with a **polysaccharide capsule** that discourages C3b binding and thus allows the bacteria to avoid ingestion by phagocytes. Uncontrolled growth of the bacteria triggers an inflammatory response, which is the cause of local tissue damage and can develop into septic shock. Inflammation of the lining that separates the brain and spinal cord from the rest of the body (menin-

BOX 7–1   A Touching Memorial

India, a country beset by as many countervailing pressures and episodes of civil strife as any other developing country, has, nonetheless, provided an inspirational example of how such a country can choose saving children over revenge. In 1984, Indira Gandhi, the prime minister of India, was assassinated by religious extremists, whose party opposed some of Gandhi's decisions on autonomy of Moslem-dominated regions. Her son, Rajiv Gandhi, succeeded his mother as prime minister. He could have launched a holy war against his mother's assassins as revenge for her death, an action that might well have sunk India into a Hindu-Moslem civil war that would have decimated parts of India as similar wars of interethnic vengeance have devastated Africa and the former Yugoslavia. But Rajiv Gandhi chose to memorialize his assassinated mother in a very different way: by stepping up efforts to immunize the children of India against polio. Polio is still very much alive in the developing world and not only deprives children of the power to walk but can deprive them of life itself. It took over 10 years for this effort to be organized, but in 1996, during a 2-day period, 121 million Indian children were given the polio vaccine. This was an incredible accomplishment in a country whose poverty is notorious worldwide.

Source: B. R. Bloom and R. Widdus. 1998. Vaccine visions and their global impact. *Nat. Med.* 4:480–484.

ges) allows the bacteria and blood components to enter spinal fluid, where the cytokines released by macrophages and other cells cause increased pressure on the brain that can lead to brain damage. Antibodies that bind to capsular polysaccharides allow phagocytes to ingest and kill the bacteria while they are still in the bloodstream and thus prevent this destructive (and frequently fatal) infection process from getting under way. Since *H. influenzae* causes meningitis primarily in children under the age of 5 years, it is necessary to immunize infants as early as possible. The problem is that infants are not able to mount a T-independent antibody response to polysaccharides. Accordingly, the *H. influenzae* b capsular polysaccharide antigens were attached covalently to a protein to produce a **conjugate vaccine.** A carbohydrate linked to a protein generates a T-cell-dependent response just like a protein. This vaccine has been highly effective and has already dramatically reduced the incidence of the type of meningitis caused by *H. influenzae.* An even newer conjugate vaccine is the vaccine against the seven types of *S. pneumoniae* that cause earache in children (Table 7–3).

To afford protection when it is most needed, a vaccine must be administered in a timely manner (Figure 7–1). For example, since meningitis due to *H. influenzae* can strike very young infants, these vaccines must be administered as early as possible. The fact that subunit vaccines must be administered several times creates a potential public health problem because it increases the likelihood that a child will not receive the full set of vaccinations in time to be adequately protected. The problem of children who do not receive the full recommended course of vaccine administration is still a formidable one even in developed countries (Box 7–2).

The Less-than-Success Stories

Not all vaccines are successful. Vaccines fail for three reasons. One is failure to elicit the anticipated protective response. Three of the great vaccine disappointments of the late 20th century have been the failure to develop effective vaccines against the bacterial diseases salmonellosis, cholera, and tuberculosis. Despite major advances in our understanding of how the bacteria that cause these diseases interact with the human body, there must still be important missing pieces in the picture because numerous candidate vaccines have failed in clinical trials to protect vaccinated people against the disease. Unsuccessful attempts to develop vaccines effective against HIV infection and malaria can be added to this list. Here too, it is frustrating and perplexing to note that the expenditure of huge amounts of money and the involvement of hundreds of scientists have not produced a better outcome. What these examples show is that throwing money at a problem does not always lead to a solution and that a high degree of scientific sophistication does not ensure success in developing successful prevention strategies. Clearly, scientists still have a lot to learn about the host-parasite interaction.

In some cases, the lack of efficacy is understandable. For example, the bacterium that causes gonorrhea is constantly changing the amino acid composition of its surface proteins, the ones targeted by opsonizing antibodies. This antigenic variability makes it very difficult to elicit the type of immunological response that will clear the bacteria from an infected person. Similarly, HIV not only enters cells from the outside but can

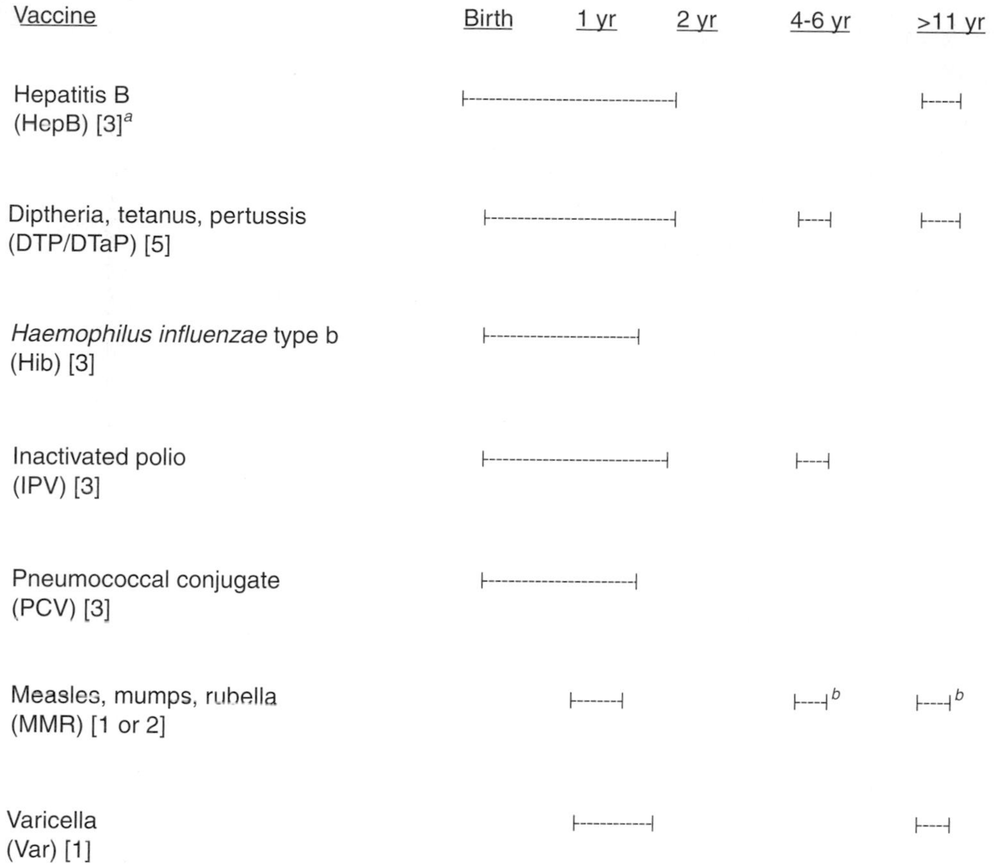

Vaccine	Birth	1 yr	2 yr	4-6 yr	>11 yr
Hepatitis B (HepB) [3][a]	├----------------------------┤				├----┤
Diptheria, tetanus, pertussis (DTP/DTaP) [5]	├----------------------------┤			├---┤	├----┤
Haemophilus influenzae type b (Hib) [3]	├--------------------┤				
Inactivated polio (IPV) [3]	├------------------------┤			├--┤	
Pneumococcal conjugate (PCV) [3]	├-------------------┤				
Measles, mumps, rubella (MMR) [1 or 2]		├------┤		├---┤[b]	├---┤[b]
Varicella (Var) [1]		├---------┤			├--┤

[a] Number of times vaccine must be given for maximal effectiveness.

[b] Vaccine must be given at entry into grade school or entry into middle (or high) school, not both.

Figure 7–1 Timing of childhood vaccinations. The bars represent the optimal time range for administering vaccines and illustrate the complexity of the vaccination program for a child. The recommendations are adjusted each year to reflect new or improved vaccines.

move from cell to cell, a mode of spread that protects it from antibodies.

A second reason for vaccine failure is side effects. This was the downfall of a vaccine against a common type of infant diarrhea caused by rotavirus. The vaccine was very effective in preventing infant diarrhea caused by rotaviruses, but a few infants developed an intestinal blockage, a side effect that caused the vaccine to be abruptly withdrawn from use. In developed countries, rotavirus diarrhea can be treated effectively by replacing fluids lost during the diarrhea period. Thus, in this case, the protection afforded by the vaccine was not sufficient to justify the risk. In developing countries, where emergency medical treatment is much more limited in availability, parents may find the vaccine more appealing than parents in developed countries because the infant death rate due to diarrheal disease is so much higher.

A third reason for vaccine failure is that the vaccine unexpectedly makes the disease worse. This is unarguably the worst nightmare for those who work long hours to develop a vaccine. The classic example of this type of vaccine failure was the respiratory syncytial virus vaccine. Respiratory syncytial virus attacks infants in their first months of life and is a major cause of hospital admissions of infants under the age of 3 months. A vaccine that showed promising results in animals was administered to infants in the early stages of clinical trials. These trials were abandoned abruptly when it became apparent that vaccinated infants were getting a more severe form of respiratory disease than unvaccinated infants. Why this happened is still not clear, but this example is another indication of how little scientists understand about the immune response despite major breakthroughs in this area. More recently, testing of a very promising vaccine against strains of *Chlamydia tra-*

BOX 7–2 Having an Effective Vaccine Is Not Enough: Missed Opportunities for Vaccination

In developed countries, the delivery of vaccines to the general public has been relatively effective. In the early 1990s, U.S. public health workers were not satisfied with the level of coverage. They established an official goal for 1996—to vaccinate at least 90% of all young children with DTP, measles-mumps-rubella vaccine (MMR), polio vaccine, and Hib, and at least 70% with HBV. A study of 1999 vaccination levels in the United States showed that among families surveyed, more than 90% of children had received the recommended number of DTP, polio vaccine, Hib, and MMR administrations by the recommended age, and 88% had received HBV vaccinations in a timely fashion. While many states have exceeded the goals, there is great state-to-state variation, thus bringing the overall U.S. vaccine coverage rate down to only 78%, which is worrisome (data from CDC, *Morb. Mortal. Wkly. Rep.* **49:**585–587, 2000).

One strategy to increase the percentage of children vaccinated is to require that vaccinations be completed before a child enters elementary school. This is not satisfactory, however, because infants and young children are the ones at highest risk for the severe form of many of these diseases. The 1999 study of vaccination levels also revealed that the percent coverage was even worse among low-income urban populations than among other populations. The study also revealed that many of the children who had not been vaccinated could have been vaccinated in a timely manner, because they had passed through the health care system as infants and young children.

Why were these opportunities missed? For one thing, not all health care providers routinely checked the vaccination status of all young patients during each visit. This was especially true when the child was brought in for treatment of an illness rather than for a routine checkup. For another thing, many health care providers seemed to think that illness precludes vaccination. There are some contraindications, but most childhood illnesses, particularly mild ones, do not preclude vaccination. Finally, health care providers did not take advantage of the fact that the vaccines listed in Table 7–3 can be administered simultaneously. Several recommendations were made to reduce these missed opportunities and to help reach the 1996 goal:

1. Accurate vaccination records should be maintained and should be easily accessible to health care providers.
2. Vaccination status should be checked for every infant and young child during every visit to a health care provider.
3. Health care providers should be made aware that mild illness does not preclude vaccination.
4. Needed vaccines should be administered simultaneously.

Once the problem of undervaccination was recognized, the CDC launched an advertising campaign to alert parents and physicians to the problem. Despite this campaign, which definitely helped raise public awareness, reports continue to come in of undervaccination of certain populations (T. A. Kenyon et al., *Pediatrics* **101:**612–616, 1998). Further investigations of the reason for the continued undervaccination rate in certain settings revealed that since physicians were not reimbursed adequately for vaccinations, even with the vaccine being provided free, they were routinely referring parents to vaccination clinics, thus necessitating another clinic visit and another wait in line. Even parents who are devoted to their children have limits—especially when they see the pediatrician acting as if vaccination were low on the scale of things to worry about.

chomatis, a bacterial pathogen that causes blindness (trachoma) in certain areas of the developing world, had to be stopped because the vaccine made the eye infections in vaccinated children worse than those in unvaccinated children.

Working on vaccine development takes the kind of courage exhibited by the earlier microbiologists who walked bravely into cholera epidemics or, in more recent times, volunteered to study HIV and multidrug-resistant tuberculosis strains. In the case of vaccine development, however, a special sort of courage is needed—the courage to face not only the possible failure of a vaccine to protect but also the possibility that it could make the disease worse. Just as the earlier discoveries that vaccination could protect people from such a devastating infectious disease as smallpox revolutionized preventive medicine, future discoveries that explain why some vaccines cause side effects or even make the symptoms of a disease worse will revolutionize vaccine development and provide a safer and surer source of new vaccines in the future.

New Directions

Fortunately, it is not necessary to end this chapter on a depressing note. Not only are there a lot of past successes to admire, but there are some new developments that are very exciting. One such development is rather pedestrian in the sense that it applies to vaccine administration, but it is an advance that will be hailed as revolutionary by physicians, parents, and children alike: the shot-free vaccination. Children, like adults, do not take kindly to being stuck with a needle. Production of a syringe by the doctor or nurse is guaranteed to raise howls of indignation and terror. The words "this won't hurt a bit" rank right up there with "the check is in the mail" in the list of definitely-not-to-be-believed statements.

Three recent developments may signal the end of the dreaded syringe. One is **nasal inoculation** of the vaccine. Nasal inoculation activates bronchial-associated lymphoid tissue, the respiratory tract equivalent of the intestinal GALT. At present, nasal inoculation with an influenza virus vaccine is being tested as a replacement for the odious shots. Stay tuned for new developments in the rapidly evolving alternative delivery field. A second development is a **patch** containing many tiny prongs. The patch is applied to the skin surface, but the prongs do not penetrate far enough to encounter the epidermal neurons, so application of the patch is completely painless.

Still another interesting development is **edible vaccines.** The ability to genetically engineer plants has made it possible to produce plants that synthesize vaccine proteins. Thus, vaccination can occur by the simple act of ingesting the plant. Currently, the edible vaccines are being produced in potato—a plant with a highly developed system for genetic manipulation. Unfortunately, most people do not rush to consume raw potatoes, and converting them into French fries may impair the efficacy of the vaccine proteins. Another easily genetically manipulatable plant, tobacco, has been passed over for obvious reasons. Banana, the plant of choice for most vaccinologists, is not so readily genetically manipulatable. In a situation of this sort, the standard procedure is to go ahead with trials of the imperfect vehicle, potato, to see if it works—a strategy called proof of principle. If the edible vaccine approach continues to look promising, more research funding will flow into genetic engineering of banana as a vehicle of edible vaccines. A major advantage of using the banana as a vehicle is that even very young children can eat raw bananas, and bananas are already fed to small children in many parts of the world.

In the foregoing text, all of the vaccines mentioned have contained either protein antigens or conjugated carbohydrate-protein antigens. A completely different approach to vaccination that has received a lot of attention recently is to inject DNA that encodes a vaccine protein into human muscle cells. These vaccines are called **naked DNA vaccines.** The DNA is first adsorbed to gold particles and injected with an air gun into muscle tissue. Incredibly enough, this results in transient production and display by the muscle cells of foreign antigens. Display of the foreign antigen lasts only a month or two, but this is long enough to evoke a robust response. Because the display is localized, side effects associated with an immune attack on the body's own cells are minimized. Also, the DNA is in differentiated cells, not in the germ line, so it will not be passed to subsequent progeny. So far, this approach has been tested mainly in animals, but the results have caused considerable excitement and human trials are already under way. This approach, if successful, would have two important advantages. First, unlike live vaccines, DNA on gold particles can be stored dry and need not be refrigerated. Second, pure DNA is much less expensive to prepare than pure protein.

Just as DNA vaccines appeared to be ready to revolutionize vaccination procedures, some troubling second thoughts began to be expressed. These second thoughts centered on a rediscovery of an old wheel: DNA is immunostimulatory. Scientists working on lupus have long suspected that this autoimmune disease is caused by the body's immune reaction to its own DNA. Articles have begun to appear that question the safety of injecting DNA into human tissue. A couple of these are cited in the "Selected Readings" at the end of the chapter. Basically, the claim is that certain DNA sequence motifs, which are found in bacterial DNA, elicit an immune response that might lead in some people to an autoimmune response, which could in turn lead to an increase in such diseases as lupus. If these concerns prove to be correct, an exciting approach to correcting human genetic disorders—gene therapy—could go down the tubes along with DNA vaccines.

A different type of vaccine problem, and one that at least in theory is more amenable to solution, is the problem of simplifying the current confusing mixture of separate inoculations of different vaccines at different times. It would help a lot to be able to administer several vaccines simultaneously in a single dose, preferably by the oral route or by inhalation, and to eliminate the need for so many booster shots. Using live viral or bacterial vaccine strains that produce antigens of more than one pathogen is a possible solution. More immediately, however, researchers are trying to determine whether DTaP, Hib, and the vaccine against hepatitis B virus (HBV) could be given in a single dose. At present, these vaccines can be administered during the same visit but are given by injection in different body sites. Orally administered forms of DTaP, Hib, and HBV are being developed, and work on administration of such vaccines by inhalation has begun. The ability to administer different vaccines in a single swallow or a single inhalation has obvious appeal.

Passive Immunization

People who have not been immunized against a particular disease can still be protected by injection of antibodies from another person or from an animal. This is called **passive immunization.** Antibodies injected into the bloodstream remain in circulation for as long as several months, apparently because antibodies are not readily degraded and excreted unless they are bound to an antigen. These antibodies opsonize bacteria or neutralize toxins and viruses just as antibodies produced by the person's own body would do. The benefits of passive immunization, unlike the benefits of vaccination (which has a memory phase) are of limited duration. Nonetheless, for an unvaccinated person with a serious condition that can be helped by antibodies, passive immunization can be a lifesaver. An example of the use of passive immunization is treatment of children who have diphtheria but have not been vaccinated—they are given antibodies that neutralize diphtheria toxin, the toxin that is responsible for the pathology of diphtheria. Passive immunization allows the child to survive the initial stages of the disease, which is self-limiting if it does not kill you. Tetanus provides another example of the power of passive vaccination. Here too, circulating toxin is responsible for the disease symptoms. Injection of antibodies that bind to and neutralize circulating tetanus toxin can save an unvaccinated person from a horrifying death. Still another example of passive immunization is the very effective use of gamma globulin (the antibody fraction of blood) to prevent hepatitis. So many people have been exposed to hepatitis A virus that a pooled fraction of serum will contain at least some antibodies that bind the hepatitis A virus and neutralize it.

Passive immunization has been receiving much more attention recently as physicians finally admit that major human killers of the preantibiotic era, such as *S. pneumoniae,* the most common cause of bacterial pneumonia, have become so resistant to antibiotics that patients infected with multidrug-resistant strains may soon not be treatable with antibiotics. Another treatment option is to provide antibodies that bind to the antiphagocytic capsule of this bacterium and thus de-

stroy its ability to evade the nonspecific host defenses. More and more often, passive immunization is being invoked as a possible clinical response to multidrug-resistant bacteria.

Passive immunization has also gained increased importance as the number of immunocompromised people has grown. These include not only people with HIV infections but also people undergoing cancer chemotherapy and organ transplant recipients. In these people, who are unable to mount an effective immune response, passive immunization may well prove to be the only option for helping them overcome life-threatening infections.

SELECTED READINGS

Albert, M. R., K. G. Ostheimer, and J. G. Breman. 2001. The last smallpox epidemic in Boston and the vaccination controversy, 1901–1903. *N. Engl. J. Med.* **344:**375–379.

Anonymous. 1998. Progress toward eliminating *Haemophilus influenzae* type b disease among infants and children—United States, 1987–1997. *Morb. Mortal. Wkly. Rep.* **47:**993–998.

Casadevall, A. 1998. Antibody-mediated protection against intracellular pathogens. *Trends Microbiol.* **6:**102–107.

Cohen, J. 1994. Bumps on the vaccine road. *Science* **265:**1371–1373.

Friedlander, E. R. 2001. Opposition to immunization: a pattern of deception. *Sci. Rev. Alt. Med.* **5:**18–23. (This article clearly presents the misinformation put out by antiimmunization groups and explains why it is incorrect.)

Glenn, G. M., M. Rao, G. R. Matyas, and C. R. Alving. 1998. Skin immunization made possible by cholera toxin. *Nature* **391:**851.

Krieg, A. M., A.-K. Yi, J. Schorr, and H. L. Davis. 1998. The role of CpG dinucleotides in DNA vaccines. *Trends Microbiol.* **6:**23–27.

Langerman, S., S. Palaszynski, A. Sadziene, C. K. Stover, and S. Koenig. 1994. Systemic and mucosal immunity induced by BCG vector expressing outer surface protein A of *Borrelia burgdorferi. Nature* **372:**552–555.

Leclerc, C., and J. Ronco. 1998. New approaches in vaccine development. *Immunol. Today* **19:**300–302.

Lipford, G. B., K. Heeg, and H. Wagner. 1998. Bacterial DNA as immune cell activator. *Trends Microbiol.* **6:**496–500.

Marwick, C. 1998. Vaccinologists aiming at less hurtful "shots." *JAMA* **280:**313.

Pisetsky, D. S. 1997. Immunostimulatory DNA: a clear and present danger? *Nat. Med.* **3:**829–830.

Robinson, H. L., H. S. Ginsberg, H. L. Davis, S. A. Johnston, and M. A. Liu. 1997. *The Scientific Future of DNA for Immunization.* Report of the American Academy of Microbiology. American Society for Microbiology, Washington, D.C.

Stephenson, J. 2000. Vaccines pose no diabetes, bowel disease risk. *JAMA* **284:**2307–2308.

Characteristics of vaccines

Antigens injected, ingested, or inhaled to induce specific defenses

Can provide lifelong immunity

Cheaper than treating disease

Prevent suffering and death

Successful vaccines

Smallpox eradicated by vaccine

DTP vaccine against diphtheria, pertussis, tetanus

    D and T are inactivated form of toxins (toxoids)—subunit vaccines

    D and T elicit only an antibody response—effective because toxins in circulation can be neutralized

    Must be administered repeatedly to generate memory cells

    P portion is whole killed cells

        May cause serious side effects

        New form is aP vaccine

            Consists of toxoid of pertussis toxin and surface adhesin of bacteria

            Fewer side effects than whole-cell vaccine

Hib vaccine

    Prevents meningitis caused by *H. influenzae* b

    Polysaccharide capsule antigens linked to protein to form conjugate vaccine

Adjuvants—stimulate immune response

Work by trapping antigens, releasing them slowly

New types encapsulate antigen, release over time—eliminate repeated injections

Alum only one licensed in United States

Cholera toxin may work via skin-associated lymphoid tissue

Time of administration of vaccines

Early for diseases that affect infants

Later for diseases that are prevented by maternal antibodies

Reasons vaccine fail

Do not elicit protective response—examples are salmonellosis, cholera, tuberculosis

Produce side effects—example is rotavirus vaccine that causes intestinal blockage

Make disease worse—examples are respiratory syncytial virus vaccine, *C. trachomatis* vaccine which makes eye infections worse

New directions

Edible, inhaled, or skin patch vaccines—eliminate shots

Naked DNA vaccines

    Injected into muscle cells

    Cause muscle cells to present desired antigen on surface

    Possible problem—DNA might cause autoimmune disease

Administer several vaccines at one time

(continued)

SUMMARY OUTLINE (*continued*)

Passive immunization

Injection of antibodies from another person or animal

Useful in several situations

Unvaccinated person with disease (e.g., diphtheria, tetanus)

Patients infected with multidrug-resistant bacteria

Immunocompromised patients

QUESTIONS

Answers to the questions can be found in Appendix 2.

1. During testing of new vaccines, it is sometimes the case that although administration of the vaccine produces high levels of antibody in serum, the vaccine recipient is not protected from infection. Explain some of the ways this could happen.

2. Vaccines often need to be administered more than once. Why is this necessary? Why is this most often the case with vaccines that are not live microbes?

3. Many modern vaccines consist of recombinant proteins. Why is this approach more attractive in many cases than using classical methods to isolate the protein from the supernatant fluid of the bacterium that produces it? What factors would have to be taken into account to make sure that the recombinant vaccine protein was suitable for use?

4. How could a vaccine possibly make a disease worse?

5. How does the existence of populations of severely immunocompromised people affect the use of live vaccine strains? Why are live vaccine strains still attractive despite this problem?

6. Why are adjuvants necessary, particularly in the case of subunit vaccines? Why might an adjuvant not be as necessary if a live vaccine strain is used?

7. Vaccines have traditionally been viewed as preventive. Yet people are now talking about "vaccine cures" in the case of such slow-developing conditions as HIV infection or tuberculosis. Explain the rationale.

8. Suppose that an effective vaccine becomes available, and this vaccine has nearly eradicated the disease worldwide. Yet there are groups that refuse vaccination on religious or philosophical grounds, and these groups arc a potential focus of infection that can move into vaccinated populations and strike the minority of children or, more likely, adults who were either not vaccinated at all or for some reason failed to develop the desired response to vaccination. Where does the right to religious freedom end and the right to have a life free of a crippling disease begin? (These questions have been much debated, and there is no right answer. Still, this question raises a very practical consideration that continues to surface in campaigns to eradicate disease.)

9. Smallpox has been eradicated through the use of the smallpox vaccine. How would such an eradication program work? Why does this great vaccine success make smallpox an attractive weapon for bioterrorists?

8

Bacterial Strategies for Evading or Surviving the Defense Systems of the Human Body

Overview of Bacterial Defense Strategies

Just as the human body has evolved multilayered strategies for defending itself against bacterial invasion, bacteria have evolved their own strategies for countering the defenses of the human body. Many of these bacterial strategies probably began evolving long before animals and humans were even a blip on the evolutionary radar screen. The majority of bacterial defense strategies studied today would have been useful for survival in natural environments (e.g., adherence to surfaces to stay close to a promising food source) or as defenses against voracious protozoa (e.g., the ability to avoid or survive phagocytosis). Perhaps the reason intact skin and the antibody response are such effective defenses is that these are very recent evolutionary developments that have no counterpart in protozoa. Even these defenses, however, have been compromised. Microbes that use insect vectors or take advantage of surgical wounds have ways to bypass the barrier of human skin, and microbes that disguise themselves by changing their surface proteins or by producing antibody-degrading enzymes have developed methods for bypassing the specific defenses.

In later chapters, you will learn how inventive individual species of bacteria have been in solving the problems posed by the defenses of the site they infect. In this chapter, we explore some common themes seen in bacterial strategies for evading the defenses of the human body. These features of disease-causing bacteria are called virulence factors. We have relegated one type of bacterial virulence factor, production of protein toxins that damage eukaryotic cells, to a chapter of its own (chapter 9).

At first glance, there would seem to be no reason to place bacterial toxins in a separate category from the virulence factors covered in this chapter. Yet, whereas the virulence factors covered in this chapter have a clear function in helping the bacteria to establish an infection, the role of toxins as an aid to bacterial infection is still unclear. There is no question that toxins cause damage to human cells. Yet this action seems in most cases to have little to do with the survival of bacteria in the human body. A classic example of this is the toxin produced by the bacterium that causes botulism (*Clostridium botulinum*). *C. botulinum* produces botulinum toxin, one of the most potent toxins known, when the bacteria multiply in food. When ingested, the clostridia do not colonize the body but pass right on through the intestinal tract. By contrast, the toxin enters the bloodstream and acts on neurons, producing a flaccid paralysis that can lead to death. What possible role could this undeniably potent toxin have in the lifestyle of *C. botulinum*? It must have some other function that has eluded investigators to date. The enigma of bacterial toxins remains one of the most intriguing unsolved mysteries of modern pathogenesis research. Before moving into the twilight zone of bacterial toxins, however, let us first cover some reassuringly explicable features of bacterial pathogens that enable them to colonize and infect the human body (Table 8–1).

Colonization and Invasion of Host Surfaces

Penetrating Intact Skin

Except for a few nematodes, there are no microbes known that can penetrate human skin unaided by surgery, catheters, or other events that breach the skin's normal integrity. It could be argued, of course, that some microbes have created their own skin trauma opportunities by colonizing biting arthropods. The bacterium that causes Lyme disease is one such pathogen. Unable to penetrate skin on its own, *Borrelia burgdorferi* enters the human body through the damaged area created by the tick that carries it. Similarly, bacteria that can survive on skin are in a good position to take advantage of surgical or catheter-induced wounds as a means of bypassing the intact skin defense.

Penetrating the Mucin Layer

In many parts of the body, mucosal cells are protected by a complex meshwork of protein and polysaccharide called **mucin.** Intestinal and vaginal mucin act as lubricants, but another vital function of mucin is to trap bacteria and prevent them from gaining access to mucosal cells. One of the least understood of all virulence factors is the ability of some bacteria to transit the mucin layer. Why do scientists interested in how bacteria cause intestinal or vaginal disease almost never consider the mucin layer or include it in their diagrams? One reason is that until recently, the procedures used to fix biological samples for microscopy collapsed the mucin layers. Photographs of intestinal sections that show a layer of bacteria lying on the epithelial cells illustrate this artifact. Yet such images have a powerful impact and have led many people to imagine all intestinal or vaginal bacteria as adhering to the mucosa. This is almost certainly an incorrect view. Most bacteria passing through the

intestine or colonizing the vagina probably never come close to the mucosal surface because they are carried along by lumen contents or get trapped in mucin, which is then replaced so that the trapped bacteria are carried out of the site. In the respiratory tract, the ciliated cells expel bacteria caught in mucin. A second reason for ignoring the mucin layer is that mucin has such a complex structure that it has been difficult to study. Moreover, tissue culture cells and organ cultures that produce mucin are only beginning to become available.

Table 8–1 Virulence factors that promote colonization and survival of infecting bacteria

Virulence factor	Function
Pili and fimbriae	Adherence to mucosal surfaces
Nonfimbrial adhesins	Tight binding to host cells
Biofilm formation	Ability to bind to surfaces and establish multilayered bacterial communities; biofilm communities have reduced susceptibility to antibiotics; bacteria in biofilms continue to seed blood
Invasins	Force nonphagocytic cells to engulf bacteria
Promotion of actin rearrangement in host cells	Forced phagocytosis, movement of bacteria within host cells, cell-to-cell spread
Binding to M cells	M cells used as natural port of entry into body
Motility and chemotaxis	Reaching mucosal surfaces (especially areas with fast flow)
sIgA proteases	Prevent trapping of bacteria in mucin
Siderophores, surface proteins that bind transferrin, lactoferrin, and other iron binding proteins	Iron acquisition
Iron abstinence	A few bacteria have replaced iron-requiring enzymes with similar ones that use manganese instead (e.g., *Borrelia burgdorferi*)
Capsules (usually polysaccharide)	Prevent phagocytic uptake; reduce complement activation
Lengthened LPS O antigen	MAC not formed; serum resistance
C5a peptidase	Interferes with signaling function of complement component C5a
Toxic proteins (toxins)	Kill phagocytes; reduce strength of oxidative burst
Variation in surface antigens	Evade antibody response

Bacteria that lack surface proteins or carbohydrates that bind mucin components could penetrate the mucin layer without being trapped. The fact that most bacteria do have mucin-binding surface molecules is what makes mucin so effective in trapping them. Mucin is also very viscous, so the ability to move through viscous materials would help bacteria reach mucosal cells. Some bacteria partially digest mucin, but this is a slow and difficult process owing to the complexity of mucin structure. Remember, mucin is designed to keep bacteria away from the mucosa, so there has been a strong selection for a structure that is resistant to enzymatic digestion.

The mucin layer is probably not a uniform layer. Mucin is expelled in thick streams from **goblet cells.** Thus, the mucin layer is probably more like a field of mucin strands than a solid mat. If so, bacteria could transit the mucin layer by moving in the spaces between the mucin strands, a trick that would also help to guide bacteria to the mucosal cell surface and keep them from wandering in the mucin layer parallel to the mucosal surface.

Another possibility is suggested by the observation that the **M cells** of the intestinal tract are the target of many of the bacteria that cause intestinal disease. The normal role of M cells is to sample the material passing through the intestine and deliver it to the immune system associated with the gastrointestinal mucosa (see chapter 6). Bacteria use the naturally phagocytic M cells as a portal through which they can transit the mucosal layer and enter underlying tissue and blood. The mucin layer over the collections of M cells (called Peyer's patches) is much thinner than the mucin layer over the rest of the mucosa. This thinner mucin layer may be one of the reasons why enteric pathogens that are not known to be active mucin-degraders use this entry port into the body.

There is one area of infectious disease research in which scientists have been forced to take the mucin layer into account: *Helicobacter pylori* infection. In the stomach, the mucin layer creates a buffer zone of nearly neutral pH that protects the mucosal cells from stomach acid. This zone also serves as a safe haven for *H. pylori*. If steps are taken to maintain the integrity of the mucin layer during sample preparation for microscopy, bacteria can be seen hanging in the mucin layer as well as adhering to the mucosa. Do the bacteria in the mucin layer contribute to the disease process, or do only those adherent to gastric mucosal cells contribute? Bacteria that produce extracellular enzymes and toxins could easily act on the mucosal cells from a distance.

Resisting Antibacterial Peptides

Peptides that intercalate into bacterial membranes, creating pores that allow essential interior molecules to escape, thus killing the bacterium, are produced in a number of body sites ranging from the base of the tongue to the crypts of the intestinal tract. First discovered in amphibians, where they were called magainins or natural antibiotics, these bactericidal peptides have now been found almost everywhere scientists have looked, and it now appears that they are an important defense of the human body. These peptides, now called defensins, are characterized by their cationic nature and by the presence of multiple cysteine residues that, through cross-linking, could give the peptides a barrel shape. This characteristic accords well with the hypothesis that the antibacterial peptides form channels in the bacterial membrane. What is hard to understand, however, is that the defensins must first transit peptidoglycan and outer membranes (in the case of gram-negative bacteria) to reach the vulnerable cytoplasmic membrane. Presumably, defensins are small enough to diffuse through porins and through the porous network formed by peptidoglycan. Evidently, they can get through because they are toxic for many types of bacteria.

Not too surprisingly, bacteria have developed ways of dealing with these peptides. Gram-negative bacteria are somewhat protected by their negatively charged LPS molecules, which bind the cationic peptides, preventing them from reaching their membrane target. This contention is supported by experiments showing that changes in LPS that make it less able or more able to bind the cationic defensins confer less or more, respectively, resistance to defensins. Another defense consists of peptidases that degrade the defensins before they can reach the cytoplasmic membrane. Cytoplasmic proteins that counter the permeabilizing effects of the defensin channels constitute still another possible defense. Potassium is an important ion that could leak out of the channels and disrupt the proton motive force. Proteins that restore the potassium balance could protect bacteria from transient exposure to defensins.

The fact that bacterial resistance to defensins can occur is discouraging, because some scientists in pharmaceutical companies have plans to develop similar peptides as antibiotics. At first glance, it would seem to be difficult if not impossible to develop resistance to peptides that form channels in phospholipid bilayer membranes. Clearly, however, bacteria have evolved more than one strategy for dealing with the toxic peptide problem.

Adherence

ROLE OF ADHERENCE. One of the dogmas of bacterial pathogenesis research is that adherence is an essential first step in the disease process. As we have just seen, however, bacteria can stay in a particular site by being trapped in the mucin layer. They need not have special organelles of adherence. Moreover, an interesting paper published by Gordon and Riley in 1992 pointed out that some strains of *Escherichia coli*—the most common cause of urinary tract infections—could divide rapidly enough in urine to stay in the bladder without adhering. Perhaps it is time to take a broader view of how bacteria stay in a site.

Why is adherence so important to bacteria? In the mouth, small intestine, and bladder, mucosal surfaces are washed by fluids, which keep down the number of bacteria in the site. In such locations, bacteria capable of adhering to mucosal cells have an advantage. Even in relatively stagnant areas, such as the colon and the vaginal tract, Brownian motion can move a bacterium that has made contact with a mucosal cell away from the surface of the cell. Virtually all known bacterial pathogens—and a lot of nonpathogenic bacteria, for that matter—have ways of attaching themselves firmly to host cells. Two of the strategies bacteria use to attach themselves to host cells are illustrated in Figure 8–1.

PILI AND FIMBRIAE. The best-understood mechanism of adherence is attachment mediated by rod-shaped protein structures called pili or fimbriae. Proteinaceous adhesins differ in thickness and length. The term **fimbriae** has been used to designate shorter, thinner structures, whereas **pili** is the term used to designate longer, thicker surface structures. In our experience, however, this convention is more often ignored than observed. In this book, where the "less is more" rule is applied in an attempt to minimize unnecessary jargon, the term "pili" will be used as the default term unless the people in a particular field have made a point of using the term "fimbriae." A pilus or fimbria is a rod-shaped structure formed by an ordered array of single subunits called **pilin.** Pilin proteins are usually about 20 kDa in size and are packed in a helical array to form a long cylindrical structure. The pilus is a long, somewhat flexible structure that extends outward from the bacterial surface and acts to establish contact between the bacterial surface and the surface of the host cell. In Figure 8–1A, pili are shown evenly distributed over the surface of the bacteria, but in some cases pili are located preferentially on one part of the bacterial surface.

The tip of the pilus attaches to a molecule on the host cell surface. Host cell receptors for pili are commonly carbohydrate residues of glycoproteins or glycolipids. Such host molecules are often involved in targeting of

A   Pili

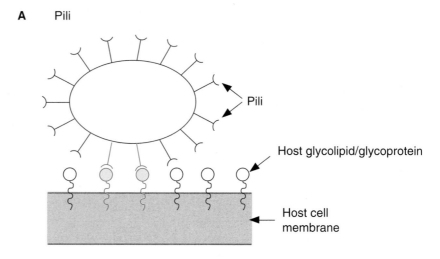

B   Afimbrial adhesins

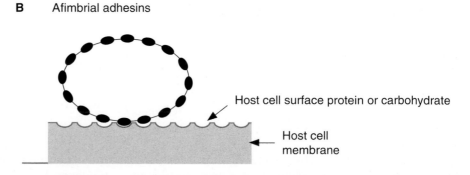

Figure 8–1 Two types of bacterial adherence mechanisms. (**A**) Pili, the rod-shaped protein structures that extend from the bacterial surface and bind to host cell surface molecules, usually carbohydrates. The tip structure is magnified in this drawing to emphasize its presence. In reality, the tip structure is much smaller than this figure would indicate. (**B**) Afimbrial adhesins, bacterial surface proteins that are not organized in a rodlike structure and mediate tight binding between bacteria and host cell.

the cell to its ultimate site, mediating cell-cell contact, or serving as part of the host cell's signal transduction mechanisms. Bacteria have subverted these host cell molecules to their own use. Binding of a pilus or fimbria to its host-cell target is quite specific. This specificity is important because the availability of suitable receptors will often determine what body site is infected by the bacterium. In at least some cases, the specific binding between the pilus tip and the host cell carbohydrate is mediated by a specialized tip structure that consists of several proteins distinct from the pilin protein. In other cases, binding of the tip appears to be mediated by pilin itself. It is not always easy to determine whether a pilus has a specialized tip structure because pilin accounts for over 99% of the protein in the pilus. Thus, minor proteins that form a specialized tip structure may be missed in the initial biochemical analysis of pilus composition. Now that DNA sequencing has become so easy, genes encoding minor proteins may be detected as unexplained genes located in operons containing the main pilin subunit gene and genes encoding proteins that assemble the pilus.

The assembly of pili by bacteria is a complex process that requires the participation of a number of auxiliary proteins. A general model for how this process occurs in gram-negative bacteria is shown in Figure 8–2. (Much has been learned about pilus assembly in recent years, leading to more and more complex models. Here we provide a simplified version of the process. In later chapters, more detailed models will be described for specific bacterial pathogens.) The first step is secretion of pilin and specialized tip proteins across the inner membrane and into the periplasmic space. In most cases, secretion of pilin and the other proteins appears to be mediated by the normal protein secretion system of the bacteria, but in some cases a special pilus-specific secretion system is used. Thus, whereas proteins that are secreted through the normal secretion machinery have an amino-terminal signal sequence which is proteolytically removed during processing, pilin subunits of some pili still have a methionine residue at their amino terminus, indicating that normal proteolytic processing did not occur. Still other types of pilin have a methyl group attached to their amino-terminal amino acid (often a phenylalanine residue) after secretion and processing.

The role of this type of modification is not known. In the periplasm, special proteins called **chaperones** prevent the pilus proteins from folding into their final configuration and convey them to an outer membrane protein complex (formed by protein C in Figure 8–2) where assembly of the pilin structure begins. The adhesive tip structure is assembled and extruded first, and then the shaft of the pilus is made by sequential addition of pilin subunits to the base of the pilus, pushing the already assembled portions outward from the bacterial surface. Finally, a periplasmic protein (H) signals the end of the extrusion process and presumably stabilizes the resulting pilus in the cell wall. How the bacteria measure the length of the growing pilus shaft and decide when it has reached the proper length remains a mystery.

Bacteria growing in the body are constantly losing and reforming pili. Continuous production of new pili is necessitated in part by the fragility of pili, which are

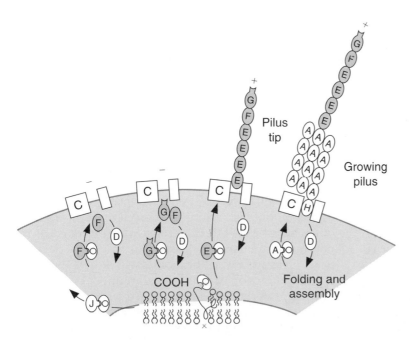

Figure 8–2 Model for assembly of pili with adhesive tip structures. As in Figure 8–1, the size of the tip structure is exaggerated to emphasize its location and its different structure compared to the pilus shaft. The adhesive tip components (E, F, and G) are assembled first, and then the main pilus subunit (A) is assembled to form the pilus shaft. Chaperones (D and J) carry out the assembly process starting from an outer membrane scaffold structure (C). (Adapted from S. L. Hultgren, S. Normark, and S. N. Abraham, *Annu. Rev. Microbiol.* **45**:383–415, 1991.)

easily broken and lost. An equally important function of pilus replacement, at least for some bacteria, is that it provides them a way to evade the host's immune response. Host antibodies that bind the tips of pili physically block the pili from binding to their host cell targets. Once the host begins to produce antibody to a particular type of pilus, that pilus type is no longer useful to the bacteria. Replacing one type of pilus with another renders the host's antibody response obsolete. Some bacteria, such as those that cause gonorrhea, can change pilin types often enough to make it virtually impossible for the host to mount an antibody response that prevents colonization.

Why do bacteria use such long, fragile structures for adherence? A plausible explanation is that, since the surfaces of bacteria and host cells are both negatively charged, pili allow the bacteria to bind host cells without getting close enough for electrostatic repulsion to prevent attachment. This cannot be the sole explanation, because bacteria are clearly capable of a much tighter form of binding that brings the bacterial surface and the host cell surface into contact with each other (see below). Possibly, pili allow the bacteria to make an initial loose contact with a host cell surface, which then triggers production of surface proteins needed to mediate tighter binding. Many pathogenic bacteria appear to use a two-step process for attachment, in which a loose association via pili is first made between bacterium and host, followed by depolymerization of the pili and a tighter binding involving surface proteins that bring the bacterial and host cell surfaces together.

SIGNAL TRANSDUCTION.　The original view of pili was that they were metabolically inert once they were formed and that their only role was to form an attachment to human or animal cell surface molecules. Recent findings have shown that human cells respond to attachment of bacteria to their surfaces by altering the expression of a number of genes. Similarly, a bacterium that has just attached itself to the surface of a mammalian cell exhibits altered expression of virulence genes, as if the act of binding triggered the activation or repression of virulence genes. One way to explain this communication is to assume that binding of the pilus tip to a eukaryotic cell surface receptor results in a physical change in the conformation of the pilus tip proteins and the host surface receptor. It is well established that conformational changes in eukaryotic cell surface molecules can trigger signaling cascades inside the eukaryotic cell. Similarly, changes in conformation in the pilus tip proteins might cause a conformational change in the shaft subunit proteins; these conformational changes move along the length of the shaft to the bacterial surface, where changes in bacterial gene expres-

sion are triggered. Thus, just as having someone grab your arm sets off certain responses in your body and in the body of the grabber, bacterium and host cell may experience reactions to the binding of pili to their target (receptor) eukaryotic molecule. If this is the case, one wonders about the attachment of bacterial LPS to CD14 on phagocytes. Certainly, the phagocyte reacts to this binding reaction in a number of ways. It will be important to learn whether the bacterium whose LPS has been attached to the phagocyte experiences a similar response to attachment.

ADHESINS OF GRAM-POSITIVE BACTERIA.　Most studies of pili have focused on gram-negative bacteria. Some gram-positive bacteria are also covered by hairlike protrusions that resemble pili, and it was natural to assume that these structures might play the same adhesive role as the pili of gram-negative bacteria. In at least one case, however, the assumption that fibrillar structures on a gram-positive bacterium are adhesins now appears to be incorrect. The gram-positive pathogen *Streptococcus pyogenes* has a **nonfibrillar adhesin** that mediates its attachment to **fibronectin,** a protein found on many host cell surfaces. Attachment to fibronectin may help *S. pyogenes* to adhere to the mucosa of the human throat when it causes strep throat or to tissue in wounds when it causes wound infections. *S. pyogenes* is covered with fibrillar structures that consist of many monomers of a protein called **M protein**. At one time, these piluslike structures were thought to mediate adherence, but we now know that they have a very different function: helping *S. pyogenes* to avoid ingestion by phagocytes (see below). Thus, physical appearance can be deceiving. In the past several years, much more information has been obtained about the adhesins of gram-positive bacteria, and some of these will be encountered in later chapters. So far, the bottom line seems to be that gram-positive bacteria, like gram-negative bacteria, have both pili-type adhesins and non-pili adhesins.

OTHER TYPES OF ADHESINS.　Some bacteria have cell surface proteins that are clearly important for adherence but that do not assemble themselves into pililike structures. These adhesins have been called **afimbrial adhesins** and are probably the proteins that mediate the tighter binding of bacteria to host cell that often follows initial binding via pili. Bacterial surface proteins are important components of the systems that allow bacteria to attach to and invade host cells (see below). The structure and function of only a small number of the afimbrial adhesins have been studied. At least some of them may recognize proteins on host cell surfaces rather than carbohydrates (Figure 8–1B).

Another type of adherence that is receiving considerable attention is attachment of bacteria to a surface and to each other to form a **biofilm**. In this case, the adherence is mediated by an extracellular polysaccharide slime that acts as a kind of glue to bind the bacteria to each other and to a surface. A biofilm is more than just a bunch of glued-together bacteria, however. The metabolism of bacteria in a biofilm shifts into an almost dormant state, making the biofilm much more refractory than free-living bacteria to disinfectants and antibiotics. At one time, scientists thought of biofilms as a uniform multilayer community of bacteria, but it is now clear that biofilms have a complex structure that looks more like islands separated by channels. The channels allow nutrients to reach most of the biofilm community.

Biofilms cause two types of medical problems. Biofilms in water towers provide a source of bacteria that can leave the biofilm, become aerosolized, and enter people's lungs. In the case of Legionnaires' disease, a new type of lung disease (see chapter 1), biofilms on the walls of air-conditioning water towers may have been the source of the aerosolized bacterium, *Legionella pneumophila*. It is very difficult to eliminate a biofilm once it is established.

A second type of medical biofilm problem is the formation of biofilms on body surfaces, on catheters that breach the skin, or on plastic implants. The **plaque** that causes dental caries or periodontal disease is actually a biofilm that becomes mineralized over time. Dislodging plaque is not a trivial task, as anyone who has visited a dentist's office for tooth cleaning or gum scraping knows very well. Biofilms also form on plastic tubing (e.g., venous catheters, urinary catheters) and on contaminated plastic implants (e.g., heart valve or hip joint replacements). Because catheters breach important defensive barriers, such as skin or the urethral sphincter, they can transmit bacteria into the body.

Although plastic is a modern human invention, bacteria rapidly adapted to this novelty and have become quite adept at forming biofilms on it. Biofilms on plastic implants, whether caused by contamination at the time of insertion or seeded by transient bacteremia (bacteria in the bloodstream) create a serious medical problem. Such biofilms are not only refractory to antibiotic treatment but give the bacteria a measure of protection against phagocytic cells. Because cells can break off from the biofilm and enter the bloodstream, biofilm-encrusted implants are ticking time bombs that may "explode" into septic shock at any moment.

Plastic implants that acquire a bacterial biofilm must usually be removed surgically and replaced surgically, because antibiotics are not effective at sterilizing them. Why bacteria that are susceptible to an antibiotic if they are free-living become more resistant to the same antibiotic when growing in a biofilm is still not well understood. The most likely explanation is that the relatively inert metabolic state of bacteria in a biofilm makes them less susceptible to antibiotics, most of which work best on rapidly growing cells. Also, those antibiotics that simply stop bacterial growth rather than killing the bacteria outright rely for effectiveness on the accessibility of the stalled bacteria to phagocytic cleanup. Because the extended size of the biofilm structure makes engulfment by phagocytes almost impossible, and because phagocytes do not move very well on plastic surfaces, such antibiotics are completely ineffective against biofilms on implants.

sIgA Proteases

Bacteria attempting to colonize mucosal surfaces have to solve the problem of how to avoid being trapped in the mucin layer. The stickiness of mucin is due in part to the presence of sIgA molecules that simultaneously bind bacterial antigens via their antigen binding sites and interact with mucin via their Fc portions. A bacterial strategy that may be designed to avoid sIgA-mediated trapping in mucin is the production of an extracellular enzyme that cleaves human IgA in the hinge region. This cleavage would separate the part of the sIgA that binds bacteria from the part that interacts with mucin. Such enzymes are remarkably specific for sIgA and have thus been called **sIgA proteases.** Most sIgA proteases are specific not only for sIgA but also for a particular human isotype, sIgA1. Another human isotype, sIgA2, which does not have the same hinge region, is not cleaved. The fact that sIgA1 is the predominant isotype in many mucosal sites may explain this specificity. The actual role of sIgA proteases in virulence is still not well understood, and there is some controversy about their importance, but the unusual specificity of these enzymes suggests that they might play some role in infection.

Iron Acquisition Mechanisms

Most articles on iron acquisition by bacteria start with the statement that iron is essential for the growth of all bacteria. It should come as no shock by now that bacteria—no respecters of human paradigms—defy this one, too. It is now becoming apparent that there are some bacteria that solve their iron acquisition problem by not using iron at all. Most pathogenic bacteria, however, do require iron and have to cope with the fact that iron concentrations in nature are generally quite low. The concentration of free iron is particularly low in the human body because **lactoferrin, transferrin, ferritin,** and **hemoglobin** bind most of the available iron. To survive in the human body, iron-requiring bacteria must have some mechanism for acquiring iron. The best-studied mechanism of bacterial iron acquisition is **siderophores.** Siderophores are low-molecular-weight compounds that chelate iron with high affinity. The structure of one type of siderophore is shown in Figure 8–3. There are two main classes of siderophores, **catechols** and **hydroxamates,** but both have the same property, namely, that they form tight chelated complexes with iron. Siderophores are excreted into the medium, and then the iron-siderophore complex is taken up by special siderophore receptors on the bacterial surface. The internalized iron-siderophore complex is cleaved to release the iron molecule inside the bacteria. Some bacteria not only produce their own siderophores but also produce receptors capable of binding siderophores produced by other organisms, the bacterial equivalent of freeloading.

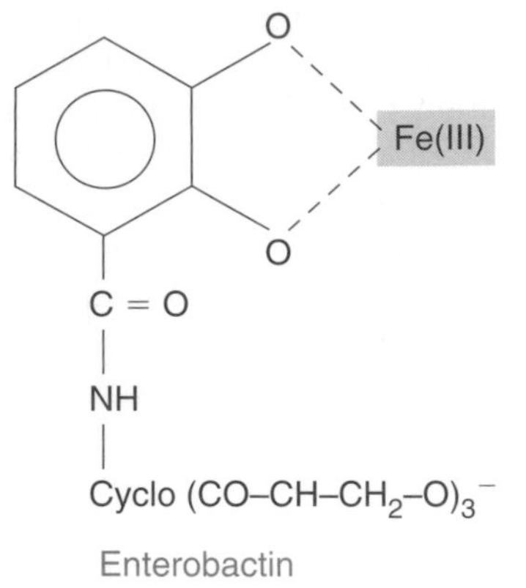

Although siderophore-based iron acquisition has been shown to contribute to the virulence of many bacterial pathogens, mutations that eliminate siderophore production or uptake by a bacterial pathogen do not always decrease virulence. This finding could be explained by the fact that bacteria often have more than one iron-sequestering system, and a mutant deficient in one system may still be able to survive by relying on the remaining system or systems. Nonetheless, it is also possible that siderophore-based iron acquisition systems are adapted mainly to survival of the bacteria outside the body, in soil and water, whereas other strategies of iron acquisition are more important in the human body. In soil and water, bacteria are probably trying to scavenge free iron, whereas in the human body virtually all of the iron is already bound to proteins such as hemoglobin, transferrin, or lactoferrin. A number of pathogenic bacteria have now been shown to be able to use transferrin, lactoferrin, or hemoglobin as a source of iron. Generally, these bacteria bind the iron-containing host molecule to their surfaces as part of the iron acquisition process. How they remove the iron from the host proteins is being investigated. As more and more pathogens are studied, it is becoming apparent that acquisition of iron from transferrin or lactoferrin, once thought to be an unusual mechanism of iron acquisition, is much more common than previously suspected.

Another possible iron acquisition strategy of bacteria is production of toxins that kill host cells. As will be seen in chapter 9, some bacterial toxins are produced only when iron levels are low. Because these toxic proteins kill host cells, they might be part of an iron acquisition strategy in which host cells are killed by the toxin to release their iron stores (primarily ferritin- or heme-

Figure 8–3 Structure of one type of bacterial siderophore (enterobactin). Siderophores differ considerably in structure but are similar in that they are basically just iron chelators with a very high affinity for iron.

bound iron), which can then be acquired by the bacteria via ferritin- or heme-binding proteins.

Still another solution to the iron problem, which would have been considered heretical a few years ago but which appears to be used by a number of bacteria, could be called **iron abstinence.** These bacteria do not require iron at all. Only a relatively small number of bacterial enzymes have iron-sulfur centers. These enzymes are mostly associated with respiratory metabolism and are dispensable for microorganisms with a nonrespiratory lifestyle. The causative agent of Lyme disease, *B. burgdorferi,* uses the iron abstinence strategy. It lacks all of the iron-dependent enzymes and instead uses manganese, a fairly abundant mineral, to replace iron as a cofactor in nondispensable enzymes.

Invasion and Intracellular Residence

Some bacteria have evolved mechanisms for entering host cells, such as epithelial cells, that are not naturally phagocytic. They do this by attaching to the host cell surface and causing changes in the host cell cytoskeleton that result in their engulfment by the host cell. In actively phagocytic cells, cytoskeletal rearrangements involving polymerization and depolymerization of actin occur as a normal part of pseudopod formation. By causing similar actin rearrangements to occur in normally nonphagocytic cells, the bacteria are in effect forcing phagocytosis by eliciting formation of pseudopod-like structures that mediate engulfment. Bacterial surface proteins that provoke phagocytic ingestion of the bacterium by host cells are called **invasins.** Some proteins that are essential for invasion of cultured cells by bacteria have now been identified, but it is not yet clear how these proteins work to promote actin rearrangements.

Bacteria can also induce their uptake by phagocytes. Bacteria ingested by phagocytes are enclosed in a membrane vesicle. Bacteria have two strategies for coping with this situation, which normally would lead to phagolysosome formation and killing of the bacteria. One strategy is to prevent phagosome-lysosome fusion. A second strategy is for the invading bacteria to escape from the phagosome by disrupting the vesicle membrane. Escape from the phagosome is mediated by a bacterial protein that disrupts membranes either by degrading membrane lipids or by forming pores in the membrane. There are many advantages to be gained by escaping the phagosome and growing in the cytoplasm of host cells. These include an abundance of nutrients, protection from antibodies and complement, and partial protection from some antibiotics that do not penetrate into mammalian cells. The only effective host defense against bacteria that can survive phagocytosis appears to be the NK cell and cytotoxic T-cell response, which kills host cells infected by the bacteria and thus exposes the bacteria to extracellular defenses such as complement and antibodies. Bacteria can also invade cells that are normally nonphagocytic and use the vesicle as a means for transiting the cell to reach the tissue below or escape the vesicle.

Bacteria that force their own ingestion by controlling host cell actin organization continue to interact with actin once they enter the cytoplasm of the host cell. Here, condensation of actin on one end of the bacterium propels the bacteria through the host cell cytoplasm and into adjacent cells. The bacteria can also move along preexisting actin filaments that give the host cell its shape. The study of the various interactions between invasive bacteria and the host cell cytoskeleton is one of the most exciting areas of current research on virulence mechanisms. One example of bacteria that interact with actin, both in the process of forced phagocytosis and for movement through the cytoplasm (*Listeria* sp.), is covered in chapter 27.

Eukaryotic cell biologists, especially those interested in the body's defense systems, view the process of invasion somewhat differently. Whereas bacteriologists see the invasion process as a process mediated by bacteria, with the purpose of entering and infecting or translocating through a human mucosal cell, gastrointestinal cell biologists view the mucosal cells as sentinels monitoring the presence of bacterial invasion. Bacterial invasion of mucosal cells triggers these cells to release chemokines and cytokines that are known to be important for mobilizing the phagocyte and immune defenses. Bacterial attachment alone is not sufficient to start the signaling process that causes the human body to mount an inflammatory response. More intimate connection, especially disruption of normal actin polymerization processes and the presence of bacteria within mucosal cells, sets off the cytokine/chemokine alarm system that initiates the inflammatory response.

Evading Complement, Phagocytes, and the Antibody Response

Capsules

A **capsule** is a loose, relatively unstructured network of polymers that covers the surface of some bacteria. Most of the well-studied capsules are composed of polysaccharides, but capsules composed of polypeptides or protein-carbohydrate mixtures have also been described. The usual role of capsules in bacterial virulence is to protect the bacteria from the host's inflammatory response (complement activation and phagocyte-mediated killing). Recall that an essential first step in the alternative pathway is assembly of C3bBb (C3 convertase) on the bacterial surface. Some capsules prevent formation of C3 convertase by failing to bind serum protein B. Other capsules have a higher affinity for serum protein H than for B. If C3b complexes with H rather than with B, it is degraded by serum protein I. Capsules that are rich in sialic acid have a high affinity for H. By preventing C3bBb formation on their surfaces, encapsulated bacteria gain some important advantages. The capsule itself is less likely to be opsonized by C3b, so bacteria will not be engulfed as efficiently by phagocytes. Some C3b may diffuse through the loose capsule network and bind to the bacterial surface under the capsule. C3 convertase may even form at this site, but the C3b molecules that attach to the bacterial surface under the capsular layer are prevented from making contact with phagocyte receptors by the thick intervening capsular network. Less C3bBb formation means that less C5b will be produced and MAC will be less likely to form on the bacterial surface, an important consideration for gram-negative bacteria. The MAC can still form on the bacterial surface that is covered by a capsule because proteins can diffuse through the loose network of most capsules. Thus, encapsulated bacteria do not automatically become serum resistant.

An effective host response against an encapsulated bacterium is to produce antibodies that bind the capsule. Antibodies bound to the capsular surface not only provide sites for phagocyte binding so that bacteria can be ingested but also support activation of complement by the classical pathway, thus increasing the amount of MAC formed. Vaccines consisting of capsular material have proved highly effective in preventing infections caused by encapsulated bacteria, such as *Haemophilus influenzae* type b. Some bacteria subvert this type of protective host response by having capsules that resemble host polysaccharides. Examples are capsules consisting of **hyaluronic acid** (a mammalian extracellular matrix polysaccharide), such as that of *S. pyogenes,* or **sialic acid** (a common component of mammalian cell glycoproteins) found in some strains of *Neisseria meningitidis.* This type of capsule is not immunogenic, and the host does not produce antibodies that opsonize the capsular surface.

Resistance to Nitric Oxide

Nitric oxide appears to play an important antibacterial role in the human body. As described in chapter 4, nitric oxide is a reactive form of nitrogen that is produced by a number of cells of the human antibacterial defense systems. Recently, scientists have begun to learn how some bacteria resist killing by nitric oxide. In *E. coli,* resistance to nitric oxide is mediated by a flavohemoglobin that is normally part of the respiratory system. This flavohemoglobin, also called nitric oxide dioxygenase, uses NADPH, FAD, and oxygen to convert nitric oxide into NO^{3-} by a reaction that is still not well understood.

Other Strategies for Circumventing Complement and Phagocytes

One of the principal targets of complement on gram-negative bacteria is LPS. LPS not only serves as a site for attachment of C3b, the signal for activation of the alternative pathway, but it also binds C5b and serves as a nucleation site for formation of the MAC. Two types of LPS modification affect this interaction between LPS and complement components. First, attachment of sialic acid to **LPS O antigen** prevents formation of C3 convertase, just as capsules, such as the one of *Neisseria gonorrhoeae,* that contain sialic acid do. Second, changes in length of the LPS O-antigen side chains prevent effective MAC formation. It is not clear how O-antigen side chain length prevents MAC killing, since C5b and some MAC components still attach. Possibly, the MAC forms too far from the bacterial outer membrane to exert a bactericidal effect. Bacteria that are not killed by the MAC are called **serum resistant.** An indication of the importance of this trait is that many of the gram-negative bacteria that cause systemic infections are serum resistant (Box 8–1).

Other strategies are designed to prevent migration of phagocytes to the site where bacteria are growing. A bacterial enzyme that specifically degrades C5a, the chemoattractant for phagocytes, has recently been found in gram-positive cocci and may be more widespread as a strategy for interfering with the signaling function of complement. Many bacteria produce toxic proteins (chapter 9) that kill phagocytes, inhibit their migration, or reduce the strength of the oxidative burst. Such toxins may protect the bacteria from phagocytes in the body.

Yet another strategy for evading complement activation and all the other reactions LPS evokes is to have an LPS-type molecule that does not elicit the sort of strong host inflammatory response normally elicited by classical *E. coli* LPS. *H. pylori* is an example of a bacterial pathogen that has such an LPS. Despite this, *H. pylori* does elicit an inflammatory response. Some possible reasons for this apparent anomaly will be explored in chapter 23.

Surviving Phagocytosis

Some bacteria have developed the ability to survive inside PMNs, monocytes, or macrophages. Such bacteria are among the most dangerous of all pathogens because they are impervious to most of the host's protection mechanisms. One strategy for surviving phagocytosis is to escape the phagosome before it fuses with the lysosome. Alternatively, bacteria may be able to prevent phagosome-lysosome fusion from occurring. Two ways of doing this are preventing acidification of the vacuole or short-circuiting the process of fusion itself. Another strategy is to acquire traits that reduce the effectiveness of the toxic compounds released into the phagolysosome after fusion occurs. Examples include resistance to killing by defensins, production of enzymes such as catalase and superoxide dismutase that detoxify reactive forms of oxygen, cell surface polysaccharides that interact with and detoxify oxygen radicals, cell surface proteins that reduce the strength of the oxidative burst, and cell walls that are refractory to destruction by lysosomal proteases and lysozyme. Because the importance of reactive nitrogen intermediates has only been recognized recently, little is known about mechanisms that might protect bacteria from these compounds. The only effective host response to bacteria that can survive inside normal phagocytes is the activated macrophage response.

Evading the Host's Antibody Response

An effective bacterial strategy for evading the host's antibody response is to change the surface antigens that are recognized by the antibody so that the antibodies no longer bind. Another way to avoid the host's antibody response is to be mistaken for a part of the host itself. Some bacterial capsules that are composed of polysaccharides do not trigger an antibody response

BOX 8–1   Bacterial Meningitis: an Example of the Power of Capsules

Bacterial meningitis is not a common disease, but it is a much-feared one because it can kill an infected person within a few days. People who manage to survive a case of meningitis frequently have irreversible neurological damage, resulting in blindness, deafness, and learning deficiencies. A striking feature of meningitis is how rapidly it develops once the infection begins. This is due to the ability of the causative bacteria to divide rapidly in blood, a trait that is due to production of antiphagocytic capsules and to the ability to avoid killing by complement. The most common causes of meningitis are *N. meningitidis* (a gram-negative bacterium that causes epidemic meningitis), *Streptococcus pneumoniae* (a gram-positive bacterium that is also a common cause of bacterial pneumonia), and *H. influenzae* type b (a gram-negative bacterium, which was the most common cause of meningitis in children until a vaccine was developed a few years ago).

What do these diverse types of bacteria have in common? All produce polysaccharide capsules, and the most dangerous strains are also serum resistant. Once the bacteria gain access to the bloodstream, the capsule protects them from killing by phagocytes. As mentioned in the text, possession of a capsule does not automatically make a bacterium serum resistant, but some strains of *N. meningitidis* become relatively serum resistant by covalently attaching sialic acid residues to their LPS molecules. *H. influenzae* b strains can also become serum resistant by modification of LPS O-antigen side chains. *S. pneumoniae*, being gram positive, is naturally serum resistant since the MAC does not form on most gram-positive bacteria owing to the lack of an LPS-type molecule that can precipitate the MAC.

A strain of *E. coli* that causes meningitis in newborns (*E. coli* K1) also produces a capsule. This capsule is composed of sialic acid residues and thus does not bind C3b. In this case, the capsule has the same ultimate effect as serum resistance because it prevents MAC components from being made in the first place. The combination of a capsule and the ability to avoid killing by complement renders ineffective all of the nonspecific defense mechanisms of serum and blood except transferrin. Unfortunately, *N. meningitidis* and *H. influenzae* can obtain iron from transferrin.

The only defense that can check the growth of these bacteria in blood and cerebral spinal fluid is the antibody response. Antibodies to capsular polysaccharides opsonize the bacteria so that phagocytes can ingest them. PMNs and macrophages readily kill all the bacteria mentioned above. People who make antibodies against capsular antigens are fully protected from the disease. In fact, the reason *H. influenzae* b is normally a disease of children (aged 5 months to 5 years) is that most people who survive past age 5 have developed an antibody response against *H. influenzae*, probably as a result of transient nasopharyngeal colonization during childhood. Newborn infants are protected by maternal antibodies. There is now an effective vaccine against *H. influenzae* b, which consists of a capsular polysaccharide component attached to a protein to make it a better antigen (see chapter 7). This vaccine is now being used to protect children in the vulnerable younger age groups. There is also a capsular polysaccharide vaccine against *S. pneumoniae* that is fairly effective. Developing a vaccine against *N. meningitidis* has proved difficult because the most common type of capsule in some parts of the world is type B, a capsule that (like the capsule of *E. coli* K1 strains) consists largely of sialic residues and thus does not evoke an antibody response. Vaccines against other types of *N. meningitidis* are available because these capsules are more immunogenic.

During outbreaks of meningitis caused by *N. meningitidis*, as many as 80% of people in an exposed population may have their noses and throats colonized by *N. meningitidis*, but only a small percentage of the population colonized by the bacteria actually develop the disease. One possible explanation is that most adult members of a population may have some level of acquired immunity to *N. meningitidis* infection.

A factor that clearly affects host susceptibility is the integrity of the mucous membranes of the nose and throat, through which the bacteria usually gain access to the bloodstream. Outbreaks of *N. meningitidis* meningitis in Africa are almost always associated with the dry season, when dry conditions undermine the protective barriers of the mucous membranes. Similarly, outbreaks in other countries appear to

(continued)

coincide with dry periods of the year. Acute viral respiratory infections such as influenza may also be a predisposing factor since such infections kill ciliated cells and undermine the integrity of the mucosal barrier. Interestingly, people with deficiencies in late complement components who are unable to form the MAC are also more prone to meningitis. Thus, although meningitis-causing strains are often somewhat serum resistant, the MAC may still exert some protective effect, at least in the case of the gram-negative pathogens.

Why do people with meningitis die so quickly? The answer is that release of bacterial cell wall components, such as LPS, teichoic acid, and peptidoglycan fragments, triggers a cascade of events leading to shock and death.

This type of bacterial toxicity is discussed in detail in chapter 3. Since the compounds that cause the symptoms of meningitis are released when bacteria lyse, the administration of antibiotics, such as penicillins and cephalosporins, that lyse bacteria can actually temporarily worsen the condition of a patient who has developed high numbers of bacteria in blood or cerebral spinal fluid. To counter this effect, which is most likely to occur in children because of the unusually high numbers reached by bacteria infecting this age group, clinicians routinely administer corticosteroids along with antibiotics in an attempt to counteract the inflammatory effect of toxic compounds released from lysing bacteria.

because they resemble carbohydrates that are ubiquitous in host tissues (sialic acid, hyaluronic acid) and thus are recognized as self. Bacteria can also hide from the immune system by coating themselves with host proteins such as fibronectin. An interesting example of this type of defense is a set of bacterial proteins (protein A of *Staphylococcus aureus*, protein G of *S. pyogenes*) that bind the Fc portion of antibodies, thus coating the bacteria with antibodies, but in a way that does not lead to opsonization of the bacteria. This antibody coat may prevent recognition of the bacteria by the immune system. It is conceivable that bacterial binding of lactoferrin, transferrin, and other host iron binding proteins serves a dual function, as a protective coat as well as a means to acquire iron from them.

The Opportunists

Bacteria that appear to possess few of the virulence factors described here can nonetheless cause infections. These bacteria are generally not able to cause infections in healthy people and preferentially infect people whose defenses are compromised in some way. Such bacteria are called **opportunists.** Opportunists can be members of the body's normal microbiota, such as *Staphylococcus epidermidis*, *Enterococcus faecalis*, oral streptococci, and *Bacteroides fragilis*, or common soil bacteria, such as *Burkholderia cepacia* and *Pseudomonas aeruginosa*.

At first, the opportunists were assumed to lack classical virulence factors. Yet, as some of these opportunistic pathogens have been studied in more detail, virulence factors have been uncovered. For example, *B. fragilis*, an anaerobe found in the colon, produces a capsule, and *S. epidermidis*, a skin bacterium, has cell-surface adhesins. In some cases, such virulence factors play a different role than they do in the classical pathogens. For example, the capsule of *B. fragilis* seems to function less to prevent phagocytosis than to elicit an inflammatory response. The surface adhesins of *S. epidermidis* allow it to bind tightly to plastic rather than to mammalian cells.

Opportunists have other features that help them to cause infection. One is that they are constantly present in the body or in the environment in relatively high numbers. That is, they are always on the spot to take advantage of any breach that occurs in the defenses of the human body. Another key feature is that many of them are able to take advantage of locations in the body that are somewhat protected from the immune system. For example, *B. fragilis* infects damaged tissue. Damaged tissue is quite anoxic and is cut off from the blood supply. Thus, neutrophils and antibodies are excluded from the site. *S. epidermidis* colonizes plastic implants, which are somewhat protected from phagocytes. An example of a very serious type of opportunistic infection, which illustrates these principles, is described in Box 8–2.

BOX 8–2　Disease without Virulence Factors: Subacute Bacterial Endocarditis

The title of this box may seem self-contradictory. After all, virulence factors are associated with microbes that cause disease. Yet this anomaly has arisen in the case of infections caused by some opportunistic pathogens. Subacute bacterial endocarditis is a good example of such an opportunistic infection and illustrates the difficulty in defining what is a "virulence factor." Endocarditis is an infection of the heart valves that can be fatal owing to destruction of the valves and surrounding heart tissue. One type of bacterial endocarditis, called subacute because it develops more slowly than endocarditis caused by more virulent bacteria, is caused by a group of streptococci that are normally found in the human mouth (alpha-hemolytic streptococci).

The alpha-hemolytic streptococci are part of the resident microbiota of the mouth and are not normally able to cause disease. However, in people with prior heart valve damage due to rheumatic fever or congenital valve defects, the alpha-hemolytic streptococci can be deadly. During dental surgery, large numbers of oral bacteria can enter the bloodstream. These bacteria, including the alpha-hemolytic streptococci, are rapidly destroyed by phagocytes in the blood. In people with heart valve abnormalities, the turbulent flow of blood near the abnormal valve causes loose clots consisting of fibrin and platelets to form on the valve surface. These clots are called "vegetation."

Oral streptococci that manage to reach the heart valve and enter these vegetations are protected from phagocytes, which cannot penetrate the protein network of the vegetation. Accordingly, the bacteria can survive and grow in these sites. It is not clear what causes the damage to the heart valve. Complement activation triggered by the bacteria may cause some damage, and phagocytes attracted to the area but unable to get to the bacteria may also cause tissue destruction. Proteases produced by the bacteria themselves may also make a contribution. Thus, an apparently "avirulent" bacterium can nonetheless cause a fatal infection in the right kind of host.

Still another feature that many opportunists have in common is their resistance to antibiotics. This not only gives them an advantage in the antibiotic-laden hospital environment, but it also makes the infections they cause difficult to treat. This is the main reason why a bacterium like *S. epidermidis* or *E. faecalis*, although not very virulent, can nonetheless kill a person if infection develops. The combination of impaired host defenses and a multidrug-resistant bacterium is a dangerous one, and one that is being seen more and more commonly in very sick hospital patients.

SELECTED READINGS

Brown, M. R., and J. Barker. 1999. Unexplored reservoirs of pathogenic bacteria: protozoa and biofilms. *Trends Microbiol.* **7:**46–48.

Cirillo, J. D. 1999. Exploring a novel perspective on pathogenic relationships. *Trends Microbiol.* **7:**96–98.

Duclos, S., and M. Desjardins. 2000. Subversion of a young phagosome: the survival strategies of intracellular pathogens. *Cell. Microbiol.* **2:**365–377.

Gordon, D. M., and M. A. Riley. 1992. A theoretical and experimental analysis of bacterial growth in the bladder. *Mol. Microbiol.* **6:**555–562.

Groisman, E. A. 1994. How bacteria resist killing by host-defense peptides. *Trends Microbiol.* **2:**444–449.

Heithoff, D. M., C. P. Conner, and M. J. Mahan. 1997. Dissecting the biology of a pathogen during infection. *Trends Microbiol.* **5:**509–513.

Kuehn, M. J. 1997. Establishing communications via gram-negative bacterial pili. *Trends Microbiol.* **5:**130–135.

Reeves, P. 1995. Role of O-antigen variation in the immune response. *Trends Microbiol.* **3:**381–386.

Smith, H. 1998. What happens to bacterial pathogens *in vivo*? *Trends Microbiol.* **6:**239–241.

Colonization of host surfaces

Penetration of intact skin
  Requires some disruption, such as surgery, catheters
  Transmission by arthropods

Penetration of mucin layer
  Some bacteria lack mucin receptors—not trapped
  Production of mucin-degrading enzymes
  Movement between mucin strands
  Mucin layer thin over M cells, which take up bacteria

Resisting antibacterial peptides (defensins)
  Act by creating pores in bacterial membranes
  LPS molecules bind defensins—prevent their reaching cytoplasmic membrane
  Peptidases degrade defensins
  Cytoplasmic proteins counter action of defensins

Adherence
  Fluids may wash bacteria away from site if they do not adhere to host cells
  Pili and fimbriae mediate attachment
    Rod-shaped protein structures on surface of bacteria
    Formed by ordered array of single subunits
    Tip structure attaches specifically to receptor on host cell (often carbohydrate residues of glycoproteins or glycolipids)
    Assembly requires actions of numerous auxiliary proteins
      In gram-negative bacteria, secretion of pilin and other proteins into periplasm usually mediated by normal protein secretion system
      Chaperones in periplasm convey pilus proteins to outer membrane where assembly of pilus begins
      Adhesive tip assembled first
      Tip forced upward by addition of pilin subunits
  Pili constantly lost and reformed
    Partially due to fragility
    Allows some bacteria to avoid host defenses by changing pilus type
    Pili allow bacteria and host cell to form initial loose contact, thus triggering mechanisms of tighter adherence
  Signal transduction
    Binding of adhesin to receptor on host cell may activate or repress virulence genes of bacterial cell
    Human cells alter expression of numerous genes in response to adhesin binding
  Adhesins of gram-positive bacteria similar to those of gram-negative bacteria
  Afimbrial adhesins
    Cell surface proteins that do not form pili
    Probably mediate tighter binding of bacterial and host cells
    May bind proteins on host cells rather than carbohydrates
  Biofilms
    Consist of bacteria binding to surfaces and each other—mediated by polysaccharide slime
    Bacterial metabolism in biofilm reduced—more refractory to disinfectants and antibiotics
    Complex structure composed of "islands" of bacteria separated by channels—allow nutrients to reach bacteria

(continued)

Biofilms cause two types of medical problems
    Source of aerosolized bacteria (e.g., *L. pneumophila*)
    Biofilms form on body surfaces (e.g., plaque on teeth)
    Biofilms form on plastic tubing (e.g., catheters) or plastic implants (e.g., heart valves, prosthetic joints)

sIgA proteases
    Cleave IgA (IgA1, specifically) at hinge region
    Break links between bacteria and mucin

Iron acquisition mechanisms
    Iron concentrations low in human body—bound to lactoferrin, transferrin, etc.
    Siderophores (catechols and hydroxamates) chelate iron
        Siderophore-iron complexes taken up by bacterial cell
        Iron cleaved from complex inside cell
    Some bacteria remove iron directly from host proteins
    Bacterial toxins kill host cells—release iron
    Iron abstinence—bacteria do not require iron; use other ions

Invasion of host cells

Bacterial surface invasins cause actin rearrangements in nonphagocytic host cells

Host cells stimulated to engulf bacteria

In professional phagocytes, bacteria taken up in phagosome
    Prevent phagosome-lysosome fusion
    Escape from phagosome into cytoplasm
        Good source of nutrients
        Protection from antibodies, complement, and some antibiotics
    Cytotoxic T-cell response only defense left against intracellular bacteria

Intracellular residence in nonprofessional phagocytes
    Actin condenses on one end of bacteria—propels bacteria into adjoining cells
    Bacteria may travel along preexisting actin filaments
    Bacteria that invade mucosal cells stimulate release of cytokines and chemokines—initiate inflammatory response

Capsules
    Network of polymers covering surface of bacteria
    Usually polysaccharides, occasionally proteins
    Protect against complement activation and phagocyte-mediated killing
    Prevent formation of C3 convertase
        Do not bind serum protein B
        Have higher affinity for H than B—degradation of C3b by serum protein I
    Effective host response—antibodies that bind capsule

Resistance to nitric oxide

LPS modification
    Sialic acid bound to O antigen prevents formation of C3 convertase
    Changes in length of O-antigen side chains prevents MAC killing (serum resistance)

Mechanisms that prevent migration of phagocytes
    Enzyme that degrades C5a
    Toxic proteins that kill phagocytes, inhibit migration, or reduce oxidative burst

(*continued*)

SUMMARY OUTLINE (*continued*)

Surviving phagocytosis
  Escape phagosome
  Prevent phagosome-lysosome fusion
  Enzymes that detoxify reactive form of oxygen or prevent burst

Evading antibody response
  Alter pilus proteins
  Capsule that resembles host molecules
  Bacteria attach host proteins to surface

Opportunists—some but not all possess typical virulence factors
  Common cause of infections in hospitalized or cancer patients
  May be members of normal microbiota or soil bacteria
  Usually present in high numbers over long periods
  Take advantage of sites protected from immune system
  Often resistant to multiple antibiotics

QUESTIONS

Answers to the questions can be found in Appendix 2.

1. Different parts of the host defense system work together to eliminate invading bacteria. Give some examples of how virulence factors could work together to make a pathogen better able to cause infection.

2. It was stated in the text that virulence factors might have arisen long before animals appeared on Earth. Of course, this is just speculation, but what arguments could be made to support this statement?

3. If the statement made in question 2 above proves to be correct, what implications could it have for the number of bacteria able to cause human disease?

4. A bacterium has pili that allow it to attach to intestinal cells, after which it can invade the body. What type of vaccine could help to prevent infections by such a pathogen?

5. Some scientists are looking into the strategy of using passive immunization to control bacteria that are resistant to many antibiotics. How would such a strategy work? (Recall that passive immunization is the injection of antibodies into a patient's bloodstream.)

6. Do vaccines necessarily work better if they target virulence factors than if they target molecules not involved in virulence? Explain why or why not.

7. This chapter did not discuss the regulation of virulence genes, but such genes are usually regulated. Why would having regulated virulence genes be an advantage to a bacterium?

8. In the case of an opportunist, what traits substitute for virulence factors? Could these traits be called virulence factors?

9

Bacterial Exotoxins: Important but Still a Mystery

Exotoxins, Toxic Proteins Produced by Bacteria

Transparent Mechanisms, Mysterious Purposes

On the surface, diseases caused by bacterial toxins would seem to be simple and easily explained. The bacterium produces a protein or protein complex that is toxic to human cells (toxin) and the toxin causes the symptoms of disease. Because many toxins, especially those studied in the early days of toxin biology, are excreted into the extracellular fluid, they are easy to purify. Modern biochemical technology has made it increasingly easy to determine the human cell receptor for a toxin and to learn the mechanism by which the toxin exerts its effect. Toxins were the first virulence factors to be identified and studied in such detail. In fact, scientists who studied toxins were the first ones to propose the concept of virulence factor—a single molecule that can cause disease symptoms. Since those early days, a large number of bacterial toxins have been studied, and it is now clear that there is a staggering diversity in toxin properties and modes of action. Toxins have proved to be useful reagents for scientists studying mammalian cell biology. Some toxins have been made into effective vaccines; the vaccines against diphtheria, tetanus, and whooping cough contain toxins, treated to render them nontoxic, as important components. Toxins have even been used to treat conditions like crossed eyes and may help children with cerebral palsy to walk.

Many different bacteria produce toxins. Not all of these toxins are directed at human cells. For example, a toxin produced by *Bacillus thuringiensis,* the so-called BT toxin, is being used widely as an insecticide in agriculture because it attacks only a small subset of harmful insects, leaving beneficial insects alone. Given the widespread production of toxins by bacteria and the number of toxins that are associated with human and animal disease, it would seem to be a foregone conclusion that toxins are important for the survival and propagation of the bacterium that produces them. There are some cases in which this is true. For example, toxins that kill neutrophils and macrophages can protect bacteria from the phagocytic cells that might kill them. Toxins that kill human cells can also release iron stores or carbon sources that the bacteria need to survive and multiply.

131

Yet there are also many cases in which the toxin has no discernible benefit for the bacterium that produces it. A classic example of this is botulinum toxin, the toxin responsible for the symptoms of the disease botulism. **Botulinum toxin** is produced when the bacteria are growing in food. It is a toxin that attacks neurons, causing paralysis and death due to collapse of the respiratory system. However, the bacteria passing through the intestine have mostly formed spores, and the spores are in the intestinal tract, not the tissue. They do not colonize the intestinal tract and so are eliminated rapidly from the human body. By the time the toxin begins to exert its effects, the bacteria are on the way out. So, why does the gram-positive bacterium, *Clostridium botulinum,* produce botulinum toxin? No good explanation of its role has been forthcoming. To make matters worse, *C. botulinum* normally lives in the soil, so a few dead people would have no discernible impact on the normal lifestyle of the bacteria. There are a number of other examples of toxins that have no clear role in the biology and ecology of the bacteria that produce them. There is a lot about bacterial toxins that we still do not understand.

The plot thickens when one considers that in many bacteria, the toxin genes are not normal components of the bacterial genome. Instead, the toxin genes are carried on lysogenic bacteriophages, which integrate into the bacterial genome. Only a bacterium that has been infected with one of these phages produces the toxin (Figure 9–1). For example, at least one type of botulinum toxin is encoded on a bacteriophage, as is diphtheria toxin, which is produced by *Corynebacterium diphtheriae,* the cause of diphtheria. Some toxin genes are found on plasmids that may have come into the bacterium from other bacterial species. The solution to these mysteries undoubtedly lies in realizing that we are almost certainly viewing toxins from the wrong perspective when we assume that they are produced with the sole aim of damaging the human body. They may well prove to have roles in the physiology of bacteria and their viruses, possibly regulation of cellular or phage functions, with their impact on the human body being merely an accidental side effect of their normal action. If this notion is correct, however, why is it that most toxins are excreted from the bacterial cell that makes them, and why are they so often specific for certain types of human cells?

Characteristics and Nomenclature

A term that has been used to designate the protein toxins of bacteria is **exotoxin.** The word "exotoxin" was chosen to emphasize the fact that the toxins are excreted from the cell, in contrast to **endotoxin (LPS),** which is

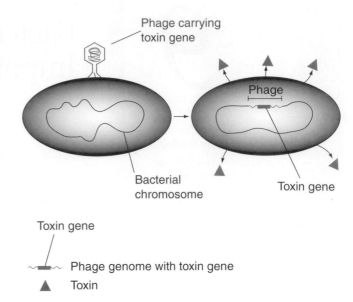

Figure 9–1 Lysogenic bacteriophages carry toxin genes that integrate into the bacterial chromosome, thus making the bacterium capable of producing the toxin.

embedded in the bacterial surface. "Exotoxin" has been falling out of use because some toxins are not excreted but rather accumulate inside the cell and are released by cell lysis. Others are injected directly into human cells, thereby bypassing the extracellular fluid entirely. For convenience, we will use the word toxin to mean the protein toxins of bacteria, whether excreted or not.

Bacterial toxins vary considerably not only in their activities but also in the host cell types they attack. Names given to different toxins reflect this diversity. Some toxins are named to indicate what type of host cells they attack. Toxins that attack a variety of cell types are called **cytotoxins,** whereas toxins that attack specific cell types can be named according to the cell type or organ affected, e.g., **neurotoxin, leukotoxin, hepatotoxin,** or **cardiotoxin.** Toxins can also be named for the bacterial species that produces them or for the disease with which they are associated. Examples are **cholera toxin,** produced by *Vibrio cholerae,* the cause of cholera; **Shiga toxin,** produced by *Shigella* species, a cause of bacterial dysentery; **diphtheria toxin,** produced by *C. diphtheriae,* the cause of diphtheria; and **tetanus toxin,** produced by *Clostridium tetani,* the cause of tetanus.

Toxins can be named for their activities, e.g., **adenylate cyclase** (a toxin produced by *Bordetella pertussis,* the cause of whooping cough) and **lecithinase** (a toxin produced by *Clostridium perfringens,* a cause of gangrene). Still other toxins are simply given letter designations, e.g., **exotoxin A** of *Pseudomonas aeruginosa.* Some toxins have more than one name. For example, a toxin produced by *Escherichia coli* O157:H7 ("killer *E.*

coli") has been called Shiga-like toxin because it is closely related to the Shiga toxin produced by *Shigella* species, or **verotoxin** because it is toxic for a tissue culture cell line called Vero. An exotoxin produced by *C. perfringens* is called both alpha-toxin and lecithinase. A notorious source of confusion for students first encountering toxin names is the term **enterotoxin.** This is a specific term that denotes protein toxins that cause diarrhea or vomiting, i.e., enteric symptoms, and should not be confused with endotoxin.

Recently, another layer has been added to the nomenclatural nightmare of toxin designations, although this one has the virtue of separating toxins based on the mechanism of action—types I to III toxins (Appendix 1). Normally, the first step in toxin action is binding to the target cell. This binding step may be followed by internalization of a portion of the toxin. **Type I toxins** bind to the host cell surface, but they are not translocated into the host cell. An example of this type of toxin is the **superantigens,** which bind to surface molecules on macrophages and T cells, forcing them into an unnatural interaction in which they produce copious amounts of toxic cytokines (see later section). **Type II toxins** are the ones that act on eukaryotic cell membranes (**phospholipases, pore-forming cytotoxins**) and exert their effect by destroying the integrity of the mammalian cell cytoplasmic membrane. **Type III toxins** are the **A-B toxins,** which have a binding region (B) that recognizes a specific receptor, a translocation region that introduces the A portion into the cell cytoplasm, and an A portion that acts on some intracellular protein.

Exotoxin Structure and Function

A-B TOXINS (TYPE III TOXINS). A-B toxins were the first toxins to be studied in detail at the molecular level, and so they have come to be the paradigm toxins. Only in more recent years have other types of toxins, such as the type I and type II toxins, come in for the same level of attention. Structures of two types of A-B toxins are illustrated in Figure 9–2. The simplest type of A-B toxin is synthesized as a single polypeptide, which has one binding (B) portion and one enzymatic (A) portion.

Frequently, the A and B portions of such toxins are separated during processing of the toxin by a proteolytic cleavage event, although the two portions remain connected by disulfide bonds (Figure 9–2). The disulfide bonds are broken when the A portion is internalized by the host cell, and this detachment of the A portion from the B portion is necessary for the A portion to become enzymatically active.

A more complex type of A-B toxin, the compound A-B toxin, has a binding (B) portion composed of multiple subunits, which are identical in some cases but not in others. The enzymatic (A) portion is a separate polypeptide (Figure 9–2). As with the simple A-B toxins, the A portion is attached to the rest of the toxin by disulfide bonds which are broken when the A subunit is internalized by the host cell.

Both the simple and compound A-B toxins bind to and enter host cells as illustrated in Figure 9–3. The B portion binds to a specific host cell surface molecule. Often, the molecule recognized by the B portion is the carbohydrate moiety of a host cell surface glycoprotein or glycolipid, but some B portions bind to proteins. The B portion determines the host cell specificity of the toxin. For example, a toxin whose B portion binds to a glycoprotein that is found only on the surfaces of neurons will function in the body as a neuron-specific toxin even though the A portion has the sort of activity that would enable it to kill other types of host cells if it could gain entry into their cytoplasm.

After the B portion attaches the toxin to the host cell, the A portion is translocated through the host cell membrane into the host cell's cytoplasm. In some cases, the bound toxin is taken up by endocytosis prior to internalization of the A portion into the cytoplasm. Acidification of the endocytic vacuole may play a role in translocation of such toxins by stimulating the separation of A and B portions and internalization of the A portion. For other toxins, endocytosis does not appear to be required; instead, the A portion translocates directly through the host cell's cytoplasmic membrane. Translocation is a complex process that is only beginning to be understood. One model posits that the B portion not only binds the host cell surface but also forms a pore

A Simple A-B toxin   **B** Compound A-B toxin

B portion

B portion

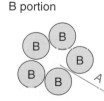

A portion

Figure 9–2 Structures of simple and compound A-B toxins. (**A**) Simple A-B toxins have one A subunit and one B subunit. (**B**) Compound A-B toxins have one A subunit and multiple B subunits.

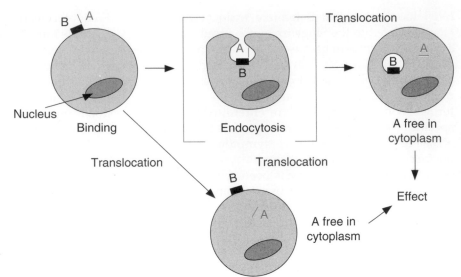

Figure 9–3 Binding and entry of A-B toxins into host cells. Endocytosis is involved in the internalization of some toxins but not others.

through which the A portion enters the host cell cytoplasm, but this model is somewhat controversial. Once the A portion has entered the host cell cytoplasm, it becomes enzymatically active and exerts its toxic effect. Incredibly enough, host cell proteins can aid in activation of the A portions of some toxins. The complex interactions between B portions and host cell receptors as well as those between A portions, the host cell proteins that activate them, and the targets they modify show how intricate the interplay of toxin and host cell actually is.

The A portions of A-B toxins may enter very different cell types, but most of them catalyze the same reaction: they remove the ADP-ribosyl group from NAD and attach it covalently to some host cell protein (Figure 9–4). **ADP-ribosylation** of the host cell protein either inactivates it or causes it to behave abnormally. The effect of this ADP-ribosylation step on the host cell depends on the role of the protein that is ADP-ribosylated. For example, the A portion of diphtheria toxin ADP-ribosylates **elongation factor-2,** a protein that plays an essential role in host cell protein synthesis. Thus, the effect of the A portion of diphtheria toxin is to kill the host cell by stopping protein synthesis. By contrast, cholera toxin A portion ADP-ribosylates a regulatory enzyme that controls cyclic AMP levels in the host cell. ADP-ribosylation keeps the enzyme from being turned off. This causes the host cell to lose control of ion flow and results in a massive loss of host cell water, which is seen macroscopically as diarrhea. Not all A-B toxins have A proteins that catalyze ADP-ribosylation of host cell proteins. Shiga toxin A subunit cleaves a host cell rRNA molecule. This results in a shutdown of protein synthesis, presumably because ribosomes containing the nicked molecule no longer carry out translation.

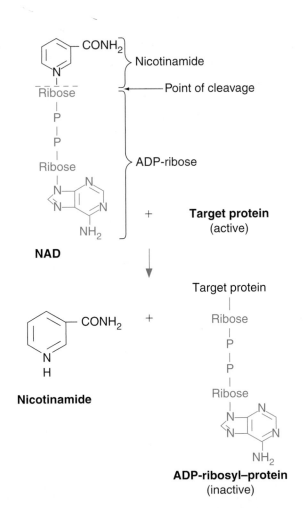

Figure 9–4 ADP-ribosylation of a target host protein. The ADP-ribosyl group is transferred from NAD (dashed line) and covalently attached to a host cell target protein.

MEMBRANE-DISRUPTING TOXINS (TYPE II TOXINS). A second class of exotoxins lyses host cells by disrupting the integrity of their cytoplasmic membranes. There are two different types of membrane-disrupting toxins (Figure 9–5). One is a protein that forms channels in the membrane. Since the osmotic strength of the host cell cytoplasm is higher than that of the surrounding environment, holes in the membrane trigger a sudden inrush of water into the cell. The cell swells and ruptures because the membrane is not strong enough to contain the sudden increase in fluid volume. The second type of membrane-disrupting toxin is an enzyme that compromises the integrity of membrane phospholipids. Such enzymes go by a variety of names, such as phospholipase, hemolysin, and cytotoxin, but they all act in the same way by destroying the integrity of host cell membrane lipids. Some phospholipases remove the charged head group from the lipid portion of the molecule. Because the charged head group stabilizes the lipid bilayer structure of the host cell cytoplasmic membrane, removal of this group destabilizes the membrane, and cell lysis occurs. Other phospholipases cleave at other sites on the phospholipid, but their effect is the same, to destabilize the host cell membrane. Membrane-active toxins are frequently called hemolysins because red blood cells are a convenient cell type to use as an assay system. However, such toxins are toxic for many types of cells because their target, the cell membrane, is part of all host cells. Membrane-disrupting toxins have at least two different roles in virulence. In some cases, their primary role appears to be killing of host cells, especially phagocytes. In others, they are used by invasive bacteria to escape from a phagosome and enter the host cell's cytoplasm.

SUPERANTIGENS (TYPE I TOXINS). An unusual type of bacterial toxin is a protein that exerts its effect by binding to the MHC class II of macrophages and the receptors on T cells that interact with the MHC. Normally, macrophages process protein antigens by cleaving them into peptides and displaying one of the resulting peptides in a complex with MHC class II on the macrophage surface (Figure 9–6). Only a few helper T cells will have receptors that recognize this particular MHC-peptide complex, so only a few T cells will be stimulated. Superantigens are not processed by proteolytic digestion but rather bind directly to MHC class II on the macrophage surface. Since they do this rather indiscriminately, many macrophages will have superantigen molecules bound to their surfaces. The superantigen also binds T-cell receptors, again rather indiscriminately, and thus forms many more macrophage-T helper cell pairs than would normally form (Figure 9–6). Thus, instead of a macrophage stimulating 1 in

10,000 T cells (the normal response to an antigen), as many as 1 in 5 T cells can be stimulated by the bridging action of superantigens. When helper T cells are stimulated by macrophages, one result is that the T cells release cytokines, especially IL-2. Superantigen action thus causes excessively high levels of IL-2 to circulate in the bloodstream, giving rise to a variety of symptoms, including nausea, vomiting, malaise, and fever. The role of superantigens in disease will be discussed in the chapters on staphylococcal and streptococcal infections. Superantigens are classified as type I toxins because they do not enter the cell.

Secretion and Excretion of Exotoxins

As already mentioned, many bacterial toxins are either excreted into the extracellular fluid or injected directly into the cytoplasm of host cells. In recent years, considerable information has been obtained about how these toxins are assembled and secreted, and just as there are types I to III toxins, there are types I to IV secretion systems, each with somewhat different properties (Appendix 1). One reason for interest in the process of toxin excretion is that a better knowledge of how toxins leave the bacterial cell might lead to the design of new types of vaccines or therapeutic agents that target the excretion machinery. In gram-positive bacteria, which have only a cytoplasmic membrane, exotoxins are presumably externalized by the general secretory pathway (Sec). Since little is known about protein secretion in gram-positive bacteria, however, this possibility remains speculative. Excretion systems that rely on the Sec-dependent secretion apparatus are called **type II secretion systems.** A and B portions of some gram-negative A-B toxins are processed by a similar route, first being secreted into the periplasm and then assembled there. Some of these toxins remain in the periplasm and are released only if the outer membrane is disrupted. In the host, where bacteria may encounter membrane-disrupting compounds, such as bile salts, leakage of toxins from the periplasm may occur readily. A-B toxins that are exported directly into the extracellular medium transit the outer membrane by a process that requires both the B portions of the exotoxin and some as-yet-uncharacterized bacterial cell components.

One of the most exciting recent developments in the toxin externalization area has been the discovery that there are bacteria that do not simply excrete their toxins into the extracellular fluid but rather inject their toxins directly into mammalian cells through a pore that opens between the bacterial cytoplasm and the host cell cytoplasm. Such secretion systems are called **type III secretion systems.** This type of secretion system will be

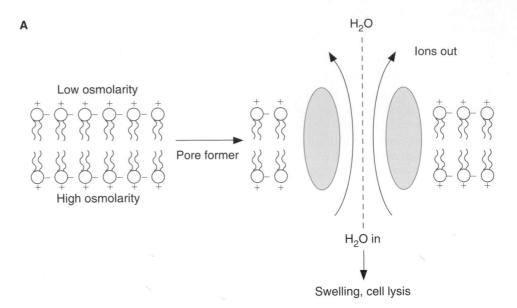

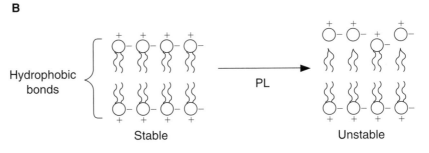

Figure 9–5 Two kinds of membrane-disrupting cyto-toxins (also called hemolysins). (**A**) A channel-forming (pore-forming) type of protein (e.g., alpha-toxin of *Staphylococcus aureus*) inserts itself into the host cell membrane and makes an open channel (pore). Formation of multiple pores causes leakage of cell interior components and an inrush of water, leading to lysis. (**B**) A phospholipid-hydrolyzing (phospholipase) kind of membrane-disrupting toxin removes the polar head group, as shown here, or otherwise compromises the phospholipid structure, destabilizing the membrane and causing the host cell to lyse.

Normal antigen presentation   **Action of superantigens**

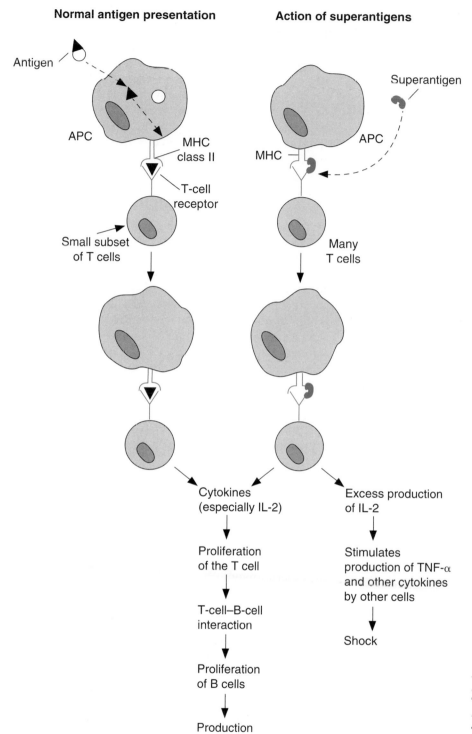

Figure 9–6 Normal interaction of a macrophage or other APC and a T-helper cell (left) compared with the interaction of an APC and a T cell mediated by superantigens (right).

described in more detail in chapter 13. First discovered in *Yersinia pestis,* the cause of plague, this mechanism of toxin delivery has proved to be surprisingly ubiquitous. The importance of this secretion strategy becomes clear when one thinks of the usual protective immune response to toxins: production of antitoxin antibodies that

prevent the toxin from binding to its target cell type. Clearly, if the toxin is injected directly into the host cell, such a protective response becomes ineffective because the toxin is never truly extracellular.

Pore-forming cytotoxins are not processed by the normal secretion system. Instead, a set of specialized proteins, often encoded in the same gene cluster as the toxin itself, mediate excretion of the toxin, possibly through a pore that spans the outer and cytoplasmic membrane. The characteristics of this type of excretion system, known as **type I secretion systems,** are currently being studied. **Type IV secretion systems,** usually associated with the conjugal transfer of DNA, can also mediate toxin excretion (see Appendix 1).

Examples of Diseases Caused by Toxins

The best way to understand how toxins participate in the disease process is to examine diseases in which toxins are the primary virulence factor. We provide here some examples of toxin-mediated diseases. Many of these examples also illustrate the continuing mystery of why bacteria produce toxins in the first place.

Diphtheria

Diphtheria is caused by *C. diphtheriae,* a gram-positive, non-spore-forming, nonmotile, aerobic rod that has a distinctive club-shaped appearance. Diphtheria is normally a disease of children and can be fatal if not treated. Diphtheria is no longer a serious public health problem in developed countries because infants are routinely vaccinated against it, but diphtheria remains a major cause of childhood death worldwide. The diphtheria vaccine is a toxoided version of diphtheria toxin, the "D" in the trivalent DTP vaccine. This vaccine has few side effects and confers long-term protection against diphtheria. With periodic booster shots, the vaccine gives life-long immunity. Unfortunately, there are still many countries where routine vaccination against diphtheria is not feasible for economic reasons. In these countries, diphtheria remains a significant cause of disease and death in infants and children. Recently, we have been reminded forcibly that diphtheria can also kill adults (Box 9–1).

Diphtheria toxin is one of the best-studied bacterial toxins and thus serves as a model for understanding how toxins act. In fact, diphtheria provided the first paradigm for a disease in which the symptoms could be explained by the action of a single molecule, diphtheria toxin. This helped to give rise to the concept of "virulence factor" and to usher in the new era of molecular analysis of bacterial disease. From that time to the present day, investigations of diphtheria toxin have continued to produce important new insights into toxin structure, function, and interaction with host cells. Also, there has long been an interest in using diphtheria toxin for targeted killing of tumor cells or, more recently, HIV-infected cells. This approach continues to attract interest despite the fact that no successful version of this therapy has yet been introduced at the clinical level.

Diphtheria starts with colonization of the throat by *C. diphtheriae.* The bacteria are acquired by inhalation of aerosols from an infected person or an asymptomatic carrier. Humans are the only known reservoir of *C. diphtheriae.* The first symptoms are relatively nonspecific: malaise, low-grade fever, sore throat, and loss of appetite. As the bacterial colonization progresses, a grayish membrane begins to form in the throat and may extend into the lung. The membrane, called a **pseudomembrane,** consists of fibrin, bacteria, and inflammatory cells. The pseudomembrane adheres to underlying tissue, and the underlying tissue bleeds when attempts are made to remove the pseudomembrane. This is a useful sign for diagnosing diphtheria, because pseudomembranes caused by other infectious agents are nonadherent. Also, the presence of the pseudomembrane and the bleeding of underlying tissue attest to the fact that bacterial colonization of the throat is causing considerable damage to the mucosal cells. The most serious form of the disease is characterized by irregular heartbeat, difficulty in swallowing, stupor, coma, and, finally, death. These symptoms indicate that damage to interior organs is also occurring. Although the throat colonization form of diphtheria is the most common, *C. diphtheriae* can also cause skin infections, and such infections are frequently seen in countries where diphtheria is endemic.

A potent toxin (diphtheria toxin) is produced by *C. diphtheriae* growing in the throat, and this toxin causes the symptoms of diphtheria. The toxin enters the bloodstream, but the bacteria remain in the throat; no bacteria are found in the blood. *C. diphtheriae* can still colonize the throats of people who have been immunized against diphtheria or who have become immune because of natural exposure to the bacteria. No pseudomembrane develops in the throats of immune people who are colonized by the bacteria. For this reason, formation of the pseudomembrane is presumed to result from killing of mucosal cells by diphtheria toxin. It is interesting that in people immunized against diphtheria, the colonizing strain of *C. diphtheriae* is usually not a toxin producer. This suggests that susceptible people are the main reservoir for the toxin-producing strains and that immunity somehow makes the toxin production counterproductive for the bacteria.

Processing of diphtheria toxin occurs in two steps. The translated form of diphtheria toxin contains a leader region that is removed by proteolytic nicking during secretion of the toxin through the cytoplasmic membrane and into the extracellular fluid, producing a 58.3-kDa secreted polypeptide. After secretion, this polypeptide is further cleaved by proteolytic nicking

BOX 9–1   Diphtheria as a Disease of Adults

In textbooks, diphtheria is generally described as a disease of children. This age distribution reflects the fact that in countries where there is no vaccination program, most people who survive infancy and childhood have acquired immunity to the disease. Under some circumstances, however, diphtheria can be a disease of adults. For example, during the diphtheria epidemics that occurred in the early days of European settlement of the Americas, both the colonists and the natives had a high adult mortality rate. George Washington is thought to have died of diphtheria at the age of 67. If most of the members of the population have had no prior exposure to diphtheria, adults do not have the protective immunity acquired by experiencing the disease in childhood. Diphtheria appears to have been a completely new disease in the Americas. Surprisingly, at least some of the European settlers also did not have protective immunity despite the fact that diphtheria was widespread in Europe.

An unpleasant reminder that diphtheria can kill adults occurred much more recently when diphtheria made an unexpected appearance during the 1990s in the former Soviet Union, causing an epidemic in which many of the victims were adults. This epidemic illustrates another set of circumstances that can shift the age range of the disease. As the former Soviet Union began to break up after the end of the cold war, and civil strife between various ethnic and religious groups became all too common, the public health programs that had been in place in previous years, including vaccination programs, were disrupted. Also, defective lots of the vaccine were probably being used even in the days before the breakdown of the Soviet Union.

The result was that many adults were not immune and were no longer protected by the herd immunity conferred by a population of vaccinated children. In some areas the fatality rate was as high for adults as for children. It would be nice to be able to report that this common enemy caused the various warring factions within the former Soviet Union to forget their national and ethnic rivalries as they struggled against a nonhuman foe, but unfortunately this did not occur. Disease-causing bacteria thrive on human stupidity.

Source: C. R. Vitek and M. Wharton. 1998. Diphtheria in the former Soviet Union: reemergence of a pandemic disease. *Emerg. Infect. Dis.* **4**:539–550.

---

into an A chain and a B chain, which remain joined by a disulfide bond (Figure 9–7). (Scientists who work on different toxins use different terms for toxin components. In the preceding section, we used the terms A and B portions to denote components of the A-B toxins. For some toxins, these are called A and B chains or A and B subunits. These terms can be used interchangeably, and whichever one is chosen by scientists working on a particular toxin has more to do with the history of the field than any real distinctions between them.)

The steps involved in binding, endocytic uptake, and translocation of the toxin are shown schematically in Figure 9–8. A domain on the B chain, called the **R domain,** binds a protein receptor on the host cell surface. This receptor has been identified as **heparin-binding epidermal growth factor (HB-EGF) precursor.** Epidermal growth factors of various types are important signals for cell growth and differentiation. Thus, it is not surprising that the receptor for the B chain of diphtheria toxin is found on so many different cell types and that

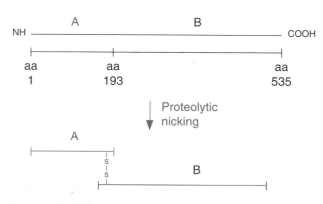

Figure 9–7 Proteolytic nicking of the secreted form of diphtheria toxin to form the A chain and B chain.

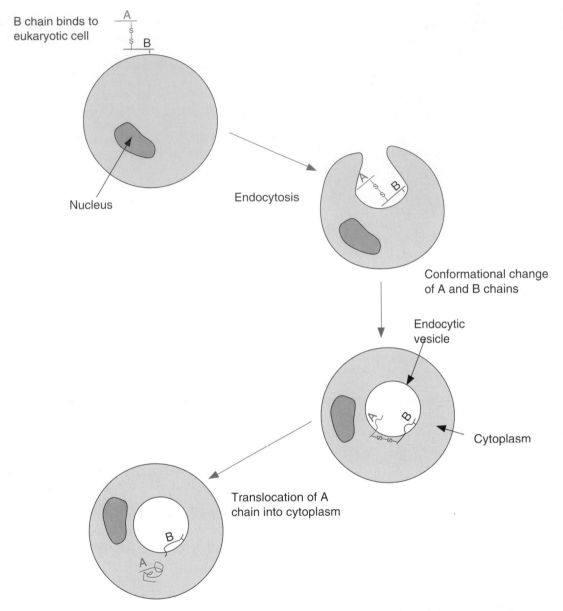

B chain binds to eukaryotic cell

Nucleus

Endocytosis

Conformational change
of A and B chains

Endocytic
vesicle

Cytoplasm

Translocation of A
chain into cytoplasm

Figure 9–8   Binding, endocytic uptake, and translocation of diphtheria toxin by eukaryotic cells.

its abundance varies so much from one cell type to another. A model for the structure of HB-EGF in the host cell membrane, which is based on the deduced amino acid sequence of the cloned gene, is shown in Figure 9–9. Now that the identity of the toxin receptor is known, it will be possible to investigate further the complex interaction that occurs between the B chain and its receptor and how this affects the interaction between the toxin and the cell membrane during the translocation step.

After the toxin has bound to the host cell receptor, the host cell takes up the toxin in an endocytic vesicle.

Endocytosis is an important step in toxin action because the decrease in pH that occurs in the endocytic vesicle after it is formed makes the translocation process possible. In the endocytic vesicle, as the pH drops to around 5, acidic amino acids are protonated, making them less hydrophilic. The change in charge distribution is associated with a change in the conformation of the toxin and also allows partial unfolding of both the A and B chains, exposing hydrophobic regions that are normally found in the interior of the toxin. The exposed hydrophobic regions, together with stretches of protonated acidic residues, allow regions of both the A and B

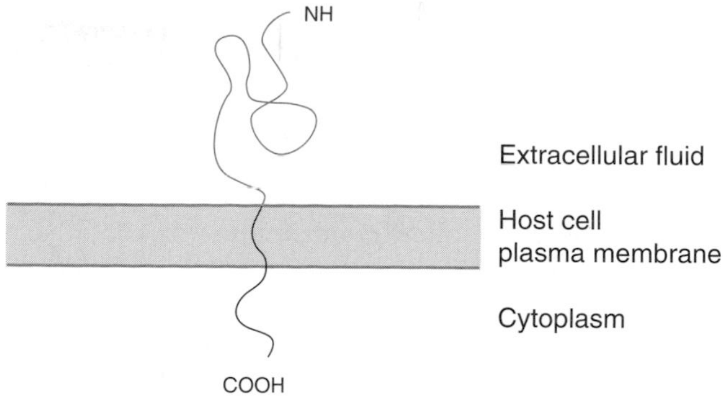

Figure 9–9 Proposed model for insertion of HB-EGF, the receptor recognized by the toxin B chain, in the host cell membrane.

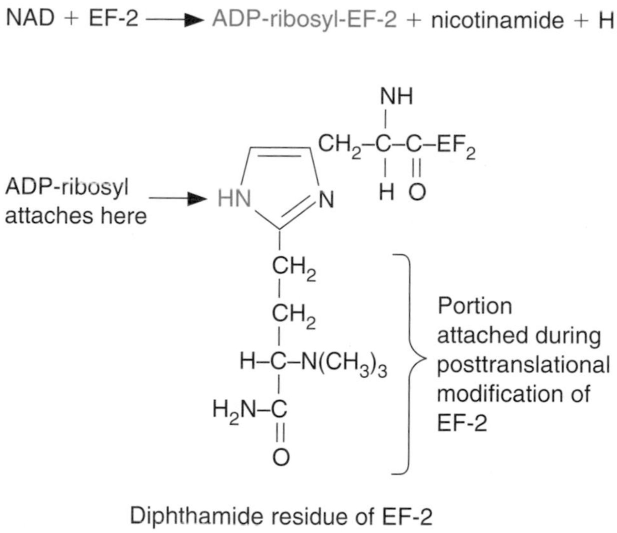

$$NAD + EF\text{-}2 \longrightarrow ADP\text{-}ribosyl\text{-}EF\text{-}2 + nicotinamide + H^+$$

Diphthamide residue of EF-2

Figure 9–10 Reaction catalyzed by the A chain of diphtheria toxin and the structure of diphthamide, the modified histidine residue of EF-2 that is ADP-ribosylated.

chains to insert into the vesicle membrane. The current model posits that this partial unfolding of the A and B chains inserts portions of both chains through the membrane and exposes the A chain on the cytoplasmic side. Reduction of the disulfide bond that joins the A and B chains then frees the A chain, releasing it into the cytoplasm.

In the cytoplasm, the A chain catalyzes the ADP-ribosylation of elongation factor 2 (EF-2), an essential factor in the protein synthesis machinery of eukaryotic cells (Figure 9–10). EF-2 participates in the elongation step of translation. Attachment of an ADP-ribosyl group to EF-2 renders it inactive. A single molecule of A chain can ADP-ribosylate enough copies of EF-2 to halt protein synthesis completely and irreversibly. Ultimately, this causes the death of the cell. Attachment of the ADP-ribosyl group occurs at an unusual derivative of histidine, called **diphthamide:** (3-carboxyamido-3(trimethylamino)propyl) histidine. The modification of this particular histidine residue to form diphthamide occurs after EF-2 is translated and occurs in all types of eukaryotic cells. The role of diphthamide is not known, but the existence of this unusual form of histidine in EF-2 but not in other cellular proteins explains why the diphtheria toxin A chain specifically inactivates EF-2.

Diphtheria toxin is an extremely potent toxin. A single molecule of A chain can kill a eukaryotic cell. Moreover, the A chain is uniformly effective in ADP-ribosylating EF-2 of all types of mammalian cells. Despite this universality of action, different mammalian cell lines differ considerably in their susceptibility to killing by exogenously added diphtheria toxin. Differences in susceptibility of different cell lines can be explained by differences in the number of toxin receptors on the cell surface. These differences also suggest why the disease has its most drastic effects on heart and nerve cells, whose surfaces contain high concentrations of the molecule bound by the B chain. Preferential attack of these tissues by the toxin produces heart failure and neurological symptoms (e.g., difficulty in swallowing), which are symptoms of the severe form of the disease.

The gene encoding diphtheria toxin is carried on a group of related **lysogenic bacteriophages (β-phage and ω-phage).** Only strains infected with these phages produce the toxin. The fact that β- and ω-phages can be induced to become lytic facilitated cloning of the toxin gene because isolation of phage DNA considerably narrowed the search for the DNA segment carrying the gene. Also, another bacteriophage was found that was closely related to β- and ω-phages but did not encode the toxin (**γ-phage**). Comparison of the three phages helped to locate the toxin gene.

Production of toxin by lysogenized *C. diphtheriae* is enhanced considerably when the bacteria are grown in low-iron medium. A repressor protein called **DtxR (diphtheria toxin regulation),** which is related to an iron regulation protein of *E. coli* called **Fur (Fe uptake repressor),** mediates regulation. The fact that synthesis of the toxin is enhanced when iron levels are low has led to the suggestion that the purpose of diphtheria toxin may be to kill host cells and thus release iron for use by the bacteria. The only problem with this explanation is that strains that do not produce toxin colonize the human throat as well as toxin-producing strains.

In many diseases, in which exotoxins are either solely responsible for, or make a major contribution to, the symptoms of the disease, antibodies to the exotoxin provide effective protection against the disease. Binding of antibodies to the B portion of the toxin physically interferes with binding of the toxin to its target cell and thus prevents the toxin from exerting its toxic activity. Before any detailed information was available about toxin structures and mechanisms of action, vaccines were created by a hit-or-miss approach involving random genetic mutations, chemical modification, or heat treatment of a toxin to render it nontoxic but still capable of eliciting antibodies that would bind and neutralize the toxin. Such preparations are called **toxoids** (chapter 7). The highly effective vaccines against diphtheria and tetanus are products of this type of approach. Today, it is possible to design toxoid vaccines in a more rational way. For example, the fact that the action of A-B toxins is dependent on binding of the B region to a host cell receptor molecule suggests that B portions, which are not toxic by themselves, would be good vaccine candidates.

Botulism and Tetanus

BOTULISM. Botulism is not an infection but an intoxication. That is, the bacteria do not colonize the human body. Rather, symptoms are caused by ingestion of a toxin, botulinum toxin, that is produced by the gram-positive sporeformer *C. botulinum* (Figure 9–11). *C. botulinum* normally grows in soil or in lake sediments. Spores of *C. botulinum* have been found in soil samples taken from all parts of the United States and are probably widely distributed in all parts of the world. Spores are also found on plants growing in feces-contaminated soil. Since bees moving from plant to plant accumulate spores along with pollen, honey frequently contains *C. botulinum* spores. The concentration of spores in honey is not high (usually fewer than seven spores per 25 g) but can be problematic for infants (see below). Contamination of human foods by *C. botulinum* spores and consequent ingestion of the spores is a common occurrence, but simple ingestion of spores is generally not sufficient to cause botulism. Germination of ingested spores may occur, especially in the colon, but *C. botulinum* is unable to compete with the resident microbiota of the adult colon and thus does not grow to high enough concentrations in the colon to cause disease.

Botulism occurs if spores have the chance to germinate in foods, leading to bacterial growth and production of botulinum toxin. Fortunately, *C. botulinum* does not grow readily in most foods. It is an obligate anaerobe, and most foods contain enough dissolved oxygen to discourage germination of the spores and growth of the bacteria. Growth is most likely to occur in foods, such as home-canned foods, that have been heated and

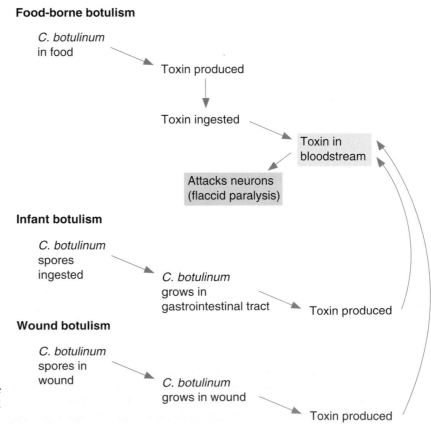

Figure 9–11 Comparison of food-borne botulism, infant botulism, and wound botulism.

then cooled and stored for long periods at room temperature. Heating reduces the solubility of oxygen, and most of the dissolved oxygen is lost. When the food is cooled, some oxygen redissolves, but lower regions can remain anaerobic enough to support the growth of *C. botulinum*.

Many cases of botulism have been associated with consumption of home-canned foods. Temperatures achievable by boiling are not high enough to kill *C. botulinum* spores. This is why pressure cookers are used to sterilize canned foods. In home canning, however, the temperature in the pressure cooker sometimes does not reach the level required to kill spores, and surviving spores can germinate in the cooled canned food. Since canned foods are prepared in jars that are filled to the top and sealed before they are cooled, the environment in the sealed jars can be quite anaerobic. Even if botulinum toxin is produced in a jar of canned food, botulism need not result, because boiling the canned food for 10–15 minutes before eating it inactivates the toxin. Thus, most cases of botulism are associated with consumption of canned food without prior heating.

Ingested botulinum toxin is absorbed from the intestine and enters the bloodstream. It is specific for neurons and attacks peripheral nerve endings. Inside the neuron, the toxin blocks neurotransmitter release. Thus, nerve impulses cannot be transmitted, and muscles connected to the nerves are not stimulated. The result is a generalized flaccid paralysis. Symptoms begin to appear 4 to 36 h after ingestion of contaminated food. The rapidity with which symptoms appear and the severity of the symptoms are directly proportional to the amount of toxin ingested. Initial symptoms include nausea and vomiting, as well as headache, double vision, slurred speech, and other neurological symptoms. Death occurs if the general flaccid paralysis is severe enough to interfere with breathing and heart function. Once botulinum toxin has bound to the surface of a neuron and entered it, external intervention becomes useless. Some nerve regeneration occurs if the affected person survives the initial onslaught of toxin, but people who survive an episode of botulism frequently sustain at least some irreversible neurological damage.

Although most cases of botulism are due to ingestion of preformed toxin, two rare forms of botulism actually involve transient colonization of the body by the bacteria, followed by toxin production: **infant botulism** and **wound botulism** (Figure 9–11). Infants less than 1 year old have not yet developed a complete colonic microbiota. Since the colon provides an anaerobic environment, *C. botulinum* can sometimes colonize the infant colon and produce a disease called infant botulism. The symptoms of infant botulism are essentially the same as those of food-borne botulism, except that nau-

sea and vomiting are not seen, and constipation, which is not a symptom of botulism, is common. Since toxin produced in the colon is absorbed more slowly than toxin passing through the stomach, infant botulism has a slower progression than food-borne botulism, but death can still occur.

C. botulinum can also colonize a deep wound, because the environment of such a wound is anaerobic enough to allow *C. botulinum* to grow (Figure 9–11). A wound becomes anaerobic because tissue destruction cuts off the blood supply to the area, and residual oxygen is rapidly depleted by body cells. Botulinum toxin leaks into the blood from the wound area and causes a disease called wound botulism, which has symptoms similar to those of food-borne botulism. Wound botulism is normally quite rare and is most often seen in wartime. The few civilian cases have occurred in people with severe, deep wounds that were heavily contaminated with soil. Wound botulism should be differentiated from tetanus, a toxin-associated disease caused by another *Clostridium* species, *C. tetani*.

BOTULINUM TOXIN. *C. botulinum* actually produces three toxins, botulinum toxin (also called **botox**), **C2 toxin,** and **C3 toxin.** Before this was understood, activities such as ADP-ribosylation, which is actually an activity of the C2 and C3 toxins, were attributed to botulinum toxin, because preparations of botulinum toxin were contaminated with these other toxins. Botulinum toxin is the only one of these three toxins that acts on neurons and is unquestionably the toxin responsible for the symptoms of the disease. It is also much more toxic than the other two toxins (50% lethal dose [LD_{50}] for mice of <0.01 ng, compared with LD_{50} values in excess of 45 ng for the other toxins). There are at least seven different serotypes of botulinum toxin (designated A, B, C, D, E, F, and G). Types A and B are the ones most commonly associated with human disease in the United States.

The specificity of botulinum toxin for peripheral neurons arises both from the specificity of toxin binding (probably to a sialic acid-containing glycoprotein or glycolipid found only on the neurons) and from the neuron-specific action of the toxin. The bound toxin is internalized and inhibits release of **acetylcholine,** a neurotransmitter (Figure 9–12). Botulinum toxin is a large protein (150 kDa) that is part of an even larger complex containing other proteins beside the toxin. The complex is called **progenitor toxin,** and the toxin itself is called **derivative toxin.** Derivative toxin is less effective than progenitor toxin when given orally but is as active as progenitor toxin when injected. This has led to the suggestion that the nontoxic components of progenitor toxin help to protect the derivative toxin from stom-

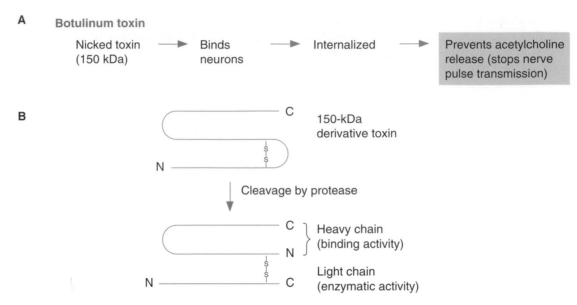

A　Botulinum toxin

Nicked toxin　⟶　Binds　⟶　Internalized　⟶　Prevents acetylcholine
(150 kDa)　　　　　neurons　　　　　　　　　　　　release (stops nerve
　　　　　　　　　　　　　　　　　　　　　　　　　　pulse transmission)

B

150-kDa
derivative toxin

Cleavage by protease

Heavy chain
(binding activity)

Light chain
(enzymatic activity)

Figure 9–12　Botulinum toxin. (**A**) Action of botulinum toxin. (**B**) Structure and processing of botulinum toxin.

ach acid and proteases. These nontoxic components could also help the toxin bind to and transit the intestinal mucosal surface. Active derivative toxin consists of two protein subunits, heavy chain (100 kDa) and light chain (50 kDa), which are connected by a disulfide bridge (Figure 9–12). Derivative toxin is originally synthesized and secreted from the bacteria as a single 150-kDa protein, which is inactive.

Proteolytic clipping of the protein to form the derivative toxin is needed for toxic activity. The proteolytic cleavage is carried out either by proteases produced by the clostridia or by gastric proteases. The binding site of the toxin is located near the carboxy terminus of the heavy chain. The amino terminus of the heavy chain is thought to form a channel in the neuronal membrane, allowing the light chain to enter the cell.

Not all strains of *C. botulinum* produce botulinum toxin. This is explained by the finding that at least in the case of types C and D toxins, the toxin gene is carried on a temperate bacteriophage. Thus, only strains lysogenized by the phage are toxin producers. Production of toxin by type G strains is correlated with the presence of an 81-MDa plasmid, but the location of the toxin on the plasmid has not been conclusively proved. Thus, type G toxin may be plasmid encoded. It is not known whether toxin types A and B are encoded on a phage or some other mobile element.

TETANUS.　Tetanus is a disease caused by another clostridium, *C. tetani*. Tetanus is also known as "lockjaw" because people with tetanus suffer muscle spasms that can lock the jaws together. In one sense, tetanus is the opposite of botulism, because whereas in botulism the

patient suffers a flaccid paralysis, in tetanus, the patient develops a spastic paralysis, in which the muscles contract and do not relax. Tetanus starts when the bacteria colonize a deep puncture wound that becomes anoxic owing to tissue damage in the area. *C. tetani*, an obligate anaerobe, can grow under these conditions and produces tetanus toxin, which diffuses away from the wound site and enters the bloodstream. The toxin acts on neurons that control the neural feedback that tells flexed muscles to relax after having performed a task. In effect, it prevents these neurons from signaling the relaxation after a muscle contraction. Hence, the spastic paralysis that characterizes tetanus.

Tetanus was never a very common disease in the developed world, but it was much feared because of its high fatality rate and gruesome symptoms. Victims develop painfully bowed spines, clenched arm and leg muscles, and locked jaws. Tetanus is almost invariably fatal. In developed countries today, tetanus is virtually unknown because of the tetanus vaccine (the "T" in DTP). Worldwide, tetanus remains a major cause of infant deaths. In any listing of the top killers of infants in the developing world, infant tetanus is right up there in the top 15, perhaps not so common as HIV or diarrheal disease but still pervasive. The custom in many parts of the world of packing the umbilical stump of a newborn with cattle dung is doubtless the major cause of this grim statistic. Possibly, animal dung prevents some other condition, but animal dung is also a prime source of *C. tetani*.

DIFFERENT TOXINS, SAME MECHANISM.　For years, botulism and tetanus were treated as completely different diseases, even though the toxins responsible for the symptoms are both neurotoxins. Thus, it came as a surprise when examination of the deduced amino acid sequences of the two toxin genes revealed that the two proteins share a considerable amount of sequence similarity. In fact, some peptides from tetanus toxin elicit antibodies that cross-react with botulinum toxin, another indication of similarity. Moreover, both toxins share amino acid sequence similarity with zinc-requiring endopeptidases. Ultimately, this insight from sequence gazing led to the discovery that both toxins are **zinc-requiring endopeptidases** that cleave a set of proteins called **synaptobrevins.** Synaptobrevins are found in synaptic vesicles of neurons, the vesicles responsible for release of neurotransmitters and inhibitory mediators.

If the two toxins have exactly the same mode of action, how could these two toxins cause such different effects (flaccid paralysis and spastic paralysis)? The answer appears to lie in the different cell specificities of the binding regions of the two toxins. Botulinum toxin targets peripheral neurons. If tetanus toxin is administered so that it only acts locally on peripheral nerves, it too causes flaccid paralysis. In high enough quantities and especially if it enters the circulation, however, tetanus toxin acts on the central nervous system and causes spastic paralysis. There is still not a satisfactory explanation for the fact that botulinum toxin seems to affect neurotransmitter release whereas different types of neuroactive compounds are affected by tetanus toxin. This difference may disappear as more is understood about how synaptic vesicles carrying these different types of neuroactive compounds are targeted and mobilized in neurons.

The discovery of the common target of these two toxins illustrates a common theme in toxin research—bacterial toxins can become powerful tools for the study of mammalian cell function. The finding that tetanus and botulinum toxins cleave synaptobrevins excited researchers interested in neurobiology because the function of the synaptobrevins had previously been unknown. Tetanus and botulinum toxins provide a new reagent that may help to understand how these proteins function. Surprisingly, another group of people to become interested in these toxins, especially botulinum toxin, was the group of scientists interested in treating certain conditions previously treated surgically (Box 9–2).

Wound Infections

In tetanus, the bacteria do little damage to the tissue in which they are dividing, but this is not generally true for bacteria that cause wound infections. Many of the bacteria that cause wound infections cause considerable damage as they proliferate in the wounded tissue. Pus, redness, pain, and tissue destruction are the result. Bacteria can cause these symptoms simply by eliciting an inflammatory response, but the ones that do the most damage are the ones that contribute directly to the destruction. An extreme form of wound infection is **gangrene,** caused by *C. perfringens*. These bacteria produce an expanding zone of dead tissue. The skin blackens and may appear swollen and cracked, as if the area had been cooked. The damage can be so severe that the limb has to be amputated. Tissue damage is caused in part by a toxin called **alpha-toxin,** which hydrolyzes the lipid lecithin in mammalian cell membranes. If the toxin enters the bloodstream, it can cause damage to organs such as the kidney.

During the 1990s, there were lurid tales about "the bacterium that ate my face." The disease was a wound infection caused by *Streptococcus pyogenes*. In some people, tissue damage was severe. In fact, this kind of streptococcal infection has been called **streptococcal gangrene.** The proper name is **necrotizing fasciitis.** *S. pyogenes* produces a variety of hydrolytic enzymes that can degrade extracellular matrix proteins and damage cell membranes. In this case, a superantigen is also suspected to be a contributor to the damage.

The toxins that disrupt bacterial membranes have a clear purpose. In the case of *C. perfringens* alpha-toxin, the toxin not only releases nutrients for the bacteria to utilize but it also creates a larger and larger area of dead tissue. Dead tissue is anoxic, an important feature for an obligate anaerobe such as *C. perfringens*. Moreover, antibiotics and the cells of the host defenses do not move into dead tissue because there is no longer a blood supply. Thus, the dead tissue becomes a protective haven for the bacteria.

To treat gangrene, it is first necessary to remove the dead tissue. Normally, this is done surgically, but surgical debridement has the disadvantage that it creates new tissue damage in the area around the excised tissue. Some physicians have turned to the lowly and despised maggot for help. Maggots eat only dead tissue and do not cause further tissue damage. Of course, family members may not like to enter a modern hospital only to see maggots swarming over Uncle Ted's wound. So a covering is supplied that keeps the maggots in place and hides them from view. After the dead tissue is removed, other treatments can be used to eliminate the remaining bacteria. One treatment is hyperbaric oxygen treatment, in which the patient is placed in a chamber that contains an atmosphere that has a higher concentration of oxygen than air. The high oxygen concentration has two effects: it helps to kill the anaerobic

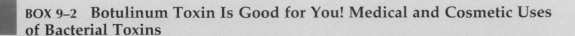

BOX 9–2 Botulinum Toxin Is Good for You! Medical and Cosmetic Uses of Bacterial Toxins

The term "toxin" has very negative connotations. Yet, scientists have managed to find beneficial uses for bacterial toxins. Since toxins often manipulate eukaryotic cell pathways that are important for reacting to external stimuli or for intracellular communication, eukaryotic cell biologists have found certain toxins to be very useful for elucidating regulatory pathways. By poisoning certain pathways, toxins allow biologists to interrupt these pathways biochemically and thereby study the importance of particular steps in the pathway for cellular functions. Studies of this type have provided much information about the functioning of eukaryotic cells, information that should prove useful in a variety of medical areas.

Several years ago, the white knight of toxin-based therapies was diphtheria toxin, and many articles appeared touting numerous innovative applications of this toxin to cure everything from HIV to cancer. These applications are still in the developmental phase, but another toxin has rushed in to fill this void: botulinum toxin. For a number of years, botulinum toxin has been used experimentally to treat painful, disabling muscle spasms of various types (dystonias). Examples of such dystonias are strabismus (crossed eyes) and painful spasms of the face and neck. Recently, the Food and Drug Administration has approved botulinum toxin therapy as a general therapy for dystonias. Dystonias were once thought to be psychosomatic in origin, but attempts to treat them using various forms of psychotherapy were unsuccessful. Their cause is still not known. Until the advent of botulinum toxin therapy, the only therapy that worked was surgical destruction of the nerve endings in the area affected by the spasms. Surgical treatment was expensive, dangerous, and not invariably successful.

Botulinum toxin therapy is generally acknowledged to be far superior to surgical destruction of nerve endings and thus represents the first successful therapy for dystonias. Since botulinum toxin prevents transmission of nerve impulses, small injections of toxin in the affected area counter the spasms and give temporary relief. The injections must be repeated at intervals, because some regeneration of the nerve endings occurs. Reportedly, attempts are currently under way to genetically engineer botulinum toxin to make it more effective at killing neurons so that a one-shot therapy with permanent effects will be feasible.

Botulinum toxin has also found favor with the cosmetic surgeons who are using it to reduce the depth of wrinkles. More recently, botulinum toxin has been administered to cerebral palsy patients in an effort to help them control the movement of their limbs. Although this use of botulinum toxin is still in the experimental phase, results are encouraging. So, the next time you read an article about bioterrorists threatening to dump botulinum toxin into your water supply remember that botulinum toxin can also be your friend.

Sources: L. L. Simpson. 1999. Botulinum toxin: potent poison, potent medicine. *Hosp. Pract.* **23**:87–91; Yahoo! Health News. 1999. Botulinum toxin helps cerebral palsy patients walk. April 19, 1999. http://www.yahoo.com.

---

bacteria still in the wound, and it decreases the ability of surviving bacteria to produce alpha-toxin.

S. pyogenes is a facultative bacterium, so it has no need for anoxic tissue, but it can use the complex array of nutrients made available by the destruction of host cells. Also, the bacteria in dead tissue are protected from the host's defense systems.

Toxins and Shock

In the 1970s a new and frightening disease appeared in young women. The disease was called toxic shock syndrome because the afflicted women developed shock-like symptoms; some of the women died. As more was learned about **toxic shock syndrome,** it became clear that the shock was caused not by gram-negative or gram-positive bacteria in the bloodstream but by a toxin that proved to be a superantigen. The toxin was produced by the gram-positive bacterium *S. aureus*. The bacteria first colonized the vagina and produced the toxin there. The toxin entered the bloodstream and spread throughout the body. The reason the disease was seen only in women was that it was associated with a type of superabsorbent tampon that could be left in place for an extended period of time. The bacteria were growing in the tampon, where conditions were conducive to toxin production. Not all strains of *S. aureus* produce this toxin, and this is one of the reasons there were not more cases of the disease. The tampons were taken off the market, and cases of toxic shock syndrome decreased significantly.

Toxic shock syndrome is still of interest, however, because it shows that protein toxins can cause a type of shock that is very like the shock induced by circulating LPS or LTA. In chapter 5, the steps in the development of shock in response to LPS or LTA were described. Excess cytokine production played a key role in this process. Although the toxic shock toxin, **toxic shock syndrome toxin (TSST),** has properties very different from those of LPS or LTA, its ability to force unnatural associations between macrophages and T cells, the hallmark of a superantigen, causes an outpouring of cytokines that triggers the shock process.

Recently, other types of toxins have been added to the list of toxins that alter cytokine production. For example, the phospholipases and pore-forming cytotoxins normally cause tissue damage by destroying the integrity of the mammalian cell membrane if they are present in high enough concentrations. At levels too low to kill mammalian cells, they can still have rather dramatic effects on these cells. One effect is the induction of cytokine production, particularly IL-1 and TNF-α. This is not too surprising in view of the important role membrane proteins play in signal transduction. An effect on cytokine production has been shown in tissue culture cells. The role of membrane-active cytotoxins in shock remains to be established, but the possibility that there could be a role is intriguing. A-B toxins have also been reported to induce cytokine production at levels too low to kill cells. Finally, some of the protein toxins, especially the superantigens, appear to act synergistically with LPS to increase the ability of LPS to elicit cytokine release.

Pasteurellosis

Pasteurella multocida is a gram-negative bacterium that is related to *E. coli*. It most often causes respiratory disease and atrophic rhinitis in animals such as pigs and laboratory rabbits, but it can cause serious disease (pasteurellosis) in humans who are exposed to infected animals. The disease caused by *P. multocida* is a complex one, but only one aspect of the disease will be covered here, bone destruction. The primary virulence factor of

P. multocida is a toxin called **PMT** (for *P. multocida* **toxin**). This toxin manages to cause an impressive variety of symptoms, ranging from destruction of the lung to bone and fat loss. How could a single toxin produce such varied effects?

PMT is a single polypeptide that binds to a ganglioside receptor on host cells and enters the cell by receptor-mediated endocytosis. Once inside the cell, the toxin interacts with a G protein, G_q, and in the process activates it. G_q controls many cellular activities and is normally activated in response to hormone stimulation. Turning G_q on permanently has many different deleterious effects on cellular metabolism. Since the ganglioside receptor is found on many cell types, PMT can enter many cells. PMT causes mitogenesis and proliferation of fibroblasts and morphological changes in epithelial cells. It also affects the balance between osteoblasts (bone builders) and osteoclasts (bone dismantlers) so as to produce the bone loss seen in infected animals. PMT's different effects on the body illustrate how varied the effects of a toxin that disrupts regulatory networks in many cell types can be.

SELECTED READINGS

Aktories, K. 1997. Rho proteins: targets for bacterial toxins. *Trends Microbiol.* **5:**282–288.

Alouf, J. E., and J. H. Freer (ed.). 1999. *The Comprehensive Sourcebook of Bacterial Protein Toxins.* Academic Press, London, England.

Bhakdi, S., I. Walev, D. Jonas, M. Palmer, U. Weller, N. Suttorp, F. Grimminger, and W. Seeger. 1996. Pathogenesis of sepsis syndrome: possible relevance of pore-forming toxins. *Curr. Top. Microbiol. Immunol.* **216:**101–116.

Henderson, B., M. Wilson, and B. Wren. 1997. Are bacterial exotoxins cytokine network regulators? *Trends Microbiol.* **5:**454–458.

Lee, C. A. 1997. Type III secretion systems: machines to deliver bacterial proteins into eukaryotic cells? *Trends Microbiol.* **5:**148–155.

Schmitt, C. K., K. C. Meysick, and A. D. O'Brien. 1999. Bacterial toxins: friends or foes? *Emerg. Infect. Dis.* **5:**224–234.

Wilson, B. A., X. Zhu, M. Ho, and L. Lu. 1997. *Pasteurella multocida* toxin activates the inositol triphosphate signaling pathway in *Xenopus* oocytes via G_q α-coupled phospholipase C-β1. *J. Biol. Chem.* **272:**1268–1275.

SUMMARY OUTLINE

Characteristics of exotoxins

Toxic bacterial proteins

Found in both gram-positive and gram-negative bacteria

Nomenclature

    Based on target (neurotoxin, leukotoxin, hepatotoxin, cardiotoxin)

    Named for species that produces them or disease they cause (cholera, Shiga, diphtheria, botulinum, tetanus toxins)

    Based on type of activity (e.g., adenylate cyclase, lecithinase)

    Designated by letter (exotoxin A of *P. aeruginosa*)

Toxin types (see also Appendix 1)

Type I

    Bind target on cell surface

    Not translocated into cell

    Example: superantigens

Type II

    Destroy integrity of eukaryotic cell membranes

    Examples: phospholipases, pore-forming cytotoxins

Type III

    A-B toxins

    May be simple or complex

    B portion binds host cell surface receptor

    Translocation region moves A portion into host cell cytoplasm

    A portion acts on host cell target; commonly ADP-ribosylates host cell protein

    Examples: diphtheria toxin, botulinum toxin

Secretion and excretion systems

Type I

    Specialized proteins mediate excretion of toxin through pore-spanning outer membrane and cytoplasmic membrane

    Mechanism used by pore-forming (type II) toxins

Type II

    Uses Sec-dependent secretion apparatus

    Toxin components secreted into periplasm; assembled there; usually released by disruption of outer membrane

    Mechanism used by A-B (type III) toxins

Type III

    Pore formed through cytoplasmic membrane of bacterial and mammalian cells

    Bacteria inject toxin directly into host cell cytoplasm

Roles of toxins in disease

Diphtheria toxin causes diphtheria

    Produced by *C. diphtheriae* (gram-positive); encoded by β- and ω-bacteriophages

    A-B (type III) toxin

    B portion targets HB-EGF on many host cell types

    A portion ADP-ribosylates diphthamide residue on EF-2; stops protein synthesis

    Pseudomembrane produced; toxin in bloodstream causes damage to heart, other organs

Botulinum toxin causes botulism

    Produced by *C. botulinum* (gram-positive sporeformer)

    A-B (type III) toxin

(continued)

SUMMARY OUTLINE (*continued*)

Targets neurons

Cleaves synaptobrevins; affects control of nerve transmission

Causes flaccid paralysis—primary effect on peripheral nerves

Tetanus toxin causes tetanus

Produced by *C. tetani* (gram-positive sporeformer)

A-B (type III) toxin

Targets neurons

Cleaves synaptobrevins; affects control of nerve transmission

Causes spastic paralysis—primary effect on central nervous system

Alpha-toxin contributes to gangrene

Produced by *C. perfringens* (gram-positive sporeformer)

Membrane-disrupting (type II) toxin

Targets many cell types

Has phospholipase activity

Kills host cells; causes tissue damage

Toxic shock syndrome toxin contributes to toxic shock syndrome

Produced by *S. aureus* (gram-positive)

Superantigen (type I)

Targets T cells and macrophages

Causes nonspecific binding of T cells and macrophages; elicits cytokine production by T cells

May potentiate effects of LPS and LTA

Helps produce fever and other symptoms of toxic shock syndrome

P. multocida toxin (PMT)

Produced by *P. multocida* (gram-negative)

Binds gangliosides on many cell types

Inactivates G_q, disrupts regulation of cellular activities

Causes bone loss, weight loss

QUESTIONS

Answers to the questions can be found in Appendix 2.

1. The B portions of A-B toxins are being used as vaccine components without any chemical treatment. Why is it safe to use B portions as they are?

2. What would happen if you injected the A chain of diphtheria toxin into your bloodstream? Could the A chain be used as a vaccine component?

3. How could you use diphtheria toxin A chain to kill cancer cells, as some scientists are trying to do? What would be the advantages of such a treatment? What would be the disadvantages?

4. Why is vaccination usually the best way to prevent diseases caused by A-B toxins?

5. Could vaccination help to prevent botulism, gangrene, or streptococcal fasciitis? Is vaccination a feasible solution to these problems?

6. Can you think of any way that botulinum toxin or tetanus toxin could aid the bacterium that produces it to live a longer and fuller life?

7. How can a toxin that has a single target inside a mammalian cell produce different symptoms? Use diphtheria and pasteurellosis as examples.

8. How do A-B toxins resemble or differ from hemolytic toxins or superantigens?

9. What is the significance of the fact that subcytotoxic doses of membrane-active toxins might contribute to septic shock?

10

Antimicrobial Compounds

Antimicrobial Compounds: the Safety Net of Modern Medicine

Importance of Antimicrobial Compounds

The nonspecific and specific defenses of the body are remarkably effective, but they are not perfect. Not only have bacteria developed ways of circumventing them, but intentional disruption of these defenses, as in surgery or cancer chemotherapy, lay the body open to infection. Such medical disruptions have great benefits if the risk of subsequent infection can be minimized. One of the greatest advances in human health during the past century was the discovery that our natural defenses could be augmented with externally provided chemical defenses: **antiseptics, disinfectants,** and **antibiotics.** Unfortunately, just as virulence factors enable bacteria to evade or undermine the natural defenses of the human body, so too the adaptability of bacteria has enabled them to devise strategies for evading these external chemical defenses. Such strategies are called mechanisms of antimicrobial resistance.

The public has come to take antiseptics, disinfectants, and antibiotics so much for granted that they have forgotten how crucial these compounds are to human well-being. Only with the appearance of antibiotic-resistant bacteria have physicians and public health officials begun to recall how essential the effectiveness of antibiotics is to modern medicine. Without antibiotics, routine nonessential surgical procedures, such as knee and hip replacement, would not be done. Essential surgical procedures, such as bypass surgery or heart valve replacement, would become a lot riskier for the patient, who would be put in the unenviable position of having to decide whether to risk death because of failure to undergo the operation or because of an overwhelming post-surgical infection. Surgical procedures have been practiced in emergency situations for centuries, but the patients often died from ensuing infections. In the 1800s and early 1900s, surgeons discovered how to reduce post-surgical infections dramatically: by using vaporized phenol (carbolic acid) in the operating room. A surgeon of that era owed his success not only to the level of his skill at wielding the knife but also to his ability to endure the effects of repeated phenol exposure. Only when antibiotics and disinfectants made phenol a thing of the past did surgery really begin to flourish and medical students to vie for admission to the specialty. Bacterial resistance to antibiotics and disinfectants could undermine these advances.

In this chapter, we will first examine the mechanisms of action of antiseptics and disinfectants. Next, we will describe how the major classes of antibiotics work. How bacteria become resistant to antibiotics is the subject of chapter 11.

Killing versus Inhibiting Growth

A key concept in antimicrobial therapy is the difference between bactericidal and bacteriostatic compounds. Some antimicrobial compounds kill bacteria—these are called **bactericidal compounds.** Others merely stop or slow the growth of bacteria—these are called **bacteriostatic compounds.** In patients with an intact immune system, bacteriostatic compounds can be very effective because the defenses of the body only need a little help in slowing the growth of bacteria so that the normal defenses can eliminate them. In people with defective defenses, however, there is much more reliance on the antimicrobial compound to effect a cure. Infections in such patients are best treated with bactericidal antibiotics.

At one time, the distinction between bactericidal and bacteriostatic antimicrobial compounds appeared very obvious. The distinction seemed to reside in the properties of the antimicrobial compound. It is now clear that properties of the bacteria can affect this distinction, too. The best example of this is bacterial biofilms. Bacteria that form biofilms change metabolically into a less active state. Such bacteria can become able to resist killing by an antibiotic that would be bactericidal if the bacteria were dividing rapidly. In other words, a bactericidal antibiotic is rendered bacteriostatic or completely ineffective by the growth state of the bacteria. This is the reason medical biofilms that form on plastic implants and catheters are so difficult to eliminate.

A second key concept in antimicrobial therapy is the distribution of the drug in the body. Some antimicrobial compounds can be used only on body surfaces or inanimate objects because they are too toxic for internal use. Antiseptics and disinfectants are examples of this type of compound. Antibiotics are compounds that can be used internally. All antibiotics are not equal inside the body, however, because each class of antibiotic has its special pharmacokinetics.

Pharmacokinetics is a term used to describe the distribution of the antimicrobial compound in the body. For example, some of the antimicrobial compounds used to treat urinary tract infections concentrate primarily in the kidneys and urine and do not disseminate widely to other parts of the body. Others are readily absorbed from the gastrointestinal tract or bloodstream and permeate tissues all over the body. Obviously, the location of the bacteria responsible for causing an infection is key to selection of the appropriate antimicrobial compound. It does not help to treat a meningitis patient with a bactericidal antibiotic if the antibiotic does not cross the blood-brain barrier. Much of the research time spent on development of new antibiotics is focused on determining how these antibiotics are localized in the body.

A third key concept in antimicrobial therapy is side effects. Although the ideal antimicrobial compound kills or inhibits the growth of bacteria specifically and does not affect human cells (differential toxicity), such an ideal compound is not always available. And even an antibiotic such as penicillin, which comes very close to this ideal, can cause severe allergic reactions in some people. Another example of a serious side effect is the ability of some of the aminoglycoside antibiotics to destroy hearing. Obviously, the state of the patient and the seriousness of the infection affect the choice of appropriate therapy. An aminoglycoside that causes deafness if administered long enough would not be considered for treatment of a relatively minor infection but might be the drug of choice for a critically ill patient whose infection can be treated only with this class of antibiotics.

All of these factors must be considered in the choice of an effective therapeutic compound. In the remainder of this chapter, the focus will be on the effects of antimicrobial compounds on the bacteria themselves, but the effects of antimicrobial compounds on the bacteria they target are only part of the treatment story.

Antiseptics and Disinfectants

Mechanisms of Action

Antiseptics and disinfectants, like antibiotics, are chemicals that kill or inhibit the growth of bacteria and other microorganisms. Most antiseptics and disinfectants are bactericidal. Most are also effective against other types of disease-causing microbes, such as viruses and protozoa. This broad coverage has a drawback, however, because the chemicals used as antiseptics and disinfectants also affect human cells and are often too toxic for internal use in humans. Accordingly, they are applied only to skin or inanimate surfaces. "Antiseptic" is the term used to describe antimicrobial compounds applied to skin, e.g., in hand-washing preparations used in hospitals and doctors' offices. "Disinfectant" is the term used to describe antimicrobial compounds applied to inanimate objects and surfaces. Some compounds, such as chlorine and quaternary ammonium compounds, fall into both categories. Others, such as phenol, are too harsh for use on skin and are only used as disinfectants. Antiseptics and disinfectants tend to attack multiple targets in microbes. For example, **halides,** such as chlorine (household bleach) and iodine, are strong oxidants that inactivate many bacterial proteins. **Hydrogen peroxide** has a similar mechanism of action. Halides and peroxide can also damage microbial DNA. **Quaternary ammonium compounds** (QACs), some of the most widely used antimicrobial compounds, intercalate into phospholipid bilayer membranes, causing cells to leak vital ions and other small molecules. These compounds also disrupt electron transport chains. Examples of QACs are cetrimide and benzalkonium chloride. Table 10–1 summarizes the mechanisms of action of these and other common disinfectants.

Antiseptics and disinfectants do best against actively replicating microorganisms. Bacterial spores are generally resistant to them, although the germination of spores can be inhibited. Otherwise, antiseptics and disinfectants are effective against a wide range of fungi, protozoa, viruses, and bacteria.

Resistance to Antiseptics and Disinfectants

The misuse of antiseptics and disinfectants has not received nearly as much attention as the misuse of antibiotics. Yet such misuse does occur (see Box 10–1) and is contributing to bacterial resistance to these important compounds. Resistance to antiseptics and disinfectants is poorly understood, but some resistance mechanisms are known. Many antiseptics and disinfectants, especially those that attack membranes (e.g., QACs), are less effective against gram-negative bacteria than against gram-positive bacteria. The reason seems to be that LPS in the outer membrane of gram-negative bacteria prevents hydrophobic molecules from intercalating into the outer membrane, while porins restrict access to the cytoplasmic membrane by limiting diffusion. Some membrane-active antiseptics, however, can breach this barrier. An interesting type of resistance to QACs has been found in staphylococci: a cytoplasmic membrane pump that pumps the QAC out of the cell cytoplasm. Why this would make the bacteria resistant to QACs, which are thought to act mainly by dissolving membranes, is still unclear. Whatever the explanation, these pumps are fairly effective in protecting the bacteria from QACs. Genes encoding QAC pumps have been found on plasmids as well as in the chromosome. The fact that resistance to antiseptics and disinfectants can

Table 10–1 Common disinfectants and their mode of killing

Disinfectant	Mode of killing
Alcohols (ethanol, isopropanol)	Denature proteins
Alkylating agents (formaldehyde, ethylene oxide)	Form epoxide bridges that inactivate proteins
Halides (I^-, Cl^-)	Oxidizing agents
Heavy metals (Hg^{2+}, Ag^+)	Bind -SH groups, thus denaturing proteins
Phenols	Denature proteins, disrupt cell membranes by intercalating in them
Quaternary ammonium compounds (QACs)	Disrupt cell membranes by intercalating in them
UV radiation	Blocks DNA replication and transcription by damaging DNA

develop is a disturbing discovery because disinfectants and antiseptics are an important line of defense against microbial infections.

Antibiotics

Characteristics of Antibiotics

Antibiotics are low-molecular-weight compounds that kill or inhibit the growth of bacteria and can be ingested or injected into the human body with minimal side effects. Table 10–2 provides a list of commonly used classes of antibiotics and their characteristics. Antibiotics can be either bactericidal or bacteriostatic. In contrast to most disinfectants and antiseptics, antibiotics generally interfere with a specific bacterial enzyme or process, such as the enzyme DNA gyrase or the enzymes that cross-link peptidoglycan.

Many antibiotics are produced by bacteria or fungi. Some of these are modified by a chemical process to make them more active or more able to override bacterial resistance mechanisms (semisynthetic antibiotics). There are also antibiotics that are completely synthetic. The fact that bacteria produce antibiotics has raised the question, what is the role of antibiotic production in nature? An obvious answer is that antibiotics are a kind of "germ warfare," in which the producing species use antimicrobial compounds to discourage microbial competitors. The problem with this widely accepted explanation is that antibiotic production by microbes growing in nature is so low that levels of antibiotics are undetectable. An alternative explanation for the role of antibiotic production in nature is that

BOX 10–1   Triclo-Insanity Hits the United States

An antiseptic compound much in the news in the late 1990s was triclosan. Despite the "tri" in its name, triclosan actually consists of two phenolic rings, one of which contains two chlorine atoms. During this period, many companies began to advertise a variety of antibacterial plastic products, ranging from cutting boards to toys. This proved to be a very effective marketing strategy, which sent millions of householders to their local stores to purchase products that were supposed to protect them from deadly bacteria. The active ingredient in these products was triclosan. The addition of triclosan was not designed to make the products safer. Instead, triclosan was impregnated into the plastic to prevent bacterial degradation of the plastics. Alert to the bacteriophobia of the times, however, advertising executives decided that they could sell products by touting the "antibacterial compound" they contained. The ads implied that these products contained a special additive other products did not have, when in fact virtually all plastic products contain it. On a scientific level, triclosan turned out to be unusual among disinfectants and antiseptics in that, unlike them, triclosan did have a specific target, an enzyme involved in fatty acid biosynthesis. A structural relative of triclosan (both chlorinated bisphenols) is hexachlorophene, the active ingredient in many deodorants (see the figure).

The popularity of products containing antibacterial compounds raised yet again the question of whether it is possible to be "too clean." The human body evolved to accommodate massive microbial populations and regular contact with a variety of disease-causing microbes. The degree of sanitation and hygiene that has become the rule in modern times—at least in developed countries—has changed drastically. In a short period of time, the amount of human exposure to disease-causing microbes has also changed. Some scientists have speculated

A Triclosan

B Hexachlorophene

Structures of triclosan (A) and hexachlorophene (B). Triclosan is routinely added to plastics to prevent microbial degradation. Hexachlorophene is an antibacterial compound used in deodorants to prevent odor-producing activities of skin bacteria.

that this change might be responsible for the rise in incidence of such conditions as asthma and inflammatory bowel disease, which are caused by a malfunctioning immune system. This rise has occurred primarily in countries that are noted for their high standards of hygiene. The argument is that an immune system that is not adequately challenged during childhood may become unbalanced or overreactive to stimuli, leading to autoimmune reactions. If this view is correct, the incorporation of antibacterial compounds in soaps and other household products will only make the situation worse.

bacteria are using these compounds as signaling molecules. Since there is no experimental basis for either the germ warfare theory or the signaling theory, however, the debate over the role of antibiotics in nature is not likely to be resolved anytime in the near future.

Several characteristics define a good antibiotic. First,

the antibiotic must have few or no side effects. That is, it must be far more toxic for bacteria than for the human body. This is known as the principle of differential toxicity. A second desirable characteristic, especially from the physician's perspective, is a broad spectrum of activity against many different types of bacteria. This is

Table 10–2   Classes of antibiotics and their mechanisms of action

Class	Mechanism of action	Resistance mechanisms	Spectrum of activity	Common names
β-Lactams (penicillins, cephalosporins, carbapenems, monobactams)	Inhibit transpeptidation step in peptidoglycan synthesis; bind penicillin-binding proteins, stimulate autolysins	Gram-negative outer membrane; porin mutations; β-lactamase; modify target (alteration of penicillin-binding protein)	Gram-positive and/or gram-negative bacteria (depends on agent)	Penicillin, ampicillin, Cefobid, Augmentin
Glycopeptides	Inhibit transglycosylation and transpeptidation steps in peptidoglycan synthesis by binding D-Ala–D-Ala	Gram-negative outer membrane; modify target (substitute D-Ala–D-lactate for D-Ala–D-Ala)	Most effective against gram-positive bacteria	Vancomycin, teichoplanin
Aminoglycosides	Bind 30S subunit of bacterial ribosome	Inactivation of antibiotic by adding groups	Broadly bactericidal	Kanamycin, gentamicin, streptomycin
Tetracyclines	Bind 30S subunit of bacterial ribosome; disrupt bacterial membrane	Inactivation of antibiotic (?); ribosome protection; efflux system	Broadly bacteriostatic; some protozoa	Tetracycline, doxycycline
Macrolides/ lincosamides	Bind 50S ribosomal subunit	Methylation of target; efflux	Bacteriostatic for most; bactericidal for some gram-positive bacteria	Erythromycin (macrolide); lincomycin, clindamycin (lincosamides)
Streptogramins	Bind 50S ribosomal subunit	Inactivation of antibiotic by removing groups	Bacteriostatic individually; bactericidal in combination; used for multidrug-resistant enterococcal infections	Synercid
Fluoroquinolones	Bind DNA gyrase	Efflux (?); reduced uptake (?); mutation in DNA gyrase	Broadly bactericidal; can enter phagocytes, kill intracellular bacteria	Ciprofloxacin, norfloxacin
Rifampin	Binds β-subunit of bacterial RNA polymerase	Mutation in RNA polymerase	Broadly antibacterial; effective against mycobacteria	Rifadin
Trimethoprim/ sulfonamides	Inhibit enzymes responsible for tetrahydrofolate production	Mutations alter affinity of target enzymes	Broadly antibacterial; some fungi (*Pneumocystis carinii*), protozoa	Bactrim, Septra
Metronidazole	Interferes with DNA replication	Decreased production of flavodoxin gene (?)	Antibacterial (mainly anaerobes); antiprotozoal	Flagyl
Oxazolidinones	Bind 50S ribosomal subunit	Mutation in 23S rRNA genes	Bacteriostatic; broad spectrum against gram-positive bacteria, mycobacteria	Zyvox

important because it is usually not possible to determine the identity of the bacterium causing an infection from the symptoms alone. Bacterial infections often have nonspecific symptoms, such as fever, malaise, and pus formation. Since it takes time to isolate and identify the bacterium responsible for an infection, it is useful to have antibiotics that are effective against the entire range of bacteria capable of producing a particular set of symptoms. Especially in the case of serious, rapidly progressing diseases, such as bacterial pneumonia and septic shock, there is not much margin for error in selection of an effective antibiotic.

Broad-spectrum antibiotics have an important drawback, which has caused scientists to take another look at this type of antibiotic. Such antibiotics not only attack the bacterium causing the infection but can also attack the resident microbiota of the body. Disruption of the normal microbiota can allow pathogens, which are normally outcompeted by the microbiota, to cause infections. An example of how the use of an antibiotic to treat a primary infection causes some patients to contract an equally serious secondary infection is described in chapter 24. A second example is yeast vaginitis in women who have taken antibiotics that disrupt their vaginal microbiota, thus allowing the yeast to overgrow and elicit an inflammatory response. Because of such experiences, more consideration is now being given to the effect of new antibiotics on the resident microbiota, with the goal of minimizing the impact of the antibiotic on the normal microbiota.

Another problematic feature of the broad-spectrum antibiotics is that even if they do not disrupt the resident microbiota significantly, they may select for resistance to the antibiotic. Some bacteria in the resident microbiota are capable of causing serious infections if they escape from the area where they normally reside. Members of the resident microbiota are a significant cause of hospital-acquired infections. An example is vancomycin-resistant *Enterococcus* species. Enterococci are common inhabitants of the human colon. The widespread use (and overuse) of vancomycin to treat or prevent infections caused by *Staphylococcus aureus* and other gram-positive pathogens has selected for *Enterococcus* strains that are resistant to vancomycin. These vancomycin-resistant enterococci are now wreaking havoc in some hospitals. Although enterococci are not very virulent pathogens, they can kill if an infection develops and is not brought under control. Infections caused by vancomycin-resistant enterococcal strains kill nearly 40% of the patients who have them.

The Process of Antibiotic Discovery

Most antibiotics have been obtained from bacteria or fungi that were isolated from soil. For many years, the pharmaceutical companies found new antibiotics primarily by screening soil isolates for antibiotic production using hypersensitive strains of bacteria. The hypersensitive bacteria were applied as a lawn to an agar plate, and various soil isolates were spotted on the plate. Then the plate was incubated to allow the lawn to become confluent. The scientists were looking for zones of no growth around a particular isolate. Isolates that produced such a zone were next checked to determine the structure of the antibiotic they produced. Experience has shown that it is relatively easy to find antibiotic-producing microbes, but finding bacteria or fungi that produce a new antibiotic is becoming harder and harder. The problem may be that if one uses the same screening method, the range of antibiotics detected by such a screen using the same hypersensitive strain as an indicator is eventually exhausted. A new screening method is needed.

If a strain producing a new antibiotic is detected, it is mutagenized or otherwise treated to boost antibiotic production to levels high enough to make antibiotic production economically feasible. The mode of action of the antibiotic is determined, and toxicity tests are done.

Today, scientists are trying new ways to discover antibiotics. One approach has been **combinatorial chemistry.** Starting with a particular core chemical structure, a large variety of chemical groups are added in a random fashion to create an array of derivatives. Scientists then test this bank of compounds, usually against a particular bacterial protein target, looking for compounds that inactivate the target. A drawback of this method is that since a molecular target is used in the screening, it is not guaranteed that a compound that inactivates or inhibits the activity of that target will be able to get to the target in an intact bacterium. To get to an intracellular target, the antibiotic has to transit the outer membrane of a gram-negative bacterium and the cytoplasmic membrane of both gram-negative and gram-positive bacteria. Also, the interior chemical milieu of the bacterial cell may not be conducive to antibiotic action. Another drawback to combinatorial chemistry is that, so far, it has not worked nearly as well as expected. No one knows why. Possibly the reason is that scientists have to choose a particular base molecular structure for chemical modification and a particular target molecule, and they do not know enough about antibiotic action to do this as well as hoped.

A second new approach is to use the crystal structure of the target molecule as a guide for design and synthesis of chemicals that will bind to the target molecule and inactivate it. This approach, called **rational drug design,** was much heralded as the salvation of the pharmaceutical companies when it was introduced. Rational drug design has some of the same drawbacks as combinatorial chemistry. Not surprisingly, the results have been very disappointing. Perhaps it is premature to give up on combinatorial chemistry and rational drug design because they are still new approaches, with which scientists have not had much experience, but it is becoming clear that neither is the miracle maker both were touted as being when they were introduced.

Yet another innovation is to look for antibiotic-producing microbes in new places. Traditionally, certain types of soil bacteria and fungi, such as bacteria of the **actinomycete** group, have been such rich sources of antibiotics that scientists have tended to focus on soil as the primary source of new antibiotic-producing microbes. This approach has started to fail in the sense that scientists keep finding microbes that produce known antibiotics, not new ones. This is true even for soils obtained in exotic locales. Perhaps isolating antibiotic-producing microbes of other types would yield new types of antibiotics. Also, changing the hypersensitive strain used to detect antibiotic production might help.

The traditionally used strains may not be hypersensitive to all antibiotics, as was tacitly assumed.

Genome sequencing of microbes has produced an unexpected finding that may have bearing on antibiotic discovery efforts: bacteria that are not actinomycetes have been found to have genes that look like antibiotic biosynthetic genes. One such bacterium is *Mycobacterium tuberculosis*, the cause of tuberculosis. Of course, no one is suggesting the use of such a dangerous bacterium to produce antibiotics, but this finding has caused scientists to wonder if there might be many antibiotic-producing bacteria that are not actinomycetes. Bolstering this suspicion, some nonactinomycete soil species have been found that produce antibiotics, such as *Flavobacterium* species.

Another important advance is that scientists working on the actinomycetes have succeeded in introducing larger and larger numbers of genes into antibiotic-producing bacteria. Antibiotic production pathways tend to require a number of proteins to assemble the antibiotic and excrete it into the medium. Being able to put new pathways into antibiotic-producing bacteria may make it possible to get the bacteria to produce hybrid antibiotics with better properties than the old ones and better activity against resistant bacteria. Previously, scientists had to modify existing antibiotics chemically to obtain new derivatives. This is an expensive procedure that runs the risk of incomplete reactions that may produce toxic products.

The Economics of Antibiotic Discovery

The foregoing description of how scientists approach antibiotic discovery is of necessity rather vague and possibly inaccurate in parts. The approaches used by pharmaceutical companies to find antibiotics are, not surprisingly, closely kept trade secrets. What is not a secret, however, is how much developing a new antibiotic costs and how long it takes to bring the antibiotic to market. A company can spend $300 million or more to bring a new antibiotic to market, and the process typically takes 10 to 20 years. At any point, a toxic side effect or a lack of sufficient efficacy may be uncovered, and the company loses its investment.

Why is bringing a drug from the research laboratory to market so expensive and time-consuming? First, the discovery and characterization process requires the efforts of a large team of highly paid scientists. Then animal trials need to be done to evaluate efficacy and safety. A promising drug will have to be patented during these early stages, a process that can be both expensive and time-consuming. But what really adds to costs and time taken is the human clinical trials. The first stage of testing in humans uses a relatively small number of healthy adults. Subsequent stages of testing are done with larger groups of volunteers representing people with a range of age and health status. Only in the last stages of clinical testing are children and pregnant women included. The larger trials are multihospital studies, so a team of administrative personnel has to be involved.

After the clinical trials are completed and the data have been analyzed, the company takes its data to the Food and Drug Administration (FDA) for approval, a process that can take months or years. This is not just bureaucrats obstructing progress. The FDA is charged with ensuring that any drug released for general use has passed a highly rigorous and thorough evaluation. Sometimes, restrictions have to be put on the patient populations to be treated or types of uses. An antibiotic that is very effective but has some toxic side effects may be acceptable if used as a last-ditch treatment for critically ill patients but not for children. The final stage, if FDA approval is obtained, is manufacturing and marketing. Sometimes, if a new antibiotic appears to be performing well, it will be used on critically ill patients on a compassionate-use basis even before clinical trials are complete.

As new antibiotics became harder to find and more expensive to develop, pharmaceutical companies became less enthusiastic about them. No antibiotic is going to be as profitable as Prozac or Viagra, drugs that are taken repeatedly over long periods. The upshot was that starting in the 1970s, when, to make matters worse, there was a glut of antibiotics on the market, the pharmaceutical companies started cutting back on their antibiotic discovery programs. Only in the 1990s has this trend been reversed, although the pharmaceutical companies are by no means as enthusiastic about getting back into the antibiotic development area as they once were.

This recent history has profound implications for public health. By the end of the 1980s, the flood of new antibiotics had slowed to a trickle. Bacteria that were becoming increasingly resistant to antibiotics were making some of the former antibiotic stars into has-beens. New antibiotics to cope with these resistant bacteria are badly needed. Yet, because of the long time it takes to bring a new antibiotic to market, results of action taken in the 1990s will not be available for years.

Mechanisms of Antibiotic Action

Targets of Antibiotic Action

The ideal antibiotic acts on a bacterial target that is either not present in eukaryotic cells or is different enough from the same molecule or process in eukaryotic cells that there is little or no cross-reactivity. A drug that attacks a vital eukaryotic cell target will have serious side effects. Although there are a number of targets that potentially satisfy this criterion, the currently used antibiotics tend to focus on only a few targets. The most used targets have been peptidoglycan synthesis, protein synthesis, DNA synthesis, and folic acid synthesis. There are two main reasons why pharmaceutical companies have focused on these targets. First, in earlier screens of antibiotics, molecules that inhibited one of these processes were the ones that were found to be effective and relatively nontoxic. Second, the expense of developing and testing a new antibiotic has become so high that administrators who approve funding for new antibiotic development feel more comfortable with a drug class and a target with which the pharmaceutical industry has had successful past experience. Reaching out for new chemical classes of antibiotics that hit new targets runs the risk that such new antibiotics could fail at the clinical trial phase because of unexpected side effects and unexpected pharmacological properties.

An example of this type of conservative thinking is the decision by some pharmaceutical companies to look for inhibitors of tRNA synthetases. As will be seen later in this chapter, tRNA synthetases (the enzymes that attach the amino acid to the appropriate tRNA) are not traditional targets for antibiotics, so at first glance tRNA synthetases would appear to be a novel target, and the tRNA synthetase inhibitors would appear to be a novel class of antibiotics. Yet, there is a little-known antibiotic called mupirocin, which is a tRNA synthetase inhibitor. Mupirocin is not appropriate for internal use because it is broken down in serum, but it has been used successfully to eliminate *S. aureus* from the noses of carriers. A hospital care worker who is a carrier of *S. aureus*, especially if the strain is one that is resistant to many antibiotics, is a danger to surgical or immunocompromised patients because *S. aureus* is a common cause of infections in such patients.

Although mupirocin itself is not appropriate for use as an internally administered antibiotic, the pharmaceutical industry nonetheless has a lot of information on its properties and pharmacokinetics. Perhaps mupirocin could be chemically modified to make it more effective internally. It is easier to convince those in control of finance to back a proven type of compound than to convince them to take a chance on a completely new type of antibiotic. This does not mean that there is no exploratory spirit in pharmaceutical companies. In fact, there is a considerable amount of innovative experimentation going on at the antibiotic development level. Nonetheless, given the huge amounts of money that have to be invested in bringing a new drug to market,

it is perhaps understandable that the familiar would have more appeal to the people responsible for financial decisions than the unfamiliar.

The obvious solution to this problem is to have exploratory research on new types of antibiotics conducted by basic scientists in academia. After all, it was the basic scientists who discovered the first anti-HIV drugs that have been appropriated so successfully by the pharmaceutical industry and have proved quite profitable to them. Here, the culture of basic science intervenes. Most academic scientists do not know much about the internal operations of pharmaceutical companies. Accordingly, they do not appreciate the economic realities that drive research decisions made within these companies. Faced with a proposal asking for funds to develop a new antibiotic class, the academic scientists who judge such proposals tend to assume, wrongly, that funding such a proposal is unnecessary; if the idea were any good, surely the pharmaceutical companies would be throwing money at it. Because of this misconception, academic research on antibiotic development has virtually ceased. This is regrettable because it has removed a measure of public control over how antibiotic discovery proceeds. The reason pharmaceutical companies rarely give money to basic research scientists is that basic research scientists insist on publishing their results, and this can compromise patent applications. Another regrettable result of the lack of public funding for antibiotic discovery is that a vital source of risk taking, which is ultimately in the public interest, is thereby eliminated.

Cell Wall Synthesis Inhibitors

β-Lactam antibiotics.   The **β-lactam antibiotics** get their name from the four-membered β-lactam ring they all have in common. This group of antibiotics now includes four main types: **penicillins, cephalosporins, carbapenems,** and **monobactams** (Figure 10–1). β-Lactam antibiotics have been among the most useful of all antibiotics. The main toxicity problem with these antibiotics is an allergic reaction that occurs because of formation of a β-lactam/serum protein conjugate, which evokes an immune response. Allergy to penicillins may result in allergy to cephalosporins as well, and vice versa. Fortunately, the monobactams are different enough in structure from penicillins and cephalosporins to be used on people who are allergic to penicillin.

How β-lactam antibiotics kill bacteria is still something of a mystery. β-Lactam antibiotics inhibit the last step in peptidoglycan synthesis, the transpeptidation reaction that cross-links the peptide side chains of the polysaccharide peptidoglycan backbone (Figure 10–2). β-Lactam antibiotics also bind to and inhibit the action

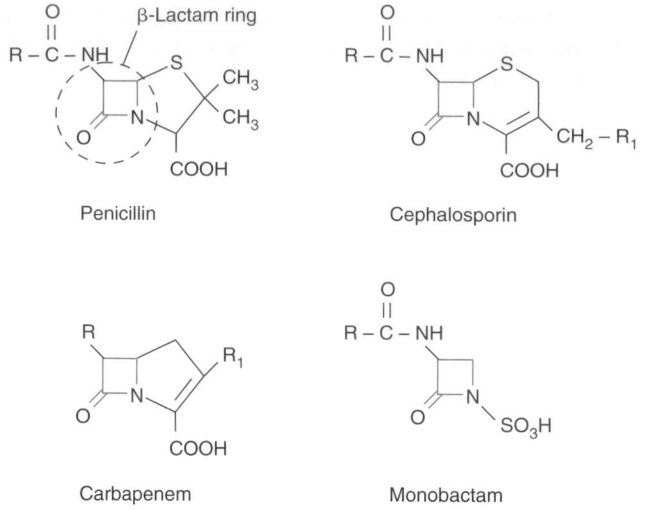

Figure 10–1 The structure of representative β-lactam antibiotics.

of other inner membrane proteins that may have a role in peptidoglycan synthesis. Transpeptidase and these other proteins are sometimes called **penicillin-binding proteins.** The net result of β-lactam binding to these proteins and inhibiting cross-linking is to trigger endogenous enzymes that degrade the peptidoglycan. Normally, these enzymes function in the turnover of peptidoglycan, which allows the bacteria to grow and divide. The action of β-lactam antibiotics apparently removes controls that normally keep these enzymes in check and stimulates their attack on peptidoglycan. Since the peptidoglycan cell wall prevents the bacteria from bursting in response to the high osmotic strength of cytoplasmic contents relative to the external medium, destruction of the cell wall leads to bacterial lysis. β-Lactam antibiotics are normally bactericidal. Occasionally, if bacteria are in a high osmolarity compartment of the body (kidney) or if environmental pH prevents activation of the hydrolytic enzymes, bacteria can escape the bactericidal effects of β-lactam antibiotics, but such cases are uncommon.

Different β-lactams differ in their spectrum of activity. Some are effective against both gram-positive and gram-negative bacteria, whereas others are much more effective against one or the other. Despite all of the time and money invested to date in studying β-lactam antibiotics, it is still not possible to predict with certainty what changes in the basic β-lactam structure will produce an effective antibiotic. β-Lactams also differ widely in their toxicity, stability in the human body, rate of clearance from blood, whether they can be taken orally, and their ability to penetrate the blood-brain barrier.

GLYCOPEPTIDES. Another group of peptidoglycan synthesis inhibitors is the **glycopeptides,** which include **vancomycin** (Figure 10–3) and **teichoplanin.** These antibiotics, especially vancomycin, have become extremely important medically because they are the last drugs that are effective against some gram-positive pathogens, such as *S. aureus* and *Enterococcus* species. Glycopeptide antibiotics bind to the D-Ala–D-Ala portion of the UDP-muramyl-pentapeptide after it is transferred out of the cell cytoplasm. Binding appears to inhibit both **transglycosylation** and **transpeptidation,** the two final steps in peptidoglycan synthesis. Vancomycin and teichoplanin are used primarily to treat infections caused by gram-positive bacteria and are not very effective against most gram-negative bacteria because they cannot penetrate the outer membrane. Despite their relatively narrow spectrum, these antibiotics are clinically important.

OTHER ANTIBIOTICS THAT INHIBIT CELL WALL SYNTHESIS. **Phosphonomycin** and **bacitracin** are two antibiotics that inhibit peptidoglycan synthesis by inhibiting earlier steps in the pathway than those inhibited by β-lactams and glycopeptides. Phosphonomycin inhibits the conversion of UDP-NAG to UDP-NAM (Figure 10–2). Phosphonomycin has had limited clinical utility but is now used to treat methicillin-resistant *S. aureus* infections. Bacitracin interferes with the recycling of bactoprenol (Figure 10–2). Bacitracin is used primarily in ointments available over the counter for preventing wound infections because it is too toxic for internal use.

Protein Synthesis Inhibitors

AMINOGLYCOSIDES. **Aminoglycosides** (e.g., **kanamycin, gentamicin**) are trisaccharides with amino groups that target the bacterial ribosome (Figure 10–4). The bacterial ribosome is a good target for antibiotics because it differs appreciably from ribosomes of mammalian cells. Aminoglycosides act by binding the 30S subunit of the bacterial ribosome. This does not prevent the 30S subunit from binding mRNA and placing a tRNA[fMet] in the P site, but the 50S subunit does not join the 30S to form the active ribosome, and no protein synthesis occurs. Aminoglycosides are bactericidal, because protein synthesis is essential for continued viability of a bacterium. Aminoglycosides are effective against a number of pathogenic bacteria, but they have side effects that limit their use. For example, prolonged use of aminoglycosides can lead to hearing loss or to impairment of kidney function.

TETRACYCLINES. **Tetracyclines,** as the name suggests, are compounds consisting of four fused cyclic six-membered rings (Figure 10–5). Tetracyclines also target

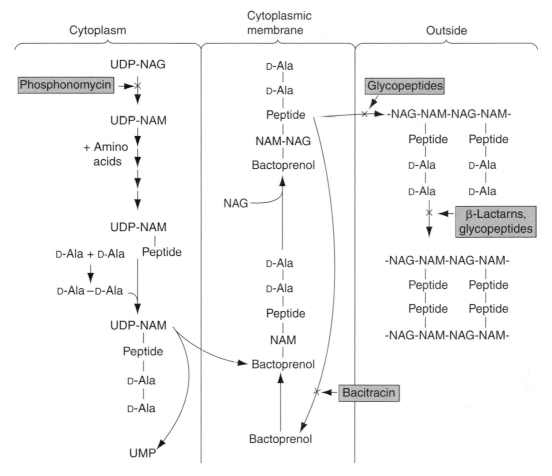

Figure 10–2   Steps in the synthesis of peptidoglycan and the effects of different classes of antibiotics. Phosphonomycin blocks the conversion of UDP-NAG to UDP-NAM. Bacitracin inhibits the dephosphorylation and recycling of bactoprenol. Glycopeptides and β-lactams block transpeptidation. Because the enzymes that carry out transpeptidation also mediate transglycosylation, these antibiotics tend to block both steps.

the bacterial ribosome and bind to the 30S subunit. The effect of binding is to distort the A site and prevent the alignment of aminoacylated tRNA with the codon on mRNA. Although most tetracyclines unquestionably act by interfering with protein synthesis, some members of the tetracycline family (e.g., **chelocardin**) appear to act instead by disrupting the bacterial membrane, not by stopping protein synthesis. At present these atypical tetracyclines are of academic interest only, because they have so far proved to be too toxic for use on humans. There is hope, however, that some nontoxic derivatives can be found. The newest tetracycline heading toward the market is **glycyl-glycine tetracycline,** a tetracycline that has a bulky glycyl-glycine side chain designed to overcome resistance to tetracycline.

Tetracyclines are generally bacteriostatic. Although tetracycline can cause discoloration of teeth if given to young children and sometimes causes nausea or pho-

totoxicity, it has been one of the least toxic antibiotics ever produced. This, together with the fact that it can be given orally, has led to overuse of tetracycline in clinical practice. Tetracycline has also been used in the treatment of acne and as a feed additive to promote growth of livestock. Not too surprisingly, tetracycline resistance is now so widespread that the utility of the tetracycline family has been considerably diminished. Nonetheless, tetracyclines still have some important uses, e.g., in the treatment of Lyme disease and some sexually transmitted bacterial diseases, such as chlamydia and gonorrhea. Scientists would like to find new members of the tetracycline family because this family of antibiotics has many good properties. It has been so widely used (and abused) precisely because it is not only effective but also nontoxic.

MACROLIDES AND LINCOSAMIDES. The **macrolide** family is another group of antibiotics that has had rela-

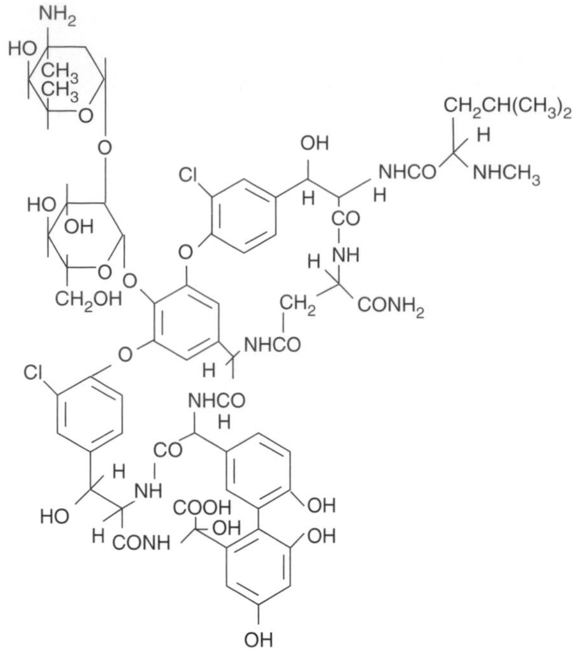

Figure 10–3   Structure of vancomycin, a glycopeptide antibiotic.

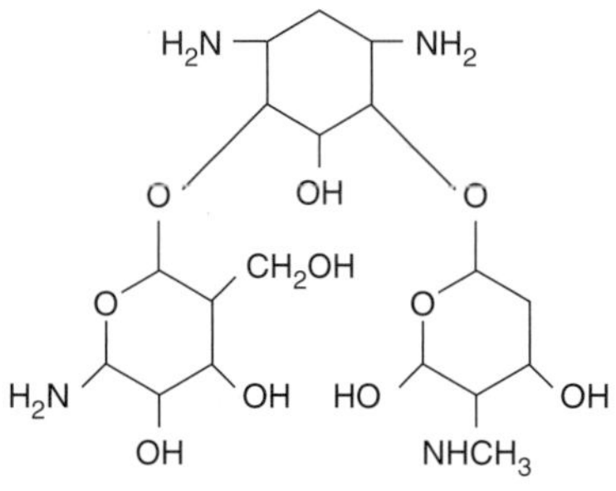

Figure 10–4   Structure of gentamicin, an aminoglycoside.

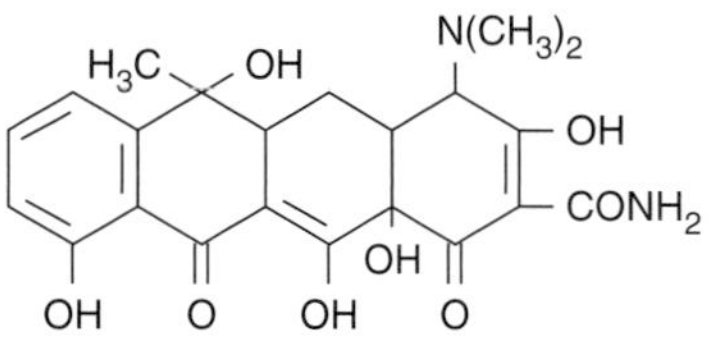

Figure 10–5   Structure of tetracycline.

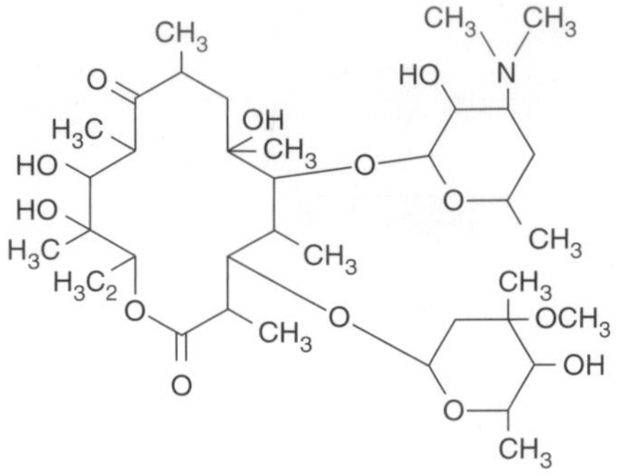

Figure 10–6   Structure of erythromycin, a macrolide.

tively few side effects (Figure 10–6). Macrolides inhibit bacterial protein synthesis by binding the 50S ribosomal subunit at a site that includes a looped segment of 23S rRNA. Binding inhibits translocation. Macrolides are bacteriostatic for most bacteria but are bactericidal for some gram-positive bacteria. Macrolides, like tetracyclines, have also been used to treat livestock, primarily to prevent shipping sickness. There is some concern, as with the tetracyclines, that this nonclinical use is contributing to the spread of bacterial resistance to this class of antibiotics.

An exciting new macrolide is **azithromycin.** Azithromycin is so effective in treating sexually transmitted bacterial diseases, such as chlamydial disease and gonorrhea, that it only needs to be administered in one or two closely spaced doses. This solves a problem that has plagued clinics that treat people with sexually transmitted diseases; the patient is given tetracycline or another antibiotic and instructed to take it daily for a week. If the patient abuses drugs or alcohol or is homeless, the entire course of antibiotic may not be taken. Also, the patient may not abstain from sexual contact until the antibiotic regimen has been completed. A patient who is treated with azithromycin in a supervised manner at a clinic will take the entire course of antibiotic, will be cured more quickly, and will thus be less likely to transmit the disease to others.

Unfortunately, azithromycin has a rather serious side effect. As a new antibiotic, still under patent protection, it is too expensive for many cash-strapped inner city clinics to use. It is also too expensive for developing countries, where resistance to tetracycline and other commonly used antibiotics in bacteria that cause sexually transmitted diseases is becoming a serious problem. This illustrates a problem that has not yet been faced successfully. Pharmaceutical companies need to make enough money from new antibiotics to pay for the expense of their development. Yet, this need is at odds with the need of vulnerable impoverished populations for cheap antibiotics.

Lincosamides differ considerably from macrolides in structure (Figure 10–7), but they have the same mechanism of action and probably bind the ribosome at or near the same site as the macrolides. Perhaps the most widely used lincosamide is clindamycin. Clindamycin has been used extensively to treat infections caused by obligately anaerobic bacteria, such as *Bacteroides* species. Clindamycin is also one of the few antibacterial compounds that are effective against disease-causing protozoa such as *Giardia* sp., a cause of a persistent and sometimes life-threatening diarrhea. Clindamycin's strength—its effectiveness against obligate anaerobes—also proved to be its downfall. Patients who took clindamycin experienced a decrease in numbers of the obligate anaerobes that constitute the major populations of the colonic microbiota. In some of these patients, this disruption of the normal microbiota allowed a pathogen, *Clostridium difficile,* to overgrow and produce powerful toxins that could kill the patient (see chapter 24).

The **streptogramins** are usually overlooked in most textbooks because they have not been used to treat human infections until very recently. The appearance of Synercid on the market changed that picture in a radical way. Synercid is a combination of two streptogramins—dalfopristin and quinupristin. Streptogramins, like macrolides and lincosamides, act by binding to ribosomes and inhibiting the translocation step in protein synthesis. Streptogramins were developed in response to the growing resistance of *Enterococcus* species and *S. aureus* to vancomycin, the last-ditch treatment of infections caused by these two gram-positive opportunists. Streptogramins would seem to be an ideal solution to the question of how to develop a new antibiotic that would be effective against the multi-resistant bacterial threats that loom in our future. Since streptogramins have not been used to treat human infections in the past, resistance would not be a problem, at least not at first, right? Well, not quite.

It turns out that streptogramins have been used widely in agriculture for a number of years. Not surprisingly, resistance to streptogramins emerged even before they were approved for human use. The CDC is now monitoring the emergence of streptogramin-resistant strains. The question remains, how linked are the consequences of agricultural use of antibiotics with the consequences of human use of antibiotics? Another complicating factor, which is covered in more detail in chapter 11, is that since the macrolides, lincosamides, and streptogramins bind to overlapping sites on the

bacterial ribosome, some of the mechanisms bacteria develop to resist the action of these antibiotics confer resistance to all three classes. This means that use of one class can select for resistance to the other classes in this triumvirate.

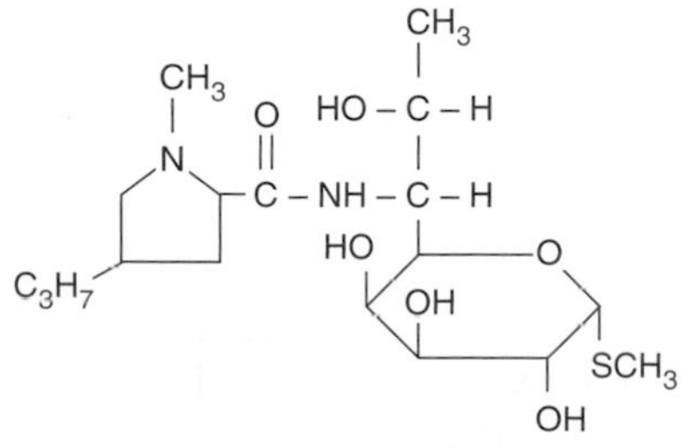

Quinolones—a Class of Antibiotics That Targets DNA Replication

Quinolones inhibit bacterial DNA replication. For a long time, the only quinolone available, nalidixic acid, was very effective in treating urinary tract infections due to gram-negative bacteria but was not particularly useful for many other types of infections. Then, scientists added a fluorine to the molecule, and a new class of antibiotics useful for humans, the fluoroquinolones, was born. This new group of antibiotics caused considerable excitement in clinical circles because of their impressive antibacterial activity and good pharmacological properties (Figure 10–8). Fluoroquinolones are bactericidal antibiotics that inhibit bacterial DNA replication by binding to and inhibiting the activity of DNA gyrase. After DNA replication, DNA supercoiling must be restored by DNA gyrase. Fluoroquinolones stop this essential process. Fluoroquinolones have poor activity against streptococci and anaerobes, which constitute a majority of the resident microflora of the mouth, colon, and vaginal tract. Thus, they are less likely than other antibiotics to disrupt the normal microbiota. Also, fluoroquinolones penetrate macrophages and PMNs better than most other antibiotics and are thus useful for curing infections caused by bacteria that survive in phagocytes.

The Achilles' heel of the fluoroquinolones is that a single mutation in DNA gyrase makes bacteria resistant to them. Overuse of fluoroquinolones in human medicine has had the predictable effect of giving rise to fluoroquinolone-resistant bacteria. Fluoroquinolones have even been approved for use in the water provided to chickens being raised in intensive chicken farming operations to prevent infections from sweeping through the bird population. The FDA's approval of this use of fluoroquinolones (recently withdrawn) was controversial from the start. No one knows how much

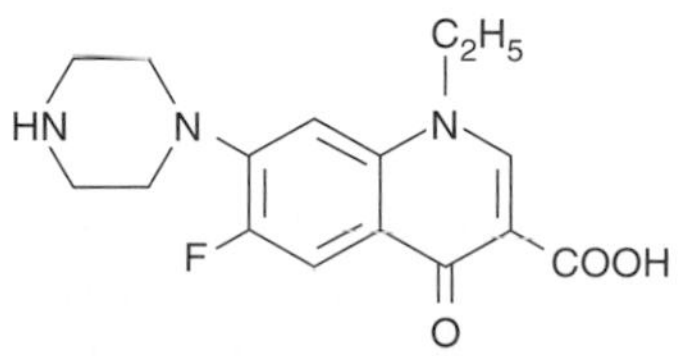

Figure 10–7 Structure of lincomycin, a lincosamide.

Figure 10–8 Structure of norfloxacin, a fluoroquinolone.

of a contribution such extensive use of fluoroquinolones might have made to resistance of bacteria such as *Salmonella* and *Campylobacter* species, which are found in the avian intestine and can cause human disease. A strain of *Salmonella enterica* serovar Typhimurium that has caused a number of outbreaks in recent years, strain DT104, is resistant to fluoroquinolones and several other antibiotic classes.

Rifampin—an Inhibitor of RNA Synthesis

Rifampin (Figure 10–9) is an antibiotic that inhibits the activity of bacterial RNA polymerase. Although rifampin has always had its clinical uses, e.g., prophylactic use during outbreaks of *Neisseria meningitidis* meningitis, and as part of the drug combinations used to treat tuberculosis, it has not received much attention until recently. The appearance of strains of *M. tuberculosis* that are resistant to isoniazid, one of the front-line antibiotics used to treat tuberculosis, caused a renewed interest in rifampin. Unfortunately, resistance to rifampin can arise fairly easily as the result of a single mutation in RNA polymerase. Nonetheless, rifampin is one of the few drugs available for treating isoniazid-resistant tuberculosis. Rifampin has also been used recently to treat some other types of bacterial infections caused by strains that are resistant to the more commonly used antibiotics.

Trimethoprim and Sulfonamides

Trimethoprim and **sulfonamides** are inhibitors of enzymes in the bacterial pathway for production of **tetrahydrofolic acid.** Tetrahydrofolic acid is an essential cofactor for 1-carbon transfer reactions that occur in pathways for synthesis of nucleic acids and formylmethionine. Mammalian cells require preformed folic acid because they do not make their own tetrahydrofolate. Thus, inhibitors of the tetrahydrofolic acid pathway do not affect them. Sulfonamides are structurally similar to *p*-**aminobenzoic acid,** a substrate for the first enzyme in the pathway, and they competitively inhibit that step (Figure 10–10). Trimethoprim is structurally similar to dihydrofolic acid and acts as a competitive inhibitor of dihydrofolate reductase, an enzyme that catalyzes the last step in the pathway (Figure 10–10).

Metronidazole

Metronidazole has become important recently because it is one of the drugs used to treat ulcers. Also, it is important for treating infections caused by anaerobic pathogens that are resistant to most antibiotics. Metronidazole, like the fluoroquinolones, interferes with

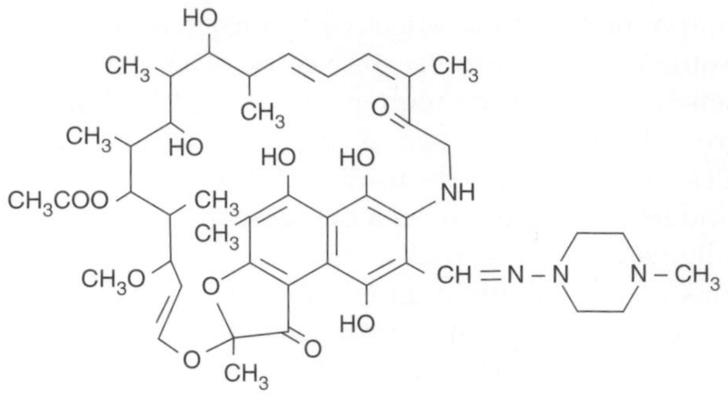

Figure 10–9   Structure of rifampin.

DNA synthesis, but it does so not by inhibiting an enzyme but by making breaks in the DNA. Metronidazole, unlike other antibiotics, must first be activated by a bacterial housekeeping protein, flavodoxin, before it can attack DNA (Figure 10–11). The ferredoxins and flavodoxins found in microaerophiles and obligate anaerobes, but not aerobes, are capable of reducing the nitro group of metronidazole to a form that interacts with DNA and causes nicks in the DNA strands. The activated form of metronidazole could be considered a mutagen. At one time, this feature of metronidazole raised questions about its safety, but since human cells do not convert metronidazole to its active form, these concerns were short-lived. In fact, metronidazole has proved to be an antibiotic that has few side effects. Since such antibiotics are increasingly rare, metronidazole is looking better every day.

Metronidazole, like the lincosamide clindamycin, is not specific for bacteria. It is also effective against certain eukaryotic pathogens, such as *Trichomonas vaginalis* (vaginitis) and *Giardia intestinalis* (diarrhea). These anaerobic protozoa have in common with anaerobic bacteria the ability to activate metronidazole to its active DNA-damaging form.

The Newest Antibiotics

A few new antibiotics have been introduced during the past several years. Two are members of known classes of antibiotics. As mentioned earlier, glycyl-glycyl tetracycline is a tetracycline derivative with a glycyl-glycyl group added. The **ketolides** are new derivatives of macrolide antibiotics. Streptogramins are a new class of antibiotics only in the sense that they have just recently been used to treat people. The structures of two streptogramins that are part of the newly licensed antibiotic Synercid are shown in Figure 10–12. The reason the mixture of **dalfopristin** and **quinupristin** is needed is that each of the drugs by itself is bacteriostatic, but together they are bactericidal.

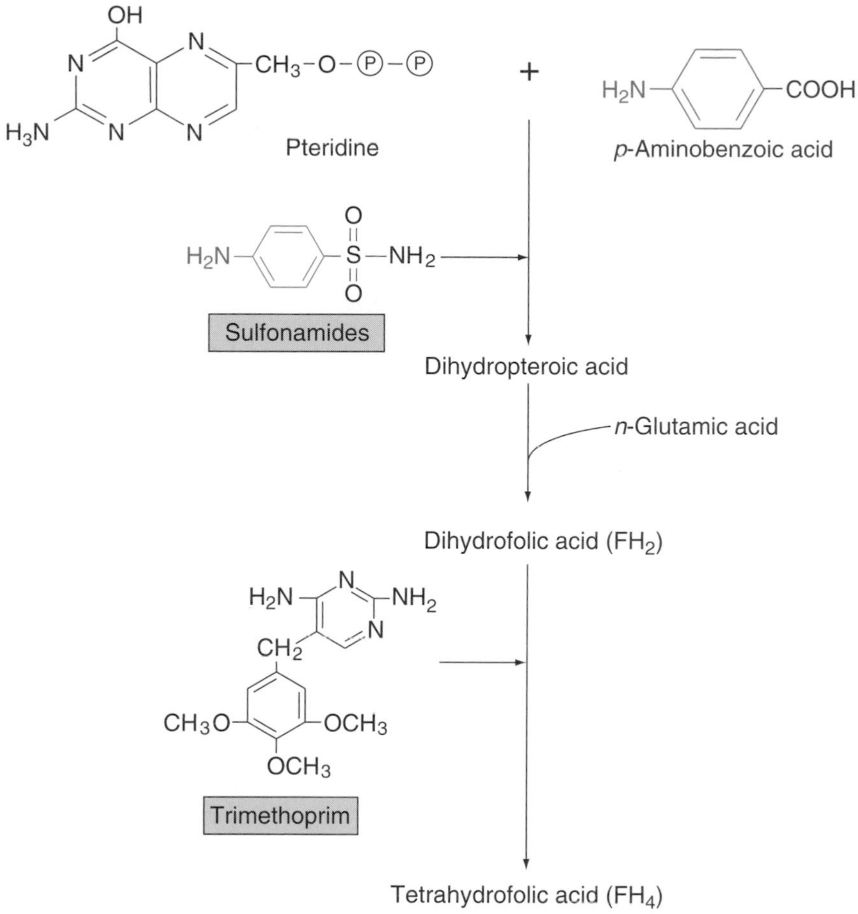

OH

Pteridine

p-Aminobenzoic acid

Sulfonamides

Dihydropteroic acid

— n-Glutamic acid

Dihydrofolic acid (FH$_2$)

Trimethoprim

Tetrahydrofolic acid (FH$_4$)

Figure 10–10   Action of trimethoprim and sulfonamides. Sulfonamides resemble *p*-aminobenzoic acid in structure and are thus able to competitively inhibit the action of the first enzyme in the tetrahydrofolate pathway. Trimethoprim resembles the substrate of a later enzyme and competitively inhibits this step in synthesis.

Streptogramins have the same mechanism of action as the macrolides and lincosamides; they bind to the same portion of the 50S rRNA molecule and prevent elongation of the peptide chain. Although this is the first use of streptogramins in human medicine, members of this class have been used for decades in agriculture, under the names virginiamycin and pristinamy-

cin, to treat and prevent disease in animals being raised in crowded conditions. Thus, it is not surprising that streptogramin-resistant bacteria are already in nature. Moreover, streptogramins have some side effects that make them less than perfect antibiotics for human use. Nonetheless, they may help in the treatment of bacteria that are resistant to all other antibiotics.

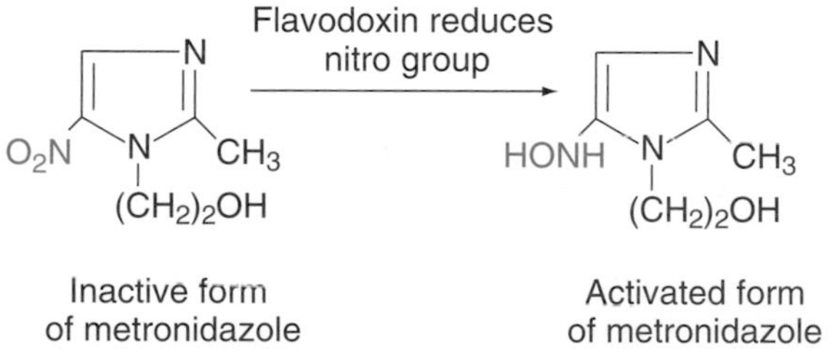

A completely new class of antibiotics, the first new class in decades, has been given the tongue-twisting name **oxazolidinones** (Figure 10–13). The name under which the first member of this class is being sold is easier to pronounce: Zyvox. The oxazolidinones bind the large ribosomal subunit near enough to where the macrolides, lincosamides, and streptogramins bind to complete with them for binding to the ribosome. Nonetheless, the oxazolidinones act earlier in the protein synthesis pathway, apparently inhibiting initiation of protein synthesis rather than the elongation step.

Flavodoxin reduces nitro group

Inactive form of metronidazole

Activated form of metronidazole

Figure 10–11   Structure and activation of metronidazole. Metronidazole is first activated by flavodoxin to a form that can attack DNA and cause strand breaks in the DNA. Exactly how the activated form of metronidazole breaks the phosphodiester backbone of a DNA strand is still not clear.

The Continuing Challenge

Although it is encouraging that new antibiotics are coming through the pipeline, they present a quandary

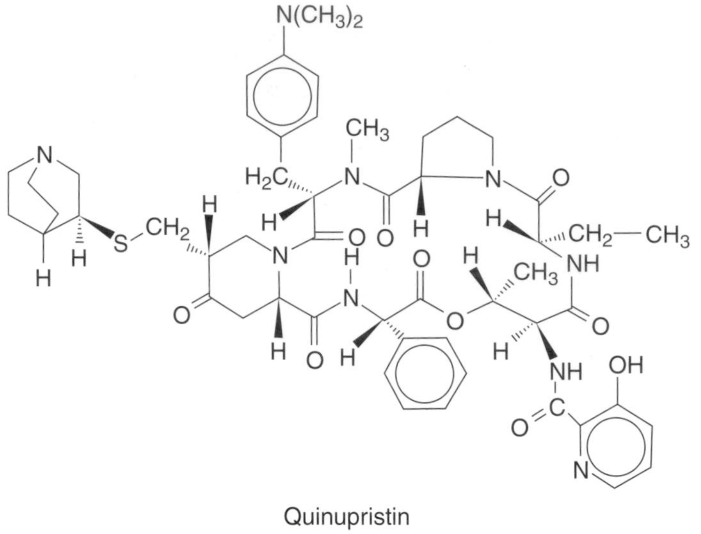

Quinupristin

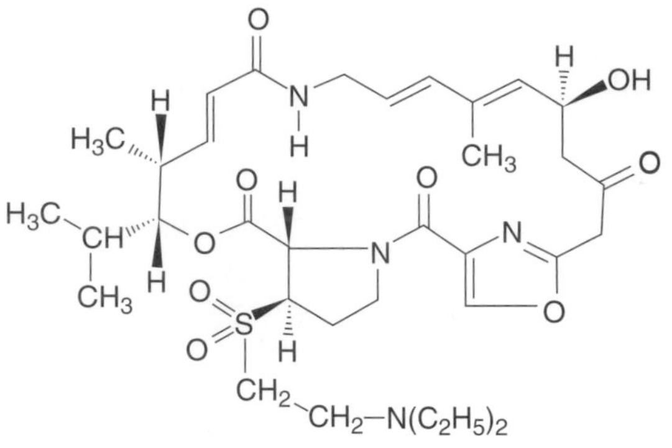

Dalfopristin

Figure 10–12 Structure of the two streptogramins in Synercid, quinupristin and dalfopristin.

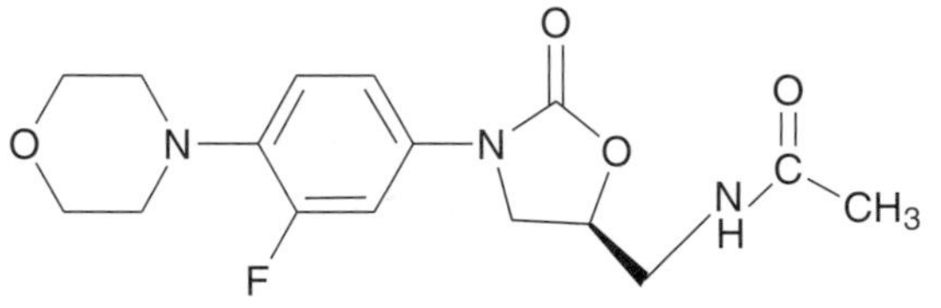

Linezolid

Figure 10–13 Structure of the oxazolidinone linezolid (Zyvox).

for physicians and the pharmaceutical companies. There is understandable pressure to reserve these new drugs for the cases in which nothing else works. Yet it is difficult to ask physicians, who have to make accurate first guesses as to what antibiotic to use on their very sick patients, to forgo the latest antibiotics, especially if multidrug-resistant bacteria have become a problem in their hospital. It is also difficult to ask the pharmaceutical companies to restrict the sales of an antibiotic that has taken hundreds of million dollars and years to develop and test. Making it difficult for pharmaceutical companies to recover their investment costs, to say nothing of making a profit, will discourage them from investing in development of the antibiotics of the future. How to preserve these new drugs is an ethical and economic challenge.

There is also the challenge of how to control the use of the older antibiotics that still work against many bacterial infections. Physicians have been accustomed to making their own decisions as to what antibiotic to prescribe, and they are already chafing at the restrictions

on medical practice being imposed by the health maintenance organizations. There are prudent use guidelines for antibiotics that have the imprimatur of the American Medical Association, but they are often ignored by physicians in everyday practice. Two of the most widely flouted guidelines are those that recommend against the use of antibiotics to treat sore throats and flu (viral infections) or to treat ear infections in children until the infections have persisted for 24 to 48 h. Physicians like to please their patients, and they have an economic as well as a psychological incentive for doing so. What does a physician do when a patient threatens to go elsewhere? Also, complaints lodged by patients against physicians can get the physician in trouble with hospital administrators. Clearly, the problem of enforcing prudent antibiotic use goes beyond scientific considerations and spills over into economic and political areas. Perhaps you, dear reader, will see the solution to these problems materialize and a new era of prudent use of antibiotics in which antibiotics are revered and conserved as the vital resource they are. We hope that you and your children will not instead witness the disastrous consequences of failure to contain abuse and overuse of antibiotics.

SELECTED READINGS

Fierer, J., and D. Guiney. 1999. Extended spectrum β-lactamases; a plague of plasmids. *JAMA* **281:**563–564.

Fung-Tomc, J. 1997. Fourth-generation cephalosporins. *Clin. Microbiol. Newsl.* **19:**129–136.

Ge, M., Z. Chen, H. R. Onishi, J. Kohler, L. L. Silver, R. Kerns, S. Fukuzawa, C. Thompson, and D. Kahne. 1999. Vancomycin derivatives that inhibit peptidoglycan biosynthesis without binding D-Ala–D-Ala. *Science* **284:**508–512.

Lin, A. H., R. W. Murray, T. J. Vidmar, and K. R. Marotti. 1997. The oxazolidinone cperezolid binds to the 50S ribosomal subunit and competes with binding of chloramphenicol and lincomycin. *Antimicrob. Agents Chemother.* **41:**2127–2131.

McDonnell, G., and D. Russell. 1999. Antiseptics and disinfectants: activity, action and resistance. *Clin. Microbiol. Rev.* **12:**147–179.

Mingeot-Leclercq, M.-P., Y. Glupczynski, and P. M. Tulkens. 1999. Aminoglycosides: activity and resistance. *Antimicrob. Agents Chemother.* **43:**727–737.

Silver, L. L., and K. A. Bostian. 1993. Discovery and development of new antibiotics: the problem of antibiotic resistance. *Antimicrob. Agents Chemother.* **37:**377–383.

Witte, W. 1998. Medical consequences of antibiotic use in agriculture. *Science* **279:**996–997.

SUMMARY OUTLINE

Antiseptics and disinfectants

Must be used externally because of toxicity

Most kill bacteria (bactericidal)

Some inhibit growth of bacteria (bacteriostatic)

Antiseptics
  Applied to skin
  Examples: hexachlorophene, alcohols

Disinfectants
  Applied to inanimate objects
  Examples: halides, hydrogen peroxide, QACs

Resistance to antiseptics and disinfectants
  LPS prevents binding of QACs
  Cytoplasmic membrane pumps remove QACs

Antibiotics

Can be ingested or injected into human body

Minimal side effects

Many produced by bacteria or fungi

Characteristics of a good antibiotic
  Few or no side effects
  Broad spectrum of activity
  Good distribution in the body
  Minimal effect on microbiota

Discovery process
  Produced biologically by soil microbes
    Screened on hypersensitive strains
    Becoming more difficult to find
  Chemical synthesis (synthetic antibiotics)
  Chemical modification of biologically produced antibiotics (semisynthetic antibiotics)
  Combinatorial chemistry
    Chemical groups added to basic antibiotic structure
    New antibiotic may not get to target inside bacterial cell
  Rational drug design
    Synthesize chemicals that will bind target molecule based on target structure
    Results disappointing so far

(continued)

Antibiotics that inhibit cell wall synthesis
    β-Lactams
        Examples: penicillins, cephalosporins, carbapenems, monobactams
        Usually bactericidal
        Inhibit last step in peptidoglycan synthesis (transpeptidation)
        May trigger endogenous enzymes that degrade peptidoglycan
        Spectrum of different β-lactams varies
    Glycopeptides
        Examples: vancomycin, teichoplanin
        Bind D-Ala–D-Ala portion of UDP-NAM pentapeptide
        Prevent transglycosylation and transpeptidation
        More effective against gram-positive bacteria than gram-negative bacteria
        Medically important use against multidrug-resistant bacteria
    Phosphonomycin
        Inhibits conversion of UDP-NAG to UDP-NAM
        Used in treatment of methicillin-resistant *S. aureus*
    Bacitracin
        Interferes with recycling of bactoprenol
        Used topically because of toxicity
Protein synthesis inhibitors
    Aminoglycosides
        Examples: kanamycin, gentamicin
        Bind 30S ribosomal subunit; prevent protein synthesis
        Bactericidal
    Tetracyclines
        Examples: tetracycline, doxycycline
        Bind 30S ribosomal subunit; prevent protein synthesis
        Generally bacteriostatic
    Macrolides
        Examples: erythromycin, azithromycin
        Bind 50S ribosomal subunits; prevent elongation of peptide chain
        Bacteriostatic for most bacteria; bactericidal for some gram-positive bacteria
    Lincosamides
        Examples: lincomycin, clindamycin
        Bind 50S ribosomal subunit; prevent elongation of peptide chain
        Bacteriostatic for most bacteria; bactericidal for some gram-positive bacteria
    Streptogramins (ketolides)
        Example: Synercid (mixture of dalfopristin and quinupristin)
        Bind 50S ribosomal subunit; prevent elongation of peptide chain
        Individual components bacteriostatic; mixture bactericidal
Inhibition of nucleic acid synthesis or replication
    Quinolones
        Examples: ciprofloxacin, norfloxacin
        Bind DNA gyrase; prevent DNA supercoiling
        Broad bactericidal activity; effective against some intracellular bacteria
    Metronidazole
        Example: Flagyl
        Interferes with DNA replication; creates breaks in DNA
        Must be activated by flavodoxin or ferredoxin of host cell
        Effective against anaerobic and microaerophilic bacteria, some protozoa

(*continued*)

SUMMARY OUTLINE (*continued*)

Rifampin
   Example: Rifadin
   Binds β-subunit of bacterial RNA polymerase
   Broad spectrum

Trimethoprim and sulfonamides
   Examples: Bactrim, Septra
   Inhibit enzymes in tetrahydrofolate biosynthetic pathway
   Broad spectrum against bacteria, some fungi (*Pneumocystis carinii*), and protozoa

QUESTIONS

Answers to the questions can be found in Appendix 2.

1. How do antiseptics, disinfectants, and antibiotics differ from each other?

2. Why might it be harder for a bacterium to become resistant to a disinfectant than to an antibiotic?

3. Many of the antibiotics described in this chapter have a similar type of action: they bind to an important bacterial target and inhibit its activity. Are there exceptions to this rule?

4. The pharmaceutical industry has been trying to develop antibiotics by solving the crystal structure of a protein target and designing molecules that fit into the active site of this target (rational drug design). So far, this strategy has not been nearly as successful as expected. Why did scientists think this would be superior to the old ways of finding antibiotics and what are some of the reasons this approach might fail?

5. Many of the aminoglycoside antibiotics are much less effective against *Escherichia coli* under anaerobic conditions than under aerobic conditions. Assume that the rates of protein synthesis are about the same in both cases and that the antibiotic inhibits protein synthesis in vitro. How would you explain the reduced effectiveness under anaerobic conditions?

6. Although in vitro tests of susceptibility to antibiotics are widely used and considered useful, there have been cases in which the in vitro tests have not predicted how well the drug would work when administered to humans. This works both ways. Some antibiotics that are effective in vitro fail when administered to humans, and some antibiotics that test resistant in vitro actually work when used therapeutically. Give some explanations for both of these outcomes.

7. In the quest for new antibiotics, what are the pharmaceutical companies trying to do? What criteria would you use to judge whether to develop a new antibiotic? What is the attraction of sticking with known antibiotics and trying to modify their structures rather than looking for new antibiotic targets?

11

How Bacteria Become Resistant to Antibiotics

The Dawning of Awareness

The 1990s were the decade when the public first began to take real notice of antibiotic-resistant bacteria. Prior to this, physicians had tended to downplay the importance of antibiotic-resistant strains of disease-causing bacteria because in virtually all cases there were still antibiotics—sometimes many antibiotics—that worked. But a shift in attitude had already begun to appear. At one time, having to turn to a second antibiotic was considered a treatment failure. Gradually, the definition of treatment failure shifted to failure to find a successful antibiotic after trying several antibiotics. As long as the physician finally hit upon an effective antibiotic, the treatment was a success. Patients did not always agree. Patients with serious systemic infections sometimes suffered irreversible damage to important organs or suffered a stroke because the infection was not brought under control quickly enough.

Arguably, among the first to become publicly concerned about antibiotic-resistant bacteria were the officials of health insurance companies and health maintenance organizations. Infections caused by resistant bacteria were proving to be expensive (Box 11–1). Resistant bacteria were also costing state and local governments money. It cost New York City nearly a billion dollars to bring the multidrug-resistant tuberculosis outbreak of the mid-1990s under control. About this same time, the New York Chamber of Commerce approached the state legislators to ask what was being done about antibiotic resistance. Even in the absence of a high-profile epidemic, businesses were losing money because of employee days lost from work and higher health care costs, and there appeared to be no end to this problem. In the Senate, Senators Kennedy and Frist held hearings about antibiotic-resistant bacteria and their potential impact on human health.

Predictably, the media fell on the issue with gusto. Headlines such as "The End of Antibiotics" and "Return to the Preantibiotic Era" began to appear in the news magazines. Not surprisingly, the content of most of these articles was sensational and frightening. Even the normally staid journal *Science* sported a cover that made the mainstream media seem conservative by comparison. On the cover of that issue of *Science* was a diptych. The left panel was a painting by

BOX 11–1   The Cot of Antibiotic Resistance—a Telling Example

During the 1990s, *S. aureus* became one of the most common causes of hospital-acquired infections in the United States and other developed countries. Hospital-acquired infections, especially postsurgical infections, are much more common than they should be. It has been estimated that in the United States alone, about 2 million hospital patients will acquire such an infection. *S. aureus*, a common cause of nosocomial infections, has become more and more resistant to a variety of antibiotics, with the methicillin-resistant *S. aureus* (MRSA) strains being the ones that are currently the most troublesome. Actually, the acronym MRSA would be more accurately rendered as multiply resistant *S. aureus* because these strains are usually resistant to several antibiotics in addition to methicillin. The only drug currently able to control MRSA infections is vancomycin, and isolated reports of MRSA strains with reduced susceptibility to vancomycin have begun to appear.

In a recent study, Rubin and colleagues attempted to estimate the costs of MRSA infections in New York City in 1995. They found that about 21% of all *S. aureus* infections acquired in hospitals or in the community were caused by MRSA strains. In the case of community-acquired infections, the additional cost per patient to treat these infections was about $2,500. Frequently, these patients had to be hospitalized. For hospital-acquired infections, the additional cost was higher—$3,700 per patient—probably because the patients involved were sicker than the community

patients and were thus less able to control the disease.

The higher cost of treating MRSA infections was due to a variety of factors. First, vancomycin is more expensive than the drugs normally used to treat *S. aureus* infections. Second, it is often necessary to isolate patients to keep them from infecting other patients. Third, patients with MRSA infection stay longer in the hospital. The increased financial cost was not the only toll taken by MRSA. The death rate for patients with MRSA infections was a shocking 21%, about 2.5 times higher than the death rate due to infections caused by susceptible *S. aureus* strains. The resistant strains are not necessarily more virulent than the susceptible ones, but their resistance makes it harder to control them with antibiotics. Thus, the increased death rate attributed to MRSA strains is largely due to antibiotic resistance.

Not included in the economic estimates were costs to the patient. Longer hospital stays mean more days lost at work and more disruption of family life. Patients who die obviously pay the highest price, but even patients who survive could leave the hospital with irreversible damage to vital organs such as the brain, lung, and kidney. Keep in mind that MRSA strains are still treatable with vancomycin. Imagine the carnage if vancomycin-resistant MRSA strains appear.

Source: R. J. Rubin, C. A. Harrington, A. Poon, K. Dietrich, J. A. Greene, and A. Moiduddin. 1999. The economic impact of *Staphylococcus aureus* infection in New York City hospitals. *Emerg. Infect. Dis.* **5**:9–17.

Brueghel that depicted skeletons piling up during the plague years of the Middle Ages and being taken away to wherever skeletons go. The right panel was painted by a modern painter. It showed an inner city scene in which skeletons consorted with the living (but clearly not long for this world), and fires loomed in the background.

The media soon discovered the widespread agricultural use of antibiotics, and the possible impact of this use on human health began to be the subject of news articles and TV programs. Environmental advocacy groups began to consider antibiotic use and antibiotic resistance an issue on which they needed to take a

stand. Humane societies got involved because their members realized that severely restricting the use of antibiotics in agriculture might force improved hygiene and reduced crowding in large-animal production facilities, changes that would improve the quality of life for the animals being raised there.

Ironically, the one group that seemed to be left out of the growing awareness of the problem was the scientific community. Many scientists felt that the intensive research effort mounted in the 1980s to define the mechanisms of resistance to antibiotics and to characterize the transmissible elements that carry antibiotic resistance genes had uncovered all that was worth knowing about antibiotic-resistant bacteria. The funding agencies, following the lead of the scientific community, deemphasized funding for research in the area. The field of antibiotic resistance research came to be viewed as somewhat old-fashioned, and the number of scientists continuing to work in this area declined to a perilously low level.

Unfortunately, a daunting number of important questions remained unanswered. When the gram-positive cocci began to resume prominence as the most serious causes of human infections, it became evident that virtually nothing was known about their mechanisms of resistance or mechanisms of transfer of resistance genes. Moreover, many of the questions that began to dominate the debate over antibiotic use patterns and possible preventive strategies in human medicine and agriculture turned out to be questions about the ecology of antibiotic-resistant bacteria and their genes. This area had been almost untouched even in the heyday of research on antibiotic-resistant bacteria. The tide is beginning to turn. In 2001, the National Institutes of Health, the CDC, and other federal agencies announced a combined task force for public action on antimicrobial resistance, an effort that may help to solve the resistance problem.

Mechanisms of Antibiotic Resistance

Overview of Resistance Mechanisms

Mechanisms of antibiotic resistance can be grouped into four main categories. One is restricted access of the antibiotic to its target. Examples of this are the porins of gram-negative bacteria that restrict diffusion of antibiotic across the outer membrane and the efflux pumps in the cytoplasmic membrane that pump antibiotics out of the bacterial cytoplasm. (Some scientists divide this category into two further categories, restricted uptake of the antibiotic and accelerated loss of the antibiotic due to efflux pumps.) A second category of resistance mechanisms is enzymes that inactivate the antibiotic, either by hydrolyzing it or by adding chemical groups to some important part of the antibiotic. A third category is modification of the antibiotic target. For example, in response to pressure from an antibiotic that binds to ribosomes and stops protein synthesis, the bacteria modify an rRNA that is critical to the binding of the antibiotic so that the antibiotic no longer binds. Or the bacteria introduce mutations into a gene encoding a target protein so that the protein still works but no longer binds the antibiotic. The fourth category, failure to activate the antibiotic, contains only one member so far: metronidazole resistance. Metronidazole must be acti-

vated before it can attack bacterial DNA. If the bacteria do not activate the antibiotic, it is harmless.

An interesting feature of many resistance mechanisms is that they are mediated by proteins that are related to bacterial housekeeping proteins. For example, enzymes that inactivate penicillin are related to and may have evolved from the enzymes that carry out the cross-linking of peptidoglycan, enzymes that are inactivated by penicillin. Apparently, bacteria sometimes adapt the target of an antibiotic to become an offensive weapon against the antibiotic. Although the different types of resistance mechanisms will be considered individually here, it is important to realize that bacteria can combine more than one mechanism of resistance to increase the efficacy of their defensive shield against an antibiotic.

Limiting Access of the Antibiotic

OUTER MEMBRANE PORINS. Antibiotics must first reach their target in order to have an effect. β-Lactam antibiotics must transit the gram-negative outer membrane to reach the cytoplasmic membrane where the penicillin-binding proteins are located. In gram-negative bacteria, the outer membrane can function as a barrier to antibiotic entry. The reason vancomycin, which is very effective against gram-positive bacteria, is not effective against most gram-negative bacteria is that it is too bulky to diffuse through the outer membrane porins. The natural advantage that restrictive porins give to gram-negative bacteria can be increased by mutations in porins that further limit diffusion of the antibiotic. And since some types of porins are relatively nonselective, a single porin mutation can confer resistance to more than one type of antibiotic. For a long time, the importance of porin mutations as a mechanism of resistance was underappreciated because this type of resistance usually confers increases in resistance of only 5- to 10-fold, whereas other types of resistance can confer 50- to 100-fold increases in resistance. However, in clinical settings, where the highest concentration of antibiotic achievable at the site of infection is sometimes less than 5 times the level required to kill or inhibit growth of the bacteria, a 10-fold increase in resistance can be as disastrous as a 100-fold increase.

REDUCED UPTAKE ACROSS THE CYTOPLASMIC MEMBRANE. An obvious way for bacteria to resist the action of an antibiotic that has a target in the bacterial cytoplasm (e.g., the ribosome or DNA gyrase) is to fail to transport the antibiotic across the cytoplasmic membrane. Yet, this is not a common mechanism of resistance, so far as we know. In some cases, the lack of such a mechanism of resistance is understandable. Tetracycline, for example, diffuses readily through membranes because it is a hydrophobic compound. Penicillin and other β-lactam antibiotics do not need to reach the cytoplasm. Nonetheless, there are other antibiotics, such as the aminoglycosides, that appear to use a specific transporter to enter the cell. Possibly the transporter, whose identity is still unknown, is too important to the bacteria to be mutated to prevent aminoglycoside uptake. An interesting but little-known fact is that some bacteria become much more resistant to aminoglycosides when they are growing under anaerobic conditions. *Escherichia coli* becomes almost 10 times more resistant to aminoglycosides when growing anaerobically and many anaerobes are totally resistant to aminoglycosides. In both cases, the resistance appears to be due to drastically reduced uptake of the antibiotic.

Enzymatic Inactivation of the Antibiotic

β-LACTAMASES. A major mechanism of resistance to β-lactam antibiotics, especially among gram-negative bacteria, is **β-lactamase,** an enzyme that cleaves the β-lactam ring and renders the antibiotic inactive (Figure 11–1). β-Lactamases are secreted into the periplasmic space by gram-negative bacteria and into the extracellular fluid by gram-positive bacteria. Because the gram-negative bacteria confine their β-lactamases to the periplasm and have porins that restrict the entry of β-lactams into this region, they can achieve the same level of resistance with a lower level of enzyme than gram-positive bacteria. Unlike porin mutations, which confer resistance to many different antibiotics, β-lactamases are much more specific and are usually active only against a subset of β-lactam antibiotics. The main reason for the large number of β-lactam antibiotics now on the market is the need for new β-lactam antibiotics that are not cleaved by existing β-lactamases. So far, the appearance of each new β-lactam on the market has been followed not long after by the first report of a new β-lactamase that inactivates it.

A strategy for countering β-lactamases is to mix the β-lactam antibiotic with a β-lactamase inhibitor, such as **clavulanic acid** (Figure 11–1) or **sulbactam.** Clavulanic acid and sulbactam do not kill bacteria but prevent β-lactamase from inactivating the antibiotic, which can then proceed to kill the bacteria. Predictably, there are now β-lactamases that are resistant to both clavulanic acid and sulbactam inhibition, but in general the β-lactamase inhibitors have expanded the spectrum and renewed the use of some old β-lactams, such as ampicillin, that were in danger of becoming obsolete. Recently, another bacterial mechanism for resisting clavulanic acid–β-lactam mixtures has been reported: a chromosomal gene encoding β-lactamase was dupli-

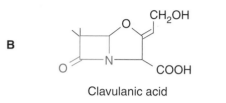

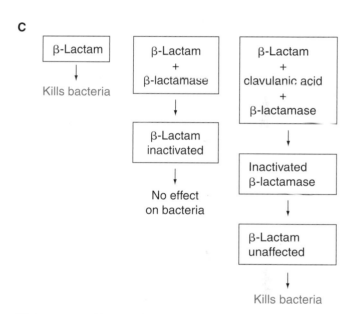

Figure 11–1 The mode of action of β-lactamase (**A**) and the structure of clavulanic acid (**B**), an inhibitor of β-lactamase. (**C**) Clavulanic acid inactivates the β-lactamase so that β-lactam antibiotic can then kill the bacteria.

cated many times to give a much higher level of β-lactamase production. Apparently, the excess β-lactamase was able to bind enough clavulanic acid to allow the remaining β-lactamase to inactivate the antibiotic.

AMINOGLYCOSIDE-MODIFYING ENZYMES. The main mechanism of aminoglycoside resistance is inactivation of the antibiotic. In contrast to β-lactamases, which cleave a C-N bond in the antibiotic, aminoglycoside-modifying enzymes inactivate the antibiotic by adding groups (phosphoryl, adenyl, or acetyl groups) to the antibiotic (Figure 11–2). In gram-negative bacteria, the

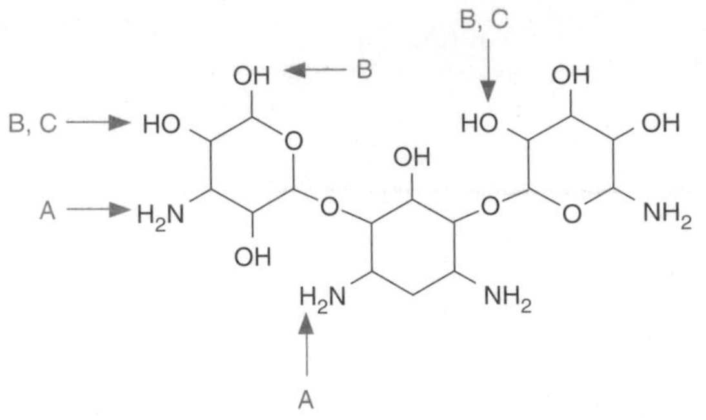

A, acetyl; B, adenyl; C, phosphoryl

Figure 11–2 Action of aminoglycoside-inactivating enzymes.

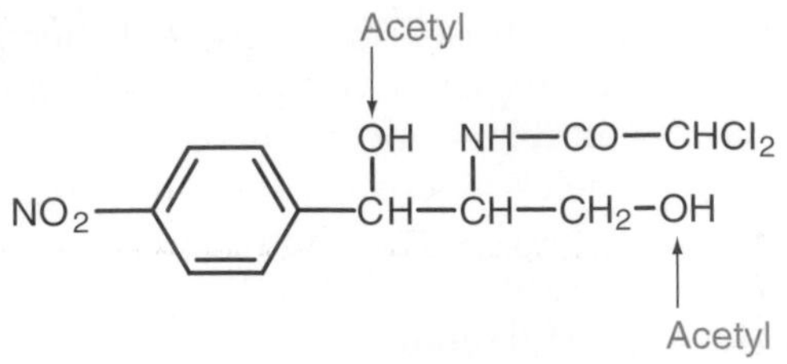

Chloramphenicol

Figure 11–3 Action of chloramphenicol transacetylase. The addition of acetyl groups to chloramphenicol prevents it from binding to the 50S subunit of the ribosome.

aminoglycoside-modifying enzymes are thought to be located on the outside of the cytoplasmic membrane. Modification of the antibiotic reduces its transport into the cell. The location of gram-positive aminoglycoside-modifying enzymes has not been established, but they must either be released into the extracellular fluid or tethered to the cytoplasmic membrane.

CHLORAMPHENICOL ACETYLTRANSFERASE. A mechanism of resistance to chloramphenicol is an enzyme that adds an acetyl group to chloramphenicol, thus inactivating it (Figure 11–3). The enzyme is called **chloramphenicol acetyltransferase** because it transfers an acetyl group from *S*-adenosylmethionine, a compound used in many housekeeping methyl transfer reactions, to chloramphenicol.

STREPTOGRAMIN ACETYLTRANSFERASE. Although streptogramins have only been in use to treat human infections for a short time, resistance is already beginning to be seen. Acetyltransferases that inactivate streptogramins are encoded by *vat* and *sat* genes. These genes have been found in staphylococci and enterococci.

OXIDATION OF TETRACYCLINE. A novel enzyme has been discovered that uses chemical modification to inactivate tetracycline. The nature of the modification is not known, but the reaction requires oxygen and thus works only in aerobically growing bacteria. It is not clear how widespread the gene encoding this resistance, *tetX,* is in nature, but it may not be of much clinical relevance. Most body sites are relatively low in free oxygen because oxygen is bound to hemoglobin. An odd feature of this resistance is that the gene was found originally in an obligate anaerobe (*Bacteroides fragilis*), despite the fact that the resistance mechanism cannot work in this type of organism. This finding highlights the potential for further surprises from nature.

Active Efflux of the Antibiotic

RESISTANCE TO TETRACYCLINES. Many antibiotics currently in use inhibit protein synthesis. For these antibiotics to work, they must enter the cell cytoplasm and accumulate to a concentration sufficient to allow them to bind the ribosome. A bacterial strategy that prevents antibiotics from reaching a high enough concentration in the cytoplasm is to pump the antibiotic out of the cytoplasm as rapidly as it is taken up. These protein pumps are called **efflux pumps.** The first efflux mechanism to be discovered mediated resistance to tetracyclines. The resistance protein was a cytoplasmic membrane protein that catalyzes energy-dependent transport of tetracycline out of the bacterium (Figure 11–4). Since tetracycline is removed as rapidly as it is taken up, the intracellular concentration of tetracycline remains too low to inhibit protein synthesis. Genes encoding tetracycline efflux proteins have been found in gram-negative bacteria (*tetA* to *tetG*) and in gram-positive bacteria (*tetK, tetL*). For a long time, efflux was thought to be the only mechanism of resistance to tetracycline, but another and possibly more widespread type of resistance has now been identified—target protection.

RESISTANCE TO MACROLIDES. An ATP-dependent efflux system that pumps macrolides out of the cell has been found in *Staphylococcus* species. This efflux system works only on some of the macrolides. The deduced amino acid sequence of the gene shares homology with known ATP-dependent transport proteins.

RESISTANCE TO QUINOLONES. There is some evidence for an efflux system that expels fluoroquinolones, although no efflux protein has yet been identified. Since the efflux activity was too low to explain the full range of observed resistance, it was suggested that fluoroquinolone efflux must occur together with some other

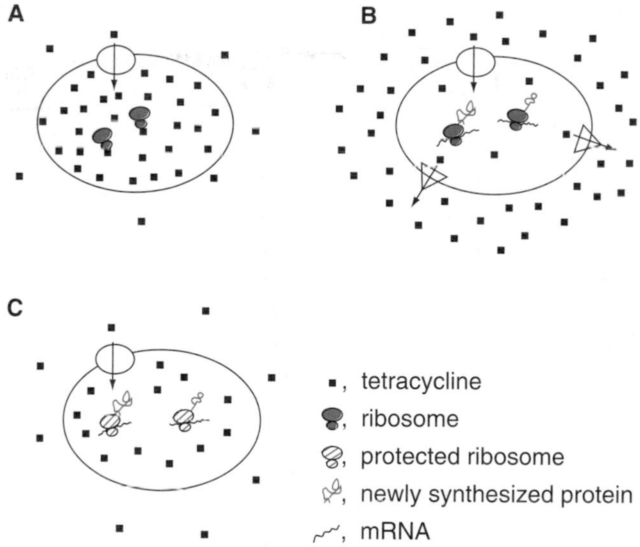

Figure 11–4 Mechanisms of tetracycline resistance. (**A**) Tetracycline (black squares) is taken up by a transporter (open ellipse); intracellular concentration becomes higher than extracellular concentration; tetracycline binds to ribosomes and stops protein synthesis. (**B**) Cytoplasmic membrane protein (open triangle) pumps tetracycline out of the cell as fast as the transporter takes it up; intracellular concentration remains too low for effective binding to ribosomes. (**C**) Tetracycline accumulation within cell is similar to that in sensitive cell, but ribosome is protected (hatching), so tetracycline no longer binds to it.

resistance mechanism, such as lessened uptake of the fluoroquinolones.

RESISTANCE TO STREPTOGRAMINS. Efflux pumps that pump streptogramins out of the cell have been found in staphylococci.

Modification or Protection of the Antibiotic Target

RESISTANCE TO β-LACTAMS. Alteration of the target of the antibiotic is a second mechanism of resistance to β-lactam antibiotics. In this case, the binding specificity of the **penicillin-binding proteins** is altered so that they no longer bind the β-lactam antibiotic. This type of resistance is particularly common among gram-positive bacteria and is currently the type of β-lactam resistance that is causing the most problems clinically. β-Lactamase inhibitors can counter resistance due to β-lactamase, but this fix does not work for resistance due to alteration in the penicillin-binding proteins. Probably the best-characterized resistance gene of this type is *mecA,* a gene encoding resistance to methicillin

that is found in *Staphylococcus aureus*. This resistance gene encodes a mutant β-lactam binding protein (also called penicillin-binding protein 2′, or **PBP2′**) that is not inhibited as readily by methicillin as the bacterium's normal β-lactam binding proteins are. Apparently, this new protein replaces the normal transpeptidase and allows peptidoglycan cross-linking to occur in the presence of the β-lactam antibiotic.

RESISTANCE TO GLYCOPEPTIDE ANTIBIOTICS. Since vancomycin prevents cross-linking of peptidoglycan by binding to the D-Ala–D-Ala of the muramyl-peptide (NAM), an obvious strategy for becoming resistant to vancomycin is to replace this dipeptide with a group that does not bind vancomycin. Most gram-positive bacteria that have become resistant to vancomycin replace the D-Ala–D-Ala with D-Ala–D-lactate, which does not bind vancomycin. There are three essential enzymes needed for this resistance phenotype (Figure 11–5). One is encoded either by *vanA* or *vanB*. It encodes a ligase that makes the D-Ala–D-lactate from D-Ala and D-lactate. A second gene, *vanH,* encodes a lactate dehydrogenase that makes lactate from pyruvate. These two enzymes make it possible for the bacteria to make the substitute part of the muramyl dipeptide, but as long as the bacteria still produce the original D-Ala–D-Ala form, they will remain susceptible to vancomycin. This is where the third gene, *vanX,* comes into the picture. VanX is an enzyme that cleaves D-Ala–D-Ala but not D-Ala–D-lactate. The mechanism of vancomycin resistance is the most complex resistance mechanism known and shows how resourceful bacteria can be when it comes to protecting themselves from antibiotics.

The origin of the vancomycin resistance genes is still a mystery. They could have come from the vancomycin-producing bacteria, such as *Amycolatopsis coloradensis,* although the currently circulating resistance genes share only 54 to 61% amino acid identity with the corresponding genes of *A. coloradensis*. Another possible source is naturally vancomycin-resistant bacteria, such as *Lactobacillus* species, that do not use the D-Ala–D-Ala dipeptide as part of their muramyl dipeptide.

RESISTANCE TO TETRACYCLINES. A second clinically important type of resistance to tetracycline, called **ribosome protection,** is conferred by a cytoplasmic protein that somehow protects the ribosomes from tetracycline (Figure 11–4). When the protein is present in the bacterial cytoplasm, tetracycline no longer binds to the ribosome. How the resistance protein does this is not clear, but there appears to be no covalent modification of the ribosome. An interesting feature of this type of resistance protein is that it has a GTPase activity and shares high amino acid similarity in its amino terminal

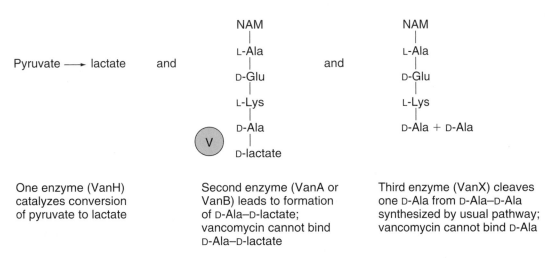

A Susceptible bacteria

Normal cross-linking
in peptidoglycan

Vancomycin (V) binds to
D-Ala–D-Ala preventing
cross-linking

B Resistant bacteria

Pyruvate ⟶ lactate   and   ...   and   ...

One enzyme (VanH)
catalyzes conversion
of pyruvate to lactate

Second enzyme (VanA or
VanB) leads to formation
of D-Ala–D-lactate;
vancomycin cannot bind
D-Ala–D-lactate

Third enzyme (VanX) cleaves
one D-Ala from D-Ala–D-Ala
synthesized by usual pathway;
vancomycin cannot bind D-Ala

Figure 11–5   Mechanism of vancomycin resistance. (**A**) Action of vancomycin in susceptible bacteria. (**B**) Mechanisms that prevent vancomycin binding in resistant bacteria; three enzymes are involved, one (VanH) that catalyzes conversion of pyruvate to lactate, a second one (VanA or VanB) that catalyzes the synthesis of D-Ala–D-lactate instead of D-Ala–D-Ala, and a third one (Van X) that cleaves the terminal D-Ala from the D-Ala–D-Ala that is synthesized by the normal pathway.

region with bacterial elongation factors involved in protein synthesis. Although tetracycline efflux has been studied for decades, the ribosome protection type of resistance was discovered only recently. Nonetheless, this type of resistance is quite widespread among a number of different groups of bacteria, including gram-positive bacteria, mycoplasmas, and some gram-negative genera, such as *Neisseria, Haemophilus,* and *Bacteroides.* Several genes encoding this type of resistance have now been identified. Examples are *tetM, tetO,* and *tetQ.*

RESISTANCE TO MACROLIDES, STREPTOGRAMINS, AND LINCOSAMIDES.   An enzyme that methylates an adenine on 23S rRNA mediates a widespread type of resistance to macrolides, streptogramins, and lincosamides. This enzyme is called **rRNA methylase.** The methylated adenine lies within a region that serves as a binding site for all three of these classes of antibiotics. Thus, acquisition of a single resistance gene confers resistance to three structurally distinct classes of antibiotic. This type of resistance has been found mainly in gram-positive cocci and in the *Bacteroides* group. Examples are *ermA, ermB, ermF,* and *ermG.* Members of the *E. coli* group of gram-negative bacteria tend to be naturally resistant to macrolides, probably because their porins do not admit the antibiotic to the periplasm.

RESISTANCE TO QUINOLONES AND RIFAMPIN.   Resistance to quinolones commonly involves point mutations that alter the affinity of the DNA gyrase B subunit for the antibiotic. Although the mutations in DNA gyrase are in an essential gene, they appear not to have a deleterious effect on bacterial growth. Bacteria can also acquire a gyrase B gene that encodes the resistant form of the B subunit. Similarly, resistance to rifampin results from mutations in RNA polymerase that reduce the affinity of the enzyme for the antibiotic.

RESISTANCE TO TRIMETHOPRIM AND SULFONAMIDES. Resistance to trimethoprim and sulfonamides arises from mutations in the enzymes inhibited by these antibiotics. The mutant form of the enzyme no longer binds the antibiotic with a higher affinity than its natural substrate. Mutations conferring resistance to sulfonamides or to trimethoprim occur rather frequently, but simultaneous double mutations that confer resistance to both types of antibiotic occur only rarely. For this reason, a combination of trimethoprim and one of the sulfonamides is currently used for antibacterial therapy.

Failure to Activate an Antibiotic

Resistance to metronidazole is poorly understood, but in at least some cases, mutations that lower expression of the gene encoding flavodoxin, the protein that activates metronidazole, seem to be responsible for metronidazole resistance. This topic will be covered in more depth in the chapter on *Helicobacter pylori* (chapter 23). Metronidazole is one of the antibiotics used to treat ulcers. The appearance of resistance to metronidazole by *H. pylori,* the cause of ulcers, is an ominous development for future ulcer sufferers.

Regulation of Resistance Genes

REPRESSORS. Since bacteria need resistance genes only when they encounter antibiotics, it makes sense that many antibiotic resistance genes are regulated. The first type of regulation described was repressor-mediated regulation of the efflux-type tetracycline resistance genes. In this type of regulation, the gene encoding the repressor (*tetR*) and the gene encoding the structural gene (*tetB*) are transcribed from divergent promoters (Figure 11–6). In the absence of tetracycline,

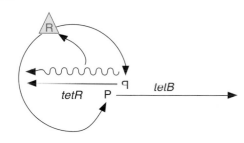
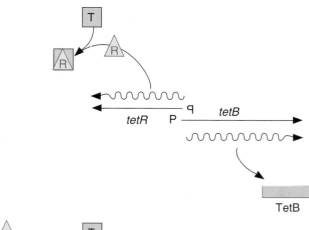

Figure 11–6   Repressor-mediated regulation of the efflux type of tetracycline resistance genes.

the repressor stops transcription of both genes. When tetracycline enters the cell and binds the repressor, the repressor-tetracycline complex is unable to bind the promoter region of the structural gene, so the structural gene (*tetB*) is transcribed. The repressor continues to be produced, but until all the tetracycline is titrated by the repressor, synthesis of the resistance gene continues. Although many β-lactamase genes are expressed constitutively, some of these genes are regulated by a repressor type of mechanism. This type of regulation has been found in *S. aureus.* An interesting feature of this regulation is that the β-lactam exerts its regulatory effect from the periplasm, presumably by interacting with a cytoplasmic membrane repressor protein, which in turn conveys the regulatory signal to the DNA.

ATTENUATION.   Another common type of regulation of resistance genes, first described for erythromycin resistance (*erm*) genes of gram-positive bacteria, is a form of **attenuation** (Figure 11–7). The mRNA for the resistance gene starts nearly 100 bp upstream of the start

No erythromycin

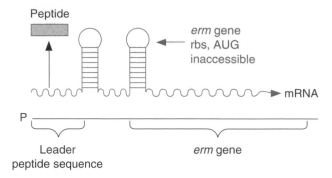

Erythromycin

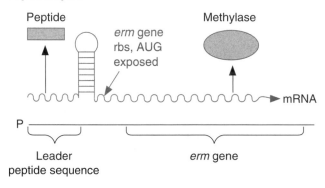

Figure 11–7   Regulation of resistance genes by attenuation. rbs, ribosome binding site.

codon for the resistance protein. This 100 bp encodes a short peptide (**leader peptide**). In the absence of the macrolide, ribosomes move rapidly along the mRNA. Under these conditions, **stem-loop structures** form in the mRNA in such a way that the ribosome binding site and start codon of the *erm* gene are hidden in the stem-loop. If erythromycin is present, most of the bacterium's ribosomes cannot translocate and thus do not move along the mRNA. This allows a different stem-loop structure to form and exposes the ribosome binding site and start codon for the *erm* structural gene. A small fraction of the ribosomes are modified at any given time (because of occasional production of the methylase despite the first stem-loop structure). These ribosomes translate the *erm* message and produce the methylase. The methylase then modifies all the bacterium's ribosomes, allowing normal growth to resume.

ACTIVATORS.   Regulation of resistance genes by **transcriptional activators** has also been reported. Vancomycin resistance genes from *Enterococcus* species are activated by a two-component regulatory system that senses vancomycin. Some β-lactamase genes found in *Enterobacter* and *Pseudomonas* species also appear to be controlled by transcriptional activators, but not much is known about the details of the mechanism.

INSERTION SEQUENCES AND PROMOTER MUTATIONS. Although transcriptional regulation mechanisms are usually reversible, so that expression of a gene can be turned off as well as on, there is a type of increased transcription that might be considered regulatory although it results in a permanent alteration. Mutations in a promoter region or insertion of an insertion sequence upstream of a resistance gene increase the expression of the resistance gene and thus the level of resistance. An example is the *ampC* gene of *Enterobacter* sp. This gene was originally expressed at such a low level that it did not make the bacteria resistant to ampicillin. Gradually, under continued selection by antibiotic use, the gene acquired promoter mutations that increased its expression to the point that it has become a serious contributor to antibiotic resistance.

Other resistance genes, which were originally silent when they entered a new host, acquired an insertion sequence in their promoter region that caused the gene to be expressed. Most insertion sequences have promoters that point outward from their ends. Thus, when they insert into a region upstream of an open reading frame, they provide a promoter that now controls expression of the gene. An example of this is a plasmid-borne erythromycin resistance gene in *Bacteroides* species, *ermF*, which is expressed because it has acquired a promoter from an insertion sequence. Since there are many such examples of promoter mutations or insertion of an insertion sequence that activate the expression of a gene, scientists now consider that any resistance gene that enters a bacterial strain, whether it is expressed initially or not, is of concern because it can be activated at any time.

Cross-Resistance and Linkage

The first resistance mechanisms to be described conferred resistance to a single class of antibiotics. For example, β-lactamases confer resistance to members of the penicillin-cephalosporin family but not to protein synthesis inhibitors. Two exceptions to this rule have appeared in recent years. The first is the **multidrug efflux pumps,** which pump out antibiotics of more than one type. How such pumps work is still a mystery because they are nonspecific in the sense that they export more than one antibiotic class, but they are specific in that they do not export small molecules essential to the bacterium. The second exception is the macrolide-streptogramin-lincosamide type of erythromycin resistance, which makes a bacterium resistant to three different classes of antibiotics. This is possible because these three types of antibiotics bind to the same site on the ribosome that is modified by the resistance protein.

A distinct—but similar—problem is the development of multidrug resistance due to genetically linked resistance genes. These genetic linkages can develop when two or more resistance genes are picked up by a plasmid or other transmissible agent. Two mechanisms by which resistance genes can move onto plasmids are transposons and integrons, described below.

Both the multidrug resistance mechanisms and the development of genetically linked resistance gene clusters create a troubling problem. In bacterial strains where either occurs, selection by one class of antibiotic can hold in place resistance genes that confer resistance to unrelated antibiotics. Thus, for example, if a plasmid contains both a tetracycline resistance gene and a macrolide resistance gene, exposure of that strain to tetracycline selects not only for maintenance of the tetracycline resistance gene but also for maintenance of the erythromycin resistance gene.

Many physicians have assumed that use of a particular class of antibiotic selects for resistance to only that particular class of antibiotic. If this were true, cessation of use of a type of antibiotic should allow resistance to that antibiotic to decrease or disappear. The multidrug resistance genes and the linkages of genes ensure that this desirable outcome will not occur in some cases because of cross-selection. To make matters worse, there are some cases in which disinfectant resistance genes have proved to be linked genetically to antibiotic resistance genes. In such cases, disinfectant use could select for the maintenance of the antibiotic resistance genes. Whereas we had all hoped that disinfectants and antiseptics would help protect us from antibiotic-resistant bacteria, they may in some cases have exactly the opposite effect. Fortunately, such cases are rare so far.

Antibiotic Tolerance

The antibiotics that inhibit cell wall synthesis are bactericidal because the bacterium participates in its own destruction; bacterial enzymes that normally participate in cell wall turnover (lytic enzymes or autolysins) degrade the peptidoglycan, leaving the bacterium without the protection of its cell wall. Bacteria that can prevent their autolysins from destroying their peptidoglycan or that are located in an area of the body where they can survive without a cell wall can avoid killing by the antibiotic. This type of response to antibiotics is called **tolerance.** Tolerance differs from resistance because a tolerant bacterium stops growing when the antibiotic is present, but it is not killed so it has a chance to recover when levels of the antibiotic fall. By contrast, a resistant

bacterium continues to grow in the presence of the antibiotic.

Tolerance of vancomycin has developed in *Streptococcus pneumoniae,* a leading cause of bacterial pneumonia and meningitis. The mechanism of tolerance is a modification in the two-component regulatory system (*vncR, vncS*) that represses autolysis. Normally, VncS phosphorylates VncR, and phosphorylated VncR represses autolysis. VncS can also dephosphorylate VncR, thus allowing autolysins to be made. In strains of *S. pneumoniae* that are tolerant of vancomycin, mutations have abolished production of VncS, the sensor. Apparently, VncR in such strains is phosphorylated by some other sensor and is less likely to be dephosphorylated. Thus, lysis is repressed most of the time. This model is still somewhat hypothetical but it illustrates a way in which a bacterium could become tolerant. The bacteria would stop growing because vancomycin inhibits formation of a new cell wall, but the bacteria survive because they do not lyse.

A different type of tolerance has been seen in the case of *E. coli* strains that cause kidney infections. Since the kidney filters blood and excretes wastes in urine, the concentration of salts in the kidney is higher than that in other tissues. Thus, when *E. coli* loses its cell wall because penicillin stops cell wall synthesis and autolysins degrade the existing cell wall, the osmotic strength of the fluid in which the bacteria are bathed is high enough to keep the bacteria from lysing due to internal turgor pressure. Forms of *E. coli* and other bacteria that lack a cell wall have been called L forms.

Transfer of Resistance Genes

Why Mutation Is Often Not the Preferred Solution

Bacteria can become resistant to antibiotics by mutation of existing genes, but this strategy is very expensive for the bacteria. In the process of testing different mutations, many bacteria will die. Sometimes a single mutation is sufficient to confer resistance. This is the case with fluoroquinolone resistance; one mutation in the bacterial DNA gyrase can make the enzyme unable to bind the antibiotic and make the bacterium resistant to the fluoroquinolone. In such cases, mutation to resistance is a feasible option for the bacterium. In other cases, such as resistance to penicillins or tetracyclines, many mutations are needed, and development of resistance by mutation can take a long time. A much easier, quicker, and safer way for a bacterium to become resistant to an antibiotic is to acquire a resistance gene or genes from some other bacterium. Scientists believe that the most common mode of acquiring resistance genes, especially when the donor is a member of a different species, is by conjugation.

Although bacteria can acquire new genes by bacteriophage **transduction** or by **transformation** (uptake of DNA from the external environment), these types of transfer tend to occur mainly between members of the same species or between members of very closely related species. The reason is that, in phage transduction, the bacteria need the right phage receptor on their surfaces, a trait that is usually restricted to a closely related group of bacteria. In the case of natural transformation, linear single-stranded fragments of DNA are taken up by a specialized set of proteins. In both cases, the DNA must integrate into the genome by homologous recombination. Thus, bacteria must be close enough to each other genetically for homologous recombination to be possible. Conjugation has no such limitations.

Narrow-host-range resistance gene transfer, such as that mediated by phage transduction or transformation, can be important clinically. For example, transformation may be transferring from other streptococci the mutant penicillin-binding proteins that make *S. pneumoniae* resistant to penicillin. However, the spread of resistance genes, especially between members of different species, is a much more serious general threat. Accordingly, attention has tended to focus on transfer of resistance genes by conjugation. **Conjugation** is the direct cell-to-cell transfer of DNA through a protein complex that transits the membranes of two bacteria. There are two types of conjugative elements: plasmids and conjugative transposons.

Plasmids

The best-studied type of conjugative element is the conjugative **plasmid** (Figure 11–8). Not all plasmids are ca-

pable of self-transfer. Plasmids that transfer themselves by conjugation must carry a number of genes encoding proteins needed for the conjugation process (*tra* genes). Thus, **self-transmissible plasmids** are usually at least 25 kbp in size. Some plasmids that cannot transfer themselves can still be mobilized by self-transmissible plasmids. These are called **mobilizable plasmids** and can be much smaller than self-transmissible plasmids because they need only one or two genes (*mob genes*) to take advantage of the transfer machinery provided by the other plasmid.

Clinical isolates resistant to many different types of antibiotics are being seen with increasing frequency. This multidrug resistance can arise in two ways. First, some types of resistance mechanisms, such as mutations in gram-negative porins or some types of antibiotic efflux, confer resistance to more than one type of antibiotic. Second, mobile genetic elements, such as plasmids, can acquire multiple resistance genes. Thus, acquisition of a single plasmid can make the recipient resistant to multiple drugs. (Later, it will be seen that multiple virulence determinants can also be transferred by plasmids.) Many examples of plasmids carrying multiple resistance genes have been reported, but until recently it was not clear how such plasmids arose.

Transposons and Integrons

A plasmid can pick up more than one resistance gene if the resistance genes are carried on **transposons,** DNA segments that can insert into a chromosome or plasmid independently of homologous recombination. Transposons are flanked by DNA segments known as **insertion sequences,** which encode the enzyme that catalyzes transposition (**transposase**) and provide the ends recognized by transposase when it cuts and pastes the DNA during an insertion event (Figure 11–9). Insertion sequences have structural similarities that make it possible to recognize them from their DNA sequences even when transposition activity cannot be demonstrated. Between the insertion sequences are resistance genes or other genes not involved in transposition that are carried by the transposon. Some multiresistance plasmids

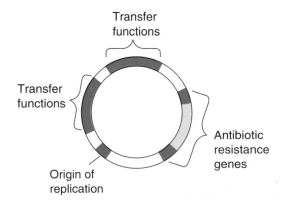

Figure 11–8 Examples of functions associated with conjugative plasmids.

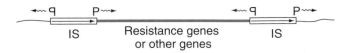

Figure 11–9 Structure of a transposon. A transposon is composed of two insertion sequences (IS) and intervening DNA, which can carry antibiotic resistance genes or genes conferring other traits. The insertion sequences and the DNA they flank move as a single unit.

may have arisen by acquiring sequential transposon insertions. However, most multiresistance plasmids appear to have arisen by a different mechanism.

Another type of element, called an **integron,** is probably responsible for the evolution of many of the plasmids that carry multiple resistance genes. Integrons are usually transposons, but they have an extra feature. They contain an **integrase** gene and an **attachment (*att*) site.** Integrase integrates circular DNA segments containing a promoterless single open reading frame (gene cassettes) into the *att* site (Figure 11–10). In effect, integrons create operons by sequential integration of the gene cassettes. Next to the *att* site is a promoter provided by the integron that will allow the integrated genes to be expressed.

Conjugative Transposons

A second type of conjugative element is the **conjugative transposon.** Conjugative transposons are normally located in the bacterial chromosome but can excise and transfer themselves from the chromosome of the donor to the chromosome of the recipient. They can also integrate into plasmids. They excise themselves from the donor genome by a process of nearly precise excision (Figure 11–11). The transfer intermediate is a covalently closed circle that does not replicate but transfers similarly to a plasmid. In the recipient, the circular intermediate integrates in the chromosome by a mechanism that does not duplicate the target site. Thus, they differ

in a number of ways from standard transposons, phages, and plasmids.

Conjugative transposons are probably responsible for at least as much resistance gene transfer as plasmids, especially among gram-positive bacteria. Also, they have a broader host range than most plasmids. Conjugative transposons can transfer not only among species within the gram-positive group or within the gram-negative group but between gram-positive and gram-negative bacteria. Conjugative transposons were overlooked for a long time because they are located in the chromosome and thus cannot be isolated and identified as easily as plasmids. Now that scientists are looking for them, conjugative transposons have been found in

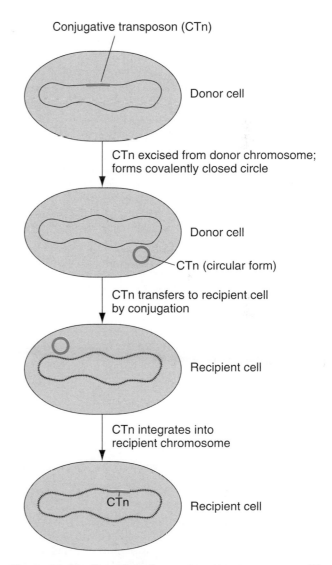

Figure 11–11   Transfer of a conjugative transposon. The transposon, which is integrated into the genome of the donor cell, excises itself to form a circular intermediate. The intermediate form transfers by conjugation into the recipient, where it integrates into the recipient's genome.

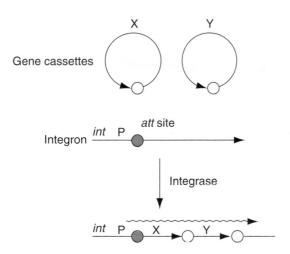

Figure 11–10   Integration of two gene cassettes, carrying promoterless resistance genes X and Y, into an integron. The integron supplies the promoter (P) and an integrase gene (*int*). The gene cassettes insert site-specifically and direction-specifically into the integron *att* site. Although two genes are shown here, some integrons accumulate many genes.

many bacteria, including such familiar genera as *Salmonella, Vibrio, Rhizobium,* and *Agrobacterium.*

A recent study of resistance gene transfers among *Bacteroides* species in the human colon has revealed that conjugal transfers of resistance genes mediated by conjugative transposons occur more frequently than expected (Box 11–2).

Will We Return to the Preantibiotic Era?

A scenario portrayed in some of the more lurid news stories about antibiotic-resistant bacteria is the return to a world much like that of the 1800s, when there were no antibiotics, and people commonly died of diseases such as pneumonia and wound infections. Surgery would once more become an intervention of last resort with a high mortality rate due to untreatable postsurgical infections. Is this likely to happen? Not very. First, it is highly unlikely that all antibiotics will become in-

effective against all bacteria. There are some bacteria, such as *Streptococcus pyogenes,* once a dreaded cause of wound infections and maternal mortality, that have remained susceptible to most antibiotics. Why this continued susceptibility is seen in some—unfortunately, not many—bacteria is not clear, but it gives room for hope that there will still be some treatable diseases.

A second consideration is that we have learned a lot about bacterial infections since the 1800s. Passive immunization—the injection of antibodies into a person who is not immune to a particular type of infection—could be used to treat infections caused by highly drug-resistant bacteria such as *S. aureus.* For certain high-risk groups, such as the elderly, vaccines may offer some measure of protection. A third consideration is that advances continue to be made in surgical procedures that make them less invasive. Laser surgery, which does not create huge surgical wounds, will not be nearly as conducive to the development of postsurgical infections as

---

BOX 11–2   How Common Is Horizontal Resistance Gene Transfer in Nature?

Plasmids or conjugative transposons that have been isolated recently from bacteria in nature generally transfer in the laboratory at very low frequencies. In a mating between a donor and a recipient, only one recipient in a million will acquire the plasmid or conjugative transposon. If this is the frequency of transfer under optimal laboratory conditions, wouldn't transfer in nature, where conditions are presumed to be less ideal, be a very rare event?

To answer this question, scientists focused on *Bacteroides* species in the human colon. *Bacteroides* is one of the numerically major genera in the human colon, accounting for about 25% of all colon isolates. *Bacteroides* species are known to have plasmids and conjugative transposons, both of which are capable of transferring antibiotic resistance genes. If the colon is perforated during surgery or other abdominal trauma, *Bacteroides* sp. can cause life-threatening infections of tissue and blood. This group of bacteria has become resistant to most antibiotics.

The scientists doing this study had access to a collection of *Bacteroides* strains that had been isolated before 1970 and to another collection of strains that had been isolated in the late 1990s. They found that before 1970, about 25% of the

strains were resistant to tetracycline, and none were resistant to erythromycin. By the late 1990s, over 80% of the *Bacteroides* strains were resistant to tetracycline, and nearly one-third were resistant to erythromycin. By using DNA hybridization and DNA sequence analysis, the scientists were able to determine that the big increase in tetracycline resistance was due to a single resistance gene, *tetQ,* which had been spread to many different *Bacteroides* species. The increase in erythromycin resistance was due primarily to the spread of two genes, *ermF* and *ermG.* The DNA sequences of the *tetQ* and *erm* genes found in different species were over 95% identical, a finding that suggested that the genes had been transferred by horizontal transfer and did not arise by independent mutational events. Finally, the investigators were able to show that *tetQ* and probably the *erm* genes as well were carried on conjugative transposons. The results of this study suggest that horizontal gene transfer by conjugation occurs very readily in the human colon.

Source: N. B. Shoemaker, H. Vlamakis, K. Hayes, and A. A. Salyers. 2001. Evidence for extensive resistance gene transfer among *Bacteroides* and other genera in the human colon. *Appl. Environ. Microbiol.* **67:**561–568.

cut-and-stitch surgery. Good hygienic practices, such as hand washing and sterilizing of surfaces, will prevent many infections if these practices are observed rigorously. As long as we do not lose disinfectants, a great deal can be done to prevent infections from occurring in the first place. And bacteria, inventive little devils that they are, are not likely to become resistant to autoclaving. There may be other preventive measures that will allow people to protect themselves from developing the predisposing conditions that increase the risk of infection. People with uncontrolled diabetes are one such high-risk group for bacterial infections. Improvements in the control of diabetes could reduce this risk. Similarly, new methods for bolstering the flagging immune systems of the elderly could make them less vulnerable to disease.

The much-maligned pharmaceutical industry should not be overlooked. Although current market forces discourage antibiotic development, the pharmaceutical industry has had a brilliant past record of discovering and developing new antibiotics. Finding ways to speed up the approval of new antibiotics would help a lot. This means, however, that the public is going to have to accept a higher level of risk of side effects if the clinical trials that cost so much time and money are abbreviated. Faced with the alternative of dying, however, people may find that side effects are acceptable after all. AIDS patients have already made this psychological transition from insisting on completely risk-free treatments to a willingness to take chances on new therapies.

Finally, there is hope of a sort in the fact that we still understand relatively little about how the most familiar antibiotics really work. We know their main mechanism of action, but there are secondary effects of most antibiotics that are deleterious to microbes that might be exploited if they were better understood. Antibiotic combinations also hold new promise. This brings us back to a theme that was introduced in chapter 4 on the nonspecific defenses: the human mind is one of the most important defenses against disease. If scientists and the public put their minds to the resistance problem instead of ignoring it as they have until recently, surprising and wonderful things could happen.

Perhaps the biggest casualty of bacterial diseases that become incurable may be confidence in the medical establishment. The public is disgruntled because scientists have not come up with a better cure for cancer or a cure for HIV infection, but at least we were never in a position in the past to cure these diseases. How will the public react if a point comes when parents have to watch children die of infections that were once curable? No one knows what the psychological fallout of lost

cures will be. Moreover, as parts of the developing world, which has been largely left out of the antibiotic revolution, become more prosperous, how will people in those countries feel about those in developed countries who squandered the miracle drugs people in developing countries are finally in a position to afford?

It doesn't take a rocket scientist to figure out that the best solution is not to lose antibiotics but to conserve this precious resource by curbing the reckless abuse and overuse of antibiotics by physicians whose habits have been shaped by the demand of patients. We don't need paintings of skeletons, such as those that graced the cover of *Science*, to evoke images of a coming plague. Instead, we need images of responsible behavior by patients and physicians alike, both dedicated to the preservation of antibiotics for the next generations.

SELECTED READINGS

Anderson, R. M. 1999. The pandemic of antibiotic resistance. *Nat. Med.* **5:**147–149.

Cockerill, F. R. 1999. Genetic methods for assessing antibiotic resistance. *Antimicrob. Agents Chemother.* **43:**199–212.

Collis, C. M., and R. M. Hall. 1992. Site-specific deletion and rearrangement of integron insert genes catalyzed by the integron DNA integrase. *J. Bacteriol.* **174:**1574–1585.

Davies, J. 1996. Bacteria on the rampage. *Nature* **383:**219–220.

Fierer, J., and D. Guiney. 1999. Extended spectrum β-lactamases: a plague of plasmids. *JAMA* **281:**563–564.

Fung-Tomc, J. 1997. Fourth-generation cephalosporins. *Clin. Microbiol. Newsl.* **19:**129–136.

Ge, M., Z. Chen, H. R. Onishi, J. Kohler, L. L. Silver, R. Kerns, S. Fukuzawa, C. Thompson, and D. Kahne. 1999. Vancomycin derivatives that inhibit peptidoglycan biosynthesis without binding D-Ala–D-Ala. *Science* **284:**508–512.

Mingeot-Leclercq, M.-P., Y. Glupczynski, and P. M. Tulkens. 1999. Aminoglycosides: activity and resistance. *Antimicrob. Agents Chemother.* **43:**727–737.

Novak, R., B. Henriques, E. Charpentier, S. Normark, and E. Tuomanen. 1999. Emergence of vancomycin tolerance in *Streptococcus pneumoniae*. *Nature* **399:**590–593.

Salyers, A. A., and N. B. Shoemaker. 1997. Conjugative transposons, p. 89–99. *In* J. K. Setlow (ed.), *Genetic Engineering*, vol. 19. Plenum Press, New York, N.Y.

Salyers, A. A., and C. F. Amabile-Cuevas. 1997. Why are antibiotic resistance genes so resistant to elimination? *Antimicrob. Agents Chemother.* **41:**2321–2325.

Silver, L. L., and K. A. Bostian. 1993. Discovery and development of new antibiotics: the problem of antibiotic resistance. *Antimicrob. Agents Chemother.* **37:**377–383.

Witte, W. 1998. Medical consequences of antibiotic use in agriculture. *Science* **279:**996–997.

SUMMARY OUTLINE

Antibiotic resistance mechanisms

Limiting access of the antibiotic
    Outer membrane porins of gram-negative bacteria
        Act as barriers to entry of antibiotics
        Mutations can restrict entry of more than one type of antibiotic
    Reduced uptake across cytoplasmic membrane—not a common mechanism

Enzymatic inactivation of antibiotics
    β-Lactamases
        Cleave β-lactam ring
        Usually specific to small subset of β-lactams
        Effect countered by adding β-lactamase inhibitors (e.g., clavulanic acid, sulbactam)
    Aminoglycoside-modifying enzymes
        Act by adding groups (phosphoryl, adenyl, acetyl) to antibiotic
        Are located outside cytoplasmic membrane in gram-negative bacteria
    Acetyl transferases add acetyl group to antibiotic
        Chloramphenicol acetyltransferase
        Streptogramin acetyltransferases
    Oxidation of tetracycline—mechanism unknown

Active efflux of antibiotic
    Efflux pumps confer resistance to tetracycline
    Found in gram-positive and gram-negative bacteria
    ATP-dependent efflux pumps confer resistance to some macrolides
    Fluoroquinolones may be expelled by pumps
    Streptogramin efflux pumps found in staphylococci

Modification or protection of antibiotic target
    Penicillin-binding proteins modified; β-lactams no longer able to bind
    Changing D-Ala–D-Ala to D-Ala–D-lactate prevents binding of glycopeptides; requires three enzymes
        VanA or VanB ligates D-Ala to D-lactate
        Van H (lactate dehydrogenase) catalyzes conversion of pyruvate to lactate
        VanX cleaves D-Ala–D-Ala but not D-Ala–D-lactate
    Ribosome protection
        Cytoplasmic protein prevents tetracycline binding to ribosome
        High amino acid homology to elongation factors
    rRNA methylase
        Methylates adenine on 23S rRNA
        Confers resistance to macrolides, streptogramins, lincosamides
    Point mutations that alter affinity of enzyme for antibiotics
        Altered DNA gyrase B subunit prevents binding of quinolones
        Altered RNA polymerase reduces affinity for rifampin
        Altered enzymes in tetrahydrofolate synthetic pathway block activity of trimethoprim and sulfonamides
    Failure to activate an antibiotic—decreased production of flavodoxin by host prevents activation of metronidazole

(continued)

SUMMARY OUTLINE (*continued*)

    Regulation of resistance genes
        Repressors
            Tetracycline efflux pumps
                Tetracycline plus repressor complex unable to bind promoter region of resistance gene (*tetB*)
                TetB produced while tetracycline is present
            β-Lactamase in *S. aureus*
        Attenuation
            Stem-loop structure formed when erythromycin present
            Ribosomes cannot move along mRNA
            Different stem-loop forms
                Allows translation of *erm* genes (methylase)
                Ribosome methylated
                Bacteria able to grow
        Transcriptional activators
            Vancomycin resistance genes in *Enterococcus* sp.
            Some β-lactamase genes in *Enterobacter* and *Pseudomonas* spp.
        Insertion sequences and promoter mutations
            Can increase expression of resistance gene if located upstream of the gene
            Examples are *ampC* gene of *Enterobacter* sp. and *ermF* of *Bacteroides* sp.
    Cross-resistance and linkage
    Multidrug efflux pumps excrete different types of antibiotics
    Modification of ribosomal binding site used by different types of antibiotics
    Multiple resistance genes linked on plasmid

Antibiotic tolerance

Bacterium stops growing when antibiotic is present

Growth resumes when antibiotic levels decrease

Vancomycin tolerance is found in *S. pneumoniae*

Transfer of resistance genes—quick way for bacterium to acquire resistance mechanisms

    Conjugative plasmids
        Plasmids transfer themselves
        Plasmid may carry several resistance genes

    Mobilizable plasmids
        Need fewer genes for transfer
        Use transfer machinery of self-transmissible plasmids

    Transposons
        DNA segments that can integrate into chromosome independent of homologous recombination
        Resistance genes or other genes flanked by insertion sequences (encode transposase)

    Integrons
        Usually transposons that carry integrase gene and *att* site
        Create operons by sequential integration of gene cassettes

    Conjugative transposons
        Normally located in bacterial chromosome
        Transfer themselves from chromosome of donor to chromosome of recipient
        Can integrate into plasmids

QUESTIONS

Answers to the questions can be found in Appendix 2.

1. Explain how mutant porins could help to make β-lactamases more effective. Could mutant porins team up with other types of resistance mechanisms to increase the effectiveness of the resistance mechanism?

2. Efflux pumps seem very energy inefficient. Why don't bacteria simply fail to take up antibiotics into the cytoplasm?

3. Efflux pumps only reduce the level of intracellular antibiotic; they do not eliminate the antibiotic completely. Why does this make the bacteria resistant to the antibiotic?

4. Some target modifications require only one or a few mutations (e.g., resistance to fluoroquinolones). Yet others, such as protection of the ribosome by methylation of rRNA, require new enzymes. Explain the difference.

5. Why does mutation to resistance occur within a short time in some cases and over a period of decades in other cases?

6. In the case of gram-negative bacteria, efflux pumps are generally coupled to outer membrane proteins. Why is this necessary?

7. Why can transfer of DNA by conjugation cross genus lines, whereas transfer of DNA by natural transformation or phage transduction is usually limited to a few closely related organisms?

8. Integrons have been found that contain disinfectant resistance genes or mercury resistance genes as well as antibiotic resistance genes. What is the potential significance of this association?

II

Specific Bacterial Pathogens

A MAJOR SCIENTIFIC DISCOVERY occurred close to the end of the 20th century: that the vast majority of biodiversity on Earth was contained in the microbial world. Carl Woese, the scientist behind this discovery, is cited in the dedication of this book. As early as the 1800s, microbiologists had suspected that this might be the case, but only with the development of DNA sequencing and other powerful molecular methods could the true extent of microbial diversity be documented. Although the bacteria that cause human disease are a small minority of the total bacterial population of the Earth, the disease-causing bacteria reflect the diversity of the larger bacterial population.

In part II, we explore diseases caused by different species of bacteria. These examples illustrate the variety of ways in which bacteria can counter human defenses and interact with human cells to produce disease symptoms. In many cases, humans are not the only hosts infected by the bacteria. Other hosts can be insects, nonhuman animals, and even amoebae. Depending on the number of hosts a bacterium infects, the ecology of a bacterial disease can be quite complex. An important theme running through the chapters of part II is the special ecology of each disease. Understanding disease ecology is particularly important for development of effective strategies of disease prevention.

The chapters of part II are organized roughly along the lines of the parts of the human body they infect. Chapters 12 to 16 focus on bacteria that enter the body through breaches in the skin. In some cases, the breach is created by an insect bite. In others, the bacteria take advantage of wounds or burns. *Pseudomonas aeruginosa* (chapter 16) serves as a bridge to the next major area of entry, the lungs. *P. aeruginosa* not only takes advantage of wounds and burns but can also cause serious lung infections. In chapters 17 to 22, other pulmonary pathogens are introduced. In chapters 23 to 28, bacteria that target the intestinal tract are featured, and in chapters 29 to 31, examples of bacteria that target the urogenital tract are provided. We grouped the chapters in this way because each site has a different array of special defenses, and the strategies of bacterial pathogens that target each site reflect the special challenges posed by the host defenses of the site. As will become evident from the contents of these chapters, it can be difficult to classify bacteria by the site of infection. Although some bacteria are site specific, such as *Helicobacter pylori* (stomach and upper intestinal tract), others, such as *Staphylococcus aureus* and *Bacillus anthracis*, can infect more than one body site. Each of the bacteria covered has its own special biology, a fact that makes designing effective preventive strategies a challenging undertaking.

It is important to realize that the bacteria covered in part II represent only a sampling of the infectious disease spectrum. Many bacteria that cause disease have not been studied enough to merit a chapter of their own. Also not represented are those bacterial pathogens that remain to be discovered. Perusal of a list of bacteria responsible for pulmonary or intestinal infections will reveal that "unknown etiology" remains a substantial category. Moreover, conditions such as heart disease, arthritis, Alzheimer's disease, cancer, and inflammatory bowel disease, which had not been considered infectious diseases in the past, are now being reexamined to determine whether bacteria or other infectious microbes are causative agents. The reason for this new interest in possible infectious causes of chronic diseases is that, if a disease is caused by microbes, it becomes possible to prevent or cure it. Gastric ulcers can now be cured with a short course of antibiotics, with the additional side benefit of drastically reducing one's risk of gastric cancer. Cervical cancer can be prevented by cauterizing genital warts caused by papillomavirus. The new hepatitis B vaccine will prevent not only hepatitis but also liver cancer. The public is hungry for cures, not empty promises such as those that have been abundant in recent years as hype artists promise miracles from the human genome sequence or stem cell research. Bacteriologists, by contrast, stand on a solid record of producing cures, and we should be proud of that. The bottom line is that in another decade, future editions of this book—if it is still around—may stretch to multiple volumes. There is much to be done, and we hope that this book inspires undergraduate and graduate readers to enter the field of infectious disease research.

12

The Spirochetes:
Borrelia burgdorferi and *Treponema pallidum*

KEY FEATURES

Borrelia burgdorferi

DESCRIPTION
Spirochete, corkscrew motility
Periplasmic flagella covered by outer sheath
Gram-negative cell wall but no LPS
No requirement for iron (iron abstinence)
Visualized by dark-field microscopy

DISEASE
Lyme disease

RESERVOIR
White-footed mouse
Transmitted to humans by deer tick
Humans are accidental hosts

MAJOR VIRULENCE FACTORS
Outer surface proteins—bind host molecules
Motility may aid movement out of bloodstream
Most virulence factors still unknown

PREVENTION AND TREATMENT
Avoid tick-infested areas, remove ticks
Antibiotics effective in early Lyme disease (doxycycline, amoxicillin)

In 1975, a woman in Old Lyme, Connecticut, called state health authorities wanting to know why so many children in her town had arthritis. She was alarmed by the fact that 12 cases of juvenile arthritis (a relatively rare disease) had been diagnosed in a town with a population of only 5,000. Subsequent investigations of these and similar cases led to the discovery of Lyme disease and to the identification of the causative bacterium, *Borrelia burgdorferi*. Although the disease was first discovered in the United States, in the sense that all the symptoms were recognized as being part of the same disease caused by a single infectious agent, different aspects of the disease had been described long before by European physicians. European physicians were also the first to suspect that the causative agent was a bacterium and

187

were treating the disease successfully with antibiotics well before U.S. physicians (who thought the disease was caused by a virus) accepted this therapy.

Lyme Disease

Lyme disease proceeds in three phases. The first is the skin phase, which follows inoculation of the bacteria into the skin by a tick as it takes a blood meal. The *Ixodes* ticks that transmit Lyme disease to humans are pool feeders. That is, they do not inject the bacteria directly into the bloodstream but create a lesion into which blood flows. Thus, the bacteria are originally introduced into the lower layers of skin. Many of them remain in the skin and move through it for a period of days, as is evident from the spreading annular rash that is such a common symptom of the disease. The rash is caused by inflammation induced by the bacteria. This initial skin phase may give the bacteria some protection from the neutrophils that patrol the bloodstream. The ability to move away from the region where inflammation is occurring may also play a protective role.

The bacteria next invade the bloodstream, leading to further dissemination throughout the body. The presence of bacteria in the bloodstream may explain some of the diffuse flulike symptoms experienced by most infected people. Bacteria that reach joints cause the inflammatory arthritis seen in many people with Lyme disease. Some bacteria can also invade nervous tissue, producing Bell's palsy and other neurological symptoms. *B. burgdorferi* does not do very well when faced with the formidable combination of blood defenses—phagocytic cells and antibodies. The bacteria are rapidly cleared from the bloodstream, and at that point the infection would be brought under control if not for the ability of the bacteria to leave the bloodstream and enter tissues such as joints and the nervous system.

The third stage of the infection begins when the bacteria enter tissues throughout the body. At that point, the bacteria become more difficult to find and may enter a quiescent phase with lowered metabolic activity, which makes them less likely to attract the cells of the host's defense systems. Also, bacteria within mammalian cells or joint fluid are somewhat protected from antibodies and phagocytic cells, especially if their antigens do not appear on the surface of the mammalian cell. The symptoms of chronic Lyme disease—fatigue, chronic arthritis, neurological damage, and vision impairment—all appear during this third stage of infection, which occurs in only a fraction of infected people. Once the disease reaches this third phase, it is very difficult to treat effectively with antibiotics, possibly because the body has mounted an autoimmune response.

Features of *B. burgdorferi*

B. burgdorferi is the *Borrelia* species that causes most cases of Lyme disease in the United States. In Europe, other species of *Borrelia* cause the disease as well as *B. burgdorferi*, but those species have many of the same properties as *B. burgdorferi*. In recognition of the variety of *Borrelia* species that can cause Lyme disease, scientists use the term *sensu stricto* to indicate that the species name *B. burgdorferi* is being used to mean only that one species. Since *B. burgdorferi* is so similar to these other species with respect to symptoms of the disease, the species name is often used *sensu lato* to mean *B. burgdorferi* plus other similar species.

Morphology and Physiology

B. burgdorferi is a spirochete. **Spirochetes** are spiral-shaped organisms that have a gram-negative cell wall architecture consisting of two membranes, between which is sandwiched the peptidoglycan layer (Figure 12–1). The spirochetes belong to a phylogenetic group separate from the phylogenetic groups containing the gram-negative and gram-positive bacteria covered elsewhere in this book (Figure 12–2). This genetic dis-

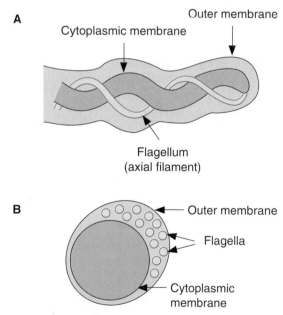

Figure 12–1 Characteristics of *B. burgdorferi*. (**A**) Structure of a typical spirochete showing flagella wrapped about the cell inside the space between the cytoplasmic membrane and the outer membrane. (**B**) Cross-section through the bacterial cell showing multiple flagella. (Panel B is adapted from M. M. Simon, U. E. Schaible, R. Wallich, and M. D. Kramer. 1991. A mouse model for *Borrelia burgdorferi* infection: approach to a vaccine against Lyme disease. *Immunol. Today* **12**:11–16.)

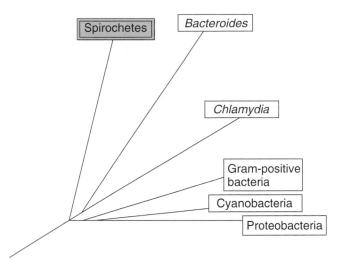

Figure 12–2 Phylogenetic relationship of the spirochetes to other groups of bacteria. The spirochetes belong to a separate phylogenetic group. The proteobacteria group contains *Escherichia coli, Pseudomonas* species, and other genera of familiar gram-negative bacteria.

Table 12–1 Features of major surface proteins of *Borrelia burgdorferi* and control of their expression

Protein	Features and control of expression
OspA	Upregulated in tick larva as it becomes a nymph
	Downregulated in nymph as it takes a blood meal
	Not expressed on bacteria in mammal until late in infection
OspB	Similar to OspA (53% amino acid sequence identity)
	ospA gene in operon with *ospB* on linear plasmid
OspC	Upregulated as bacteria migrate from midgut to salivary gland in tick
	Production stimulated by increase in temperature and factors in blood
	Present on bacteria in mammal
Erps (OspD-related proteins)	Produced early during infection of mammal
	Induced in vitro by increasing temperature of incubation from 23° to 35°C
DbpA (decorin-binding protein)	Binds mammalian protein decorin
	Produced by bacteria in a mammal
VlsE	Surface protein that varies antigenically, similar to variable membrane proteins (Vmps) found in *Borrelia hermsii* (the cause of relapsing fever)

tance is evident in some features of their surfaces. *Borrelia* spp. do not have LPS in their outer membranes. Instead, the outer membrane contains a number of lipoproteins, some of which are designated Osp, for outer surface proteins (Table 12–1). To date, four of these lipoproteins have received the most attention—**OspA, OspB, OspC,** and **OspD**—but other Osp-like proteins have also been identified. OspA and OspB, the two most abundant lipoproteins, are encoded by two genes organized as an operon. They share an amino acid sequence identity of 53%, and some antibodies cross-react with both proteins.

Recently, other surface proteins, such as **OspE-related proteins (Erps), decorin-binding proteins,** and antigenically variable proteins called **Vls proteins,** have been identified. Proteins exposed on the surface are of particular interest to microbiologists seeking to develop vaccines against Lyme disease because binding of antibodies to the surface of *B. burgdorferi* activates complement and kills the bacteria. Although *Borrelia* species do not have LPS, their surfaces elicit the same type of inflammatory response as LPS. The Osp lipoproteins are probably the mediators of the inflammatory response elicited by the bacteria.

B. burgdorferi is unusually long and thin, about 0.2 μm in diameter and 20 to 30 μm in length, with 4 to 20 coils. The bacteria are actively motile, but the flagella do not extend outward from the surface of the bacterium like those of most gram-negative bacteria. Rather, the flagella are embedded into the two ends of the spirochete and are wrapped around it inside the space be-

tween the cytoplasmic membrane and the outer membrane (Figure 12–1). Periodic contractions of these internal flagella (also called **axial filaments**) cause the outer surface to rotate, producing a corkscrew-type motility. This type of motility is most effective in viscous solutions and may be responsible for the ability of the spirochetes to move out of skin into the bloodstream and out of the bloodstream into tissues.

Borrelia species are not visible by phase-contrast microscopy because of their small diameter. They can be viewed by using a dark-field microscope. A dark-field microscope is a microscope adapted with a special condenser that allows the microscopist to see light reflected off the bacteria. The bacteria are seen as bright objects against a black background. Spirochetes can also be visualized using a type of microscopy called fluorescence microscopy, in which the specimen is treated with labeled fluorescent antibodies directed against the OspA proteins. When the fluorescent label is activated by light of a certain intensity, the bacteria appear as bright spirals against a dark background (Figure 12–3).

BOX 12–1   Spirochetes Make Triathlons Tougher for Athletes

Athletes who participate in triathlons now need more than strength, speed, and endurance. They also need a robust immune system. In 1998, athletes participating in triathlons in Wisconsin and Illinois developed an acute febrile disease during the weeks following the competition. At first, only a few cases surfaced, but further interviews with participants in one or both of these events revealed that 12% of participants interviewed (74 athletes) reported symptoms suggesting that they too had been infected. The state public health laboratories, working in conjunction with the CDC, quickly identified the causative agent as the spirochete *Leptospira interrogans*. *L. interrogans* enters the bloodstream, eliciting an inflammatory response. From blood, *L. interrogans* can enter and damage organs. At least one of the stricken athletes suffered acute renal failure.

The diagnosis of leptospirosis came as something of a shock because leptospirosis was thought to be very uncommon in developed countries. It has been associated mainly with field workers in developing countries who come into frequent contact with crops contaminated with rodent urine. *L. interrogans* is excreted in urine because it is so thin that it can pass through the filtration system of the kidney, a barrier that blocks excretion of other microorganisms. Its corkscrew motility may also help it tunnel through the kidney tissue. Apparently, rodents in the vicinity of the lakes in Wisconsin and Illinois that were the site of the swimming portion of the triathlon were infected with the leptospires and were shedding them into lake water. Presumably, swimmers acquired the bacteria by unintentionally ingesting lake water or through small cuts or abrasions.

Borrelia Plasmids

Borrelia species have linear plasmids as well as the conventional circular plasmids. Linear plasmids were first discovered by scientists studying *B. burgdorferi*, and for a while it was thought that linear plasmids were a unique feature of this genus. In recent years, however, linear plasmids and chromosomes have been found in a number of other bacterial groups. The two strands of the double-stranded linear plasmids are covalently closed at the ends (Figure 12–4) and have sequences similar to the **telomeres** that are found on eukaryotic chromosomes (which are also linear). The mechanism by which the linear plasmids of spirochetes replicate is still unknown.

It is not unusual for bacteria to have plasmids, but *B. burgdorferi* has more plasmids than most bacteria. In one strain that has been studied, there are 12 linear and 9 circular plasmids. The portion of the genome found in plasmid DNA is about 0.6 Mbp, a little more than one-third of the DNA that resides in the bacterial genome (1.52 Mbp). Results of comparisons of DNA carried on these plasmids suggest that there is extensive recombination between different plasmids, leading to rearrangements in plasmid DNA. What role this variability of plasmid-borne genes plays in adaptation of the bacteria to its various hosts remains to be determined. It is interesting to note that few of the genes carried on the *Borrelia* plasmids have homologs in the sequence databases. They seem to be specific to *Borrelia* and thus may hold many clues to the unique virulence factors that allow the bacteria to have such a complex lifestyle.

Progress toward developing methods for genetically manipulating *B. burgdorferi* has been slow and tortuous, but in recent years some promising gains have been made. For example, it is now possible to introduce plasmid DNA into *B. burgdorferi* by transformation. Oddly enough, a plasmid, pGK12, that was originally isolated from a gram-positive bacterium also replicates in *B. burgdorferi*.

The *Borrelia* Genome Sequence— Some Clues but Still Many Mysteries

The sequence of the genome of *B. burgdorferi* is now available. In many ways, it has been less informative than was hoped, but this is probably an artifact of the small amount of information that is available about *Borrelia* virulence factors. Searches for homologs of known virulence factors from other bacteria drew a blank. Clearly, the virulence factors of *Borrelia* spp., and perhaps other pathogenic spirochetes as well, are different from those of *E. coli* and other well-studied bacterial pathogens. The sequence did give information about the metabolism of *B. burgdorferi*, however. For one thing, it settled the controversy over whether *Borrelia* spp. had LPS; there were no genes for LPS biosynthesis in the *Borrelia* genome sequence. Hence, no LPS.

Also absent were any genes encoding cytochromes or tricarboxylic acid (TCA) cycle enzymes. This is con-

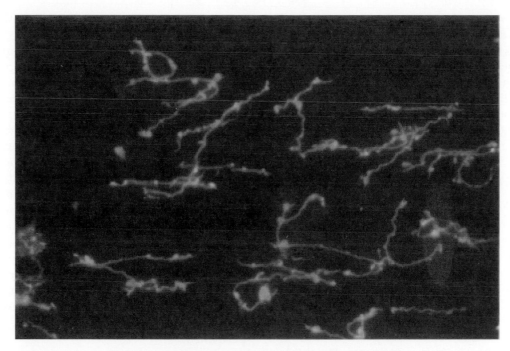

Figure 12–3 Indirect immunofluorescence of *B. burgdorferi*. Spirochetes were fixed in methanol on a slide and then incubated with a fluorescently labeled monoclonal antibody directed against the OspA protein. (From A. G. Barbour. 1988. Laboratory aspects of Lyme borreliosis. *Clin. Microbiol. Rev.* **1**:399–414.)

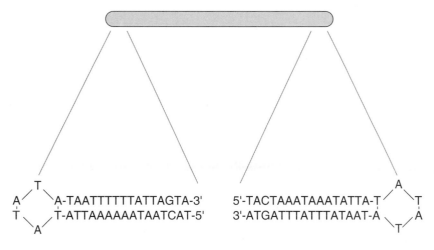

Figure 12–4 Structure of a linear *Borrelia* plasmid. The sequences from two ends of one such plasmid are shown. End sequences of different plasmids are similar but not identical. They are also similar to the ends of the vaccinia virus genome, which are known to function as telomeres. The linear plasmids probably replicate from the center outward via an expanding bubble-type structure. The genes for many of the outer surface protein genes (*osp* genes) are located on linear plasmids.

sistent with the observation that, although *B. burgdorferi* can grow in the presence of oxygen, it seems not to need oxygen for growth. Because the bacteria lack a TCA cycle, they cannot make any of the amino acids whose synthesis requires TCA cycle intermediates. Given this, it appeared odd at first that there were few genes encoding amino acid transport proteins. This is consistent, however, with the observation that the bacteria preferentially take up peptides rather than individual amino acids.

One surprising trait of *B. burgdorferi* that was sug-

gested by the genome sequence was its novel strategy for coping with the low concentration of free iron in the human body. A survey of the genome sequence revealed that none of the genes encoding iron-requiring proteins were present. This led to the hypothesis that *B. burgdorferi* solves the iron limitation problem by not using iron at all. Subsequent studies have shown that indeed *B. burgdorferi* uses manganese instead of iron for proteins, such as superoxide dismutase, that normally require iron. Given that most research papers on iron utilization begin with a statement to the effect that all living creatures require iron, this contention that *B. burgdorferi* did not was met with some skepticism. Earlier studies showed that *Lactobacillus* species also do not use iron, but the suggestion that a mammalian pathogen would have this trait was hard for many to accept. It now seems likely, however, that there are other bacteria that do not require iron. How many species will prove to have this trait remains to be seen.

The Tick-Mammal Cycle

At the time Lyme disease was first described, it was viewed as a new disease, both in the United States and Europe. But as the ecology of *B. burgdorferi* was better understood, it became clear that the disease was not new at all. *B. burgdorferi* normally infects wild animals and is spread to humans by the bite of a tick. In the northeastern United States, *Ixodes* ticks are the transmitters of *B. burgdorferi*, but in California, another Lyme disease hot spot, other tick species play the same role. The tick's usual hosts are deer and mice. The tick has three developmental stages: the larval stage, the nymph stage, and the adult stage. At each stage, the tick requires a blood meal to allow it to make the next developmental step. Larvae and nymphs feed mainly on rodents, although they will also take a blood meal from other warm-blooded animals, including humans. Adult ticks feed on deer. This final blood meal is necessary for the ticks to mate and produce progeny.

B. burgdorferi inhabits the gut and salivary glands of the tick without causing any adverse effects. *B. burgdorferi* also infects mice, but the infection is benign. Since *B. burgdorferi* does not infect deer, the mouse appears to be its main reservoir in the wild. The bacteria can infect other mammals, however, such as voles and shrews. The bacterium's relationship with its vector, the tick, and its main reservoir, the white-footed mouse, is crucial because *B. burgdorferi* is not transmitted transovarially from a mother tick to its progeny. Thus, to maintain itself in the mouse population, *B. burgdorferi* must be spread constantly by ticks to new mouse hosts. Harming either the tick or the mouse would clearly not be in the best interest of *B. burgdorferi*. The larval form of the tick must be infected so that the nymph form can spread the bacterium as it feeds on uninfected mice. The role of the deer is to provide the blood meal that allows the adults to mate and produce more progeny. This complex set of tick-mammal interactions has been successful in perpetuating *B. burgdorferi* in the wild mouse population.

The human form of the disease arose when humans inadvertently inserted themselves into the ecological cycle by which *B. burgdorferi* maintains itself in the environment. People began to move with greater frequency into rural areas. At the same time, a public backlash against deer hunting led to an explosion of the white-tailed deer population. Attracted by the plants in people's yards, deer increasingly entered areas used frequently by humans, shedding their ticks as they did so. Mice, attracted to houses and the food they contain, also dropped their ticks in areas frequented by humans. Given these favorable conditions, and the fact that ticks will take a blood meal from humans if no other warm-blooded host is available, ticks infected with *B. burgdorferi* began to spread the bacteria to humans. In humans, who are not its usual host, *B. burgdorferi* causes a variety of symptoms ranging from headache and other flulike symptoms to neurological disorders, all of which are usually self-limiting. In some people, however, the disease can proceed to a more serious chronic condition that is characterized by arthritis. Death occurs only rarely, but the chronic form of the disease can be quite debilitating, and neurological damage may become permanent.

Response of *B. burgdorferi* to Its Arthropod and Mammalian Hosts

Osps

OspA AND OspC. When the bacteria enter a tick larva along with the blood ingested during a blood meal, the bacteria remain for a period in the midgut of the tick. During this stage, OspA is produced and displayed on the surface of the bacteria. When the larva develops into a nymph and the nymph takes a blood meal, the bacteria stop producing OspA and instead begin to produce a related protein, OspC. This switch from OspA production to OspC production is triggered by a change in temperature and unknown factors in blood. After the tick completes its blood meal, the bacteria migrate from the midgut to the salivary glands of the tick, where they are poised for inoculation into the next human or animal the tick bites.

ERPS. *B. burgdorferi* produces a number of surface proteins that are similar in amino acid sequence to the Osp protein OspE (Erps). These proteins are made by bacteria in the mammalian body early in the infection process and elicit a good antibody response. Since they are produced early in the infection, they could be involved in the early stages of adaptation to the mammalian host. Production of Erps can be elicited in laboratory medium by changing the temperature of incubation from 23 to 35°C, a trait that also suggests a role in adaptation to the change in hosts from an arthropod to a mammal.

Little is known about the virulence factors that mediate exit from the blood vessels and entry into host cells, but genetic studies are beginning to provide some insights into this process. The corkscrew motility of spirochetes probably makes a contribution to invasion by allowing the bacteria to bore their way through the extracellular matrix found between cells. Also, endothelial cells are not tightly bound together with proteins, as mucosal cells are. They must be able to separate in order to allow neutrophils and monocytes to exit the bloodstream. A thin spirochete should be able to pass between these cells with ease. Consistent with this, nonmotile mutants of *B. burgdorferi,* which lack the internal flagella, are deficient in the ability to transit a monolayer of **human umbilical vein endothelial cells (HUVEC).** *B. burgdorferi* also triggers the upregulation of endothelial cell surface molecules such as E-selectin, which stops the rolling motion of neutrophils through the blood vessel. ICAM-1, which aids in the binding of neutrophils to the endothelial cells prior to exiting the blood vessel, and VCAM-1, which plays a similar role for lymphocytes and monocytes, are also upregulated. Gram-negative LPS triggers a similar change in the proteins on the surface of endothelial cells, but in *B. burgdorferi* this activation is probably mediated by the Osp proteins.

OTHER SURFACE PROTEINS. An interesting group of *B. burgdorferi* surface proteins are the decorin-binding proteins. Decorin is a proteoglycan, which is a component of the intracellular matrix. A decorin-binding protein, **DbpA,** has been identified and has been shown to be produced by *B. burgdorferi* in the human body. DbpA is also a protective antigen. That is, immunization of mice with DbpA protects them from infection. DbpA appears to be accessible to antibodies, a fact that suggests it is exposed on the bacterial surface. DbpA could be a useful component of a future vaccine because it is produced early in the blood phase of the infection, at least in mice.

A type of surface protein that may help the bacteria to evade the immune system is an antigenically variable protein called VlsE. This protein was first noticed because of its amino acid sequence similarity to a surface protein of *Borrelia hermsii. B. hermsii* causes a disease called relapsing fever, which gets its name from the fact that an infected person has recurring episodes of fever. The advent of each episode of fever is associated with the appearance of a new surface protein on the bacteria that is different enough from the previous form of the protein to make the host's immune response ineffective. A new round of antibody production once again kills the bacteria but also selects for bacteria with yet another antigenic variant of the surface protein. The antigenically varying protein is called **Vmp,** for **variable membrane protein.** The newly identified VlsE protein of *B. burgdorferi* is named for Vmp-like sequence. The *vlsE*

gene is located on a 28-kbp linear plasmid, lp28–1. When this plasmid is lost, the virulence of the strain of *B. burgdorferi* is decreased significantly, so something carried on this plasmid is acting as a virulence factor.

Leaving the Bloodstream

Although the bacteria may be able to protect themselves to some extent against antibody-mediated killing by reducing the expression of some antigenic surface proteins or changing surface antigens, the combination of phagocytes and antibodies rapidly eliminates bacteria from the bloodstream. The only way the bacteria can survive and persist is to leave the bloodstream and invade host cells, establishing an intracellular residence that protects them from further harassment by antibodies, phagocytes, and complement. The ability to leave blood vessels by penetrating the layer of endothelial cells lining the blood vessels is an important virulence factor for *B. burgdorferi.* In vitro, *B. burgdorferi* transits monolayers of HUVEC. In some studies, *B. burgdorferi* has been shown to cross such endothelial monolayers by moving between endothelial cells, a property that is reminiscent of the migration of neutrophils out of blood vessels.

There are also reports of bacteria entering the endothelial cells and either replicating inside them or transiting the monolayer by transcytosis. *B. burgdorferi* can invade and grow inside cultured mammalian cells other than HUVEC, such as human skin fibroblasts. Both the ability to pass through the endothelial lining of blood vessels and the ability to invade and survive inside nonprofessional phagocytes would contribute to survival of *B. burgdorferi* in the host. The invasiveness of *B. burgdorferi* is also apparent from the fact that the bacteria can invade heart tissue, cross the blood-brain barrier, and accumulate in synovial fluid.

The Lyme Disease Vaccine

In 1998, the FDA approved a vaccine, **LYMErix,** that consists of OspA protein. As mentioned earlier, OspA is produced by bacteria growing in the tick but is not produced by bacteria growing in the human body. Because OspA is produced in abundance by *B. burgdorferi* grown in laboratory medium, scientists developing the vaccine assumed at first that it would make a good vaccine target. The OspA vaccine was rushed into clinical trials and through the FDA approval process. Only later did scientists realize that OspA is not produced when bacteria are growing in the human body. Not surprisingly, the OspA vaccine is not as effective as one would wish. What is surprising is that it is effective at all. The first two injections are given 1 month apart, and then a third is given about 12 months later. About 50% of those given two injections and about 75% of those given three injections are protected. This level of protection is disappointing when compared with other vaccines but is surprisingly high given that OspA is not found on spirochetes that enter the human body. The best explanation for this anomaly is that antibodies against OspA enter the tick's hindgut with the blood meal and prevent the bacteria from being transmitted effectively to the person being bitten. Also, bacteria injected into the human body may still have low residual amounts of antibodies complexed to OspA on their surfaces, targeting them for destruction by the phagocytic cells and complement.

Approval of the OspA vaccine generated considerable controversy. Some argued that its low efficacy made it undesirable, especially given the side effects that some vaccinated people experienced. Others argued that the side effects were generally of short duration and that a partially effective vaccine was better than none at all. People in areas where Lyme disease is endemic have opted for vaccination, apparently siding with those who argue that some protection is better than none at all. This tale is instructive because it illustrates the importance of understanding which bacterial proteins are produced at various times during the infection process. Extrapolations from bacteria grown in culture to bacteria growing in real world settings can be misleading. Currently, efforts are under way to develop a vaccine based on OspC, which should be more effective because OspC is present in the bacteria at the time they infect people.

Recently, a potential new concern about the LYME-rix vaccine has surfaced. Some studies suggest that antibodies against OspA appear in the sera of some people during late stages of the disease. Appearance of these antibodies is correlated with development of chronic Lyme arthritis. On the basis of such findings, scientists have suggested that OspA, which is a very immunogenic protein, elicits antibodies that cross-react with an antigen on leukocytes (see later section of this chapter). That is, OspA may trigger an autoimmune disease in some people. It remains to be seen whether a subset of the people vaccinated with OspA develop chronic arthritis. If the hypothesis that Lyme disease is an autoimmune disease triggered by OspA is proved, this would be reason enough for the vaccine to be withdrawn from use.

Chronic Lyme Disease

In a small number of people who contract active Lyme disease, the disease does not resolve with time but becomes chronic. Patients with chronic Lyme disease experience arthritis, neurological damage that may inter-

fere with vision, and fatigue. At this point, Lyme disease may no longer respond to antibiotic treatment or may require months-long antibiotic treatment. This chronic stage of Lyme disease has been much studied but is still poorly understood. The fact that chronic Lyme disease is difficult to treat successfully with antibiotics suggested that it might be an autoimmune disease. Recently, a theory of how chronic Lyme disease develops has been proposed. This theory is based on two observations. First, antibodies to OspA can be detected late in the disease, indicating that the bacteria may produce this lipoprotein in the mammalian host under some conditions. OspA is a very immunogenic protein. Second, T-helper cells stimulated by antigen-processing cells presenting OspA epitopes display a protein on their surfaces (**human leukocyte function-associated antigen-1 [hLFA-1]**) which contains a peptide that resembles a peptide in OspA. Antibodies against OspA could thus cross-react with hLFA-1, triggering an autoimmune response that targets a human leukocyte antigen.

As already mentioned, if this theory is correct, it raises disturbing questions about the vaccine based on OspA. Could this vaccine trigger autoimmune disease in some people? So far, no sign of such a side effect has been seen, but this possibility makes the need for an alternative vaccine even more urgent.

Other cross-reactive antibodies have been demonstrated in the serum of patients with Lyme disease. Antibodies that cross-react with neuronal tissue seem to target a 64-kDa protein, but the location of this protein in neurons has not been established. If this antigen participates in an autoimmune response, it should be exposed on the cell surface. Other proteins possibly implicated in an autoimmune response are a heat shock protein and OspB. Obviously, the longer the infection remains untreated, the more chance there is of an autoimmune response developing.

There may also be a host genetic predisposition that causes some people to be more likely to contract chronic Lyme disease. Many people who develop chronic Lyme arthritis have an MHC class II complex of the **HLA-DR4** type, the same type associated with rheumatoid arthritis. Why this particular type of MHC molecule is associated with rheumatoid arthritis is unknown. High levels of antibodies to OspA and OspB in such people are also strongly associated with development of chronic arthritis.

Variation in the Severity of the Disease—Coinfection Confounds the Problem

In some people, Lyme disease is relatively mild, whereas in others it is more severe. This could be due to genetic differences in susceptible humans or to strain-to-strain variation in the virulence of the bacteria, or both. In recent years, another explanation for differences in disease severity has surfaced—coinfection with another infectious agent. White-footed mice and *Ixodes* ticks are also reservoirs for at least two other microbial pathogens, *Ehrlichia* species and *Babesia* species. *Ehrlichia* species are intracellular bacterial pathogens that cause potentially fatal febrile diseases, **human granulocytic ehrlichiosis (HGE)** and **human monocytic ehrlichiosis (HME).** *Babesia* species are protozoal parasites related to the protozoa that cause malaria. Babesiosis has symptoms similar to those of Lyme disease and is usually not fatal. *Ehrlichia, Babesia,* and *Borrelia* species are found in the same geographical locations, and human coinfections occur more frequently than was once thought to be the case. As many as 10 to 16% of people infected with *B. burgdorferi* are coinfected with *Ehrlichia* or *Babesia* species. The coinfection phenomenon has been seen in Europe as well as in the United States. A coinfection is likely to be associated with more severe disease than infection with *B. burgdorferi* alone.

The phenomenon of coinfection makes developing a vaccine more complex in the sense that eliminating Lyme disease by vaccination will not eliminate HGE, HME, or babesiosis. It also complicates therapy. Whereas some of the same antibiotics are effective against both *B. burgdorferi* and *Ehrlichia* species (doxycycline), different antimicrobial compounds must be used to treat babesiosis (clindamycin plus quinine).

Studying Virulence Factors of *B. burgdorferi*

Special Difficulties

B. burgdorferi is still not easy to cultivate in laboratory medium. The organism has a slow growth rate (10 to 12 h per generation). Strains isolated from infected people or animals rapidly lose their virulence when passaged through laboratory medium. This characteristic has been used to identify potential virulence factors by comparing the attributes of cells that have been through many passages with those that have been passed through culture only a few times. Nonetheless, it makes life difficult for investigators because they cannot continue to pass the bacteria in laboratory medium. Some investigators have turned this trait to advantage by looking for virulence factors among those proteins that disappear when the virulence of the strain decreases.

The problem with this approach is that it does not narrow down very much the traits that account for reduction of virulence, because all the genes carried on the plasmid are lost at the same time. Recently, the ability to manipulate *B. burgdorferi* genetically has improved to the point that mutations in specific genes can be made. This will help greatly to identify virulence factors in the future. At present, however, it is important to realize that assumptions made about the importance of such proteins as DbpA or OspC may not be based on the results of experiments in which the individual gene was interrupted or deleted.

Animal Models

There are a number of useful animal models. Most strains of laboratory rodents can be infected. Rabbits develop a skin lesion when inoculated with *B. burgdorferi*, but the lesion is not of the same type as that seen in humans. **C3H SCID** (severe combined immunodeficient) mice develop arthritis similar to that seen in humans and have been used as a model for that phase of the disease. SCID mice are immunocompromised because they have lost both their T- and B-cell responses. There is also a dog model for Lyme disease that mimics many aspects of the disease in humans, but the larger size of dogs and public opposition to the use of dogs for experimentation makes them more difficult to work with than mice.

Diagnosis and Prevention of Lyme Disease

Diagnosis

In people infected with *B. burgdorferi*, the first symptoms of disease are headache, fever, chills, and malaise. These are also symptoms of a much more common viral disease, the flu. A more distinctive sign of Lyme disease, and thus a much more valuable diagnostic clue, is a ring-shaped rash centered on the site of inoculation. This annular region of inflammation (**erythema migrans**) expands and moves outward. Erythema migrans appears days to a few weeks after the bacteria are introduced into the host. It is a valuable diagnostic sign, but at least 20 to 40% of infected people do not develop this characteristic lesion. The lesion disappears spontaneously after several weeks. In 15 to 20% of cases, there are also neurological symptoms, ranging from a painful facial palsy or drooping of facial muscles (Bell's palsy) to meningitislike symptoms. In 5 to 10% of cases, heart damage occurs.

The third stage of the disease, which begins months to years after the tick bite, is characterized by inflammation of the large joints, especially the knee and elbow. About 10% of patients with this type of inflammation develop a chronic form of the arthritis, which may last for a year or longer. Chronic neurological symptoms (disabling fatigue, impaired vision, paralysis, and dementia) occur in some people.

If Lyme disease is diagnosed early enough and treated with antibiotics, the disease can be cured and the patient experiences no long-term effects. If the disease reaches the late stage, however, treatment with antibiotics is not always successful. The continued progression of symptoms that occurs in some patients despite antibiotic treatment could be due to autoimmune disease triggered by the bacteria. The currently approved regimen for Lyme disease involves administration of the antibiotic (doxycycline and amoxicillin are current drugs of choice) 2 to 4 times daily for 2 to 4 weeks. Many of the horror stories about people debilitated to the point of being almost unable to care for themselves or suffering irreversible neurological damage arose during the period before the disease was widely recognized in the United States as having a bacterial etiology and people did not receive early effective treatment.

There are a number of problems that interfere with diagnosis and prevention of the disease. Since the symptoms of Lyme disease can vary considerably from one person to another, diagnosis based on symptoms is not always straightforward. There are serological tests available, but they vary in quality. The cheapest and most commonly administered tests are those that detect antibodies to a mixture of *B. burgdorferi* antigens. Such a test can give false-positive results if antibodies in serum bind nonspecifically to antigens in the mixture. In fact, in one study of 788 patients referred by physicians to a Lyme disease clinic, 452 were found not to have Lyme disease when more stringent diagnostic criteria were applied. Of these 452 patients, 302 had a positive serological test for Lyme disease. Today the diagnosis is made even more problematic because people vaccinated with the Lyme disease vaccine may become seropositive according to currently available serological tests. Because the simple primary serological tests for Lyme disease are so unreliable, following up a positive initial test with a Western blot test is recommended for greater specificity.

Furthermore, physicians are urged to consider the preponderance of evidence rather than to rely on one symptom or the results of a serological test. A person with multiple symptoms of Lyme disease and a positive serological test result can be considered as potentially having the disease, whereas a positive serological test result in the absence of most of the Lyme disease-specific symptoms, such as the annular rash, should be treated with suspicion. Conversely, classic symptoms of Lyme disease coupled with a negative serological test

result should suggest the possibility that the patient has not been infected long enough to mount a robust immunological response or is not responding immunologically for some other reason.

Reasonable as these recommendations may sound, physicians may not follow them. Physicians, influenced by the considerable media attention given to Lyme disease and the increasing patient awareness of this disease, sometimes tend to see Lyme disease in patients who actually have other conditions. Or patients may be convinced that they have Lyme disease and demand treatment. Some physicians prescribe antibiotics to any patient who reports having been bitten by a tick. Chronic Lyme disease is even more difficult to diagnose accurately because its symptoms are so variable. Also, some cases of disease diagnosed as chronic Lyme disease do not respond to antibiotic therapy. Is this because the diagnosis is incorrect, or because the disease has progressed to such an advanced stage that eliminating the bacteria no longer eliminates the symptoms? It has been estimated that 80% of people who are diagnosed with "antibiotic-resistant" Lyme disease do not have Lyme disease.

Prevention and Treatment

Because there are multiple concerns about the available vaccine and because antibiotic treatment may not be 100% effective in treating chronic Lyme disease, preventing contact between infected ticks and humans is obviously a high priority. The most effective prevention strategy would be to eliminate deer from suburban lawns, not an easy task as anyone who has experienced a deer invasion will realize. Spraying insecticides on lawns and clearing brush away from houses to eliminate nesting sites for rodents are other options. Here, deeply ingrained societal beliefs come into play. The sort of people who are most likely to be at risk for Lyme disease are those who have come to fear and avoid insecticides.

Increased awareness of the disease by the public and by physicians in areas where Lyme disease is endemic has enhanced the likelihood that cases of Lyme disease will be diagnosed and treated in the early stages when treatment is most effective. Unfortunately, one side effect of the extensive media attention given to Lyme disease is that misconceptions about the disease have themselves become epidemic. The serological test for Lyme disease is not as reliable as an ideal test would be, but it is very useful for diagnosing the disease. There are false-positive results because of cross-reactivity between borrelial antigens and antigens of other bacteria (especially flagellar antigens). Perhaps a greater cause for concern are the false-negative results due to the long lag period before a detectable antibody response to *B. burgdorferi* occurs (3 to 6 weeks). The annular lesion is a very valuable diagnostic clue, except in the 20 to 40% of people who do not exhibit this sign of the disease. A patient history becomes most important in cases of this sort. Possible symptoms of Lyme disease, coupled with the presence of the patient in an area where Lyme disease is known to be endemic, may be the key diagnostic clues.

The search for a vaccine against Lyme disease continues. Now that OspA and OspB have been discredited to some extent as vaccine candidates because they are produced primarily in the arthropod, not in the human body, other Osps are being considered as vaccine candidates.

Syphilis and Lyme Disease: Two Spirochetal Diseases with a Similar Pathology but a Different Ecology

Progression of Syphilis

At first, Lyme disease and syphilis (another disease caused by a spirochete) might appear to be completely different diseases. Lyme disease is spread by ticks, whereas syphilis is spread by sexual intercourse. Both diseases are caused by spirochetes, but syphilis is caused by *Treponema pallidum*, a different genus and species from *B. burgdorferi*. Nonetheless, the pathogenesis of the two diseases is remarkably similar. Because syphilis has been studied much longer than Lyme disease, it is useful to review what little is known about the virulence factors that are important in syphilis, since these may provide helpful hints about what aspects of the bacterium-host interaction are important for progression of Lyme disease. Perhaps the greatest cause for concern about syphilis is that it can be transmitted transplacentally (**congenital syphilis**). Birth defects caused by congenital syphilis include malformations of the teeth and long bones, heart damage, learning disabilities, and mental retardation. Whereas transplacental transfer of Lyme disease is a rare occurrence (two cases so far reported), there are now nearly 500 cases of congenital syphilis in the United States each year.

Studying the virulence mechanisms of *T. pallidum* is even more challenging than studying the virulence mechanisms of *B. burgdorferi*. For one thing, *T. pallidum* has never been cultivated in laboratory medium, despite almost 100 years of effort. For another, there is no animal model that mimics the human form of the disease. The bacteria will grow in rabbit testicles, the primary method for culturing the bacteria, but do not cause symptoms typical of human syphilis. When injected intradermally in the back of a rabbit, lesions form, but systemic disease does not develop. Most information about the disease has come from immunological studies of people with syphilis and from studying bacteria taken directly from rabbit testicles. *T. pallidum*, like *B. burgdorferi*, will adhere to and invade monolayers of HUVEC. This has provided an in vitro system for investigating the invasiveness of *T. pallidum* and its ability to stimulate an inflammatory response.

Syphilis, like Lyme disease, has multiple stages. The early stage of syphilis (**primary syphilis**) is characterized by a lesion (called a **chancre**) that appears at the site of infection. *T. pallidum* can be seen in this lesion, and the spirochetes are infectious. Not all people develop a chancre, and some people who develop one do not notice it because it is hidden in the vagina, mouth, or anus. The chancre disappears spontaneously after a couple of weeks. The bacteria rapidly penetrate mucosal membranes and enter the bloodstream, giving rise to the second stage of the disease (**secondary syphilis**).

Symptoms of secondary-stage disease, such as fever and rash, occur in many but not all infected people. In people with a rash, treponemes can be found in the lesions as well as in the bloodstream. Inside the body, the treponemes invade the heart, musculoskeletal system, and central nervous system. The disease then enters another stage (**latent syphilis**) in which the bacteria are difficult to find but are presumably present because there is a continued antibody response to bacterial antigens. During this stage of the disease, a person becomes relatively noninfectious, and transplacental transmission is rare although it can occur. In some cases the bacteria break out of their intracellular location and cause a recurrence of the bacteremia. This occurs mainly in people who are immunocompromised. In others, the bacteria cause a slowly progressive inflammatory disease (**tertiary syphilis**). Symptoms of tertiary syphilis develop over a period of years to decades and include heart damage, neurological symptoms, disabling fatigue, and disfiguring skin lesions.

An interesting feature of *T. pallidum* is the relative paucity of proteins in its outer membrane. The genome sequence of *T. pallidum* revealed the presence of over 20 genes encoding lipoproteins similar to the ones found in the outer membrane of *B. burgdorferi*. The genome sequence also revealed that *T. pallidum* does not have genes for making nucleotides, fatty acids, most amino acids, and enzyme cofactors. This may explain why no one has yet cultivated *T. pallidum* in laboratory medium. It requires more supplements than are normally included even in rich medium. Information from the genome sequence may help to break the cultivation barrier that has hampered work on this microorganism.

The damage done to the heart, muscles, skin, and nervous system of people with late secondary and tertiary syphilis is thought to be caused by circulating immune complexes which consist of treponemal proteins, fibronectin, and host antibodies. These complexes, deposited in various body sites, elicit an inflammatory response. Fibronectin is thought to be a receptor for the structure on the treponemal surface that mediates attachment to host cells. A tightly bound treponemal antigen-fibronectin complex could cause the immune system to recognize fibronectin as a foreign antigen (much as conjugating a nonimmunogenic polysaccharide to a bacterial protein does), with the result that the immune system attacks host tissues.

Diagnosis and Treatment of Syphilis

In contrast to Lyme disease, for which the diagnostic tests are new and not entirely dependable, reliable blood tests for syphilis have been around for decades. Historically, an early syphilis diagnostic test presents an interesting example of a serological test that worked for the wrong reasons. Before much was known about the bacterium that causes syphilis, and in the absence of an animal model, immunologists had to work with the differences between people with the disease and people without the disease. A scientist named Wassermann discovered an antigen that seemed to tell these two populations apart. Originally, Wassermann thought this antigen was a bacterial antigen, but it turned out to be **cardiolipin,** a lipid found in mitochondrial membranes released from lysing mammalian cells. Presumably, the reason cardiolipin appeared to be specific for syphilis is that tissue damage associated with bacterial invasion of various host tissues and organs releases cardiolipin into the blood. Since cardiolipin is not normally seen by the immune system, it is recognized as foreign, and antibodies are made against it. These were the antibodies detected by the early (so-called nonspecific) tests. The problem with the **Wassermann test** and other tests based on anti-cardiolipin antibodies is that such antibodies are also elicited in response to other conditions, such as viral infections (e.g., mononucleosis and hepatitis), protozoal infections, autoimmune diseases, and certain malignancies.

More sensitive and specific tests for syphilis are now available. The first is a fluorescent antibody test that uses treponemes to detect anti-treponemal antibodies in the patient's blood. The second is a *T. pallidum* inactivation test based on the observation that treponemes lose motility rapidly when incubated with serum containing anti-treponemal antibodies. Both of these tests require live treponemes and sophisticated microscopes.

Thus, they are expensive and can only be done in specially equipped laboratories. The fluorescent antibody test is used more commonly than the inactivation test. Because these tests are expensive, physicians commonly treat patients on the basis of the rapid, nonspecific tests and do not order the more specific tests. This can be a problem if the person diagnosed wrongly as having syphilis is an engaged person preparing for marriage. At one time, syphilis testing was required for couples applying for a marriage license. An important reason for revoking such requirements was the psychological fallout—in low-syphilis areas—of a false-positive test.

Syphilis is treatable with penicillin. *T. pallidum* remains one of the few bacterial species in which resistance to penicillin has not yet appeared. As with Lyme disease, treatment is most successful if the disease is diagnosed early. The longer the disease goes untreated, the less likely antibiotics are to prevent irreversible damage caused by the autoimmune disease triggered by the bacterial infection. Early detection and treatment are especially important in pregnant women because of the danger of transplacental infection of the fetus.

Currently, in many parts of the developed world, syphilis has been eradicated or nearly eradicated. Efforts to eradicate the disease in the United States are currently under way. The ease with which syphilis can be diagnosed and treated makes eradication efforts feasible. Still, pockets of the disease are found in areas such as inner cities and rural areas where medical care is difficult to obtain or too expensive. Although we are facing the possibility of eradicating syphilis, we are still uncertain about the origins of the disease (Box 12–2). For centuries, scientists and historians have argued about where the disease originated.

Taking Stock

The spirochetes are a phylogenetically distinct group of disease-causing bacteria. In this chapter, three species of spirochetes were described—*B. burgdorferi, L. interrogans,* and *T. pallidum.* These are by no means the only pathogenic members of this group. *T. pertenue,* the cause of a skin disease called yaws, was mentioned in passing (Box 12–2). Oral spirochetes, such as *Treponema denticola,* are thought to play a role in periodontal disease. A spirochete called *Serpulina* sp. causes a disease in pigs that resembles human inflammatory bowel disease, and because of this is being investigated as a possible contributor to the human form of the disease. Spirochetes are abundant in nature, so it is likely that there are more spirochetal pathogens to be discovered.

BOX 12–2   The Origins of Syphilis—Still a Matter of Contention

Syphilis is the classic example of a disease that is consistently blamed on someone else. The English called it the French disease, the French called it the Italian disease, and so on. In a final attempt by Europeans to absolve themselves of all responsibility for the disease, syphilis was allegedly traced to the New World, whence it was supposedly brought back to Europe by Columbus's men. The hypothesis that syphilis was spread from the Americas to Europe had a certain appeal based on symmetry. So many devastating diseases (smallpox, measles, and tuberculosis, to name only a few) were brought to the Americas by Columbus and later explorers that it seemed only right that the Americas should have their revenge. The New World origins of syphilis have now been called into question, however. Anthropologists interested in the history of infectious diseases have discovered bone lesions indicative of syphilis in skeletal remains found in Italy and in northern England. The Italian remains were buried in the 12th century. The northern England remains came from the 1400s, before the departure of Columbus on his historic voyage. A second indication that syphilis was in Europe long before the 1400s was that the symptoms of what was then called "leprosy" bore a much closer resemblance to syphilis (in the highly virulent form it exhibited at that time) than to what we now know as leprosy.

The absence of a syphilis epidemic prior to the late 1400s could be explained by the fact that people identified as lepers were isolated in leper colonies until the 1400s, when a papal edict eliminated most of the leprosariums. In keeping with the tradition of blaming syphilis on someone else, the scientists who made this discovery, being of European and American descent, have now suggested that the disease arose in Africa. In Africa, there is a disease called yaws, which is caused by a spirochete, *Treponema pertenue*. *T. pertenue* is almost indistinguishable from *T. pallidum*. Yaws is not a sexually transmitted disease; it is transmitted by direct contact and is primarily a skin disease. How did yaws develop into syphilis, if in fact it did? A possible explanation is that in areas where yaws is endemic, adults were comparatively immune to the disease we now call syphilis. Explorers carrying the disease back to northern climates did not have this immunity, and the disease became a disease of adults, spread primarily by sexual transmission.

It is clear from the genome sequences of *B. burgdorferi* and *T. pallidum* that few of the virulence factors that are found in the more familiar gram-negative bacteria and in the gram-positive bacteria are found in the spirochetes. Or, if spirochetes possess such virulence factors as exotoxins or type III secretion systems, the genes encoding these virulence factors are so different at the nucleotide sequence level that they are not recognizable. The virulence factors of the spirochetes are still poorly understood. Moreover, in only one case, that of *B. burgdorferi*, is there a genetic system, and since it has been available for only a relatively short time, mutants lacking some of the suggested virulence factors, such as the internal flagella and the surface lipoproteins, have not been available for testing in animal models of disease. Finally, most of the known spirochetes are difficult to cultivate in laboratory medium. Given these limitations, the amount of progress made to date toward understanding how spirochetes cause disease is impressive, but it is obvious that there is still a long way to go.

SELECTED READINGS

Anguita, J., S. Samanta, B. Revilla, K. Suk, S. Das, S. W. Barthold, and E. Fikrig. 2000. *Borrelia burgdorferi* gene expression in vivo and spirochete pathogenicity. *Infect. Immun.* **68:**1222–1230.

Brown, S. L., S. L. Hansen, and J. J. Lagone. 1999. Role of serology in the diagnosis of Lyme disease. *JAMA* **282:** 62–66.

Casjens, S., N. Palmer, R. van Vugt, W. M. Huang, B. Stevenson, P. Rosa, R. Lathigra, G. Sutton, J. Peterson, R. J. Dodson, D. Haft, E. Hickey, M. Gwinn, O. White, and C. M. Fraser. 2000. A bacterial genome in flux: the twelve linear and nine circular extrachromosomal DNAs in an infectious isolate of the Lyme disease spirochete, *Borrelia burgdorferi*. *Mol. Microbiol.* **35:**490–516.

Dorward, D. W., E. R. Fische, and D. M. Brooks. 1997. Invasion and cytopathic killing of human lymphocytes by spirochetes causing Lyme disease. *Clin. Infect. Dis.* **25**(Suppl.)**:**S2–S8.

Fraser, C. M., S. J. Norris, G. M. Weinstock, O. White, G. G. Sutton, R. Dodson, M. Gwinn, E. K. Hickey, R. Clayton, K. A. Ketchum, E. Sodergren, J. M. Hardham, M. P. McLeod, S. Salzberg, J. Peterson, H. Khalak, D. Richardson, J. K. Howell, M. Chidambaram, T. Utterback, L. McDonald, P. Artiach, C. Bowman, M. D. Cotton, C. Fujii, S. Garland, B. Hatch, K. Horst, K. Roberts, M. Sandusky, J. Weidman, H. O. Smith, and J. C. Venter. 1998. Complete genome sequence of *Treponema pallidum,* the syphilis spirochete. *Science* **281:**375–379.

Gross, D. M., T. Forsthuber, M. Tary-Lehmann, C. Etling, K. Ito, Z. A. Nagy, J. A. Field, A. C. Steere, and B. T. Huber. 1998. Identification of LFA-1 as a candidate autoantigen in treatment-resistant Lyme arthritis. *Science* **281:**703–706.

Guo, B. P., E. L. Brown, D. W. Dorward, L. C. Rosenberg, and M. Hook. 1998. Decorin-binding adhesins from *Borrelia burgdorferi. Mol. Microbiol.* **30:**711–723.

JAMA. 1998. Outbreak of acute febrile illness among athletes participating in triathlons—Wisconsin and Illinois, 1998. *JAMA* **280:**1473–1474. (Editorial.)

Persing, D. H. 1997. The cold zone: a curious convergence of tick-transmitted diseases. *Clin. Infect. Dis.* **25**(Suppl.)**:** S35–S42.

Posey, J. E., and F. C. Gherardini. 2000. Lack of a role for iron in the Lyme disease pathogen. *Science* **288:**1651–1653.

Purser, J. E., and S. J. Norris. 2000. Correlation between plasmid content and infectivity in *Borrelia burgdorferi. Proc. Natl. Acad. Sci. USA* **97:**13865–13870.

Sartakova, M., E. Dobrikova, and F. C. Cabello. 2000. Development of an extrachromosomal cloning vector system for use in *Borrelia burgdorferi. Proc. Natl. Acad. Sci. USA* **97:**4850–4855.

Schwan, T. G. 1996. Ticks and *Borrelia*: model systems for investigating pathogen-arthropod interactions. *Infect. Agents Dis.* **5:**167–181.

Zhang, J.-R., J. M. Hardham, A. G. Barbour, and S. J. Norris. 1997. Antigenic variation in Lyme disease borreliae by promiscuous recombination of Vmp-like sequence cassettes. *Cell* **89:**275–285.

SUMMARY OUTLINE

B. burgdorferi

Characteristics
Spiral shape, corkscrew motility
Flagella in the periplasm between the cytoplasmic membrane and the outer sheath
Both linear and circular plasmids
Transmitted by ticks (especially *Ixodes* ticks)
White-footed mouse is intermediate host

Disease—Lyme disease
Annular rash that expands in diameter (most people)
Fever
Migrating arthritis
Chronic Lyme disease (uncommon)
Arthritis
Nerve damage
Seldom fatal

Virulence factors
Ability to grow in ticks and mammals
OspA to E—surface proteins, function unknown, but some are expressed in the tick and some in a mammalian host
Erps (OspE-related proteins)—surface proteins, function unknown
Decorin-binding protein—surface protein, binds decorin, function unknown
VlsE—surface protein, varies antigenically, similar to Vmps of *B. hermsii*
Ability to adhere to and transit layers of endothelial cells; entry into and exit from the blood vessels
Does not require iron

(continued)

SUMMARY OUTLINE (*continued*)

T. pallidum

Characteristics
- Spiral-shaped organism
- Humans are the only host
- Transmission
  - Sexual transmission
  - Mother to infant transmission, birth defects, fetal death
- Still has not been cultivated

Disease—syphilis
- Primary phase—chancre (lesion near site of inoculation)
- Secondary phase—rash (most people, but may be absent)
- Tertiary phase—neurological damage, tissue damage
- Congenital syphilis—fetus infected in uterus

Virulence factors
- Ability to transit epithelia to invade body
- Corkscrew motility, helps cross layers of tissue, enter and exit bloodstream
- Ability to cross the placenta

QUESTIONS

Answers to the questions can be found in Appendix 2.

1. Why did Lyme disease appear only in the late 20th century? In what sense is this a new disease?

2. Lyme disease has been characterized as overdiagnosed and underreported. How could both of these assessments be correct?

3. Why is it not surprising that the current serological tests for Lyme disease are so unsatisfactory?

4. Why would physicians be so quick to suspect Lyme disease even in areas where cases of the disease are uncommon?

5. *B. burgdorferi* carries a lot of genetic information on plasmids. At least some of these plasmids are lost during repeated passages in laboratory medium. What does this suggest about the adaptation of *B. burgdorferi* to new conditions?

6. So far, studies of virulence properties of *B. burgdorferi* have focused on a small number of surface-exposed lipoproteins. Why this emphasis, and what broader research priorities could you suggest for the future?

7. If you were designing a new Lyme disease vaccine, what would be your criteria for a candidate vaccine? Would you consider including more than one protein antigen? (Hint: Go back to what you learned in earlier chapters about the different host defenses and what is known about defenses that are most effective against *B. burgdorferi*.)

8. What do *B. burgdorferi* and *T. pallidum* have in common besides being spirochetes?

9. The number of syphilis cases in the United States has now dropped to the point that eradication of this disease is being contemplated by health authorities. The fact that these cases are largely limited to the southeastern United States makes eradication all the more feasible. If you were designing the eradication effort, what measures would you include in your program design?

10. Complete genome sequences are now available for *B. burgdorferi* and *T. pallidum*. What sorts of insights have been obtained from the sequence data, and what are the current limitations on interpreting this information?

13

Yersinia pestis, the Cause of Plague, and Its Relatives

KEY FEATURES

Yersinia pestis, Yersinia enterocolitica, Yersinia pseudotuberculosis

DESCRIPTION

Gram-negative coccobacillus

Nutritionally fastidious; many growth requirements

DISEASES

Y. pestis: Plague (bubonic, pneumonic)

Y. enterocolitica, Y. pseudotuberculosis: Gastroenteritis

RESERVOIRS

Y. pestis: Fleas; wild and domestic rodents, cats

Y. enterocolitica, Y. pestis: Domestic animals; spread by contaminated food, water

MAJOR VIRULENCE FACTORS

Y. pestis: Virulence plasmids (9.5 kbp, 101 kbp unique to *Y. pestis*); type III secretion system, injects toxic proteins into eukaryotic cells (70-kbp plasmid); F1 antigen—antiphagocytic; ability to obtain iron from host; ability to survive in flea, block flea digestion so that flea regurgitates bacteria

Y. enterocolitica, Y. pseudotuberculosis: Adhesins (*inv, ail, yadA*)—facilitate transit of M cells; type III secretion system (70-kbp plasmid)

PREVENTION AND TREATMENT

Y. pestis: Rodent control; monitoring disease in animal reservoirs; treatment with antibiotics

Y. enterocolitica, Y. tuberculosis: Avoid contamination of foods; cooking, pasteurization eliminate contaminating bacteria; usually not treated unless disease becomes systemic

---

The Rich and Terrible History of *Yersinia pestis*

Few diseases have captured the public imagination like bubonic plague, a disease that has come to stand as a paradigm for infectious disease disasters. This position is not entirely merited. Tuberculosis, for example, has killed far more people and is still present in epidemic proportions today. In terms of the magnitude of the disaster, the devastating effects of such diseases as smallpox and measles on the native peoples of the Americas were at least as great or greater, with death rates of 80% or more in some places. Nonetheless, plague continues to have a special mystique.

The first recorded plague pandemic began in Egypt in 542 A.D. and eventually spread to Europe, Africa, and Asia. This pandemic lasted until 600 A.D. The second plague pandemic, the one known as the Black Death, spread from Asia to Europe in the 1300s. In Europe, it raged for over 100 years before finally subsiding. The third pandemic began in China in 1855, eventually travelling to Europe and the United States. In the United States, it first appeared in San Francisco, where it ignited a storm of controversy (Box 13–1).

Today, *Y. pestis*, the cause of plague, is no longer a serious threat in developed countries because we understand how it is spread and have antibiotics that are effective in treating those few cases that occur (however, see Box 13–2). Most of the modern cases occur in East Africa, where poverty makes prevention and treatment difficult. There are isolated cases of plague in developed countries. The disruption caused by a war can also favor plague outbreaks, such as the outbreaks that occurred in Vietnam during the Vietnam War.

Plague has not disappeared even in the developed world. Every year in the western United States, for example, there are cases of bubonic plague among hikers or hunters who come into contact with infected animals. Infected cats can also spread the disease by acquiring an infection from contact with infected wild animals and bringing it home to human contacts. Plague may loom larger as a future threat, however, because it is one of the possible weapons that have attracted the attention of modern bioterrorists. Biological warfare seems very modern to us, but the first known use of *Y. pestis* as a weapon occurred centuries ago.

Biological Warfare in the 14th Century

What is possibly the first recorded case of germ warfare occurred in the Black Sea port city of Kaffa. Kaffa, a fortified city, had been besieged by Tartars for 3 years. Toward the end of that period, Tartar soldiers began dying of a mysterious disease in great enough numbers to cause their leader, Janiberg, to lift the siege and flee the area. Before leaving, however, Janiberg reportedly ordered the bodies of soldiers who had died of the disease to be catapulted into Kaffa. Although the residents of Kaffa promptly ejected the bodies, the exposure had been sufficient to spread the disease to residents of the city. Traders who had been trapped in the city during the siege left when the siege lifted, carrying the disease to Italy and eventually to other parts of Europe. Some historians have questioned the accuracy of this account

BOX 13–1   Denial Doesn't Make It Go Away

The first sign of an impending plague outbreak in San Francisco occurred in March 1900, when a Chinese worker was found dead of the disease. Although the health department soon confirmed that the man had died of plague, public officials up to the governor of the state stoutly denied that bubonic plague had appeared in San Francisco. Newspapers ridiculed the claims made by local health officials. Even the Chamber of Commerce got into the act. The San Francisco Board of Health attempted to cordon off Chinatown in hopes of containing the disease. The case quickly took on racial overtones as state and city officials instituted measures to limit travel by Asians and transfer inhabitants of Chinatown to detention camps. Eventually, the Board of Health was made to cease these actions. Ironically, the motivation for restoring the civil rights of Asian residents of the city came more from those who wished to deny the existence of plague cases than from those concerned about the violation of the rights of San Francisco inhabitants. Failure to take early, effective action may have contributed to the spread of plague in the area; by 1905, when the plague finally ended, there had been at least 121 cases and 118 deaths. To the end of his term, the governor continued to deny that there had been any cases of plague in the Golden State, claiming that the cases considered to be plague were really "syphilitic septicemia."

Source: L. G. Lipson. 1972. Plague in San Francisco in 1900. *Ann. Intern. Med.* **77**:303–310.

of the catapulted corpses, suggesting instead that rats moving between city and troops carried the disease, but we have no hesitation in passing the story on as fact. Now that historians have disproved the widespread belief that the nursery rhyme "Ring around the rosy" was about bubonic plague, thus robbing microbiology professors of a treasured anecdote, a replacement plague story is badly needed.

How likely is *Y. pestis* to be used as a biological weapon today? A major problem faced by modern bioterrorists is delivery of the bacteria to human popula-

BOX 13–2   Forget the Whales— Save the Rats!

Since public health officials know that rats and their fleas spread plague, an incipient outbreak in a major city where there are at least as many rats as people would undoubtedly trigger a frenzy of rat killing. Such a response during a plague epidemic, sensible as it sounds, might actually make the situation worse. Scientists at Cambridge University developed a population dynamics model to predict the outcome of a plague epidemic under a variety of conditions. According to their model, reducing the number of rats once an outbreak has begun could actually increase the number of cases of human disease. The reason is that rat fleas will dine preferentially on rats. They feed on humans only if there are not enough rats available. Thus, reducing the number of rats could increase the number of humans infected by fleabite. The bottom line is that if you want to reduce the rodent population in a city, do it when there is no outbreak in progress. Reducing the number of rats in this way could actually prevent an outbreak by reducing the number of susceptible rats. Once an outbreak is under way, however, spraying insecticides around human habitations would be the most effective method of preventing the spread of disease to the human populations. Also, early diagnosis and treatment of human plague cases becomes an important health measure, not just to benefit the infected people but to prevent them from developing pneumonic plague and spreading the disease to other people.

Source: M. J. Keeling and C. A. Gilligan. 2000. Metapopulation dynamics of bubonic plague. *Nature* **407**:903–906.

Modern Interest in *Y. pestis*

If plague is now just a distant memory of an infectious disease disaster, why devote a chapter to it? Because, paradoxically, *Y. pestis* has now become a positive force, yielding important new information about the interactions between bacterial pathogens and the human body. Researchers working on *Y. pestis* were the first to document the important role of iron in bacterial pathogenesis. *Y. pestis* was also an early model for how extrachromosomal elements such as plasmids can play an important role in making a microbe a pathogen. Plasmids and phages contribute to pathogenicity in other microbes, too, but the large number of genes carried on the virulence plasmids of *Y. pestis* is unusual.

A major recent discovery that has come out of research on *Y. pestis* was the discovery of **type III secretion systems,** which inject toxic proteins from the cytoplasm of the bacterium directly into the cytoplasm of a mammalian cell. Previously, the standard view of toxin production was that toxins were excreted into the extracellular medium, where they encountered mammalian cells. Attachment of the toxin to the mammalian cell was followed by entry into the cell of the active portion of the toxin, which killed or damaged the mammalian cell. The idea that bacteria could bind to mammalian cells and inject toxins directly into them changed the way scientists think about delivery of toxins. This mechanism of toxin delivery has turned out to be surprisingly widespread, not only among pathogens that infect mammalian hosts but also among pathogens that infect plants.

Finally, *Y. pestis* is of interest because it has an unusual interaction with its insect host, the rat flea. The flea can die of starvation if it becomes infected by *Y. pestis* because the bacteria block normal feeding by the flea. Most arthropods that serve as vectors for infectious microbes carry the microbe with no apparent damage to themselves, and there is often a complex set of interactions between the microbe and its arthropod host that ensures the arthropod emerges unscathed. An example of such a benign interaction was described in the chapter on *Borrelia burgdorferi,* the cause of Lyme disease. The fact that *Y. pestis* is not only spread effectively by an insect that can be killed by it, but also that the bacteria actually exploit their deleterious effect on the flea to facilitate their regurgitation and introduction into mammalian hosts, shows that the range of interactions between arthropods and the disease-causing microbes they spread can vary widely. But not all modern interest in *Y. pestis* is focused on modern issues (see Box 13–3).

Characteristics of *Y. pestis* and Plague

Yersiniae are small gram-negative coccobacilli. *Y. pestis* has many nutritional requirements, but given the right

tions. Lobbing infected corpses into New York City would not be as easy today as it was in Kaffa in the 14th century. Spraying the bacteria would require special technology to prevent the death of the bacteria, which do not survive for long outside the flea or mammalian host. Despite the difficulties in weaponizing *Y. pestis,* the U. S. government considers it a likely enough possibility to include management of plague in its "Final Bioterrorism Readiness Plan."

BOX 13–3   Only a Microbiologist Would Want To Know . . .

Most scientists have accepted for over a century the contention that the disease known as bubonic plague that devastated populations in Europe and Asia during the Middle Ages was caused by the bacterium we now know as *Y. pestis*, because the symptoms of the disease were similar to symptoms of modern cases of plague caused by *Y. pestis*. But some enterprising microbiologists were not satisfied with this leap of faith. Since scientists and physicians of earlier centuries viewed human diseases from a different perspective than we do today, reliance on described symptoms can be misleading. It is true that the symptoms of plague, such as the characteristic buboes (large swellings in the armpit or groin) and blackening around the mouth and extremities, are unusual enough to be considered good evidence for a link between today's *Y. pestis*-caused disease and the plague of earlier centuries. Nonetheless, some scientists wanted to know for sure whether the famous plague of medieval times was actually due to *Y. pestis*.

To determine whether this was the case, scientists went to graveyards where plague victims had been buried. For convenience, they focused on well-documented graves from the 16th to 18th centuries, when plague was still making the rounds but record keeping was better than in earlier centuries. Their idea was to use PCR to amplify the 16S rRNA gene of the bacterium that caused the death of these people and sequence it to determine whether the causative bacterium was, in fact, *Y. pestis*. Of course, such old remains consisted mainly of bones rather than flesh, where microbiologists would normally look for a systemic pathogen, but this did not deter these intrepid time travelers. Instead, they had the clever idea of looking at unerupted teeth in children. The pulp of teeth lasts for a very long time after death if the tooth surface is intact. Also, if a disease is caused by systemic infection, the bacteria should enter teeth that had not yet grown out of the gum. This feature of unerupted teeth ensured that the pathogen and not some contaminating exogenous bacterium would be detected.

PCR amplification was performed on unerupted teeth in children who died of plague in 16th century France. As a control, unerupted teeth from the same period, from skeletons of children who had died of other causes, were also examined. PCR amplification and sequencing of the amplified region revealed that, in fact, the bacteria in the unerupted teeth of plague victims were *Y. pestis*. No trace of *Y. pestis* was found in the unerupted teeth of the control group.

Surely, all of us can sleep more soundly knowing that this bit of the microbiological history of the human race has been rigorously confirmed. Seriously, although the results of this study may not have been too surprising, it shows how molecular techniques can be applied to diagnosing diseases in centuries-old specimens. In a sense, showing that *Y. pestis* was the cause of plague in earlier centuries was a validation of this approach to determining disease causation in very old specimens. Previously, molecular techniques such as PCR had been used to obtain segments of the genome of the virus that caused the 1918 influenza pandemic. The plague study pushed the clock back a few more centuries. Scientists have tried to analyze DNA in much earlier samples, such as those taken from the intestinal tracts of thousand-year-old mummies or even older mastodons. The problem with many of these studies is that they tend to turn up bacteria that could be contaminants from the modern environment. In the case of *Y. pestis*, this was not a serious concern. The likelihood that *Y. pestis* would be a contaminant, especially in unerupted teeth, was virtually zero.

Source: M. Drancourt, G. Aboudharam, M. Signoli, O. Dutour, and D. Raoult. 1998. Detection of 400-year old *Yersinia pestis* DNA in human dental pulp: an approach to the diagnosis of ancient septicemia. *Proc. Natl. Acad. Sci. USA* **95:**12637–12640.

medium, it grows rapidly. There is also a good genetic system in place that allows the bacteria to be manipulated genetically.

Plague is a systemic infection in mammals. Many types of mammals can be infected, and the disease is often fatal. The steps in the transmission of *Y. pestis* are illustrated in Figure 13–1. The bacteria are injected into skin by the bite of a flea, which carries the bacteria in its gut. The flea acquires the bacteria by taking a blood meal from an infected mammal. In the flea gut, the bacteria replicate by using nutrients in the ingested blood and form a clumped mass, which blocks the intestine from receiving further blood meals. The mass of bacteria is lodged in the esophageal region of the flea, ef-

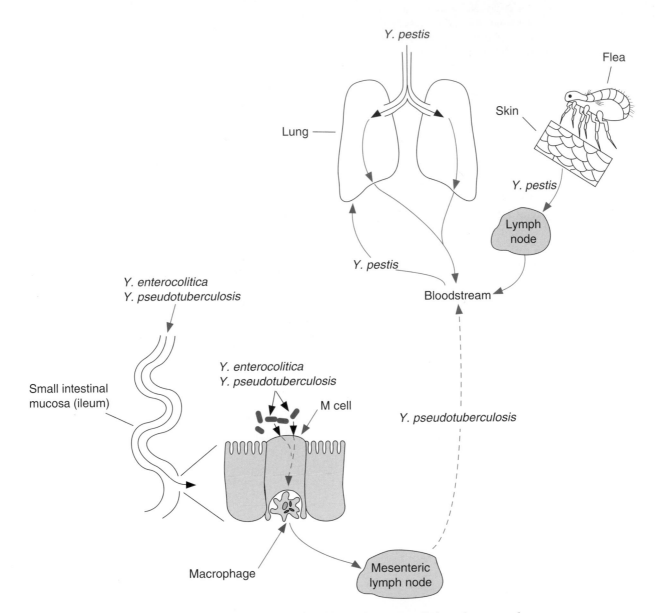

Figure 13–1 Steps in the transmission of *Yersinia* species. Infected mammals serve as the reservoir of *Y. pestis*. When an infected flea bites a human, it regurgitates fragments of the mass containing *Y. pestis*. The bacteria disseminate rapidly though the lymphatic system and the bloodstream and locate in lymph nodes, where the inflammatory response causes buboes to form (bubonic plague). At this point, *Y. pestis* may enter the bloodstream again and travel to the lungs, where it causes pneumonic plague. Pneumonic plague can be transmitted from one human to another. *Yersinia enterocolitica* and *Yersinia pseudotuberculosis* are ingested and enter the lymphatic system via the M cells of the small intestine. Rarely, *Y. pseudotuberculosis* enters the bloodstream.

fectively preventing any fluids ingested by the flea from moving into the lower gut, where nutrients are extracted. An infected flea is, in effect, a starving flea. Eventually, unless the flea can regurgitate the bacteria-laden mass, it will die.

In a mammal, bacteria injected into the wound created by the fleabite enter the bloodstream and disseminate rapidly. In the early stages of dissemination, the bacteria seem able to suppress the inflammatory response, a trait that protects them as they move into the bloodstream. Rapid dissemination to all parts of the body is probably a requirement for insect-transmitted microbes because the next insect may feed on any portion of the body. The bacteria must be widely available to infect the next flea.

Y. pestis has an affinity for lymphoid tissue and localizes in the lymph nodes (Figure 13–1). There, damage caused by the bacteria themselves and the inflammatory response they begin to elicit cause painful swellings to develop, especially in the armpit or groin. These swellings are called **buboes,** and this form of plague is called **bubonic plague.** Bacteria then move into the bloodstream. If the infected person survives the initial septicemia, the bacteria can move to the lungs. In the lungs, the bacteria multiply, causing more damage. This form of plague is called **pneumonic plague.** Bacteria in the lungs can be spread to uninfected people by aerosols. In people infected by this route, the bacteria first multiply in the lung and then move into the bloodstream. People infected by the aerosol route die within days, presumably because the bacteria they inhale are already acclimated to the human body and do not have to adapt to the change from insect host to human host. Death is due to septic shock.

Yersinia enterocolitica and *Yersinia pseudotuberculosis,* Food-Borne Relatives of *Y. pestis*

Two other species of *Yersinia* have served as model pathogens in the past: *Y. enterocolitica* and *Y. pseudotuberculosis.* These *Yersinia* species are carried by many wild and domestic animals. Bacteria from domestic animals can contaminate milk and food, which, if not adequately treated or cooked, can introduce the bacteria into the human intestinal tract (Figure 13–1). There, the bacteria exhibit an affinity for the M cells of the ileum, which they utilize as entryways into underlying lymphoid tissue. The resulting inflammatory response to the bacteria can cause pain severe enough to be mistaken for appendicitis. Infections caused by these two gastrointestinal pathogens are not very common in the United States. They are more common in Europe, especially northern Europe.

In the early days of modern pathogenesis research, both *Y. enterocolitica* and *Y. pseudotuberculosis* yielded important new insights into how bacteria attach to and invade mammalian cells. For example, the first identification of a bacterial protein adhesin (**invasin**) that specifically recognized a human cell surface antigen, **β-integrin,** was made by studying the interaction between *Y. enterocolitica* and tissue culture cells.

The invasion assay developed in these studies has become a standard assay for invasion of cultured cells by many different species of bacteria. In the invasion assay, the bacteria are first allowed to bind to the cultured cells and invade. Next, to kill any bacteria that are still outside the cells, the cultured cells are treated with an antibiotic that does not enter eukaryotic cells. The eukaryotic cells are then washed to remove the antibiotic and lysed to release bacteria that have invaded the cell, and the lysate is plated on agar medium. Although *Y. enterocolitica* and *Y. pseudotuberculosis* remain models for the study of bacterial invasion of eukaryotic cells, they appear to act as extracellular pathogens in the body.

In this chapter, the focus is on *Y. pestis,* but *Y. enterocolitica* and *Y. pseudotuberculosis* are still of interest because of the question of why these species, which are so closely related to *Y. pestis,* cause comparatively mild, localized disease whereas *Y. pestis* causes a systemic infection that is often fatal if not treated. *Y. pestis* is most closely related to *Y. pseudotuberculosis.* In fact, sequence comparisons at different genetic loci suggest that *Y. pestis* appeared only about 1,500 to 4,000 years ago, that it was derived from a strain of *Y. pseudotuberculosis,* and that it has remained nearly clonal ever since. If this is true, *Y. pestis* is an example of a pathogen that evolved to higher virulence from a less virulent ancestor. Whatever happened to generate *Y. pestis* thousands of years ago caused other major changes in the organism as well, such as its ability to be spread by insects.

Yersinia Plasmids

A possible explanation for why *Y. pestis* could change so rapidly in such a short time is suggested by the plasmids it carries. All three *Yersinia* species carry a 70-kbp plasmid (**pCD1**) (Table 13–1). This plasmid carries genes needed to produce the type III secretion system that allows bacteria bound to the mammalian cell surface to inject toxic substances into the mammalian cell. *Y. pestis* has two other plasmids not found in *Y. enterocolitica* or *Y. pseudotuberculosis,* a 9.6-kbp plasmid (**pPCP1**) and a 101-kbp plasmid (**pMT1**). Although many discussions of the virulence of *Y. pestis* focus on the 70-kbp plasmid, it seems clear that this is not where

Table 13–1 Comparison of the three *Y. pestis* virulence plasmids

Characteristic	pPCP1	pCD1[a]	pMT1
Size	9.6 kbp	70 kbp	101 kbp
Present in			
Y. pestis	Yes	Yes	Yes
Y. enterocolitica, Y. pseudotuberculosis	No	Yes	No
Virulence factors			
Plasminogen activator (pla)	+		
Adherence/invasion (unknown gene)	+		
Adherence/invasion (yadA)[b]		+	
Type III secretion system and the proteins it injects (yop, ysc, lcr genes)		+	
LcrV (lcrV)		+	
F1 capsule (caf genes)			+

[a]Designated pYV in *Y. enterocolitica* and pIB1 in *Y. pseudotuberculosis*.
[b]Inactivated in *Y. pestis*; two other invasin genes, *inv* and *ail*, which are located in the chromosome, are also inactive in *Y. pestis*.

the main action is, since the less pathogenic species also carry a very similar plasmid. All three *Y. pestis* plasmids have now been completely sequenced. The 9.6-kbp plasmid carries a gene encoding a protease that can activate plasminogen, a blood protein involved in clot resolution. The plasminogen activator appears to be important for dissemination of the bacteria.

The 101-kbp plasmid carries genes for production of the *Y. pestis* capsule plus 74 other genes, 44 of which have no homologs in the databases. This plasmid also carries a gene encoding a protein called murine toxin (see later section). The two extra plasmids carried by *Y. pestis* may explain part of the higher virulence of this species compared with *Y. enterocolitica* and *Y. pseudotuberculosis*, but acquisition of new genes may not be the full story. As will become evident later in this chapter, some of the adhesin genes carried on the 70-kbp plasmid, which are active in *Y. enterocolitica* and *Y. pseudotuberculosis*, have been inactivated in the *Y. pestis* 70-kbp plasmid. Usually, scientists think of greater virulence as arising from acquisition of genes. The possibility that *Y. pestis* may have increased in virulence because of the loss of some genes is yet another novel finding by scientists working on *Y. pestis* virulence traits.

Virulence Factors of *Y. pestis, Y. enterocolitica,* and *Y. pseudotuberculosis*

Since *Y. pestis* seems to have evolved from *Y. pseudotuberculosis*, it is useful to compare the virulence factors

of *Y. pestis* with those of *Y. pseudotuberculosis*. The virulence factors of *Y. pseudotuberculosis* have proved to be similar to those of *Y. enterocolitica*, a fact that should not be surprising in view of the fact that both of these species cause similar diseases.

YADA. The first step in infection of the small intestine by *Y. pseudotuberculosis* is attachment to and transiting of the M cells of the Peyer's patches. Originally, there were several candidates for the gene most important in this early step. One was *inv*, the gene encoding a surface protein called **invasin**. The name was suggested by the fact that invasin-producing cells could bind to and invade tissue culture cells. Studies of attachment to and invasion of tissue culture cells also identified another locus, **ail** (attachment and invasion locus). The *inv* gene was expressed preferentially at 20°C and was not expressed at 37°C. Thus, any Inv protein on the surface of the invading bacteria would be rapidly lost. The *ail* gene was expressed at 37°C, but disruption of this gene had little effect on virulence in mice. Its main role now appears to be to protect the bacteria from killing by complement. Also, there may be enough overlap in function between Ail and other surface proteins that loss of one of them is compensated for by the others, with little apparent effect on virulence.

The most important virulence determinant for *Y. enterocolitica* in the initial stages of intestinal infection has proved to be **YadA (yersinia adhesin A)**. Mutations in *yadA* significantly reduce virulence. Curiously, *yadA* is dispensable for *Y. pseudotuberculosis*, which presumably has another protein that plays the role of YadA. In *Y. pestis, yadA* is inactive, and its loss may actually enhance the virulence of *Y. pestis*. YadA is unusual in the number of its activities (Table 13–2). It binds to intestinal mucin, an activity that might help it to initiate colonization of the small intestinal mucosa. Of course, this feature of YadA could also be a drawback for the bacteria, because there is mucin all along the small intestine, whereas the M cells are clustered in the ileum near the end of the small intestine. Perhaps more important, YadA binds β1-integrins, proteins that are found on the surface of M cells. Although M cells are naturally

Table 13–2 Activities of YadA

Binds
  Intestinal mucin
  β1-integrins (cell surface adhesion proteins)
  Collagen (extracellular matrix)

Resistance to phagocytosis

Cooperates with the type III secretion system by mediating initial adherence phagocytic, YadA, like invasin, could well stimulate this phagocytic activity, creating for themselves a fast track through the intestinal mucosa.

Bacteria with YadA on their surfaces resist engulfment by PMNs, a statement that might seem contradictory to previous statements about YadA stimulation of entry into M cells. This antiphagocytic action of YadA is easily explained, however, if one takes into account that YadA prevents complement activation at the bacterial surface. Complement activation is an important factor in uptake of bacteria by phagocytes.

YadA is indeed a fascinating multifunctional protein. In addition to its antiphagocytic activity, it also binds collagen, a component of extracellular matrix. Finally, YadA can initiate binding to mammalian cells, anchoring the bacteria to the cells so that the type III secretion system can form a channel between the bacterial cytoplasm and the cytoplasm of the mammalian cell.

TYPE III SECRETION SYSTEM. As mentioned earlier, secretion systems that consist of a membrane-spanning complex through which bacteria inject proteins directly into the cytoplasm of eukaryotic cells are called type III secretion systems. All three pathogenic *Yersinia* species have type III secretion systems. Most of the genes required for the type III system and the proteins it secretes are carried on the 70-kbp plasmid, which is found in all three of the pathogenic *Yersinia* species. Most of the genes have one of three designations, which can be very confusing to a novice. The confusion arose because the genes were named before it was understood how they all functioned. The designations are *yop* (**yersinia outer membrane protein**), *lcr* (**low-calcium response**), and *ysc* (**yersinia secretion**).

A current model for how a type III secretion system works is shown in Figure 13–2. Most of the proteins make up the membrane-spanning channel that will eventually fuse with the eukaryotic cell to form the injection pore. This core of the structure can assemble in the absence of a eukaryotic cell because the genes are maximally expressed in response to 37°C temperature. The translocated proteins are not, however, expelled from the bacterial cell unless contact with a eukaryotic cell is made and the full injection apparatus is assembled.

One explanation for what keeps the channel closed in the absence of contact with a eukaryotic cell is based on a phenomenon called the low-calcium response. If ambient calcium concentrations are high, a protein gate remains closed, and no translocation of proteins out of the bacterial cytoplasm occurs (Figure 13–2). Secretion is triggered by a low-calcium environment, which causes the gated pore to open and triggers the vectorial

movement of toxic proteins through the pore and into the cytoplasm of the eukaryotic cell. The low-calcium signal may reflect the fact that the cytoplasm of a eukaryotic cell is low in free calcium because of the presence of such calcium-binding proteins as calmodulin. Exposure of the tip of the secretion apparatus to the low-calcium environment of the eukaryotic cytoplasm is thought to be the signal that causes the pore to open. Secretion is ATP dependent. The model for opening and closing the channel is based on work done in the laboratory. In the body, calcium may not be the only or even the most important trigger. What factors control whether the channel is open or closed in vivo remain to be established.

The proteins that are secreted through the secretion system have a variety of effects on the eukaryotic cell, but all cooperate to kill the cell. The type III secretion system may be primarily a defense against PMNs and macrophages. A list of the known injected proteins is provided in Table 13–3. YopB and YopD are translocated early; they form the portion of the pore that transits the membrane of the eukaryotic cell (Figure 13–2). YopE and YopH promote disassociation of cytoskeletal microfilaments or prevent formation of focal adhesions. The combination of these activities prevents the cytoskeleton-controlled changes that make it possible for a eukaryotic cell to engulf and ingest a bacterium. Thus, YopE and YopH are antiphagocytic in their effects. YopH also abrogates other antibacterial responses of PMNs, thus decreasing the effectiveness of an important antibacterial defense of the body. Other injected proteins, such as YopJ, suppress the production of cytokines. This too suppresses the ability of immune cells and phagocytic cells to mobilize a defense against the invading bacteria. Injected proteins also induce apoptosis (programmed cell death) in macrophages and thereby promote systemic infection.

An interesting feature of the type III secretion system is that the current model of its organization and appearance makes it look remarkably like the portion of the bacterial flagellum that transits the inner and outer membrane. In fact, many of the Ysc proteins share amino acid similarity with proteins that make up the base of a flagellum. It is worth noting that these similarities have aided scientists considerably in putting together a picture of how a type III secretion system might work. It is also a good example of how studies of bacterial traits that might seem at first glance to have no relevance to pathogenesis can become suddenly relevant.

Mechanisms for the biogenesis of surface organelles such as flagella and pili have been coopted to form the type III secretion system. Under some conditions, the hook region of flagella can secrete proteins, and it is

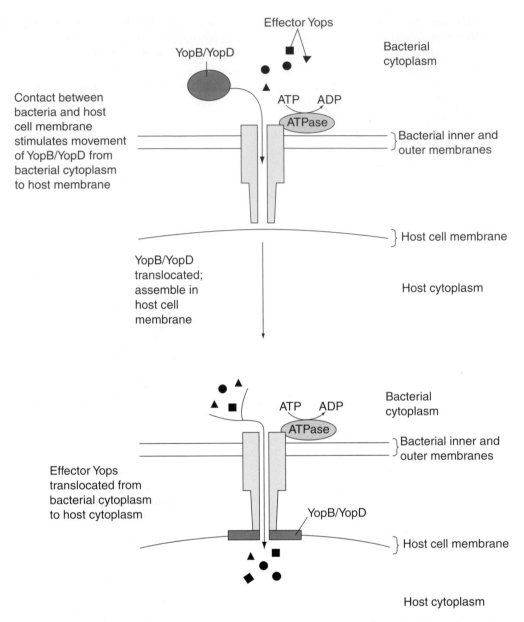

Figure 13–2 Signals regulating a type III secretion system. Once the bacteria make contact with a eukaryotic cell membrane in an appropriate environment, YopB and YopD are translocated from the bacterial cytoplasm and form a pore in the eukaryotic cell membrane. Once the pore opens, the effector Yops are secreted directly into the eukaryotic cell cytoplasm. The components of the secretion system in the eukaryotic cell membrane, designated YopB and YopD, are also referred to as Ysc proteins.

likely that the flagellar transport system may have given rise to the type III secretion system. The type II secretion system, which is responsible for exporting hydrolytic enzymes and some toxins outside the bacterial cell, has some similarities to the system for biogenesis of type IV pili and may have arisen from the pilin biogenesis system. The competence systems that take up DNA by natural transformation may have had a similar origin.

Scientists who study type III secretion systems use an interesting strategy for identifying proteins that are injected into eukaryotic cells rather than simply excreted into the medium. First, they determine if the protein, when supplied in the medium of tissue culture cells, is toxic to those cells. If not, the protein may have to be injected to cause toxicity. Second, the proteins can be introduced into the tissue culture cell by a form of transfection that temporarily disrupts the membrane so

Table 13–3 Toxic effects of Yops translocated by the type III secretion system and LcrV

YopB, YopD—form the part of the pore that transits the eukaryotic cell membrane

YopJ—a cysteine protease that prevents activation of mitogen-activated protein kinases and NF-κB, two regulators of eukaryotic gene expression; target is macrophages

LcrV—released into the medium by type III system; secreted into host cells independently of type III system; also regulates opening of the type III channel (formed by YopB and YopD) and is essential for injection of Yops

YopE—disruption of actin filaments by inhibiting host cell Rho GTPases; target cell unknown

YopT—disruption of actin filaments by inactivation of Rho factor; target cell unknown

YopH—inhibits antibacterial response by PMNs; tyrosine phosphatase activity; inhibits assembly of focal adhesins; blocks early Ca²⁺ signaling in PMNs

that the proteins can enter. If they are toxic under these conditions, they may be injected proteins. Third, scientists fuse the gene encoding the protein of interest with the gene encoding adenylate cyclase from the bacterium *Bordetella pertussis* (chapter 17). The *B. pertussis* adenylate cyclase requires calmodulin for activation and thus is active only in the cytoplasm of a eukaryotic cell. If such a fusion protein raises the cyclic AMP content of a tissue culture cell, it is probably being injected into the cell.

LcrV. A protein that appears to be excreted to the extracellular medium rather than excreted by the type III secretion system is **LcrV.** LcrV is involved in opening the channel and translocating the Yops into the eukaryotic cell. LcrV can act on eukaryotic cells, but this activity is independent of the type III secretion system. Antibodies to LcrV appear in people and in laboratory animals infected with *Y. pestis,* and antibodies against LcrV are protective. Thus, LcrV is accessible on the bacterial surface, indicating that it is not one of the proteins that are injected into the mammalian cell cytoplasm.

ADHESINS AND INVASINS. The 70-kbp virulence plasmid that carries the genes necessary for the type III secretion system and the proteins it injects also carries the gene encoding the adhesin YadA. The genes encoding two other invasion proteins, Inv (invasin) and Ail (accessory invasion locus) are located on the chromosome, not on one of the virulence plasmids.

Why are active forms of adhesin and invasin genes such as *inv, ail,* and *yadA* found in *Y. enterocolitica* and *Y. pseudotuberculosis,* which are spread by ingestion, but

not in *Y. pestis,* which is spread by fleas? *Y. enterocolitica* and *Y. pseudotuberculosis* target the naturally phagocytic M cells of the follicles and Peyer's patches. The adherence-invasion proteins these genes encode may stimulate transfer of the bacteria through the cells of the Peyer's patches.

IRON ACQUISITION. Scientists have demonstrated that *Y. pestis* has at least three mechanisms for obtaining inorganic iron and one for obtaining iron from heme and heme proteins. Inspection of the *Y. pestis* genome sequence indicates that there may be even more than these four systems. Why are there so many iron sequestration systems? One explanation is that different ones are used at different points in the infection process. For example, an iron-binding siderophore called **yersiniabactin** may be important in the early steps in the infection process in animals. The genes encoding proteins that assemble yersiniabactin are located in the chromosome on a **pathogenicity island.** This island is found in *Y. pestis,* in *Y. pseudotuberculosis,* and in some of the more virulent strains of *Y. enterocolitica.* Other iron sequestration systems may come into play later in the infection process, although some of them, such as **Yfe** and **Yfu** iron transporter systems, are clearly expendable in laboratory medium and in mice.

The heme utilization system (**Hmu** or **Hms**) that enables the bacteria to obtain iron from hemin might seem to be important for bacteria in a mammal because heme and heme proteins are ubiquitous in the body. Nonetheless, this system is not required for virulence in mice.

At room temperature, *Y. pestis* exhibits a phenomenon called **hemin storage.** This phenomenon, which is mediated by the Hmu proteins, involves the tight binding of hemin to the surface of the bacteria. So much heme is bound that colonies of bacteria producing Hmu on an agar plate that contains heme become a dark blackish brown. Yet, it is now clear that this hemin is not nutritionally available to the bacteria, which appear to become iron-starved in the presence of a glut of heme. Thus, Hmu may not be important in the flea, either.

Virulence Factors Unique to *Y. pestis*

THE FLEA–*Y. PESTIS* INTERACTION. Plague is most often spread from animals to humans by fleas. *Y. pestis* can infect a variety of flea species, rather than having the sort of species-specific association seen in the case of *B. burgdorferi,* the cause of Lyme disease (see chapter 12). One reason for this is that *Y. pestis* has a rather unusual mode of ensuring that the flea transmits it. *Y. pestis* in the blood of the animal is ingested by the flea when the flea takes a blood meal. In the gut of the flea, the bacteria agglutinate to form a plug that keeps the flea from feeding again. This process is called **blocking.** In Figure 13–3, a diagram of the flea gut is shown. The block occurs in the proventriculus, a spine-covered region between the crop and the midgut. In a blocked flea, the blood meal accumulates in the upper part of the digestive tract and cannot reach the midgut, where the blood meal normally goes. A blocked flea will starve to death if it cannot eliminate the blockage. To take another blood meal, the flea must first regurgitate the agglutinated bacteria to clear its gut for reception of new food. In this way, the bacteria are injected into the wound made by the flea on the animal on which it is feeding. A blocked flea is also likely to feed more frequently in an attempt to compensate for the partial blockage that remains. Clearly, fleas that are more successful at regurgitating and thus partially clearing the bacterial bolus are more likely to live longer and infect more mammalian hosts. Thus, blocking, which at first looks like a counterproductive strategy for the bacteria, actually promotes more efficient spread.

Little is known about the factors that allow *Y. pestis* to colonize fleas, but one characteristic that contributes to blocking has been identified. Oddly enough, the gene that promotes flea colonization was originally identified as a gene encoding a murine toxin. This explains its gene designation, *ymt,* for *Yersinia* **murine toxin.** More recent studies have shown that *ymt* has no role in pathogenesis in mammalian hosts, and it is not clear why the protein it encodes initially appeared to be toxic for mice. Ymt protein does appear to be important for bacterial colonization of the flea gut, although the specific role it plays in colonization has not been identified. The *ymt* gene is carried on the 100-kbp plasmid found in *Y. pestis* but not in *Y. enterocolitica* and *Y. pseudotuberculosis.*

Hmu (or Hms) also appears to be important for survival in the insect, but the mechanism by which the Hmu system promotes survival in the insect is still unclear.

Survival in the Mammalian Body

ANTIPHAGOCYTIC MECHANISMS. A *Y. pestis*-specific strategy that appears to promote its dissemination early in the infection process is to produce surface proteins that are antiphagocytic. An example is the capsular protein **F1,** encoded by the *caf1* (**capsular antigen fraction 1**) gene. This gene is carried on the 101-kbp plasmid that is unique to *Y. pestis.* F1 protein forms fibrillar structures on the bacterial surface and appears to prevent phagocytosis in vitro. Its role in pathogenesis is still unclear, however. Mutants that lack it have the same LD_{50} in mice as wild-type *Y. pestis.* Yet antibodies against F1 are protective in animal models, and it is an

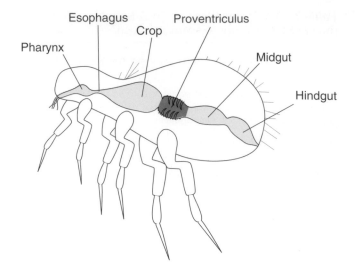

Figure 13–3 Anatomy of the flea digestive tract. When the flea takes up blood containing *Y. pestis*, the bacteria aggregate to form a macrocolony in the proventriculus. This prevents the blood from entering the midgut, where it would normally be digested. If the flea does not regurgitate the clot, it will be unable to feed and will die.

immunodominant component of the plague vaccine. A possible explanation is that it plays no role in virulence, but antibodies to it help phagocytic cells to ingest the bacteria. If so, however, why hasn't *Y. pestis* lost this gene the way it lost the active adhesin and invasin genes? Perhaps there is a special role for F1 in humans that is not so evident in mouse models of the infection.

Still another difference between *Y. pestis* and the food-borne yersiniae is the 9.6-kbp plasmid of *Y. pestis.* This plasmid carries the gene *pla,* which encodes an outer membrane protease that can activate plasminogen (Table 13–1). In addition to a possible role in adhering to and invading cells, **Pla** appears to prevent chemotaxis of PMNs to the site of inoculation, but how a protein attached to the bacterial cell does this is not clear. Pla seems to be important fairly early in the infection, because loss of the *pla* gene has a greater effect on the virulence of bacteria injected by fleabite than on bacteria injected by syringe into the bloodstream.

ANIMAL RESERVOIRS. Humans are an accidental host for *Y. pestis.* The natural reservoir for *Y. pestis* is rodents and a variety of other animals. Since *Y. pestis* can kill its rodent host, it is imperative that the bacteria be spread efficiently to new hosts to maintain itself in the population. In the western United States, *Y. pestis* has been found not only in ground squirrels and other rodents but also in cats and antelopes. Dogs, by contrast, are relatively resistant to infection and so are not as likely as cats to spread the infection to humans. In the western United States, mice and voles are important reservoirs because they are relatively resistant to the disease and thus are more likely to survive infection and maintain *Y. pestis* in nature.

Flea transmission is not the only route of transmission from animals to humans, although it is undoubtedly the most effective one. Transmission from antelopes to humans, for example, has occurred only in the case of hunters, who probably acquired the infection in the process of skinning and butchering the animal. Whether the bacteria entered the body through small cuts and abrasions or were inhaled in aerosols, or both, is not known. Humans can acquire *Y. pestis* from infected pets by inhaling aerosols rather than from fleabites. Humans in the late stages of an uncontrolled *Y. pestis* infection can also spread the bacteria to other humans by aerosols that carry bacteria that have made it to the person's lung. This type of plague, which is called pneumonic plague, is particularly lethal, probably because the bacteria are already adapted to the mammalian body. After the flea-to-human transition, *Y. pestis* has to undergo changes that make it able to survive in a mammalian host.

Future Directions

In the past, research on *Y. pestis* virulence factors has focused primarily on the virulence plasmids. This is understandable, because plasmids are smaller and thus more manageable than the chromosome. Yet, there are likely to be important chromosomal genes that influence survival in the insect or survival in the human body. One chromosomal pathogenicity island has already been identified, the island that contains the iron acquisition genes (for yersiniabactin). A comparison of the genome sequences of *Y. pestis* and *Y. pseudotuberculosis* will identify regions of the *Y. pestis* genome that differ in the two species. Although the sequences of these regions might not reveal their functions, they would at least identify targets for further study. The known virulence factors also need further study. Many of the statements made about their possible role in the animal are still highly speculative and need to be backed up with in-depth studies of how various virulence factors function in the insect and the mammal. Finally, the mechanism by which a type III secretion system injects proteins into a eukaryotic cell is still in the early phases of understanding. Similarly, work has only begun on the proteins that are translocated and how they affect the cell into which they are injected.

SELECTED READINGS

Achtman, M., K. Zurth, G. Morelli, G. Torrea, A. Guiyoule, and E. Carniel. 1999. *Yersinia pestis,* the cause of plague, is a recently emerged clone of *Yersinia pseudotuberculosis. Proc. Natl. Acad. Sci. USA* **96:**14043–14048.

Blocker, A., D. Holden, and G. Cornelis. 2000. Type III secretion systems: what is the translocator and what is translocated? *Cell. Microbiol.* **2:**387–390.

Chanteau, S., M. Ratsitorahina, L. Rahalison, B. Rasoamanana, F. Chan, P. Boisier, D. Rabeson, and J. Roux. 2000. Current epidemiology of human plague in Madagascar. *Microb. Infect.* **2:**25–31. (A description of an ongoing outbreak of plague in Madagascar.)

Cornelis, G. R. 2000. Molecular and cell biology aspects of plague. *Proc. Natl. Acad. Sci. USA* **97:**8778–8783.

Cowan, C., H. A. Jones, Y. H. Kaya, R. D. Perry, and S. C. Straley. 2000. Invasion of epithelial cells by *Yersinia pestis:* evidence for a *Y. pestis*-specific invasin. *Infect. Immun.* **68:**4523–4530.

Iriarte, M., and G. R. Cornelis. 1999. The 70-kilobase virulence plasmid of Yersiniae, p. 91–126. *In* J. B. Kaper and J. Hacker (ed.), *Pathogenicity Islands and Other Mobile Virulence Elements.* American Society for Microbiology, Washington, D.C.

Karlen, A. 1995. *Man and Microbes,* p. 86–87. Simon & Schuster, New York, N.Y.

Perry, R. D., and J. D. Fetherston. 1997. *Yersinia pestis*—etiologic agent of plague. *Clin. Microbiol. Rev.* **10:**35–66.

Rakin, A., S. Schubert, C. Pelludat, D. Brem, and J. Heesemann. 1999. The high-pathogenicity island of Yersiniae, p. 77–90. *In* J. B. Kaper and J. Hacker (ed.), *Pathogenicity Islands and Other Mobile Virulence Elements.* American Society for Microbiology, Washington, D.C.

Straley, S. C., and M. N. Starnbach. 2000. *Yersinia:* strategies that thwart immune defenses, p. 71–92. *In* M. W. Cunningham and R. S. Fujinami (ed.), *Effects of Microbes on the Immune System.* Lippincott, Williams & Wilkins, Philadelphia, Pa.

Fiction

Bubonic plague has been the subject of a number of books. Some of them are listed here.

Camus, A. *The Plague.* (There are many editions of this book available. A fictionalized account based on a modern plague epidemic in Algeria. Great to read back-to-back with the Defoe book for a real high-octane shot of plague lore.)

Defoe, D. *Journal of the Plague Year.* (There are many editions of this classic book. It contains a fictionalized account of the 1665 plague epidemic in London but was written in 1721 by an author who was born soon after the epidemic occurred.)

Hillerman, T. 1999. *The First Eagle.* Harper & Row, Publishers, Inc., New York, N.Y. (A mystery novel in which one of the victims was trapping fleas in a plague study on a Navajo reservation in the southwestern United States.)

Y. pestis

Characteristics

Gram-negative coccobacillus

Nonmotile

Can survive in flea or human

Transmitted by vector

Causes blocking in the flea, forces regurgitation of the bacteria

Rodents are main reservoir; other animals and humans can also serve as hosts

Transmitted to humans by flea or by aerosol from a person or pet with pneumonic plague

Disease—plague

Flea injects bacteria into skin

Bacteria enter blood and move to lymph nodes (buboes) (bubonic plague)

Bacteria can invade lung (pneumonic plague)

Death caused by septic shock

Virulence factors

Common to all three pathogenic species

70-kbp virulence plasmid

Type III secretion system

Inject toxic Yops, suppress cytokine production, disrupt cytoskeletal structure (anti-phagocytic)

LPS, septic shock

Yersiniabactin, iron acquisition

Unique to *Y. pestis*

9.6-kbp and 101-kbp plasmids

Plasminogen activator (Pla), dissolves clots, may help bacteria spread in the body

F1 capsule (*caf1*), antiphagocytic

Factors important for survival in insect, "*Yersinia* murine toxin" (Ymt), function unknown

Inactive *inv*, *ail*, *yadA* adhesin genes, may aid spread in the body by decreasing attachment to PMNs

Y. enterocolitica, Y. pseudotuberculosis

Characteristics

Similar to *Y. pestis* in appearance

Spread by contaminated food and water

No insect vector

Many domestic and wild animal reservoirs

Disease—gastroenteritis

Invade Peyer's patches in small intestine

Replicate in submucosal tissue

Rarely spread to bloodstream

Cause local inflammation

Self-limiting, treatment usually not needed

Virulence factors

Adhesins, invasins (*inv*, *ail*, *yadA*)

Ability to cause inflammation

Ability to avoid phagocytosis via type III system, toxic Yops

QUESTIONS

Answers to the questions can be found in Appendix 2.

1. Try to frame an explanation for the fact that plague is so different from the food-borne illnesses caused by *Y. enterocolitica* or *Y. pseudotuberculosis*. What evidence is still missing?

2. Why would the loss of functional copies of the genes *inv, ail*, and *yadA* increase the virulence of *Y. pestis*? Why might *Y. enterocolitica* and *Y. pseudotuberculosis* need these genes in a functional form?

3. What does the fact that all three pathogenic species have the same 70-kbp plasmid say about possible gene exchange among these species? Given the lifestyles of these species, how likely is horizontal gene transfer to occur?

4. Compare and contrast *Y. pestis* and *B. burgdorferi* (chapter 12).

5. Why would disrupting the human cell cytoskeleton have an antiphagocytic effect? How does this differ from the antiphagocytic effect of the F1 capsule?

6. Why is it unlikely that there will be a massive outbreak of plague in the United States or Europe similar to the ones that ravaged Europe and Asia in the Middle Ages? The rats are available, especially in big cities, and the bacteria are available.

7. What are the implications of a type III secretion system for development of a vaccine against *Y. pestis*?

8. There are a number of laboratories in which people work every day with large quantities of *Y. pestis*. Yet laboratory-acquired infections are almost unknown. Why is this not surprising? Suppose you are still leery of working with these bacteria. How could you do so in complete safety?

14

Staphylococcus Species

KEY FEATURES

Staphylococcus aureus, Staphylococcus epidermidis, Staphylococcus saprophyticus

DESCRIPTION

Gram-positive cocci

S. aureus colonies have a golden color on complex media

Coagulase positive (*S. aureus*), coagulase negative (*S. epidermidis, S. saprophyticus*)

DISEASES

S. aureus: Toxinoses and infections at many different sites; septicemia

S. epidermidis: Catheter-associated infections; biofilms on plastic implants; endocarditis

S. saprophyticus: Urinary tract infections

RESERVOIRS

Human body, environment: *S. aureus*—nose, skin; *S. epidermidis*—skin; *S. saprophyticus*—ubiquitous in the environment

MAJOR VIRULENCE FACTORS

S. aureus: Protein toxins; lipoteichoic acid; surface adhesins; capsule; resistance to antibiotics

S. epidermidis: Forms biofilms on plastic (surface slime, adhesins); elicits an inflammatory response; resistance to antibiotics

S. saprophyticus: Attaches to bladder cells; elicits an inflammatory response

PREVENTION AND TREATMENT

Hand washing, disinfectants

Reduce length of catheter use

Vaccine for *S. aureus* under development

Passive immunization

Antibiotics

The Many Types of Staphylococcal Infections

Staphylococci are gram-positive cocci that are common causes of human infections. *Staphylococcus aureus*, in particular, is a leading cause of disease ranging from skin infections and food poisoning to life-threatening postsurgical infections. Another *Staphylococcus* species, *S. epidermidis*, a member of the normal skin microbiota, has also become a threat to human health, especially in hospitals. Both *S. aureus* and *S. epidermidis* can cause life-threatening septicemia. Now that members of these two species have developed resistance to many antibiotics, they are much-dreaded visitors to hospital wards and nursing homes. Most diseases caused by *S. aureus* and *S. epidermidis* originate when the bacteria take advantage of breaches in skin to enter the bloodstream. These breaches can be natural ones, such as hair follicles, where *S. aureus* causes pimplelike lesions and boils (also called furuncles). Many children develop impetigo, a blisterlike skin infection whose most common cause is *S. aureus*. *S. aureus* is also the main cause of sties, which are knobby swellings of the eyelids that form when the bacteria infect eyelash follicles and create abscesses.

Boils, furuncles, impetigo, and sties can be temporarily disfiguring and even painful, but they are seldom life threatening. More serious breaches of skin, such as burns, wounds, catheters, and surgical incisions, are settings for the most serious types of staphylococcal infection, in which the staphylococci not only cause considerable local tissue damage but also can enter the bloodstream and cause septic shock. A third pathogenic *Staphylococcus* species, *S. saprophyticus*, is an emerging cause of urinary tract infections, especially in sexually active women.

S. aureus

As already noted, *S. aureus* is a common cause of skin infections. Usually, these skin infections appear as localized lesions, such as boils, furuncles, impetigo, and sties. There is, however, one skin condition caused by *S. aureus* that has a more generalized distribution—scalded skin syndrome. **Scalded skin syndrome** occurs primarily in infants and gives the infant the appearance of having been scalded by hot water. Superficial layers of the skin peel off because of a toxin produced by the bacteria that may be located in a wound or in the bloodstream. The toxin disrupts connections between skin cells, allowing patches of skin to be displaced and sloughed off. Scalded skin syndrome is now a very uncommon disease and, when it occurs, usually does not have serious consequences.

S. aureus was identified as early as 1880 as a cause of serious infections, such as wound infections and septic shock, but it was undoubtedly a problem long before that. Historians have observed that prior to World War II, wound infections killed many more soldiers than the weapons used in combat. *S. aureus* was almost certainly a major contributor to this carnage. What changed with World War II was the introduction of antibiotics to the battlefield armamentarium. A famous advertisement from that time shows a drawing of a fallen soldier. The caption was: "He will come home, thanks to penicillin."

S. aureus was later found to be responsible for an impressive variety of diseases, including infections of the heart (endocarditis), infections of bone (osteomyelitis), central nervous system infections such as brain abscesses, and pneumonia (Table 14–1). *S. aureus* is also a common cause of a toxin-mediated food poisoning. During the 1970s, yet another toxin-mediated condition caused by *S. aureus* was added to scalded skin syndrome and food poisoning—toxic shock syndrome.

Toxic shock syndrome came about as a result of the introduction of tampons that were absorbent enough to be left in place much longer than regular tampons. Strains of *S. aureus* grew on the tampon surface and excreted a toxin, **toxic shock syndrome toxin (TSST).** The toxin was absorbed through the vaginal epithelium and entered the bloodstream, causing a cascade of events that ended in shock and death. Once the source of the problem was identified and the tampons associated with the syndrome were removed from the market, the incidence of toxic shock syndrome decreased significantly, and it is now a relatively uncommon disease.

Another type of toxic shock syndrome can occur in cosmetic surgery patients who are having their noses restructured. Such cases probably arise because of the practice of packing the nose with dressings designed to stop the flow of blood. The most common site of *S. aureus* colonization of the human body is the nose (Figure 14–1). This creates a situation remarkably similar to that created by superabsorbent tampons. Such cases have been rare, but they provide an example of the way a disease presentation can change.

Coagulase-Negative Staphylococci: *S. epidermidis* and *S. saprophyticus*

Coagulase is a surface protein produced by *S. aureus* that causes blood to clump. This reaction is the basis for the coagulase test, which has been used widely to differentiate *S. aureus* from other species of staphylococci. Although no role in pathogenesis is known for coagulase, "coagulase positive" was for a long time synonymous with "virulent." Starting in the 1970s, however, the coagulase-negative staphylococci began to be identified as a cause of human infection. This was the result of new medical procedures, especially the increased use of plastic implants, and an increasingly immunocompromised patient population. *S. epidermidis*, a common inhabitant of skin, was recognized as a significant cause of hospital-acquired infections. Although plastic is a recent human innovation, *S. epidermidis* proved to be

Table 14–1 Types of diseases caused by *S. aureus*

Food-borne disease

Soft tissue infections

Impetigo

Toxic shock syndrome

Septicemia

Pneumonia

Osteomyelitis

Infections of plastic implants

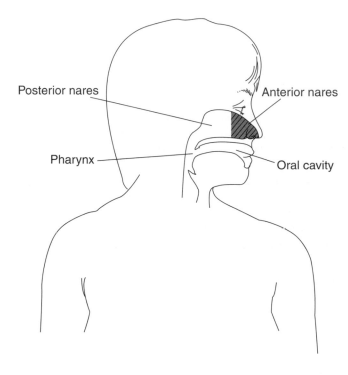

, *S. aureus* colonization

Figure 14–1 Anatomy of the human nasopharynx. The shaded area indicates the anterior nares, where *S. aureus* is found in greatest abundance.

adept at forming biofilms on its surface. Plastic venous catheters, used to introduce nutrients or pharmaceutical compounds into the veins of hospital patients, served as a conduit for *S. epidermidis* to enter the bloodstream. *S. epidermidis* also colonized plastic heart valves and became a common cause of **endocarditis.** *S. epidermidis* can also cause endocarditis in people who do not have plastic valves, but it is most often associated with valves that are damaged in some way. There are now

estimated to be 500,000 cases of sepsis each year in the United States alone. *S. aureus* and *S. epidermidis* are leading causes of hospital-acquired bacteremia and sepsis.

More recently, *S. saprophyticus* has been added to the list of staphylococci that cause human infections. *S. saprophyticus*, like *S. epidermidis*, was once thought to be a harmless commensal but is now the leading cause of urinary tract infections caused by gram-positive bacteria. *S. saprophyticus* is found widely in the environment and in various areas of the human body. The disease is seen most commonly in sexually active women between 15 and 35 years of age and may have emerged because of increased sexual activity by women in this age group. As many as one-fifth of the urinary tract infections experienced by members of this group are caused by *S. saprophyticus*.

Emerging Antibiotic Resistance, a Developing Horror Story

From the forgoing examples, it is evident that *Staphylococcus* species, especially *S. aureus*, are versatile human pathogens that are quick to take advantage of changing human practices. They have also adapted to antibiotics by becoming resistant to many of them. *S. aureus* and *S. epidermidis* have become notorious for resistance to many antimicrobial compounds. In recent years, strains of *S. aureus* have emerged that are resistant to virtually all antibiotics except vancomycin. These have been called **methicillin-resistant *S. aureus* (MRSA)** strains, but the description "multiply resistant *S. aureus* strains" would be more appropriate, because many MRSA strains are also resistant to tetracyclines, macrolides, lincosamides, fluoroquinolones, and aminoglycosides. Resistance to trimethoprim/sulfamethoxazole is also becoming common in MRSA strains. In some hospitals, nearly 90% of *S. aureus* isolates are MRSA. Given that MRSA was rare before 1975, the growing incidence of MRSA is an impressive and chilling development.

Not only is the incidence of MRSA strains changing, but the nomenclature used to designate these strains is changing too. Because methicillin is no longer used for treatment and has been replaced in testing by oxacillin, another β-lactam antibiotic, strains formerly called MRSA are now being called **oxacillin-resistant *S. aureus* (ORSA)** strains. As will become evident later in this section, the changing nomenclature used to label resistant strains of *S. aureus* is not limited to strains resistant to β-lactam antibiotics. To get some idea of how dangerous the increasing incidence of multidrug-resistant *S. aureus* could become, consider the fact that prior to

Posterior nares

Anterior nares

Pharynx

Oral cavity

218 *Chapter 14*

the availability of antibiotics, the mortality rate for sepsis patients was over 80%. Even today, as many as one-third of sepsis patients die despite aggressive antibiotic treatment. For a long time, MRSA strains were thought to be confined to hospitals, but recent studies of *S. aureus* strains carried by healthy people in the community have revealed that MRSA strains can be found in this population. The first community-acquired MRSA infections were reported in the 1990s.

The most ominous recent development has been the appearance of MRSA (or ORSA) strains with decreased susceptibility to vancomycin, a glycopeptide antibiotic that is being used to treat infections caused by multiply resistant strains of *S. aureus*. Most of these strains have MIC values for vancomycin that do not yet place them in the resistant category but are nearing that breakpoint between susceptibility and resistance. They have been called **VISA** (for **vancomycin intermediate susceptibility *S. aureus***) or **GISA (glycopeptide intermediate susceptibility *S. aureus*)** strains. In the laboratory, it is possible by stepwise selection to select strains of *S. aureus* that are resistant to high concentrations of vancomycin, suggesting that there is no metabolic barrier to the development of high-level vancomycin resistance in *S. aureus* strains.

Multidrug-resistant staphylococci are costing patients and health maintenance organizations money—lots of money. This is due not only to longer hospital stays, as doctors try to bring a recalcitrant staphylococcal infection under control, but also to health costs related to permanent damage to such important organs as the heart, lungs, and kidneys caused by septic shock.

Characteristics of Staphylococci

Colonization of the Human Body

Before turning to the virulence factors of the staphylococci, let us consider some traits that are not, strictly speaking, virulence factors. These traits are important, however, because they increase the opportunity for a bacterium to take advantage of any breaches that occur in host defenses. As in real estate, the three most important characteristics of bacteria that cause opportunistic infections are location, location, and location. Bacteria that normally colonize the human body are in an ideal position to take advantage of the breaches of skin and mucosal surfaces that will inevitably occur in the lives of even the most healthy people. *S. aureus* is found in many areas of the body but is present in highest numbers in the nose. About one-third of all adults are colonized with *S. aureus* at any point in time; about 25% are colonized persistently. Sooner or later, however,

virtually everyone is colonized with *S. aureus*. Thus, *S. aureus* is a fact of life for all of us.

Carriage of *S. aureus*, especially multiply resistant strains, by health care workers is a serious problem for hospitals. From the nose, *S. aureus* makes its way to hands, including the gloved hands of hospital workers. Staff-to-patient transmission is the main vehicle of transmission of multidrug-resistant *S. aureus* strains in hospitals because the resident strains colonizing staff workers, who are constantly exposed to antibiotics, are more likely to be resistant to antibiotics than strains found on the patient.

A patient can also be infected with his or her own resident strains of bacteria. This is the main reason for being concerned about community strains of MRSA. In some hospitals, MRSA has been brought into the hospital by patients and then spread within the hospital. Because of the expense of testing incoming patients for MRSA, and then isolating those who are colonized and trying to clear carriage of the strain, hospitals generally do not take such preventive measures. In the future, if vancomycin resistance appears in MRSA strains, however, screening of patients and staff members may become essential.

A person or staff worker who carries *S. aureus*, even MRSA strains, can usually be cleared of colonization by using an antibiotic called mupirocin. **Mupirocin** is not used as an injected antibiotic, because enzymes in serum rapidly metabolize it, but it can be applied topically to the interior of the nose. Today, pharmaceutical companies have become very interested in mupirocin, both because many MRSA strains are susceptible to it and because it attacks a novel antibacterial target, tRNA synthetases. Scientists hope to find analogs of mupirocin that can be used internally. Predictably, resistance to mupirocin has emerged, so one future need is for analogs of mupirocin that are active against the resistant strains.

Key Features of the Staphylococci

S. aureus gets its name from the golden color of its colonies ("aureus" derives from the Latin word for gold). Another distinguishing feature is the tendency of *S. aureus* cells to grow as clusters. In fact, the word "staphyle" from which the genus name is derived is Greek for grape cluster. This characteristic is the result of the division pattern of *S. aureus*. Dividing *S. aureus* cells begin to divide again in a different division plane before the first cells are separated.

A feature of *S. aureus* that has been used traditionally to differentiate it from the other species of staphylococci is the coagulase test. *S. aureus* strains produce coagulase. Although the name suggests an enzyme activity, coagulase is actually a surface protein that binds a blood protein, prothrombin, which is part of the coagulation cascade. Binding of prothrombin causes blood to clump (coagulate). Strains of *S. epidermidis* and *S. saprophyticus* do not produce coagulase. Accordingly, they are called **coagulase-negative staphylococci (CNS).**

A trait of *S. aureus* that contributes to its persistence in the environment is its ability to survive for long periods of time outside the human body. *S. epidermidis* is even more hardy than *S. aureus*, as is evident from the fact that it is hardy enough to survive the dry, inhospitable environment of human skin. The small white colonies formed by *S. epidermidis* are unpleasantly familiar to scientists who work with bacteria. *S. epidermidis* moves quickly to take advantage of poor aseptic technique, whether in the laboratory or in a clinical setting, and is often found growing on agar plates where it is not wanted.

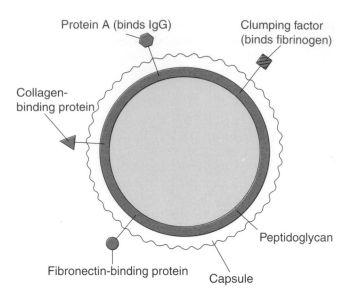

Figure 14–2 Cell surface proteins of *S. aureus*, called MSCRAMMs, mediate attachment to host proteins.

Virulence Factors of *S. aureus*

Virulence Factors

OVERVIEW. *S. aureus* strains produce a variety of virulence factors. Different strains produce different virulence factors, but in the aggregate, the diversity of virulence factors is impressive. Although daunting in their number, the virulence factors of *S. aureus* strains can be organized into a few classes of factors defined by their cellular location and their presumed function. Some virulence factors are proteins that are attached to peptidoglycan and exposed on the cell surface (Figure 14–2). These proteins mediate attachment of the bacteria to certain blood proteins such as immunoglobulin G (IgG) and fibrinogen or to extracellular matrix proteins such as fibronectin and collagen. The surface adhesins that bind to extracellular matrix proteins have been given the tongue-twisting acronym **MSCRAMMs,** which stands for **microbial surface components recognizing adhesive matrix molecules.**

At least two possible roles for the adhesive surface proteins of *S. aureus* have been proposed. One is that covering the bacteria with components of blood or tissue could help the bacteria to appear like self and thus hide from the immune system. A second proposed role is attachment to tissue. Attachment to tissue could be a prelude to invasion of host cells. Alternatively, it places the bacteria in a good position to degrade the extracellular matrix that holds host cells together, thus making it easier for the bacteria to move between host cells in tissue. Destroying tissue would also release nutrients for the bacteria and create an area of dead tissue that

functions as a safe haven for the bacteria, since cutting off an area from the blood supply makes it difficult for phagocytic cells, antibodies, and antibiotics to reach the site. The surface adhesins may also be responsible for the initial binding of *S. aureus* to plastic. In the body, plastic implants or catheters are rapidly covered with a coating of blood and tissue proteins, such as fibronectin, collagen, and fibrinogen. Once the initial layer of cells is formed, the carbohydrate slime of *S. aureus* allows a thicker biofilm to form. It may be significant that the plastics colonizer par excellence, *S. epidermidis*, also has surface proteins that bind blood and extracellular matrix proteins.

A second category of *S. aureus* virulence factors is extracellular protein toxins such as pore-forming proteins and hydrolytic enzymes. Some of these toxins may be responsible for the shock that develops in patients with uncontrolled staphylococcal bacteremia. Others could be directed against neutrophils, lessening the ability of these phagocytic cells to engulf and kill the bacteria. The cell wall itself undoubtedly contributes to virulence. Bacteria release fragments of peptidoglycan and lipoteichoic acid when they lyse. These molecules produce an inflammatory response similar to that caused by the LPS of gram-negative bacteria and can cause septic shock by activating various inflammatory cells to release cytokines.

MSCRAMMS AND OTHER SURFACE ADHESINS. Although the first MSCRAMMs were identified on the basis of their ability to bind to human proteins such as fibronectin, fibrinogen, or collagen, a certain amino acid sequence motif has emerged that may make it easier to recognize potential MSCRAMMs. Scientists analyzing the genome sequence of *S. aureus* have found over 100 proteins with this motif. (The genome sequence of one *S. aureus* strain is available in the public domain [http://www.genome.ou.edu/staph.html]. Reportedly, the genomes of other *S. aureus* strains have been sequenced by the pharmaceutical companies, but these are not available to the public.) The human proteins bound by some of the best-studied MSCRAMMs and other surface adhesins are listed in Table 14–2. MSCRAMMs are secreted through the cytoplasmic membrane. Many are then attached covalently to the pentaglycine cross-link of peptidoglycan by an enzyme called **sortase.** Neither the MSCRAMM proteins nor the enzyme sortase are peculiar to *S. aureus;* both are now being found in a number of gram-positive bacteria. This is good news for scientists who want to develop antimicrobial compounds that target MSCRAMMs or sortase.

The steps in secretion and attachment to peptidoglycan are shown in Figure 14–3. The signal sequence at the N-terminal end of the adhesin protein targets the protein for secretion. The signal sequence is removed during the secretion process by a signal peptidase. The secreted protein is still attached to the cell by a membrane-spanning region located at the C-terminal end of the protein. Proteins that are processed by the enzyme sortase have an amino acid sequence motif, Leu-Pro-X-Thr-Gly (**LPXTG,** where X can be any amino acid). This sequence lies between the membrane-spanning region and a region that will span the peptidoglycan cell wall. Sortase cleaves this LPXTG segment of the protein between the threonine (T) and glycine (G) residues and transfers the N-terminal end of the cleaved protein to the end of an uncross-linked pentaglycine bridge on a peptidoglycan subunit, which is then attached to the growing peptidoglycan chain. This leaves the protein exposed on the cell surface but tethered to the cell wall.

Given the exposed nature of the surface adhesins and their putative role in virulence, it might seem likely that they would be good targets for the immune system. Yet people or animals who have been infected with *S. aureus* do not become immune to reinfection, even though they make antibodies to *S. aureus* surface proteins. One explanation is suggested by a feature of antibodies to the **fibronectin-binding protein (FnBP).** These antibodies do not block binding of the staphylococcal protein FnBP to fibronectin. Rather, they bind to FnBP after it has attached to fibronectin. This sort of misdirection of the antibody response could be a protective mechanism for the bacteria. It remains to be seen if this is true for other surface proteins. In the case of the IgG-binding protein, **protein A,** the protein binds the Fc portion of the anti-

Table 14–2 Adhesins of *S. aureus* and their targets

Adhesin	Target
Fibronectin-binding protein (FnBP)	Fibronectin (component of extracellular matrix)
Protein A	Fc portion of IgG
Poly-*n*-succinyl-β-1,6 glucosamine (PNSG)	Plastic; possibly protein of extracellular matrix
Collagen-binding protein	Collagen
Coagulase	Prothrombin
Clumping factor	Fibrinogen

body (Figure 14–4A), so that this portion of the antibody cannot bind receptors on phagocytic cells. That is, antibody binding does not opsonize the bacteria. This is another type of misdirection that might help the bacteria to evade the immune response.

Protein A, the IgG-binding protein, has proved useful to scientists in a variety of fields. If a scientist is interested in whether protein X interacts with protein Y in a prokaryotic or eukaryotic cell, one approach to determining if such interactions occur is to mix cell extracts with antibodies to protein X. Then agarose beads coated with *S. aureus* protein A are added. The protein A traps the Fc portion of the antibodies bound to protein X and any other protein that is bound to protein X (Figure 14–4B). The beads are then allowed to settle and are washed to remove all unbound protein. If protein Y is bound to protein X, it will be trapped on the bead along with protein X.

Not all surface adhesins are proteins. At least one is a polysaccharide, **poly-*n*-succinyl-β-1,6 glucosamine (PNSG).** PNSG has attracted attention because it is produced in vivo during an infection, and one study has found that antibodies against it are protective. Moreover, all strains of *S. aureus* tested produced this surface polysaccharide. It is also produced by *S. epidermidis* strains, a fact that makes it even more attractive as a vaccine candidate. The genes encoding the enzymes that synthesize this polysaccharide are called *ica,* for intercellular adhesin locus (*icaA, icaB, icaC, icaD*). The name comes from the fact that the adhesin allows bacteria to adhere to one another. The adhesin may also promote adherence to other molecules, such as extracellular matrix components. The utility of this antigen as a vaccine target, however, remains to be proved.

INVASION OF ENDOTHELIAL CELLS. *S. aureus* strains adhere to, invade, and grow within tissue culture cells,

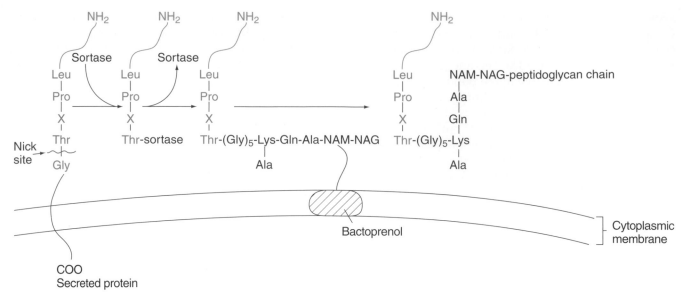

Figure 14–3 Sortase recognizes an LPXTG motif in a secreted protein as a nick site and transfers the cleaved protein to the peptide subunit of peptidoglycan. Leu, leucine; Pro, proline; X, any amino acid; Thr, threonine; Gly, glycine; Lys, lysine; Gln, glutamine; NAM, *N*-acetylmuramic acid residue of peptidoglycan; NAG, *N*-acetylglutamic acid residue of peptidoglycan. (Adapted from R. P. Novick. 2000. *Trends Microbiol.* **8:**148–151.)

including endothelial cells. *S. aureus* has not been considered to be an intracellular pathogen, because in pathology specimens it is always seen outside of host cells. Transient invasion of host cells might be important, however, if it helps to explain the ability of *S. aureus* cells to enter the bloodstream. Bacteria do not have to be invasive to enter the bloodstream, because just the ability to produce local inflammation can create enough damage to endothelial cells to allow access to a blood vessel. Nonetheless, the ability to invade and pass through endothelial cells would facilitate considerably transit from tissues to blood. Thus, invasion of host cells may play a role in dissemination of the bacteria in the body.

SUPERANTIGENS. Recall from chapter 9 that superantigens are proteins that force an association between MHC complexes on antigen-presenting cells and the T-cell receptor that would not normally occur. This association is tight enough to trigger cytokine release by both cell types. If many such complexes form, enough cytokine release can occur to trigger the shock process. *S. aureus* produces two classes of superantigens, TSST and **staphylococcal enterotoxin (SE).** There are now seven types of SEs—**SEA, SEB, SEC1, SEC2, SEC3, SED,** and **SEE.** TSST, encoded by the *tst* gene, is the toxin responsible for the symptoms of toxic shock syndrome. Not only did the superabsorbent tampons pro-

vide a special environment where *S. aureus* could multiply, but they also contained air pockets that provided the oxygen necessary for expression of the *tst* gene.

TSST in the bloodstream can trigger a massive release of cytokines that cause shock and death. In animals, TSST makes the animal hypersusceptible to LPS, which may enter the bloodstream regularly in small amounts because of lysis of gram-negative bacteria in the intestine. Whether this is true in humans is not known. LPS might not even be the most important molecule whose action is potentiated by TSST. One would expect the action of lipoteichoic acid of gram-positive bacteria to be potentiated in the same way, but this possibility has not been explored.

An unanswered question is, What is the true function of TSST? Production of a toxin in the vaginal tract that has its pathogenic effect only when it leaves the site and enters the bloodstream is clearly not doing anything of obvious benefit to the bacteria. A possible role could be to block mucosal immunity. TSST may interfere with the T cells found in sites where the mucosal immune system is located and prevent efficient development of an effective sIgA response.

SEs are responsible for the symptoms of a staphylococcal disease that is a lot more common than toxic shock syndrome and a lot less lethal—food poisoning. SEs, which are encoded by genes called *ent* (for **enterotoxin**), are produced by bacteria in the food. The toxin is ingested with the food. In the stomach, the SE stim-

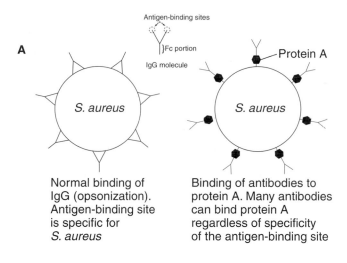

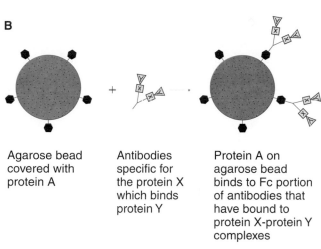

Figure 14–4   Binding of IgG by protein A. (**A**) Protein A binds IgG by the Fc region rather than by the antigen-binding sites in the normal way. (**B**) Use of protein A attached to agarose beads to harvest IgG attached to other proteins.

ulates the vagus nerve endings, which control the vomiting reflex. Projectile vomiting and abdominal pain are the hallmarks of *S. aureus* food poisoning. This type of food poisoning is usually not fatal, although people who have suffered it report wanting to die during the symptomatic period. Also, there have been cases in which pilots of small planes or people in similarly vulnerable positions have begun to experience the symptoms and come close to having a fatal accident.

The disease has a rapid onset, usually a few hours after eating contaminated food, and symptoms subside in a day or two, as expected from the fact that this is a toxinosis, not a bacterial infection. Once again, there is the mystery of why *S. aureus* produces SEs since they confer no apparent benefit on the bacteria, which are rapidly eliminated. The picture gets even stranger

when you consider that both TSST and SEs are single-chain polypeptides with some sequence similarity, raising the possibility that they are members of the same protein superfamily. The *entA* gene is carried on a bacteriophage, another similarity to *tst*, but other SE genes (e.g., *entC* and *entD*) are carried on plasmids.

OTHER TOXIC PROTEINS.   Although the role of the superantigens in the biology of *S. aureus* is uncertain, other toxic exoproteins make a clearer contribution to the survival and spread of the bacteria in the human body. An example of an exoprotein that may promote spread of the bacteria is a group of proteases called **exfoliative toxins (ETs).** As mentioned earlier, some *S. aureus* strains cause skin conditions such as scalded skin syndrome in infants, a disease in which the infant develops the sort of red, peeling appearance that resembles a bad scald. These same strains have also been implicated in **bullous impetigo,** a type of skin infection that produces blisterlike lesions. In both cases, the epidermis is separated from the underlying tissue. The ETs are responsible for this exfoliation or separation of skin layers.

The best-studied ET is **ETA.** The target for the protease activity of ETA has now been identified. It is a protein found on the surfaces of epidermal cells called **desmoglein-1 (Dsg-1).** Dsg-1 is produced only in the skin, a fact that would explain the localized effect of ETA. The role of Dsg-1 is to maintain keratinocyte cell-cell adhesion. Cleavage of Dsg-1 would lead to separation of skin keratinocytes, a result that would lead to the sort of separation of layers of epidermal tissue seen in scalded skin syndrome and bullous impetigo.

Another exoprotein that contributes to spread of the bacteria is **staphylokinase (Sak).** Sak dissolves clots. To understand how Sak does this, consider the process by which the body normally breaks down clots as part of the wound healing process. Clots are made up of platelets held together by a fibrin mesh. One of the components of this mesh is the protein plasminogen. Normally, during dissolution of a clot, endothelial cells secrete a protein called **tissue plasminogen activator (tPA).** It interacts with plasminogen, activating it to a form called plasmin that degrades the fibrin mesh, dissolving the clot. This is a carefully controlled process that is confined to the clot. Free plasmin is rapidly degraded in blood. Sak activates plasminogen, but not in a controlled way. Sak activity could help to destroy not only clots but also the extracellular matrix and fibrin fibers that hold cells together, thus allowing the bacteria to move through tissue. It could even help the bacteria escape from abscesses, walled-off regions of dead tissue that provide nutrients for bacteria within them but also confine bacteria to the site.

The extracellular matrix consists of a mixture of

224 ■ *Chapter 14*

proteins and polysaccharides (e.g., hyaluronic acid). *S. aureus* produces proteases and a hyaluronidase that may, along with Sak, contribute to local dissolution of the extracellular matrix.

A second function of exoproteins is to kill or limit the ability of neutrophils to attack the bacteria. **Alpha-toxin,** an exoprotein that forms pores in human cell membranes, could serve as a defense against neutrophils. Also, by inducing cellular damage that triggers cytokine production, alpha-toxin might contribute to shock. Alpha-toxin used to be called alpha-hemolysin because it could lyse red blood cells. Some strains of *S. aureus* also produce other hemolysins—beta-hemolysin, delta-hemolysin, and gamma-hemolysin. These hemolysins can damage membranes of cells other than red cells and may well have a role similar to that of alpha-toxin.

Yet another extracellular toxin, **leukocidin,** also damages mammalian cell membranes. Its name arises from the fact that it can kill leukocytes (of which neutrophils are one type). Leukocidin consists of two protein components, **S** and **F** (Figure 14–5). The S component is like the B part of an A-B toxin in that it binds to G_{M1} gangliosides. However, it also has an enzymatic activity, ADP-ribosylating a protein involved in phospholipid metabolism. F, too, has enzymatic activity. It ADP-ribosylates a protein that controls phosphatidylinositol metabolism. **Phosphatidylinositol,** an important signaling molecule in eukaryotic cells, controls a number of cellular processes. Thus, the action of this unusual two-component toxin appears to alter phospholipid metabolism and cause disruption of normal cellular activities. Scientists have now shown that all three proteins responsible for gamma-hemolysin activity (HlyA, HlyB, and HlyC) are virtually identical in sequence to leukocidin components S and F. Thus gamma-hemolysin may act similarly to leukocidin.

CAPSULE. At least three-fourths of *S. aureus* strains have a polysaccharide capsule. This capsule is distinct from the PNSG surface carbohydrate involved in adherence and biofilm formation. In fact, the capsule interferes with binding to some cell types. This capsule could help to prevent phagocytosis, but to date its role in the virulence of *S. aureus* has not been established. Nonetheless, recent studies have shown that a conjugated form of the capsular polysaccharide may have promise as a vaccine that could provide hope for preventing MRSA infections. About two-thirds of MRSA strains have one of two capsule serotypes, a feature that makes the conjugated vaccine approach attractive.

IRON ACQUISITION. *S. aureus* can bind the human iron-binding protein **transferrin** and remove iron from it. The bacterial transferrin receptor has now been identified, and its identity was a surprise. This surface-

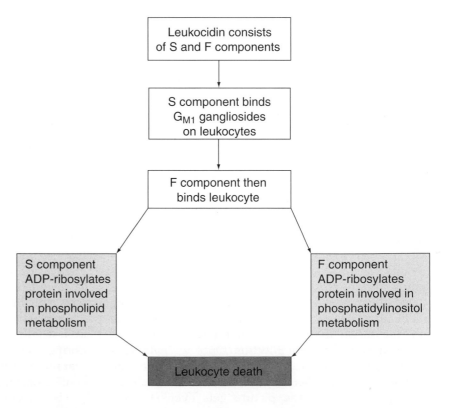

Figure 14–5 Structure and action of leukocidin.

exposed protein turned out to be **glyceraldehyde-3-phosphate dehydrogenase (GAPDH),** an enzyme usually associated with glycolysis. What is an enzyme that should be in the cytoplasm doing on the surface of *S. aureus,* and how is it involved in stripping iron off transferrin? The answer to this is still far from clear, but it appears that GAPDH is a more versatile protein than anyone suspected. The current model for iron acquisition by GAPDH is that tetramers of the protein bind to transferrin and somehow remove iron from it. The iron is transferred to a surface lipoprotein, which in turn conveys the iron to a transport protein that conveys it into the cell. *S. aureus* also has a siderophore-based mechanism for iron acquisition, but GAPDH is by far the most fascinating mechanism at the moment.

ANTIBIOTIC RESISTANCE. It is impossible to discuss *S. aureus* without going more deeply into the already-mentioned problem of antibiotic resistance. The first report of penicillin resistance in *S. aureus* was published about a year after the first use of penicillin to treat human infections (see Box 14–1 for the mechanism by which penicillin kills bacteria). Ever since, strains of *S. aureus* have become resistant to more and more antibiotics until some strains are only treatable with vancomycin or, more recently, two new antibiotics: a combination of two streptogramins (Synercid) and another class of protein synthesis inhibitors, the linezolids (e.g., Zyvox). The streptogramins have been known for years as protein synthesis inhibitors that prevent translocation of the ribosome, but the linezolids, which interfere with a very early step in protein synthesis, constitute a completely new class of antibiotic.

The MRSA strains, among the most dangerous strains of *S. aureus,* were introduced earlier in the chapter. In MRSA strains, methicillin resistance is conferred by the *mecA* gene, which encodes a mutant **penicillin-binding protein, PBP2a,** which has a very low affinity for β-lactam antibiotics. *S. aureus* strains also produce β-lactamases, but the *mecA* type of resistance seems to be causing the most problems. In particular, whereas the β-lactamases are effective against only a narrow spectrum of β-lactam antibiotics, PBP2a confers resistance to virtually all of them. Scientists believe that *mecA* may have come from a *Staphylococcus* species, *S. sciuri,* which is found primarily in squirrels. If this is the case, the riddle of how a squirrel staphylococcal gene migrated into the human *S. aureus* strains will be a fascinating one to solve. A possible scenario is suggested by the fact that although *S. aureus* and *S. epidermidis* are often portrayed as human-specific pathogens, they can also be isolated from dogs and from cattle. Possibly, it is in one of these animal reservoirs that a squirrel staphylococcal strain and *S. aureus* met and became friendly enough to exchange DNA.

Another curious feature of *mecA* is that when most *mecA*-carrying *S. aureus* strains are grown in culture, only a subset of the cells expresses *mecA,* leading to a phenomenon called **heterogeneous resistance.** The cells expressing *mecA* are rapidly selected for when the culture is exposed to methicillin.

Scientists are anxiously watching MRSA strains to see whether they will become resistant to glycopeptide antibiotics such as vancomycin. Decreased susceptibility to glycopeptides has been described in some clinical isolates. Synercid resistance may not be long in coming, either. Synercid is a combination of two streptogramin antibiotics. Streptogramins have never been used in human medicine before, but an analog of Synercid, **virginiamycin,** has been widely used as a feed additive in agriculture. Reports of streptogramin-resistant *S. aureus* are already beginning to appear.

For some time, MRSA was thought to be a hospital-specific phenomenon, and victims of hospital-acquired MRSA generally had underlying conditions that reduced their ability to combat infections. More recently, however, there have been cases of MRSA infections that were acquired in the community and occurred in children, not usually considered to be a high-risk group for MRSA infections. MRSA is clearly loose in the community as well as in hospitals. Before the discovery of penicillin, *S. aureus* was a common cause of death in surgical patients and soldiers with battle wounds. The arrival of virtually untreatable *S. aureus* strains might lead hospitals to curtail surgical procedures that are not needed to respond to medical emergencies. People have become used to having access to a range of surgical options, such as bypass surgery or knee surgery, that improve the quality of life but are not essential. How the public would respond to reduced access to such surgical options is not something health officials like to think about.

REGULATION OF VIRULENCE GENES. Many of the *S. aureus* virulence genes, especially those encoding surface adhesins and exoproteins, are regulated by a quorum sensing system. When cells are in the early stages of growth, the adhesin genes are preferentially expressed. Once the bacteria enter late exponential phase and reach a high population density, adhesin production is decreased and exoprotein production is increased. This progression makes sense because the exoproteins from many bacteria all localized in the same

BOX 14–1   *S. aureus* Helps Scientists To Answer the 50-Year-Old Question of How Penicillin Kills Bacteria

Although this book focuses on mechanisms by which bacteria cause disease, the importance of antibiotics in the treatment of disease has made antibiotic action and antibiotic resistance more and more relevant to an understanding of the bacterium-host interaction. Accordingly, we include a description of some recent studies in which *S. aureus* served as the model organism used to answer a question that had been unanswered for over 50 years: how does penicillin kill bacteria? For a long time, one answer to this question predominated. It has been known for a long time that the most immediate effect of penicillin is to inhibit cross-linking of the peptidoglycan. But could this alone kill bacteria? It might weaken the peptidoglycan, but numerous studies showed that bacteria could survive such weakening without lysing.

The next hypothesis was that autolysins are either activated or get out of sync with the cell wall cross-linking enzymes in such a way as to cause stripping of the cell wall, leading to cell death and lysis. This explanation had such an intuitive appeal that for a long time few were bothered by the fact that there was virtually no evidence to support it. In fact, there was evidence suggesting that bulk autolysin production had very little to do with penicillin killing.

Recent studies of how penicillin kills staphylococci have shown that killing is a two-step process (see the figure). Shortly after exposure to penicillin, susceptible cells rapidly lose viability. Lysis, the second step, occurs much later. A possible explanation for the early step arose from studies of a cluster of genes that appeared to be involved in the early loss of viability. These genes were identified as *lytS* and *lytR*, a two-component regulatory system that controls expression of the two other nearby genes, *lrgA* and *lrgB*. The signal recognized by the LytSR system is not known. LrgA was shown to have sequence similarity to a family of phage proteins called holins. **Holins,** as the name implies, form pores in the bacterial membrane, collapsing the proton motive force. This led to the hypothesis that there are bacterial holins that, in the presence of penicillin, form pores that collapse the proton motive force and lead to the

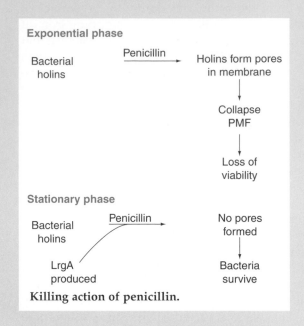

Killing action of penicillin.

rapid loss of viability in penicillin-exposed cells. LrgA could function normally as an antiholin that prevents pore formation by bacterial holins. Why would bacteria want to kill themselves by producing holins in the first place? Possibly the holin-antiholin system, which apparently affects murein hydrolase activity, is a means of regulating lysis due to the murein hydrolases. It is interesting that LrgA is produced maximally during the transition from exponential to stationary phase. It has been noted that biofilms of *S. aureus* become tolerant to penicillin. That is, the minimum bactericidal concentration (MBC) of penicillin becomes much higher than the minimal inhibitory concentration (MIC) in stationary phase. In stationary phase, the MIC-MBC ratio is more than 1:32, whereas in exponential phase it is usually less than 1:4. High production of LrgA as cells enter stationary phase could protect the bacteria from the initial killing phase of penicillin.

Source: K. W. Bayles. 2000. The bactericidal action of penicillin: New clues to an unsolved mystery. *Trends Microbiol.* **8:**274–278.

place will have a much greater effect than exoproteins from a few isolated bacteria. *S. aureus* wound infections are often characterized by large pus-filled lesions. This is the kind of damage that is produced by multiple bacteria acting in concert.

The current view of this regulatory system is shown in Figure 14–6. The center of the regulatory system is a set of genes called *agr*, for **accessory gene regulator.** Another regulatory gene is *sarA*. The *sarA* gene encodes a protein, SarA, that binds to sequences upstream of *agr* gene promoters and stimulates their expression. Expression of the *agr* genes is dependent on growth phase. In exponential phase, the bacteria produce only low levels of the Agr proteins. **AgrD** is secreted by **AgrB,** a cytoplasmic membrane protein, and cleaved to produce an AgrD-derived cyclic peptide, **thiolactone** (Figure 14–7). This peptide serves as an autoinducer. The structure of the autoinducer is very different from the structures of autoinducers produced by gram-negative bacteria and does not diffuse readily through membranes (Figure 14–7). To act, it must interact with a cytoplasmic membrane sensor, **AgrC.** When the concentration of this peptide is high enough, its interaction with ArgC causes AgrC to become phosphorylated. The phosphorylated form of AgrC phosphorylates AgrA. Phosphorylated AgrA activates production of an RNA molecule called **RNAIII.** (The peptide autoinducer has also been called **RAP,** for **RNAIII activator peptide.**) The RNAIII molecule is responsible for downregulation of many genes encoding MSCRAMMs and upregulation of genes encoding exotoxins such as TSST, the hemolysins, and SEB. Thus, as the bacteria increase in density, they switch from an adherence strategy to a toxin strategy, causing tissue damage in the process.

Virulence Factors of the Coagulase-Negative Staphylococci

S. epidermidis

Virulence factors of *S. epidermidis* have been much less studied than those of *S. aureus*. One feature that undoubtedly contributes to the virulence of *S. epidermidis* strains is their ability to adhere to plastic and form a biofilm. After the initial layer of bacteria has bound to the plastic, a polysaccharide capsule allows other bacteria to bind to this first layer to form the multilayer biofilm. The capsule, called **polysaccharide intercellular adhesin (PIA),** consists of a sulfated polysaccharide. Bacteria in a biofilm are protected to some extent from phagocytes. Moreover, bacteria in a biofilm are generally far less susceptible to antibiotics than are free-

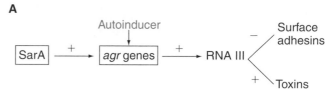

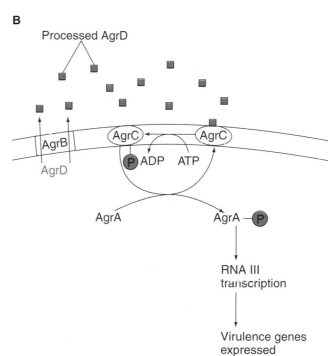

Figure 14–6 Regulation of surface adhesin and exoprotein genes. (**A**) Overview of regulation. SarA is necessary for production of the Agr proteins, but details of how it acts are still under investigation. The Agr proteins in turn form a regulatory cascade (shown in panel B) that causes a regulatory RNA molecule, RNAIII, to be produced. RNAIII suppresses production of surface adhesins and enhances production of toxins. +, causes increased gene expression; –, causes decreased gene expression. (**B**) A closer look at the interaction between the autoinducer (processed segment of AgrD) and the AgrAC two-component regulatory system. AgrD is secreted by AgrB and processed to form the cyclic peptide autoinducer (small squares). The autoinducer does not diffuse through membranes but instead, when the concentration reaches high enough levels, interacts with AgrC to stimulate its phosphorylation. Phosphorylated AgrC in turn phosphorylates AgrA, which activates transcription of RNAIII. (Adapted from Balaban and Novick [1995].)

living cells. The lower susceptibility of biofilm bacteria to antibiotics is thought to be due to a combination of the lower metabolic activity of biofilm bacteria and impaired diffusion of the antibiotic. Since *S. epidermidis*, even in the free-living form, is already resistant to many antibiotics, this added level of resistance makes biofilms

A Gram-positive bacteria: cyclic thiolactone peptide

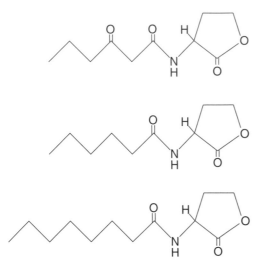

B Gram-negative bacteria: homoserine lactones

Figure 14–7 Comparison of the structure of the cyclic thiolactone peptide autoinducer of *S. aureus* (**A**) with the structures of homoserine lactone autoinducers produced by some gram-negative bacteria (**B**).

on plastic implants virtually impossible to treat with antibiotics. Because of this, if colonization of an implant occurs, the device must be removed surgically and replaced. In the case of venous catheters, removing the catheter can sometimes lead to control of the infection unless the bacteria have colonized some interior site, such as a defective heart valve or a plastic implant.

Why has *S. epidermidis* become resistant to antibiotics? Normally, one thinks of intestinal bacteria as the bacteria most affected by antibiotic use. Recently, scientists showed that some antibiotics are exuded in sweat. Thus, skin bacteria may be exposed just as much to antibiotics being taken internally as bacteria in the intestinal tract or the vaginal tract.

S. epidermidis has a cell wall transferrin-binding protein like that of *S. aureus* that presumably helps the bacteria obtain iron from transferrin. It, too, has GAPDH activity.

S. saprophyticus

A protein that binds fibronectin may serve as an adhesin that allows *S. saprophyticus* to attach to urethral cells so that it is not washed out of the bladder during urination. The protein also is a hemagglutinin, which allows *S. saprophyticus* to bind to red blood cells. The two activities seem to be associated with different parts of the protein. To determine which of these activities allows *S. saprophyticus* to bind to urinary bladder cells, sections of ureters were incubated with either red blood cell membranes (which would block the hemagglutinin part of the protein) or fibronectin (which would block the fibronectin-binding activity); then, *S. saprophyticus* cells were added. The red blood cell membranes, but not fibronectin, prevented attachment of *S. saprophyticus* to the human ureters, so the hemagglutinin activity is probably the one that is most critical for binding to bladder cells. Both *S. aureus* and *S. epidermidis* have a similar hemagglutinin, although this protein has not been shown to be important for the virulence of either of these species. Possibly, the ability of *S. saprophyticus* to colonize the vaginal tract is the answer to the question of why this protein may have a role in the virulence of *S. saprophyticus* but not that of the other staphylococci. *S. saprophyticus* has more opportunities to gain access to the bladder because of its location.

Future Directions

Much progress has been made toward defining the virulence strategies of the staphylococci, especially *S. aureus*. Clearly, a better understanding of these important pathogens, especially *S. aureus* and *S. epidermidis*, has major practical importance because of the seriousness of diseases caused by these bacteria and because of the increasing difficulty in managing them due to increasing antibiotic resistance. A vaccine against *S. aureus* (StaphVAX), which consists of conjugated capsular polysaccharides, is currently being tested in clinical trials. These trials have been focused on kidney dialysis patients, a group of patients at high risk for development of serious staphylococcal infections. In this group, the vaccine has resulted in a 57% reduction in *S. aureus* infections. But even if this vaccine is successful, it will not prevent all staphylococcal infections, since it represents only a subset of capsular serotypes.

There is every reason to think that future progress will be rapid and satisfying. Both *S. aureus* and *S. epidermidis* are easy to cultivate and can be manipulated genetically. There is genome sequence information for at least one strain of *S. aureus*, and sequence information for one strain of *S. epidermidis* is in the offing. The DNA sequence will be useful for designing microarrays that can be used to monitor gene expression under a variety of environmental conditions. (For an explanation of microarrays, see chapter 3.) Perhaps most important, however, is the change of attitude in the scientific community about the importance of studying these pathogens at a basic level. For a long time, the staphylococci were neglected (even in the first edition of this book), in part because of the assumption that not much novel basic science information would be found by studying them. This assumption has been shown to be completely wrong, and enough novel findings have already emerged to whet the appetites of scientists interested in new virulence paradigms.

SELECTED READINGS

Amagai, M., N. Matsuyoshi, Z. Wang, C. Andl, and J. R. Stanley. 2000. Toxin in bullous impetigo and scalded skin syndrome targets desmoglein. *Nat. Med.* **6:**1275–1277.

Balaban, N., and R. P. Novick. 1995. Autocrine regulation of toxin synthesis by *Staphylococcus aureus. Proc. Natl. Acad. Sci. USA* **92:**1619–1623.

Chakrabarti, S. K., and T. K. Misra. 2000. SarA represses *agr* operon expression in a purified in vitro *Staphylococcus aureus* transcription system. *J. Bacteriol.* **182:**5893–5897.

Foster, T. J., and M. Hook. 1998. Surface protein adhesins of *Staphylococcus aureus. Trends Microbiol.* **6:**484–488.

Ji, G., R. Beavis, and R. P. Novick. 1997. Bacterial interference caused by autoinducing peptide variants. *Science* **276:**2027–2030.

Lowy, F. D. 1998. *Staphylococcus aureus* infections. *N. Engl. J. Med.* **339:**520–532.

Mazmanian, S. K., G. Liu, H. Ton-That, and O. Schneewind. 1999. *Staphylococcus aureus* sortase, an enzyme that anchors surface proteins to the cell wall. *Science* **285:**760–763.

Meyer, H. G., U. Wengler-Becker, and S. G. Gatermann. 1996. The hemagglutinin of *Staphylococcus saprophyticus* is a major adhesin for uroepithelial cells. *Infect. Immun.* **64:**3893–3896.

Novick, R. P. 2000. Sortase: the surface protein anchoring transpeptidase and the LPXTG motif. *Trends Microbiol.* **8:**148–151.

Projan, S. J., and R. P. Novick. 1997. The molecular basis of pathogenicity, p. 55–81. *In* K. B. Crossley and G. L. Archer (ed.), *The Staphylococci in Human Disease.* Churchill Livingstone, London, England.

SUMMARY OUTLINE

S. aureus

Characteristics
   Gram-positive cocci, grow in clusters; yellow colonies
   Coagulase positive, nonmotile
   Hardy; some strains resistant to many antibiotics
   Normal location is the anterior nares, about one-third of people colonized

Diseases
   Food-borne disease—vomiting and pain caused by a toxin (SE); no infection
   Impetigo, boils, and scalded skin syndrome—limited to skin
   Toxic shock syndrome—now uncommon
   Wound infections
   Implant infections
   Endocarditis (heart damage)
   Bone infection (osteomyelitis)
   Sepsis

Virulence factors
   MSCRAMMs—bacterial surface proteins that bind to human proteins; may aid adherence to
      tissue or serum-coated plastic surfaces
   Capsule—formation of biofilms; adherence to plastic
   Toxins
      ETA—associated with bullous impetigo and scalded skin syndrome; protease that cleaves a
         protein that normally mediates adherence of keratinocytes to one another
      TSST—superantigen involved in toxic shock syndrome; produced in vagina (tampon),
         enters bloodstream
      SE—superantigen related to TSST, responsible for symptoms of food-borne toxinosis

(continued)

SUMMARY OUTLINE (*continued*)

Lipoteichoic acid—contributes to shock
Alpha-toxin, a pore-forming protein
Leukocidin, a two-component cytotoxin

Hydrolytic enzymes—may aid spreading in tissue; contribute to host tissue damage
Membrane damage
Cell destruction, spreading in body

Resistance to antibiotics
MRSA (*mecA*, encodes a mutant PBP)
VISA, GISA strains, less susceptible to the glycopeptide antibiotics such as vancomycin

S. epidermidis

Characteristics
White colonies
Coagulase negative
Very hardy
Component of the skin microbiota
Resistant to many antibiotics

Diseases
Infections associated with venous catheters
Endocarditis
Sepsis in hospitalized patients

Virulence factors
Lipoteichoic acid
Polysaccharide slime, biofilm formation

S. saprophyticus

Characteristics
Ubiquitous in the environment, colonizes skin and vaginal tract

Disease
Urinary tract infections in sexually active women

Virulence factors
Surface adhesin, mediates attachment to bladder cells
Ability to elicit an inflammatory response

QUESTIONS

Answers to the questions can be found in Appendix 2.

1. Why would a pathogen like *S. aureus* have so many different virulence factors, some of which seem redundant?

2. The succession of virulence factors controlled by Sar and Agr proteins makes sense for a biofilm. Would the same type of regulatory pattern make sense for bacteria circulating in the bloodstream?

3. The connection between quorum sensing and a two-component regulatory system is unusual. In the gram-negative bacteria studied to date, the autoinducer is thought to interact directly with the regulatory proteins that bind to DNA (although this has been questioned recently in some cases). Why would *S. aureus* need a two-component regulatory system to sense its thiolactone peptide autoinducer? (Hint: The homoserine lactone compounds produced by gram-negative bacteria with autoinducing systems diffuse readily through membranes.)

4. *S. aureus* and *S. epidermidis* appear to be much more similar to each other in terms of virulence factors than either is to *S. saprophyticus*. Why does this make sense in terms of the types of diseases caused by these three *Staphylococcus* species?

5. Make an educated guess as to why *S. saprophyticus,* which now appears to be a fairly common cause of urinary tract infections in young women, was missed for so long.

6. Why are people working on vaccines attracted to PNSG as a vaccine target? Why is it important that this polysaccharide surface adhesin is produced by *S. epidermidis* as well as by *S. aureus*?

7. *S. aureus* growing in a biofilm is less susceptible not just to penicillin but also to vancomycin. What are the clinical implications of this fact?

8. In 1990, a northeastern U.S. hospital noted an unusually high incidence of *S. epidermidis* infections in their cardiac patients. The source of this miniepidemic proved to be a surgeon. How might this episode have happened? (Hints: The surgeon had dermatitis. Also, in cardiac surgery, it is necessary to saw through the rib cage, creating many sharp bone fragments.)

9. Why are health officials so worried about strains of *S. aureus* that are only less susceptible to vancomycin, not outright resistant?

15

Group A and Group B Streptococci and Enterococci

KEY FEATURES

Group A and Group B Streptococci and Enterococci

CHARACTERISTICS

Gram-positive cocci, fermentative metabolism

Nonmotile

Hemolysis pattern—beta-hemolytic (groups A and B streptococci), gamma-hemolytic (enterococci)

Also differentiated on the basis of surface antigens

DISEASES

Streptococcus pyogenes (group A streptococci)—variety of infections ranging from wound infections to pneumonia and postpartum maternal infections

Streptococcus agalactiae (group B streptococci)—neonatal meningitis, wound infections, and pneumonia in adults

Enterococcus faecium, Enterococcus faecalis—wound infections and sepsis in hospitalized (especially immunocompromised) patients

RESERVOIRS

Human body: Mouth, throat—*S. pyogenes;* gastrointestinal tract—*S. agalactiae;* colon—*Enterococcus* species

Can colonize other parts of the body

Animal reservoirs: *S. agalactiae, Enterococcus* species

MAIN VIRULENCE FACTORS

S. pyogenes—protein toxins (superantigens and hydrolytic enzymes), lipoteichoic acid

S. agalactiae—polysaccharide capsule, others poorly characterized

Enterococcus species—poorly characterized; hardy, able to persist in the environment

PREVENTION AND TREATMENT

Good hygiene (e.g., hand washing)

No vaccine available

Antibiotics, but resistance is a serious problem in the case of the enterococci

The groups A and B streptococci and the enterococci are nonmotile gram-positive cocci with a fermentative metabolism. They tolerate oxygen, but many of them grow better under anaerobic conditions. A commonly used test for the initial classification of streptococci is the hemolysis test. Some streptococci growing on blood agar plates create a zone of clearing by completely lysing nearby blood cells. This type of hemolysis is called **beta-hemolysis**. Less complete lysis of blood cells by other streptococci, causing a green zone to form, is called **alpha-hemolysis**. No zone of hemolysis is called **gamma-hemolysis**. The bacterial species covered in this chapter are beta- or gamma-hemolytic. A very important species of alpha-hemolytic streptococci, *Streptococcus pneumoniae*, is covered in a later chapter. Other alpha-hemolytic streptococci include the oral streptococci, such as *Streptococcus sanguis*, some of which play a role in the formation of dental caries.

The beta-hemolytic streptococci are further classified on the basis of surface carbohydrate antigens. This classification system, called the Lancefield grouping, is still used today to identify streptococci. The original Lancefield grouping divided the streptococci into groups A through G. Group A streptococci are mostly members of the species *Streptococcus pyogenes*. Most group B streptococci belong to the species *Streptococcus agalactiae*, which not only causes disease in humans but also causes mastitis in cattle. Most of the beta-hemolytic streptococci that cause serious human infections belong to one of these two groups. The bacteria now known as *Enterococcus* species were classified initially as group D streptococci. Only later were many members of the group D streptococci given their own separate genus. Enterococci are usually gamma-hemolytic. Enterococci are most likely to be seen growing as single cells or as diplococci, whereas streptococci usually form chains of cells. Enterococci are more resistant to heat, drying, salt, and antibiotics than are the streptococci.

The bacterial species covered in this chapter are notable for their ability to cause wound infections and are significant causes of nosocomial wound infections. *S. pyogenes* strains (group A streptococci) also cause pneumonia, septicemia, and endocarditis. This disease spectrum is not surprising in view of the fact that *S. pyogenes* colonizes the mouth, throat, and upper respiratory tract. *S. pyogenes* is also found in the vaginal tract. *S. agalactiae* strains (group B streptococci) were once most commonly associated with meningitis in infants but have recently become prominent causes of nosocomial infections, including pneumonia and wound infections in adults. Enterococci were earlier considered to be innocuous members of the colonic microbiota. However, with the advent of intensive care units and increasingly larger populations of immunocompromised patients in

hospitals and nursing homes, two *Enterococcus* species, *E. faecium* and *E. faecalis*, have emerged as causes of life-threatening diseases such as endocarditis, sepsis, and infections of surgical wounds.

A Closer Look at Diseases Caused by Streptococci

The Changing Spectrum of Group A Streptococcal Disease

S. pyogenes is the most pathogenic of the species covered in this chapter—and the most variable. Group A streptococci have had an incredible history of changing disease patterns (Table 15–1). In the 1700s and 1800s, *S. pyogenes* was a major cause of maternal deaths, because it gave rise to a disease called puerperal fever. Bacteria in the vaginal tract infected the uterus either before birth or during birth, and the infection rapidly became systemic. In those days, and in earlier centuries, death of the mother after childbirth was much more common than it is today, and group A streptococci were a major contributor to the maternal death toll. As described in chapter 4, it was the differences in mortality between women in different wards of the Vienna Lying-in Hospital that first alerted Semmelweis to the importance of hand washing. Today, puerperal fever is virtually unknown in developed countries and is be-

Table 15–1 Changing disease patterns of *Streptococcus pyogenes*

Time period	Prevalent diseases
18th and 19th centuries	Puerperal fever in women
	Streptococcal fasciitis in wounded soldiers
	"Blood poisoning" in children and adults (systemic disease)
Late 19th to early 20th century	Scarlet fever; rheumatic fever
	Wound infections
1940s to present	Scarlet fever and rheumatic fever virtually disappear
Late 20th century	Some scarlet fever outbreaks seen
	Invasive systemic infections
	Toxic shock-like syndrome
	Outbreaks of fasciitis cases
	Nosocomial infections of wounds
	Pneumonia
	Endocarditis

coming more uncommon in most developing countries because of improved sanitation.

During wartime, *S. pyogenes* surfaced as a dreaded cause of wound infections. Up until World War II, wound infections were responsible for far more deaths among soldiers than the trauma caused by the wounds themselves. In particular, *S. pyogenes* caused an invasive and destructive type of wound infection called **streptococcal gangrene (necrotizing fasciitis).** Large areas of skin were destroyed, followed by entry of the bacteria into the bloodstream and death due to septic shock. In the 1980s and 1990s, a small number of cases of this type of streptococcal disease reappeared, this time in the civilian population (Box 15–1). The tabloids quickly picked up on the scary aspects of this type of infection and ran such headlines as "The bacterium that ate my face." Fortunately, streptococcal fasciitis cases remain rare, thanks to improved sanitation and prompt effective treatment of wound infections.

Another type of wound infection caused by *S. pyogenes,* known popularly as "blood poisoning," had less spectacular symptoms but could be just as deadly. Once again, the infection started in a wounded area. The inflammatory response was characterized by red streaks radiating out from the wounded area, and there was considerable pain in the affected region. Although the amount of skin damage was minimal, the bacteria could enter the bloodstream, causing fatal septic shock.

In the late 1800s, *S. pyogenes* manifested itself in another guise: **scarlet fever.** A diffuse red rash characterized this disease, which was spread by airborne or foodborne transmission of the bacteria. Scarlet fever was primarily a disease of children and at this stage in its history could be rapidly fatal. Families lost one child after another to this disease. Fumigators, who came into affected houses and sprayed with carbolic acid, became much sought after. Unfortunately, this treatment was usually unsuccessful, because the bacteria were carried by people who resided in the house, not by bed linens and other inanimate objects. As time passed, scarlet fever became less virulent, and by the 1940s it was considered a mild childhood disease. Then it disappeared almost entirely. During the 1990s, there were some outbreaks of the less serious form of scarlet fever among schoolchildren, but the number of cases is still far smaller than it was in the earlier part of the 20th century.

From the 1940s onward, *S. pyogenes* showed up more commonly in connection with another type of disease—glomerulonephritis and rheumatic fever. These diseases occurred at least as commonly in adults as in children. A group A streptococcal skin infection triggered in some people a condition called **glomerulonephritis** (inflammation of the kidney). A "strep throat" infection caused by group A streptococci sometimes leads to a febrile disease (**rheumatic fever**), which could progress to damage to the heart valves (**rheumatic heart disease**). Although glomerulonephritis is unpleasant, being characterized by malaise and generalized swelling due to impaired excretion of fluids, it is self-limiting and does not cause any long-term kidney damage. By contrast, rheumatic heart disease can cause permanent damage to heart valves, which leads to death due to heart failure or, if not immediately fatal, predisposes the person to later, potentially fatal, infections of the heart valve (endocarditis). Rheumatic fever and rheumatic heart disease have largely disappeared from developed countries. No one knows why, although it is possible that widespread use of antibiotics played a role. Glomerulonephritis, however, is still nearly as common as it was in the 1940s. Thus, if antibiotics were responsible for the demise of rheumatic heart disease, they affected certain strains of *S. pyogenes* disproportionately.

In the late 20th century, there were small isolated outbreaks of scarlet fever and invasive systemic *S. pyogenes* infections. One type was labeled toxic shock-like syndrome because its symptoms resembled those of the toxic shock syndrome caused by *Staphylococcus aureus.* A rapidly fatal pneumonia caused by *S. pyogenes* was also seen. The most famous case of group A streptococcal pneumonia occurred in Jim Henson, the creator of the popular puppet characters the Muppets. Although otherwise healthy, Henson developed bacterial pneumonia and died within a matter of weeks despite intensive medical treatment. Today, *S. pyogenes* is a threat mainly to patients with surgical wounds or indwelling catheters. Even in this group, it a less common cause of infection than staphylococci.

A distinctive feature of *S. pyogenes* strains, which may explain why this once-great human scourge seems to have been tamed, is that it is one of the few species of bacteria that have remained susceptible to most antibiotics. Why this should be the case, when its near relatives, the group B streptococci and enterococci, have become increasingly resistant to antibiotics, is unclear. Given its long lethal history, no one should complain about the continued susceptibility of *S. pyogenes* to antibiotics. Nor should we take this serious human pathogen for granted—it could become resistant to antibiotics at any time. Physicians were complacent about *S. pneumoniae* (see chapter 18), which remained susceptible to penicillin much longer than most bacteria, only to become resistant to multiple antibiotics in the last decades of the 20th century.

Understanding Disease Diversity

How are we to understand the incredible variety of seemingly different diseases caused by *S. pyogenes,* a

BOX 15–1   The New Invasive Form of *S. pyogenes* Disease: an Outbreak in Ontario, Canada, 1987 to 1991

The first case of severe invasive *S. pyogenes* infection was seen in early 1987. Then a few sporadic cases occurred in 1988 and 1989, followed by a sizeable increase in the number of cases in 1990 and 1991, resulting in a total of 50 cases during the 1987 to 1991 period. In part, the increase in identified cases could have been due to increased awareness of the disease, but there seems to have been a real increase in incidence of the disease in 1990 and 1991 compared with previous years. The 50 cases were evenly divided between men and women. The median age was 40 to 50 years, although patients ranged in age from 4 to 100 years. In all cases, *S. pyogenes* was isolated from blood or body fluids, and symptoms of shock were evident. *S. pyogenes* is an occasional cause of hospital-acquired infections, but only a fraction of the patients appeared to have acquired the infection in this way. Nor were the patients severely immune compromised. Half of them had no known underlying conditions that would compromise host defenses, and only a few had severe underlying conditions such as AIDS. The disease thus appears capable of striking otherwise healthy adults and can be community acquired. Thirty-eight patients had some focus of infection when admitted to the hospital, usually a soft tissue infection, but 12 had no sign of prior infection, and only one-third of the patients recalled an injury (scratch, wound, fall) that could have precipitated the infection. Of the patients who recalled an injury, only one thought the injury was serious enough to seek immediate medical attention. Thus, for most of the patients, there were no early warning signs of the disease. In cases in which the injury was recalled, the time from injury to development of hypotension was less than a week. In patients who had an identifiable focus of initial infection, such as a soft tissue infection, an unusual degree of pain at the site of infection was the most frequent symptom that distinguished these infections from ordinary wound infections. Some patients complained of a flulike illness several days prior to hospitalization. Approximately half of the patients with this new disease died, some within a day of admission to the hospital. In cases in which the precipitating event could be identified, the time between the event and development of hypotension was 3 to 7 days. The high fatality rate may have been due to the fact that the insidious development of the disease allowed it to be identified only after the disease had progressed to the point where shock had already begun. The characteristics of the patients, the absence of clear-cut early warning signs in most cases, and the high fatality rate of the disease seen in this study have also been seen in other outbreaks in the United States and Europe.

Source: B. Demers, A. E. Simor, H. Vellend, P. M. Schlievert, S. Byrne, F. Jamieson, S. Walmsley, and D. E. Low. 1993. Severe invasive group A streptococcal infections in Ontario, Canada: 1987–1991. *Clin. Infect. Dis.* **16:**792–800.

record unrivaled by any other bacteria except *Escherichia coli* and *S. aureus*? As more is learned about *S. pyogenes*, it seems likely that the answer lies in two related areas. First, there are strain-to-strain differences in the possession of various virulence factors. This is certainly true for *E. coli* strains that cause diseases as diverse as urinary tract infections, gastroenteritis, meningitis, and sepsis, and appears likely to be true for *S. aureus* strains as well. A second source of variation is regulation of virulence genes. As will become evident in a later section of this chapter, *S. pyogenes* has a number of regulatory circuits that control the expression of virulence genes. Variation in the presence of these regulators and variations in signals in different parts of the body that stimulate them to activate or repress virulence gene expression would lead to different patterns of behavior for organisms in different body sites. The amount of strain-to-strain variation as manifested by the markedly different disease states caused by different strains raises the question of whether it is appropriate to speak of *S. pyogenes* as a single entity. For simplicity, it is tempting to treat *S. pyogenes* as if it were a monolithic unit. But as our understanding of this remarkable species increases, such a view will likely become obsolete, although some common virulence traits may emerge. The strain-to-strain variation needs to be taken into account when one is reading the scientific literature on *S. pyogenes* virulence factors. Apparent contradictions between findings of different laboratories may simply be due to the decision to focus on different strains.

Group B Streptococci and Enterococci— Emerging Human Pathogens

Group B Streptococci

Infections due to both **group B streptococci (GBS)** and **enterococci** can be thought of as modern diseases. Only during the last few decades, with the proliferation of surgical interventions and intensive care units, have these two groups of bacteria been seen as significant causes of human infections. Now enterococci, especially *E. faecalis*, are leading causes of nosocomial infections. Group B streptococci do not cause infections as often, but the pattern of these infections is changing. Group B streptococci emerged originally as a cause of serious disease in very young infants. The infant acquired the bacteria during birth by passing through the vaginal tract of a woman colonized by these bacteria (Figure 15–1). Since about 40% of pregnant women are colonized in their gastrointestinal tracts with group B streptococci, introduction of the bacteria into the vaginal tract is probably not a rare event. Two consequences of the surface inoculation of the infant and inhalation of the bacteria by the infant are pneumonia and meningitis, both very serious conditions.

Group B streptococci can also cause invasive disease in pregnant and nonpregnant adults. In a 1992–1993 survey of cases of invasive group B streptococcal disease in Atlanta, Georgia, 40% occurred in nonpregnant adults, 17% in pregnant women, and 43% in infants. The incidence of adult cases was highest in older age groups, but there were also some cases in the 15- to 60-year age group. The number of cases seen in 1992–1993 had increased significantly for all three age groups compared with earlier years. This increase was disturbing, especially in the case of infants, because major improvements in diagnosis and prevention of neonatal infections had been available since the mid-1980s, and it had been hoped that these improvements would cause a decline in the incidence of the disease in this age group. In the mid-1990s, consensus guidelines were published that recommended routine screening and treatment of pregnant women as part of prenatal care. This has paid off for infants. The incidence in neonatal infections dropped between 1992 and 1998 but is still unaccepta-

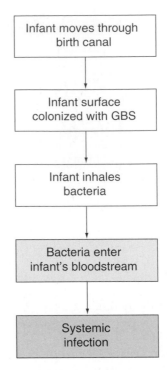

Figure 15–1 Progression of group B streptococcal infection in infants. GBS, group B streptococci.

bly high. The incidence in nonpregnant adults did not change, so this caused a shift in the age distribution of group B streptococcal infections. In 1998, 66% of infections occurred in nonpregnant adults, 4% in pregnant women, and 30% in infants.

Group B streptococcal invasive disease is serious for adults, but it is even more serious for infants. Infants in the first days of life are especially vulnerable to infectious diseases. Moreover, even infants who recover from a group B streptococcus infection can be left with long-term disabilities, especially if the disease takes the form of meningitis. Because of the seriousness of neonatal infections, the preferred strategy is prevention. There are now rapid tests to detect vaginal colonization of women close to term. Such women can be treated during labor with antibiotics to reduce the risk that the infant will be exposed to an infectious dose of viable bacteria. Administration at the onset of labor also has the advantage that possible effects of the antibiotic on the infant are minimized.

A perusal of the literature will show that neonatal meningitis and pneumonia caused by group B streptococci was noticed only in the last few decades of the 20th century. Does this mean that group B neonatal infection is a modern disease or simply that our ability to diagnose it is a recent event? No one knows the answer to this question. Some invoke the curious fact that group B streptococcal infant infections seem to be relatively uncommon in developing countries compared with developed countries, an observation that would support claims for a recent emergence of the disease in developed countries. A caveat is in order, however. In times and regions where most childbirths occur at home and not in hospitals, the cause of death of an infant soon after birth is less likely to be determined. Most group B streptococcal infections occur during the first days of life. Since infants die for so many reasons, a fairly high incidence of group B streptococcal meningitis could be hidden in the high background of infant deaths in general. There is much less doubt that group B streptococcal infections in nonpregnant adults are a recent development.

Enterococcal Infections

Just as there is little doubt that group B streptococcal infections in nonpregnant adults are a recent phenomenon associated with invasive medical procedures, so too is the same trend evident in the case of the *Enterococcus* species. Enterococci, as the species names *E. faecium* and *E. faecalis* suggest, are normally residents of the human colon. Enterococci are among the numerically minor populations of colonic bacteria, being present in approximately the same concentrations as *E. coli*, but their constant presence throughout life places them in a good position to cause infection if an opportunity presents itself. At one time, enterococci were thought to be innocuous because they do not cause infections in healthy people. Today, in the United States, they are the leading cause of hospital-acquired bacteremia and one of two leading causes, second only to *S. aureus*, of nosocomial infections in general. Enterococci cause a variety of infections, including urinary tract infections, wound infections, endocarditis, and catheter-associated infections.

The enterococci are true opportunists, bacteria that require some breaches in the host defenses—such as surgical wounds, underlying immunosuppression, or indwelling catheters—to cause infection. For a time, it was fashionable in some circles to dismiss enterococci as "just opportunists," not worthy of study because (presumably) they were not "true" pathogens. We have it on the highest medical authority, however, that a person who dies of an enterococcal infection is just as dead as someone who dies of plague or cholera. Since citizens of developed countries are far more likely to die of enterococcal infection than a disease such as plague or cholera, this point is worth taking seriously. In fact, surveys done during the early 1990s showed that at that time enterococci were already responsible annually for over 100,000 urinary tract infections, 25,000 cases of bac-

teremia, 40,000 cases of wound infections, and over 1,000 cases of endocarditis in the United States alone. These numbers have increased rather than decreased in recent years.

The fact that enterococci are exceptionally hardy bacteria gives them an important edge, because they can persist for long periods of time on the hands of hospital staff members and in the hospital environment. It is important to note that fecal aerosols are a not uncommon occurrence in hospitals, especially in intensive care wards where patients are more likely to require bed pans and experience diarrhea. Superficial cleaning of the patient's bed and the hands of staff members may not remove all the bacteria. Predictably, rigorous application of disinfectant soaps, thorough hand washing, and replacement of gloves when moving from one patient to another has proved to be the most effective way of preventing or stopping outbreaks of enterococcal infections in the hospital environment.

About 80% of enterococcal infections are caused by *E. faecalis*, with *E. faecium* responsible for the remainder, a statistic that suggests *E. faecalis* is the more serious pathogen of the two. **Vancomycin-resistant enterococci (VRE)** have made appearances in many U.S. hospitals and have proved to be difficult or impossible to treat. So far, the VRE strains have almost all been *E. faecium*. VRE infections have been considered a hospital-specific phenomenon, caused by heavy use of vancomycin in hospitals. This is the case in the United States but not in Europe, where for a variety of reasons vancomycin has been used much more sparingly to treat human infections. This has not made Europeans free of VRE, however (see Box 15–2).

Virulence Factors

Group A Streptococci

The virulence factors of group A streptococci are better understood than those of group B streptococci or enterococci, largely because it has been easier to identify such factors in a virulent pathogen such as *S. pyogenes* than in opportunists such as the group B streptococci and the enterococci. Some of the virulence factors of *S. pyogenes* that have been identified to date are listed in Table 15–2.

ADHESINS. A number of these factors are surface proteins that mediate adhesion of *S. pyogenes* to human cells or blood proteins. Like *S. aureus*, *S. pyogenes* is loaded with surface-exposed protein adhesins called **MSCRAMMs** (see chapter 14). These include **M protein, M-related proteins** (which have a similar amino acid sequence to M protein), **F1** and **F2 (fibronectin-**

BOX 15–2   VRE, a Food-Borne Disease Problem?

In 1996, concerns about the safety of genetically modified plants were beginning to make the news. All of these safety concerns were, and still are, hypothetical, but they were being taken seriously, especially in Europe. One of these concerns was that antibiotic resistance marker genes introduced on cloning vectors into the plants along with the gene of interest might somehow be released from the plant during digestion and enter intestinal bacteria of humans and animals. Although this is extremely unlikely to occur and would not be medically significant if it did, European opponents of plant biotechnology promoted this possibility as a serious safety concern. Ironically, their preoccupation with this issue may have contributed indirectly to another regulatory decision that may have serious future health consequences.

During the antibiotechnology hysteria, with virtually no debate and no media attention, the European Union approved the use of an antibiotic called avoparcin as a growth promoter for chickens and pigs. Avoparcin is a glycopeptide that cross-selects for resistance to vancomycin. What happened next was not surprising. Vancomycin-resistant strains of *E. faecium* began to appear in animal intestines and were then isolated from the unpasteurized cheeses, smoked meat products, and other products that were being offered for sale in food stores.

The question then arose as to whether the animal strains of VRE could colonize the human intestine. Or, if not, could they transfer their vancomycin resistance genes to human enterococci? Reports of isolation of VRE from the intestines of urban Europeans suggested that one or the other of these outcomes was in fact possible. In the United States, avoparcin was never approved for use in agriculture, and the few surveys done to date of intestinal enterococci from U.S. adults failed to find VRE. Since European hospitals have remained relatively free of VRE, it seems likely that agricultural use of vancomycin was responsible for the VRE being found in the intestines of healthy humans. VRE, unlike the classical food-borne pathogens, does not cause immediate intestinal disease. People colonized with VRE, however, are at increased risk for developing a serious and difficult-to-treat postsurgical infection if they have to have surgery. How high this risk actually is has been the subject of much debate, but at least this risk is a real one.

Once these facts came to light, the European Union abruptly cancelled approval for agricultural use not only of avoparcin but also of other antibiotics that cross-selected for resistance to front-line human antibiotics. In Germany, colonization of urban adults by VRE promptly fell from 12% to 3%. Whether VRE will disappear completely from this population remains to be seen. This story illustrates two important principles. First, it has shown how distracting public attention from real public health issues with endless debates over hypothetical future problems can have potentially serious public health consequences. Second, the experience with vancomycin and food-borne VRE in Europe has changed the way scientists and regulatory officials think about microbiological safety of food. For the first time, antibiotic-resistant bacteria are being considered as a possible food-borne hazard. In earlier years, this concern would have been considered frivolous. But with the increasing incidence of diseases caused by multiply resistant bacteria, such as VRE, that are found both in the animal intestine as well as in the human intestine, concern about antibiotic-resistant bacteria in the food supply has become a more serious one.

Source: H. C. Wegener, F. M. Aarestrup, L. B. Jensen, A. M. Hammerum, and F. Bager. 1999. Use of antimicrobial growth promoters in food animals and *Enterococcus faecium* resistance to therapeutic antimicrobial drugs in Europe. *Emerg. Infect. Dis.* **5:**329–335.

binding proteins), and **Epa** (a collagen-binding protein). M and M-like proteins bind to extracellular matrix proteins such as collagen and fibronectin, and to blood proteins such as factor H, IgA, IgG, and fibrinogen. Binding to antibodies is not the normal type of antibody binding in which the antigen-binding sites interact with a bacterial surface protein. Rather, the bacterial surface proteins bind the Fc portion of the antibodies, so that the antigen-binding sites are pointing away from the cell surface (Figure 15–2). Binding to the extracellular matrix proteins could help the bacteria to adhere to tissue.

Table 15–2   Virulence factors of *Streptococcus pyogenes* and their role in the host

Virulence factor	Role in the host
Adhesins	
M protein	Binds extracellular matrix proteins (collagen, fibrinogen)
	Binds Fc portion of IgG
M-related proteins	Bind extracellular matrix proteins
	Bind to antibodies (by Fc portion)
F1 and F2	Bind fibronectin
Epa	Binds collagen
Extracellular enzymes	
Streptolysin O (SLO)	Lyses red blood cells
Streptolysin S (SLS)	Lyses red blood cells
Streptokinase	Activates plasminogen to plasmin; dissolves fibrin clots
Antiphagocytic factors	
M protein	Binds fibrinogen and the Fc portion of IgG
	Binds complement factor H
Hyaluronic acid capsule	Discourages C3b binding; makes bacteria look like "self"
C5a peptidase	Reduces concentration of C5a; decreases chemotactic signals for neutrophils
Sic	Interferes in formation of membrane attack complex of complement cascade
Superantigens (SpeA–J)	
SpeA	Found in strains that cause toxic shock-like syndrome and lethal invasive infections
SpeB	Cysteine protease; may aid spread of bacteria
Others less well studied	
Lipoteichoic acid (LTA)	Can activate cytokine production, leads to septic shock; may act synergistically with superantigens

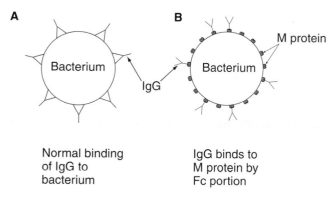

Figure 15–2   One antiphagocytic action of M protein. (**A**) Normally, IgG binds to bacterial cells by the antigen-binding site. (**B**) Streptococcal M protein binds to the Fc portion of IgG.

M protein is the best studied of the protein adhesins and is probably the most important of these proteins. M protein is highly variable antigenically. There are over 80 serotypes of M protein. This feature makes M protein unattractive as a vaccine candidate unless subsections of the protein can be identified that are more highly conserved. As with the *S. aureus* MSCRAMMs,

M protein has the LPXTG motif and is attached to peptidoglycan by a sortaselike enzyme. M protein is interesting because it functions as a virulence factor in at least two ways. Binding to fibrinogen could be considered an adhesive property. Covering the bacteria with the host protein fibrinogen could also function to make the bacteria look like "self" and prevent them from being engulfed and killed by phagocytes. M protein also binds the Fc portion of IgG, another host protein. Still another antiphagocytic role of M protein is that it binds complement factor H, an activity that discourages the binding of C3b to the bacterial surface (see chapter 5). Thus, M protein is antiphagocytic in at least two ways as well as serving as a possible adhesin.

M protein has yet another role in the virulence of strains that cause rheumatic heart disease. Some antibodies against M protein cross-react with heart tissue (Figure 15–3). This has led to the hypothesis that rheumatic heart disease is caused by certain strains of group A streptococci that colonize the throat, causing the severe inflammation. During this infection, antigens from the bacteria, such as M protein, enter the bloodstream and elicit an antibody response (Figure 15–4). In some people, the antibodies cross-react with heart valve tis-

A Streptococcal M5 peptide B2   TIGTLKKILDETVKDKIA
Human cardiac myosin   LEDLKRQLEEEVKAKNA

B Streptococcal NT4 peptide   GLKTENEGLKTENEGLKTE
Human cardiac myosin   KLQTENGE

C Streptococcal M6 protein   LTDQNKNLTTEN
Human cardiac myosin   LTSQRAKLQTEN

Figure 15–3 Comparison of amino acid sequences of streptococcal M protein and myosin. Similar amino acid sequence regions found in three different M proteins and human heart tissue may explain the cross-reactivity of anti-M antibodies with heart tissue. Two dots, identical residues; one dot, conserved substitutions. (Reprinted from M. W. Cunningham, S. M. Antone, M. Smart, R. Liu, and S. Kosanke. 1997. Molecular analysis of human cardiac myosin-cross-reactive B- and T-cell epitopes of the group A streptococcal M5 protein. *Infect. Immun.* **65:**3913–3923, with permission from the publisher.)

sues, causing an autoimmune response that damages the heart valves.

ENZYMES. *S. pyogenes* produces a variety of extracellular proteins that interact with blood cells or blood proteins. These include two hemolysins, **streptolysin O (SLO)** and **streptolysin S (SLS)**. These hemolysins lyse red blood cells by forming pores in the red blood cell membrane. They are the basis for the classic identification test for this species: the hemolysins create large zones of clearing (beta-hemolysis) around colonies growing on blood agar plates. Group A streptococci are sometimes called beta-hemolytic streptococci because of this trait. Other groups of streptococci are either not hemolytic or form a greenish zone of incomplete hemolysis. The zone of beta-hemolysis is enhanced considerably if the plates are incubated in a candle jar. The plates are placed in a glass container, a candle is placed in the container and lighted, and then the jar is sealed. The candle uses up most of the oxygen. This probably helps increase the zone of hemolysis because streptolysin O is sensitive to oxygen.

An enzyme called **streptokinase** activates the blood protein plasminogen to plasmin. Plasmin then dissolves fibrin clots. Scientists have taken advantage of this activity of streptokinase, and it is now given to many patients in the early stages of a heart attack in hopes of preventing the formation of clots. The role of streptokinase in virulence is still unclear.

COMBATING PHAGOCYTOSIS. The antiphagocytic effects of M protein have been mentioned along with its possible role as an adhesin. M protein not only makes the bacteria look like "self" by covering the bacteria with host proteins but also binds complement factor H, which leads to a cascade of events that prevent activated complement component C3b from binding to the bacterial surface. *S. pyogenes* has other backup strategies for preventing phagocytes from engulfing and killing it. Other virulence factors include an antiphagocytic capsule composed of hyaluronic acid. **Hyaluronic acid** is a component of human intracellular matrix. Thus, the capsule not only prevents phagocytosis by the usual route of discouraging C3b binding but makes the bacteria look like "self" to the immune system. *S. pyogenes* also produces a **C5a peptidase** that may prevent neutrophil migration to the site of infection by reducing the concentration of C5a, which guides the neutrophils to their target.

A recently identified secreted protein called **streptococcal inhibitor of complement (Sic)** is incorporated in the membrane attack complex of the complement system in vitro, thus disrupting this protective response of the host. The importance of the Sic proteins is evident from a phenomenon observed in strains responsible for epidemic waves of group A streptococcal infections. Sic is a hypervariable protein. During an epidemic or during colonization of the nasal mucosa of mice, the number of variants increases considerably. This variation may arise from pressure from the immune system that makes it expedient for the bacteria to change their surface antigens. M protein also varies, but this variation does not seem to be as important. These findings call

Figure 15–4 Two theories explaining aspects of the progression of rheumatic fever and rheumatic heart disease.

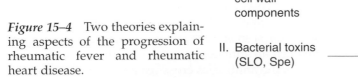

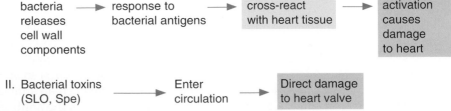

into question a widespread belief about epidemics of group A streptococcal infections—that they are caused by a single clone of group A streptococci. A single clone may start the epidemic, but variants rapidly arise.

SUPERANTIGENS AND OTHER TOXIC COMPONENTS.   Finally, *S. pyogenes* strains produce a superantigen called **Spe.** There are now seven known variants of Spe—SpeA through SpeJ (excluding SpeD, E, and I). **SpeA** seems to be the most important superantigen and is produced by the recently emerging strains that cause toxic shock-like syndrome and rapidly lethal invasive infections. **SpeB** is a cysteine protease that may aid in the spread of the bacteria in tissue by cleaving host proteins. Destruction of extracellular matrix and cells would make it easier for the bacteria, which are not motile, to diffuse through tissue to new sites.

Of course, because *S. pyogenes* is a gram-positive bacterium, its cell wall contains **lipoteichoic acid (LTA),** which, like the LPS of gram-negative bacteria, can activate the cascade of steps that lead to septic shock. LPS can act synergistically with the superantigen of *S. aureus,* the toxin associated with toxic shock syndrome, to induce septic shock. So, possibly LTA activates the steps in septic shock in a similar manner by acting synergistically with the superantigens of the gram-positive bacteria such as *S. pyogenes* and *S. aureus.* This would seem logical because there is likely to be some lysis of the bacteria during an infection.

Regulation of Virulence Factors

Of all the virulence factors, the roles of M protein and the hyaluronic acid capsule in an infection are best established. Group A streptococci isolated from people with invasive streptococcal infections exhibit increased production of both of these virulence factors. The importance of some of the other putative virulence factors is suggested by the fact that they are coregulated with the M protein gene or the genes encoding proteins responsible for synthesis of the hyaluronic acid capsule. For example, genes encoding the M-like proteins, the C5a peptidase, and Sic are all regulated by a protein called **multiple gene regulator in group A streptococci (Mga)** (Figure 15–5). The synthesis of Mga is regulated in turn by the carbon dioxide concentration of the medium and possibly other signals that remain to be identified. Expression of *mga* is also regulated by **Nra,** a regulatory protein that also controls expression of *prtF2,* the gene that encodes fibronectin-binding protein F2, and *cpa,* which encodes the collagen-binding protein Cpa.

Similarly, a two-component regulatory system, **CovR** and **CovS** (formerly CsrR and CsrS), represses the synthesis of not only the *has* genes, which encode the enzymes responsible for the synthesis of the hyaluronic acid capsule, but also genes encoding streptolysin and streptokinase (Figure 15–5). It is not clear what signal is triggering production of CovR and CovS, but the fact that these regulatory proteins control production of bacterial proteins that interact with human blood components suggests that some blood factor might be the signal. It is also the case, however, that some of the proteins controlled by this regulatory system vary in abundance with growth phase, so a trigger that is coupled to growth phase regulation cannot be ruled out.

All of this suggests a complex concerted pattern of gene expression directed against defenses of blood and tissue, which could explain why group A streptococci are so skillful in causing serious infections if they gain access to internal tissues and the bloodstream. The complex network of regulatory cascades that is gradually emerging could also explain why different strains of *S. pyogenes* can cause such different diseases.

Virulence Factors of Group B Streptococci

Much less is known about the virulence factors of the group B streptococci. Clearly, the ability of this group to colonize the vaginal tract is a major factor. Very young infants are especially vulnerable to infections, since their defense systems are not yet fully developed. Moreover, advances in the ability of obstetricians to save preterm infants, who are even more vulnerable, has created an ultrasusceptible population of neonates. In fact, premature birth is one of the main risk factors for acquiring group B neonatal infections.

CAPSULE.   Group B streptococci produce a capsule that is poorly characterized but may contribute to virulence. Some studies have identified low levels of maternal antibody to capsular polysaccharide as a risk factor for neonatal infections. Whether this affects vaginal colonization or transplacentally transferred IgG to the infant, or both, is not clear. Another factor that points to the importance of the polysaccharide capsule is the fact that some capsular serotypes seem to predominate as causes of infections. For example, a recent study identified serotype V as the most common serotype in infections involving nonpregnant adults, whereas other serotypes predominated in the case of early-onset neonatal infections. In other streptococci, such as *S. pneumoniae,* which is the main cause of bacterial pneumonia in adults and earache in children, a similar pattern is seen—the predominance of certain capsular serotypes. Such patterns make designing vaccines easier, especially when there are a large number of serotypes seen

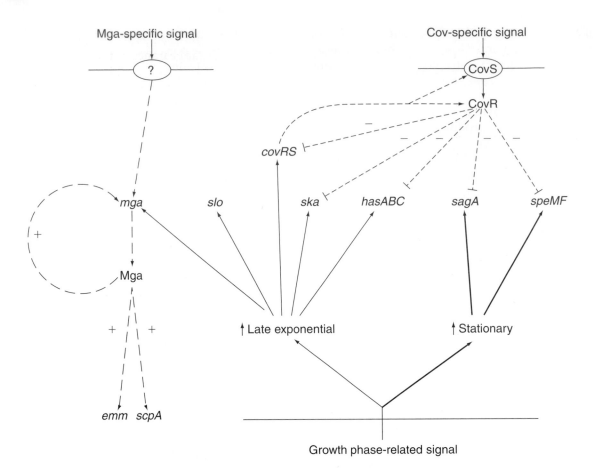

Figure 15–5 Regulation of virulence factors of group A streptococci. Positive regulation is indicated by +, and negative regulation is indicated by –. Lines with short dashes represent CovR-mediated regulation, and lines with long dashes represent regulation by Mga. Solid lines indicate regulation correlated with growth phase either in exponential phase (light lines) or stationary phase (heavy lines). (Reprinted from M. J. Federle, K. S. McIver, and J. R. Scott. 1999. A response regulator that represses transcription of several virulence operons in the group A streptococci. *J. Bacteriol.* **181:**3649–3657, with permission from the publisher.)

in isolates, but they also indicate that there is something important about subtle differences in capsular polysaccharides that has eluded scientists so far.

PERSPECTIVE. Research on group B streptococci has tended to focus on the immediate clinical aspects of the disease rather than the molecular basis of virulence. This is understandable, given that the consequences of the disease for infants are so serious. At least the group A streptococci are temporarily in abeyance, giving us the feeling that we can afford esoteric studies of virulence factors. In the case of the group B streptococci, however, studies of virulence factors can seem almost frivolous in the face of the real threat the disease poses to the small scraps of life that are its main victims. This view could be shortsighted, however. A better understanding of the virulence factors of the group B strep-

tococci could suggest vaccines or other intervention strategies that are more effective than identifying lists of risk factors that many obstetricians ignore anyway. The fact that an embarrassingly large number of women have more than one infant that develops a group B streptococcal infection shows that the current approach to preventing group B streptococcal infections is still not working very well.

Enterococcus Virulence Factors

PROBLEMS WITH STUDYING ENTEROCOCCAL VIRULENCE FACTORS. As with the group B streptococci, not much is known about the characteristics that allow *E. faecium* and *E. faecalis* to cause infection. This is due to several factors. First, until recently, those who were true believers in the notion that there is a sharp distinction between "true pathogens" and "opportunists" had managed to block funding for research on the opportunists such as enterococci. Their position had some merit in the sense that if it is difficult to discern the virulence factors of a highly pathogenic bacterium, it will be far more difficult to sort out the virulence factors of an opportunist. From a purely scientific point of view, studies of the most virulent pathogens, which cause infections in otherwise healthy humans or animals, will be far more likely to yield unambiguous answers than studies of opportunists. Yet, this view may prove to be misguided. There is almost certainly a continuum of host-parasite interactions. If so, focusing exclusively on one end of this continuum will produce a very misleading picture.

From a practical point of view, the opportunists are a major current health problem. Given the magnitude of the problem, something has to be done about understanding their characteristics, however scientifically unsatisfying the search might be. Moreover, it is entirely possible that the rigid distinction between "true" pathogens and opportunists has kept scientists from learning about the more subtle but nonetheless important interactions between the human body and the bacteria it normally harbors. After all, enterococci are found in the intestinal tracts of virtually all humans. Yet, under certain conditions, these bacteria can cause infections, and the body mounts an antibody response against the invaders. At the very least, something about how the body distinguishes between friend and foe might be learned. Also, the need for new antibiotic targets has become acute enough to make public health officials more enthusiastic about research on enterococci.

ANIMAL MODEL.   Some of the difficulties encountered in attempting to study an opportunist like E. faecalis are evident from a description of an animal model—the mouse peritonitis model. In this model, large numbers of the bacteria (ca. 10^8) are injected directly into the peritoneal cavity of a mouse. The LD_{50} of E. faecalis in mice is high enough to make this necessary. With such a high LD_{50}, it is difficult to see the effects of mutations that might affect virulence by looking for increases in the LD_{50}. One solution to this problem is to use increases in time to death as an indicator of lower virulence. A second solution is to inject the bacteria in a mixture with sterile rat fecal extract to decrease the LD_{50} somewhat. This trick has been used in developing animal models for a number of bacteria that are not very pathogenic for laboratory rodents. The fecal extract probably works by eliciting an inflammatory response that causes some tissue damage. The proteins in the extract may even protect the injected bacteria temporarily, giving them a chance to gain a foothold in the animal. Still another solution is to use a competition assay. In the animal model, the mutant being tested is introduced along with wild type. Disappearance of the mutant after a certain period of time indicates that in the animal, the mutant was not able to compete successfully with the wild type. This type of competition assay is far more sensitive than a comparison of LD_{50} values.

VIRULENCE FACTORS FOUND SO FAR.   Oddly enough, what little has been learned about enterococci makes them look more and more like S. aureus from the virulence point of view. E. faecalis produces a cytolysin that ruptures a variety of mammalian cell types, and both species of enterococci are able to bind to proteins of the extracellular matrix. The cytolysin is a homolog of S. aureus Cna, a protein that mediates binding to collagen. In E. faecalis, this protein is called **Ace** (for **adhesin of collagen from enterococci**). Ace is interesting for another reason: it was discovered by searching the newly available genome sequence of E. faecalis for proteins with amino acid sequence similarity to proteins known to be important for the virulence of such well-studied pathogens as S. aureus. This approach to identifying potential virulence genes allows scientists to bypass the years it used to take to find virulence genes by mutagenesis studies. Of course, this approach limits the investigator to surveying for proteins already known, thus potentially missing novel mechanisms, but it is certainly a powerful new tool in pathogenesis research.

In another screen of genes in the E. faecalis genome sequence, scientists identified some genes, called fsr genes, that encode proteins that are homologs of the Agr proteins of S. aureus. The Agr proteins control some key S. aureus virulence genes (see chapter 14). In E. faecalis, the proteins encoded by the fsr genes appear to control genes encoding two proteases, a **gelatinase (GelE)** and a **serine protease (SprE)**. The sprE gene has been shown to contribute to virulence in the mouse peritonitis model.

The fact that scientists studying the E. faecalis genome sequence are finding homologs of S. aureus virulence genes raises the question of why enterococci are not more pathogenic than they are in otherwise healthy people. An interesting observation suggests that the answer might have something to do with regulation. Scientists found that E. faecalis clinical isolates could bind to extracellular matrix proteins such as laminin and collagen, but only when they had been grown at 45°C. Those grown at 37°C showed much less ability to adhere to these proteins. Since enterococci colonize the human body, which maintains a constant temperature (37°C), this suggested that what the scientists were really seeing was not so much a temperature effect as a stress effect; in fact, the bacteria grew much more slowly at 45°C than at 37°C. One interpretation of these results, and a very tentative interpretation, is that *S. aureus* is more able to respond in a carefully modulated way to conditions encountered within the human body, whereas enterococci are simply responding to an unaccustomed stress. (Or possibly, enterococci are simply more laid-back microbes that are harder to rile than the finicky staphylococci. No harm in a little anthropomorphizing.) Such a response would be expected to be less efficient than one that was better modulated to a complex set of conditions. Nonetheless, the fact that enterococci are now a significant cause of diseases ranging from endocarditis to sepsis, with *E. faecalis* being the third most common cause of endocarditis, should make us take them seriously as human pathogens.

VANCOMYCIN RESISTANCE. Although antibiotic resistance is not usually considered a virulence factor, it could be argued that in the case of opportunists like the enterococci, resistance to antibiotics as the ultimate arbiter between survival and death should be given some status. It was in the enterococci that horizontally transferred vancomycin resistance was first discovered. This was an important breakthrough for two reasons. First, vancomycin has become one of the last antibiotics that can be used to treat infections caused by some important gram-positive pathogens. Second, in contrast to other resistance mechanisms, in which only one or two genes were involved, vancomycin resistance in the enterococci proved to be due to multiple genes that in effect modified the pathway of peptidoglycan biosynthesis. This complex resistance mechanism gave scientists a new appreciation for how far bacteria can go to become resistant to antibiotics.

The mechanism of vancomycin resistance discovered in enterococci is described in chapter 11 (Figure 11–5). Normally, the bacteria have a peptidoglycan peptide that ends in D-Ala–D-Ala. This is the dipeptide to which vancomycin binds. Binding of vancomycin blocks interaction of the dipeptide with the cross-linking transpeptidase, thus effectively stopping the cross-linking of peptidoglycan. To counter this, enterococci have evolved a strategy that changes the D-Ala–D-Ala to another compound, such as D-Ala–D-lactate, to which vancomycin is unable to bind. To accomplish this aim, the bacteria must produce an enzyme that produces the lactate and ligates it to the peptide cross-link. In addition, the bacteria have to destroy any D-Ala–D-Ala that is made by the normal bacterial enzymes. Thus, the resistance pathway has to include a gene encoding an enzyme that cleaves D-Ala–D-Ala. This alternative pathway for synthesis of the cross-linking peptide is now carried on a transposon in one case (VanA-type resistance) and on a conjugative transposon in another (VanC-type resistance). Thus, the resistance pathway has become transmissible from one bacterium to another.

A somewhat surprising finding has been that, although in the laboratory this type of vancomycin resistance can be transferred by conjugation to *S. aureus*, where the pathway is functional, the vancomycin resistance that is emerging in *S. aureus* is not the enterococcal one but something completely different. Work is still under way to determine how the vancomycin intermediate susceptibility *S. aureus* (VISA) strains have become less susceptible to vancomycin, but it is already clear that they are doing this their own way and not simply acquiring the resistance genes from enterococci, as everyone thought they would do. This may have something to do with the effect of vancomycin resistance on the fitness of the strain.

The vancomycin-resistant enterococci have become such a problem that in 1995, the U.S. Department of Health and Human Services released a set of recommendations for preventing the spread of vancomycin-resistant enterococci in hospitals; some of them are listed in Table 15–3. Note that developing effective recommendations of this sort requires a knowledge of the main types of transmission. Epidemiological studies

Table 15–3 Recommendations for preventing spread of vancomycin-resistant enterococci in hospitals[a]

Prudent vancomycin use
  Know situations where use is acceptable
  Know situations where use should be discouraged

Education programs
  Include physicians, residents, students, pharmacists, nurses, and laboratory personnel

Take advantage of microbiology laboratory in detection, reporting, and control of vancomycin resistance, i.e., enhance communication between lab and other health care workers

Identify enterococci

Test antimicrobial susceptibility of all clinical isolates

Develop screening procedures in hospitals where VRE have not previously been found

Prevent and control nosocomial transmission of VRE
  Inform staff of cases of VRE
  Isolate infected patients
  Require staff to wear gowns and gloves
  Require staff to wash hands
  Dedicate equipment (e.g., stethoscopes) to VRE patients
  Restrict number of staff members who interact with VRE patients
  Screen staff for carriage

Detect and report all isolates of *S. aureus* and *S. epidermidis* that become insensitive to vancomycin

[a] Adapted from Hospital Infection Control Practices Advisory Committee. Recommendations for preventing the spread of vancomycin resistance. 1995. *Morb. Mortal. Wkly. Rep.* **44**(R12):1–13.

had found that enterococci are probably spread mainly through contamination of clothing and other parts of the hospital environment. This is not surprising given the well-known hardiness of enterococci, including their ability to tolerate dry conditions for long periods of time. Bacteria from these sources are available to be picked up by the hands of hospital personnel and carried to susceptible patients. Because of this mode of spread, careful attention to disinfection of surfaces, glove changes, and regular hand washing is of great importance. Since susceptible patients tend to be located in intensive care wards, prevention efforts are focused on those areas of the hospital. Information transfer also plays a large part in the recommendations. It is difficult for staff members to be on "red alert" day in and day out. Thus, informing staff members that a case of VRE has occurred or that the hospital has a continuing problem with VRE helps staff members adjust their behavior to reflect greater caution.

SELECTED READINGS

Blumberg, H. M., D. S. Stephens, M. Modansky, M. Erin, J. Elliot, R. R. Facklam, A. Schuchat, W. Baughman, and M. M. Farley. 1996. Invasive group B streptococcal disease: the emergence of serotype V. *J. Infect. Dis.* **173:**365–373.

Cunningham, M. W. 2000. Pathogenesis of group A streptococcal infections. *Clin. Microbiol. Rev.* **13:**470–511.

Federle, M. J., K. S. McIver, and J. R. Scott. 1999. A response regulator that represses transcription of several virulence operons in the group A streptococci. *J. Bacteriol.* **181:**3649–3657.

Hoe, N. P., K. Nakashima, S. Lukomski, D. Grigsby, M. Liu, P. Kordari, S. J. Dou, X. Pan, J. Vuopio-Varkila, S. Salmenlinna, A. McGeer, D. W. Low, B. Schwartz, A. Schuchat, S. Naidich, D. DeLorenzo, F. Yun-Xin, and J. M. Musser. 1999. Rapid selection of structural variants of group A *Streptococcus* sustains and enlarges serotype M1 epidemic waves. *Nat. Med.* **5:**924–929.

Hospital Infection Control Practices Advisory Committee (HICPAC). 1995. Recommendations for preventing the spread of vancomycin resistance. *Morb. Mortal. Wkly. Rep.* **44**(RR12)**:**1–13.

Schuchat, A. 1998. Epidemiology of group B streptococcal disease in the United States: shifting paradigms. *Clin. Microbiol. Rev.* **11:**497–513.

Schuchat, A. 2001. Group B streptococcal disease: from trials and tribulations to triumph and trepidation. *Clin. Infect. Dis.* **33:**751–756.

Stollerman, G. H. 2001. Rheumatic fever in the 21st century. *Clin. Infect. Dis.* **33:**806–814.

Wessels, M. R. 1999. Regulation of virulence factor expression in group A streptococcus. *Trends Microbiol.* **7:**428–430.

SUMMARY OUTLINE

Comparison of group A and group B streptococci and enterococci

	S. pyogenes (group A)	*S. agalactiae* (group B)	*Enterococcus*
Characteristics	Gram-positive cocci, chains or pairs	Gram-positive cocci chains or pairs	Gram-positive cocci, single cells or pairs
	Nonmotile	Nonmotile	Nonmotile
Hemolytic reaction	Beta-hemolytic	Mostly beta-hemolytic, but some are alpha- or nonhemolytic	Mostly nonhemolytic
Antibiotic resistance	Susceptible to most antibiotics	Increasingly resistant to antibiotics	Resistant to many antibiotics
Normal location	Mouth, throat	Gastrointestinal tract; also found in nonhuman animals	Colon; humans and other animals
Infections	Strep throat (rheumatic heart disease, glomerulonephritis), scarlet fever, impetigo, cellulitis, toxic shock-like syndrome, wound infections, bacteremia	Infant meningitis and pneumonia; nosocomial pneumonia, bacteremia	Nosocomial wound infections, bacteremia, urinary tract infections; endocarditis

(continued)

Comparison of group A and group B streptococci and enterococci (*continued*)

	S. pyogenes (group A)	*S. agalactiae* (group B)	*Enterococcus*
Virulence factors	Adhesins, hydrolytic enzymes (SLO, SLS, streptokinase), antiphagocytic factors (M protein, capsule, C5a peptidase, Sic); autoimmune response (antibodies to M protein cross-react with heart tissue); superantigens (SpeA–J)	Capsule, colonization of vaginal tract	Hardy, colonization of colon, some similar to those of *S. aureus*
Regulation of virulence factors	Mga, CovR, S	Unknown	Similar to *S. aureus* (?)

QUESTIONS

Answers to the questions can be found in Appendix 2.

1. What are some of the factors that explain the extraordinary fluctuations in the incidence and nature of streptococcal infections that have occurred over the past 100 years or more?

2. Is it likely that the changes in streptococcal disease patterns fluctuated nearly as much in the centuries prior to the 19th century? Explain.

3. Try to make sense of the multitude of virulence factors that have been identified for the group A streptococci. In the case of an infection that starts with a skin wound and ends with systemic infection, what factors would you expect to be important at each stage of dissemination?

4. If you managed to answer 3, first publish your answer so that we can all benefit, and then try to make sense of what is known about the regulation of *S. pyogenes* virulence genes. How could they be orchestrating the development of disease?

5. If *S. pyogenes* has so many impressive virulence factors, why is it that some strains cause only minor skin disease, such as impetigo, whereas others cause lethal infections?

6. Group B streptococci can kill you just as certainly as group A streptococci. Yet, the group B streptococci seem to have a much more limited repertoire of virulence genes than the group A streptococci. How do you explain this?

7. Why are group B streptococcal infections shifting from being a problem mainly in infants to being just as big a problem in nonpregnant adults?

8. Why are some people so concerned about enterococci in the food supply, when these bacteria do not cause gastrointestinal disease? Could there be parallel examples not involving the food supply?

9. *Enterococcus* strains seem to have some of the same virulence genes as *S. aureus*. Yet, enterococci do not infect healthy people the way that *S. aureus* can. How do you explain this anomaly?

10. Given that both group B streptococci and enterococci have become increasingly resistant to antibiotics, why have the group A streptococci remained susceptible to antibiotics?

16

Pseudomonas aeruginosa and Related Species, a Lesson in Versatility

---

KEY FEATURES

Pseudomonas aeruginosa and Related Species

CHARACTERISTICS

Gram-negative, motile rods

Oxidase positive

Respiratory metabolism

Wide range of substrates utilized

DISEASES

Variety of opportunistic infections ranging from eye infections in contact lens wearers to burn and wound infections leading to septic shock

Lung infections in cystic fibrosis patients

RESERVOIRS

Ubiquitous in the environment in water, in soil, and on plants

Transient colonization of the human body

MAJOR VIRULENCE FACTORS

Adhesins

LPS

Type III secretion system

ExoS and ExoU—toxins injected by the type III system

Other toxins—elastase, exotoxin A (similar to diphtheria toxin)

Alginate production, biofilm formation (cystic fibrosis patients)

PREVENTION AND TREATMENT

Hygiene

Resistant to many antibiotics

No vaccine available

A Consummate Opportunist

Pseudomonas aeruginosa is a ubiquitous soil microbe that can cause infections in humans and plants. Although this chapter will focus on the infectious side of *P. aeruginosa*, it is worth noting that *Pseudomonas* species are not all bad. Not only do they play an important role in the ecology of soil, but their ability to degrade an impressive variety of organic compounds, including some toxic wastes, has made them useful for bioremediation applications. Some *Pseudomonas* species produce fungicidal compounds and are thus able to protect plants from certain types of fungal infections. *P. aeruginosa* is a classic example of an innocuous—even beneficial—bacterium that has taken advantage of breaches in host defenses to become a human pathogen. Serious burns that decimate the defenses of skin are readily infected by *P. aeruginosa*. Cystic fibrosis patients have impaired lung defense functions, a fact that makes them an open target for opportunists like *P. aeruginosa*. In modern times, a variety of new practices, such as surgery and wearing contact lenses, have created breaches that enable *P. aeruginosa* to cause infections not seen previously. Infections caused by *P. aeruginosa* are particularly problematic, not only because of the ubiquitous nature of this opportunistic pathogen but also because of its resistance to most antibiotics.

A close relative of *P. aeruginosa, Burkholderia* (formerly *Pseudomonas*) *cepacia* also causes human infections. Like *P. aeruginosa,* it is ubiquitous in soil. Normally considered a friend of humans, it has been used widely as a biopesticide. An example of how this ubiquitous species can become a problem in hospitals was provided by a 1998 outbreak of lung infections, some of which were fatal, in an intensive care unit. None of the usual sources, such as hands of health care workers or bed rails and linens, turned out to be the source of this outbreak. Instead, the outbreak was finally traced to mouthwash. Comatose and other seriously ill patients who cannot take care of their own dental hygiene routinely have their teeth and gums swabbed with mouthwash by health care workers. This practice prevents a buildup of bacterial biofilms in the mouth that can be fatal because they shed bacteria that enter the lungs. But if the mouthwash itself is contaminated—in this case by *B. cepacia*—this very effective preventive strategy can turn deadly. After much analysis of the various stages of the preparation and administration of the mouthwash, the CDC determined that the contamination event occurred at the plant that produced the mouthwash. Normally, the alcohol in most mouthwashes prevents bacteria from multiplying, but in this case, the alcohol-free mouthwash (designed to prevent drying of gum tissue) allowed bacterial contaminants to proliferate. The average person or even the average hospital patient would not have experienced any problems with the contaminated mouthwash, but the very sick—partially immunocompromised—patients in the intensive care unit were unusually susceptible to infection. This is yet another example of how insidious and how unpredictable opportunistic infections can be.

Characteristics of *P. aeruginosa*

P. aeruginosa is a gram-negative motile rod with an oxidative metabolism. Pseudomonads in a drop of liquid are very entertaining to watch under a microscope because they are so actively motile and move with astonishing speed across the microscope field. The Gram stain procedure kills and immobilizes them, robbing them of their most endearing trait. *P. aeruginosa* is sometimes described as an obligate aerobe, but this description is misleading because most strains can grow under anoxic conditions with nitrate as a terminal electron acceptor. *P. aeruginosa* cannot grow fermentatively, however, and for this reason it is referred to in the clinical literature as a "nonfermenter." The high activity of the pseudomonad electron transport machinery has given rise to a rapid diagnostic test, the **oxidase test.** Pseudomonads, including *P. aeruginosa*, have electron transport components that can oxidize a variety of compounds, including the dye *N,N,N',N'*-tetramethyl-*p*-phenylenediamine dihydrochloride. The change in color of this dye from colorless to blue, when a portion of a colony is applied to paper impregnated with it, is a useful test for a presumptive identification of *P. aeruginosa* and related species.

The nutritional versatility of pseudomonads is phenomenal. It is almost accurate to say that if you can draw a chemical structure containing carbon, oxygen, and hydrogen, some pseudomonad can degrade it, given oxygen or nitrate and enough time. An important clinical consequence of this versatility is that *P. aeruginosa* can be found almost anywhere in a hospital. It has even been found growing in mop water and dilute disinfectant solutions. *B. cepacia* has a similar metabolic versatility.

P. aeruginosa is not just colorful because of its motility and metabolic diversity. It is also literally colorful on agar medium. Colonies of *P. aeruginosa* have a distinctive blue-green color. This color is due to the production of the pigment **pyocyanin.** For the medical implications of this, see Box 16–1. This pigment illustrates another feature of *P. aeruginosa,* its production of secondary metabolites. **Secondary metabolites** are compounds produced by an organism that appear to have no direct role in energy metabolism or the biosynthetic reactions that are essential for life. Antibiotics are another example of a microbial secondary metabolite. The roles of secondary metabolites in the life of the microbe and during the course of an infection caused by it remain controversial, but these compounds are often produced at considerable expense—energetically speaking—and surely have some important role that remains to be discovered. Whatever the role of pyocyanin in the metabolism and virulence of *P. aeruginosa*, the bacteria can produce copious amounts of this pigment.

P. aeruginosa is also notable for its ability to form biofilms and has been used as a model organism for studying biofilm formation and structure. **Biofilms** are thick

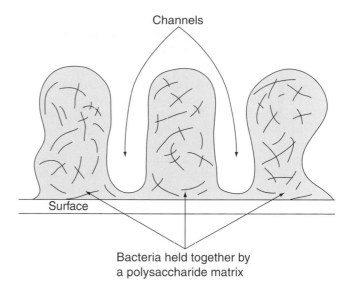

Figure 16–1 Structure of a mature bacterial biofilm.

Types of Infections

P. aeruginosa is capable of transiently colonizing the skin and intestinal tract of humans and animals, and because it is ubiquitous in the environment it is constantly available for recolonization. The ability to colonize the human body, even if only transiently, places *P. aeruginosa* in a good position to take advantage of any breaches in human defense systems. For an example of how dangerous transient colonization of the hands and nails can be, see Box 16–2. *P. aeruginosa* is a consummate opportunist. It does not infect healthy adults, but given an opening in the defenses of the human body, it can cause a surprising variety of infections. Some of these are listed in Table 16–1. *P. aeruginosa* is best known for its ability to infect burns and to cause lung infections in cystic fibrosis patients. *P. aeruginosa* is the main cause of death in burn patients who survive the initial trauma of the burn. In a badly burned area, the normal defenses of skin have been almost completely destroyed, and the once dry area becomes moist as blood fluids seep out of the burned tissue. These patients may also acquire lung infections if they sustained airway and lung damage due to inhaling fire-heated air. Better management of burn patients has reduced the risk of infection, but such infections still occur.

P. aeruginosa is now the major cause of death in cystic fibrosis patients. In earlier decades, a child with cystic fibrosis died very young because of the defect in pancreatic function that prevented proper absorption of nutrients. This problem was solved by using special dietary regimens. As children with cystic fibrosis began to live longer, another problem emerged. They were almost certain to have recurrent lung infections that ul-

layers composed of bacteria linked together by a polysaccharide matrix. At one time, biofilms were thought to be relatively simple, unstructured assemblages, consisting of many layers of bacteria. Recent work has shown, however, that biofilms exhibit a developmental sequence and have a complex architecture. This architecture is characterized by mushroom-shaped assemblages of bacteria separated by channels that convey nutrients to the thick biofilm (Figure 16–1). Biofilms are a medical problem because bacteria in a biofilm are less metabolically active and far less susceptible to antibiotics than free-living bacteria.

It is not clear how relevant the ability of *P. aeruginosa* to form biofilms is to the ability of *P. aeruginosa* to cause disease. Biofilm formation is thought to be a factor in lung infections of cystic fibrosis patients, because the bacteria appear to form biofilmlike assemblages in the lung, but relevance for other pseudomonad infections has not been established. It is true that bacterial biofilms on intravenous catheters, urinary catheters, and plastic implants have become a major medical problem. Yet, these biofilms are usually caused by gram-positive cocci such as the staphylococci (see chapter 14), not *P. aeruginosa*.

BOX 16–2   Outbreak of *P. aeruginosa* Infections in a Neonatal Intensive Care Ward

In 1998, in a 50-bed neonatal intensive care ward, the infants began to develop infections at a higher rate than usual. The culprit proved to be *P. aeruginosa*. A critically important question that had to be answered as soon as possible was the mode of spread of the bacteria. Since babies in an intensive care ward are handled constantly by staff members, transmission of bacteria on the hands of clinicians and nurses was one of the first possibilities considered. A microbiological investigation revealed that 5% of the clinicians and 10% of nurses working in this ward had *P. aeruginosa* on their hands. Moreover, half of the infants in the ward had become colonized, either in their respiratory tracts or in their gastrointestinal tracts. This meant that they were tiny ticking time bombs for future infections made possible by the many breaches in their defense systems. What brought this case to the attention of the health care community was that one of the main factors associated with carriage of *P. aeruginosa* was artificial nails or nail wraps. In this case, molecular fingerprinting revealed that the strain found in most of the colonized babies was identical to a strain carried by a nurse who did not have artificial nails. Nonetheless, the realization that artificial nails (and, by associa-

tion, long nails) might increase the risk of colonization of hands with *P. aeruginosa* has led to the recommendation that long nails, whether artificial or not, be discouraged among staff working in a neonatal intensive care ward. The rationale for the association between colonization and fingernails is that long nails are less likely to be thoroughly cleansed during hand washing than shorter ones. So far, this stricture is purely advisory, not enforced, but the people who work in neonatal intensive care wards are so dedicated to the health of the very vulnerable little lives in their charge, that it is likely the recommendation will be taken very seriously, even though the evidence that supports it is not very strong.

If long nails are in fact a contributor to carriage of *P. aeruginosa*, this is yet another example of how insidious the pseudomonad problem is for hospitals. The bacteria can come from anywhere—air, water, disinfectant solutions, hands, bed linens, and who knows where else.

Source: M. Foca, K. Jakob, S. Whittier, P. Della Latta, S. Factor, D. Rubenstein, L. Saiman, and S. Jones. 2000. Endemic *Pseudomonas aeruginosa* infection in a neonatal intensive care ward. *N. Engl. J. Med.* **343**:695–700.

Table 16–1 Examples of *P. aeruginosa* infections and the predisposing conditions that favor them

Disease	Predisposing condition
Dermatitis	Hot tubs; loofah sponge use
Burn infections	Third-degree burns
Eye infections (ulcerative keratitis)	Long-wear soft contact lenses
Lung infections	Cystic fibrosis
	Inhalation of hot air during a fire
	Patients intubated to support breathing (ventilator-associated pneumonia)
Nosocomial septicemia	Surgical wounds
	Infants in an intensive care ward
Nosocomial urinary tract infections	Indwelling urinary catheter

timately produced enough lung damage to kill them. *P. aeruginosa* is the most common cause of these lung infections. *B. cepacia* is also a significant cause of lung infection in cystic fibrosis patients. Improved measures for preventing and treating lung infections in these patients have greatly extended their life expectancies.

P. aeruginosa is also a concern of contact lens wearers. Small scratches on the cornea, caused by improper use of contact lenses, give *P. aeruginosa* a window of opportunity to infect the scratched area. The resulting infections can become quite serious if they are not treated promptly and effectively. *P. aeruginosa* has even found opportunities to infect members of the spa set, causing dermatitis in hot tub aficionados. Expanded pores may be the explanation for the occasional reports of skin infections in devotees of hot tubs. Users of loofah sponges have also suffered a similar fate, possibly because the sponges impair the protective barrier of skin. There has even been one report of a *Pseudomonas* infection associated with mud wrestling.

On a more serious note, *P. aeruginosa* is a well-known cause of hospital-acquired infections. It causes urinary tract infections in patients with indwelling catheters, bloodstream infections in surgery patients, and lung infections in patients with a tube placed in their airway to support breathing (ventilator patients). What makes these infections particularly troublesome is that *P. aeruginosa* has become resistant to many antibiotics. The genome sequence, which has recently been released, suggests an explanation. In the genome sequence are many sequences that appear to encode efflux pumps such as those known to confer resistance to a variety of antibiotics (see chapter 11). Not all strains of *P. aeruginosa* are able to cause systemic infections. Some seem to be unable to cope with the defenses of blood and are confined to areas of tissue near where the infection began. This is true of the strains that cause infections in cystic fibrosis patients, because although lung infections in these patients can be quite destructive, sepsis is uncommon. Nonetheless, the amount of lung damage done by recurrent lung infections caused by pseudomonads can be sufficient to kill the infected person.

Virulence Factors

Measuring Virulence—Model Systems Raise Exciting New Possibilities

In the case of most bacteria described in this book, the range of animal models is fairly circumscribed. Usually, the animal model of choice is a laboratory rodent. Occasionally, something more exotic, such as a guinea pig or a ferret, is used, but all have in common that they are furry mammals. This is not the case for *P. aeruginosa*. Of course, there is a mouse model, the "burned mouse" model for skin infections. An area on the back of an anesthetized mouse is shaved and burned with an ethanol flame. The bacteria are injected subcutaneously in the burned area. The LD_{50} for wild-type *P. aeruginosa* in this model is less than 100. If the area were not burned, the LD_{50} would be over 10^8, another example of the importance of impaired host defenses in *P. aeruginosa* infections. Some people have expressed concerns about the ethics of this model because of the pain inflicted on the animals, and attempts are being made to replace this model entirely or at least limit its use. For studies of lung infections, there is a guinea pig or rat model. The bacteria are injected into the airway of the animal.

In recent years, some more exotic models have been introduced. One is the plant *Arabidopsis*. The bacteria are inoculated into the leaves, where they produce visible lesions. The power of this model is that *Arabidopsis* has been used as the premier model system for studying plant biology, and as a result many mutant strains of the plant are available. Moreover, the genome sequence for *Arabidopsis* has been determined. In other words, this is a model that is better characterized than most mammalian models, a fact that makes it possible to probe host-microbe interactions at a very advanced level. Don't have any *Arabidopsis* on hand? No problem. You could also use lettuce leaves, another version of the plant model. The drawback to this cheaper and more expedient plant model is that there is not nearly so much genetic information about lettuce as about *Arabidopsis*.

A second nonmammalian model is the nematode *Caenorhabditis elegans*. The origin and fate of every cell of this tiny worm has been mapped, making it an excellent model for studies of development. Now it is being used to study host-bacterium interactions. The unsuspecting worms are fed *P. aeruginosa*. The results depend on how the bacteria are grown prior to inoculation. If they are grown in high-salt medium, the bacteria produce a **phenazine** toxin that kills the worm within 24 h (**fast killing**). If the bacteria are grown in low-salt medium, they do not produce this toxin and kill the worm more slowly, in 1 to 2 days, by a mechanism that appears to involve invasion of tissues by the bacteria (**slow killing**). The two types of killing are probably independent of each other, because mutant pseudomonads that no longer cause fast killing seem to be unaffected in their ability to carry out the slow killing process.

You may be wondering what all of this plant-worm business has to do with human disease. Prepare for an exciting surprise. So far, it appears that many of the mutations that reduce virulence in the *Arabidopsis* or *C. elegans* systems also reduce virulence in the burned mouse model. Accordingly, the plant or worm model can be used for preliminary studies, reducing the need for studies involving mice. Also, many more mutations can be screened in a shorter period of time. This should facilitate progress toward finding new virulence factors. *B. cepacia* and *Salmonella enterica* serovar Typhimurium also cause infections in these hosts, so the plant and nematode models should be of even wider importance than for *P. aeruginosa* alone.

The fact that plants and nematodes can be infected by *P. aeruginosa* is consistent with a larger theme that has been developing from studies outside the *P. aeruginosa* field—the theme of unexpected similarities between the defense systems of animals and plants (Box 16–3). The moral of this developing story seems to be that if you refer to someone as a vegetable or a worm, you are being more scientifically accurate than you realize.

What type of genes are required for virulence in or-

BOX 16–3   Do Plants Have an Immune System?

In many areas, plants and animals seem to have solved problems in different ways. For example, plants live by converting light energy into chemical energy and by fixing atmospheric carbon dioxide to produce cell carbon. Animals obtain energy by eating plants and each other, preformed carbon and energy sources. Plants resist insects by producing potent insecticidal compounds, such as alkaloids, whereas animals simply run away or protect themselves with thick fur coats. Given the large number of differences between plants and animals, it has come as something of a surprise that animals have more in common with plants than was previously thought—at least in their defenses against bacterial infections. When bacteria infect plants, a common symptom is a dark, dry area composed of dead plant cells. This is called the **plant hypersensitive response.** Special plant-produced proteins, called R proteins, which recognize specific bacterial proteins called Avr proteins, trigger the hyper-

sensitive response. The name Avr comes from "avirulence" because the ability of the plant to recognize these proteins makes the bacteria unable to cause serious infection. Many plant pathogenic bacteria inject their proteins into plants using a type III secretion system, a strategy also used by many human pathogens. The plant R proteins have evolved to recognize these proteins and bind to them, similar to an antibody-antigen interaction. The R protein-Avr interaction stimulates a signal transduction cascade that activates the hypersensitive response. Although this response results in the local killing of plant cells, it limits bacterial growth in much the same way that a successful mammalian response walls off an infection, and prevents the bacteria from moving throughout the plant, an outcome that is lethal for the plant.

Source: J. M. McDowell and J. L. Dangl. 2000. Signal transduction in the plant immune response. Trends Biochem. Sci. **25**:79–82.

---

ganisms as diverse as plants, nematodes, and mammals? So far, most of them have proved to be "housekeeping genes," which serve ordinary cellular functions and do not appear to be associated specifically with classical virulence genes, such as toxin genes. One such gene is *dsbA,* which encodes a periplasmic disulfide-forming enzyme that is important in the maturation of periplasmic enzymes. Another such gene is *hrpM,* a homolog of the *Escherichia coli mdoH* gene, which encodes an enzyme involved in synthesis of membrane-derived oligosaccharides. The membrane-derived oligosaccharides are periplasmic oligosaccharides that are part of the bacterium's response to changes in osmolarity. There are also *gacS* and *gacA,* which appear to encode a two-component regulatory system that may control synthesis of secondary metabolites. Finally, there is a gene that might be involved in production of the storage polymer poly-β-hydroxybutyrate. Finding that these genes are important for virulence suggests the possibility that the most fundamental and conserved virulence factors are not necessarily those that cause toxic effects or that target cells and proteins of the host defenses but are proteins that help the bacteria to survive and divide in the plant or animal.

Overview of the Disease Process

The different types of infections caused by *P. aeruginosa* occur in very different settings and progress in different ways. For example, in burn infections, the bacteria cause local inflammation and then disseminate into the bloodstream. In lung infections, the bacteria are growing in a very different environment and face different challenges; a dissemination into the bloodstream is uncommon. In the eye, where the bacteria colonize scratches, they are interacting with the multiple layers of epithelial cells that compose the cornea. Given this, it is not surprising that *P. aeruginosa* has many virulence factors and a complex system for controlling production of these virulence factors.

P. aeruginosa has several general types of virulence factors, which will be described in more detail in the next sections. First, there are the adhesins. Both pili and nonpilus adhesins play a role in adherence. Second, *P. aeruginosa* invades human cells in some cases. Third, there is a type III secretion system that injects toxic proteins into host cells. The injected proteins are toxic for PMNs and macrophages and thus play a role in protecting the bacteria from the host defenses. The proteins can also increase the production of inflammatory cytokines, which may contribute to tissue damage, especially in the lung. Other toxic proteins are excreted into the medium. Some of these excreted proteins are proteases that can degrade tissue proteins or host defense molecules, such as complement components and antibodies. There is also a secreted glycolipid with hemolytic activity that may contribute to lung damage. Finally, the bacteria can produce a polysaccharide slime (**mucoidy**) that is involved in biofilm formation. This trait is thought to be particularly important in the pathogenesis of lung infections in cystic fibrosis patients. Genes encoding these factors are scattered over the chromosome. The distribution of some of the important virulence genes is shown in Figure 16–2.

Adhesins

The ability to adhere to host cells appears to be quite important for colonization of the lung or of a burned or wounded area, because mutations that affect adherence decrease virulence in animal models for burn and lung infections. *P. aeruginosa* produces at least two types of protein adhesins pili and adhesive cell surface components (**nonpilus adhesins**). The pili of *P. aeruginosa* are **type 4 pili,** which are characterized by having a methylated phenylalanine as the first amino acid of the processed pilin subunit. The *P. aeruginosa* pili bind preferentially to asialoG$_{M1}$ gangliosides on host cells. Generally, G$_{M1}$ gangliosides contain a sialic acid moiety. *P. aeruginosa* produces a neuraminidase which removes sialic acid residues from G$_{M1}$ to form the asialoG$_{M1}$, which is a better receptor for the pili. The pili are located at one pole of the cell and, when attached to a host cell, cause a twitching motility that allows the bacteria to move along the cell surface.

Production of pili involves a number of genes, including not only *pilA* (the pilin structural gene) but also *pilB* and *pilC* (two genes involved in pilin assembly) and a group of genes, called **xcp** genes, that encode a transport system designed to excrete proteins to the cell surface. A secretion system called **Xcp,** which is also responsible for secreting some of the toxic exoproteins, is probably needed for proper localization of PilB and PilC, since PilA is secreted through the inner membrane by the normal secretion machinery. A transcriptional activator, PilR controls expression of the pilin structural gene, which is most similar to NtrC, the activator that controls expression of nitrogen-regulated genes, such as the gene for glutamine synthetase (Figure 16–3). In fact, pilin synthesis depends on the nitrogen-specific sigma factor σ^{54}, just as does synthesis of NtrC-controlled genes. The similarity to NtrC and the dependence on σ^{54} suggest that pilin synthesis is regulated at

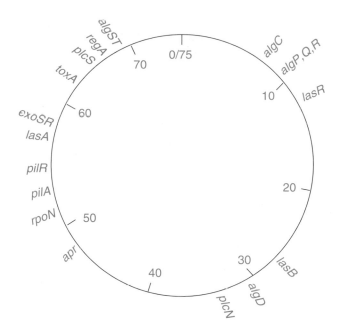

algC: alginate biosynthetic gene
algD: cluster of alginate biosynthetic genes
algP,Q,R,ST: regulatory genes controlling alginate synthesis
apr: gene for alkaline protease
exoS,R: genes required for ExoS and ExoR production, not structural genes
lasA,B: structural genes for elastase
lasR: regulatory gene controlling *lasA,B*
pilA: pilin structural gene
pilR: regulatory gene controlling *pilA*
plcS: gene for hemolytic phospholipase C
regA: regulatory gene controlling *toxA* expression
rpoN: gene for σ^{54}
toxA: gene for exotoxin A

Figure 16–2 Approximate map locations of some *P. aeruginosa* virulence genes. Genes are scattered over the chromosome, not clustered in one location.

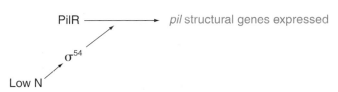

Figure 16–3 Presumed nitrogen regulation of pilin biosynthetic genes. Nitrogen starvation leads to expression of the sigma factor σ^{54} and activation of *pil* gene expression.

some level by nitrogen starvation. Also, since NtrC is one component of a two-component regulatory system, PilR is presumed to be the transcriptional activator component of such a system as well. The sensor component of this system remains to be identified. Production of the nonpilus adhesins also appears to require σ⁵⁴ and is presumably controlled by nitrogen, but the regulatory loci responsible for this control have not been identified.

Although **neuraminidase** is thought to be involved in adherence, neuraminidase production is regulated by osmolarity, not nitrogen levels, and is highest in medium with high osmotic strength. Neuraminidase production is controlled by some of the same regulatory genes that control production of alginate, a polysaccharide that may have a role in biofilm formation as well as in protection of the bacteria from phagocytes (see below).

The pili of *P. aeruginosa* mediate binding to epithelial cells, but not to mucin. *P. aeruginosa* is capable of binding to mucin, however. This binding is mediated by the nonpilus adhesins. There appear to be two of these, one that mediates binding to both mucin and epithelial cells and one that mediates binding to mucin only. The nonpilus mucin-binding adhesin has not been identified and characterized by biochemical means, and the main evidence for its existence comes from studies of mutants. It may be important for lung infections in cystic fibrosis patients, because bacteria bind more effectively to mucin from people with cystic fibrosis.

Another nonpilus adhesin is LPS. *P. aeruginosa* adheres to a chloride channel protein called **CFTR (cystic fibrosis transmembrane conductance regulator).** The gene encoding this protein is mutated in many cystic fibrosis patients. The core polysaccharide of LPS attaches the bacteria to CFTR. *P. aeruginosa* bound to lung cells in this way can then invade them. This is not necessarily good for the bacteria because the epithelial cells are sloughed very readily, and constant elimination of infected cells may actually help to clear the upper airway of bacteria, as the bacteria-laden epithelial cells are propelled out of the airway by the ciliated cells.

The binding of *P. aeruginosa* to normal CFTR and invasion of host cells may make a contribution to virulence in another setting, the human eye. The cornea is composed of many layers of epithelial cells, but only the cells in the lower layers produce CFTR. A scratch would expose these cells, allowing *P. aeruginosa* to attach to and invade them. In this case, since the lower layer cells are not sloughed as are the epithelial cells of the lining of the airway, the bacteria would stay in the site, causing tissue damage because they produce toxic proteins and elicit an inflammatory response.

The Type III Secretion System

Like many other human and plant pathogens, *P. aeruginosa* has a **type III secretion system** that injects toxic proteins directly from the bacterial cytoplasm into the cytoplasm of the host cell (see chapter 9). This mode of toxin delivery is more efficient than relying on extracellular toxin molecules that diffuse away from the bacterial cell. Moreover, the toxic proteins are protected from antibodies that might bind to and neutralize them. Two toxins that are injected by the type III system are **exoenzyme S (ExoS)** and **exoenzyme U (ExoU)**. This strategy is probably aimed at reducing the effectiveness of the phagocyte defense, because ExoS is toxic for PMNs and ExoU is toxic for macrophages.

ExoS and ExoU

Initially, ExoS was something of a mystery. It had ADP-ribosylating activity similar to that of many protein exotoxins, but exogenously applied ExoS did not injure tissue culture cells. Most exotoxins have a binding as well as an enzymatic component that allows them to bind to host cells and internalize their enzymatic component. This mystery was solved when scientists discovered that ExoS is injected into host cells by a type III secretion system. Possibly, the name should now be changed to exotoxin S, but the term exoenzyme has been around so long that such a name change is unlikely.

In vitro, ExoS ADP-ribosylates a number of host cell proteins, including the intermediate filaments of cytoskeleton (a poor substrate) and GTP-binding proteins, such as Ras, which are involved in host cell signal transduction systems. It now appears that the GTP-binding proteins are the main target of this enzyme in vivo. ADP-ribosylation of G proteins is also a feature of other bacterial toxins, e.g., cholera toxin and pertussis toxin. ExoS must be activated by a host cell protein to achieve full enzymatic activity (Figure 16–4A). This host protein has been purified and was originally named **FAS (factor-activating ExoS)**. It is now called **14-3-3 zeta protein.** Normally, 14-3-3 zeta protein interacts with cell proteins, such as Raf, that are part of the cell's signal transduction system. ExoS recruits it for its own activation.

ExoS is clearly important for virulence. Disruption of the gene encoding it raises the LD_{50} in the burned mouse model from 30 to over 10^5 bacteria. The ExoS-minus mutant strain colonized the burned area as well as the wild type but was less able to cause deeper infection. In infections with wild-type *P. aeruginosa*, ExoS is produced by the bacteria growing in the burned area and is detectable in blood before the bacteria are. An ExoS-minus mutant colonized the lungs of rats but did

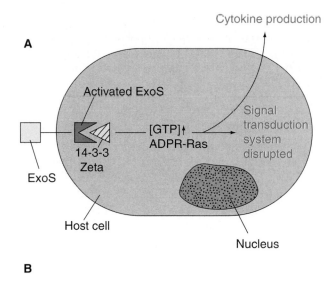

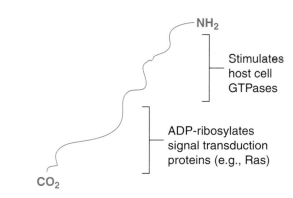

Figure 16–4 (**A**) Activation of ExoS by host cell protein 14-3-3 zeta protein. (**B**) The two domains of activated ExoS have two different functions; the N-terminal portion stimulates GTPases, and the C-terminal portion ADP-ribosylates the regulatory protein Ras.

not cause the extensive damage caused by the wild type. This could be due either to impairment of phagocytic killing of the bacteria, leading to continued infiltration of phagocytes into the area, or to some more direct toxic effect of ExoS on the lungs themselves.

ExoS has a second activity. It upregulates the production of cytokines and chemokines by cells that produce these proinflammatory proteins. This activity is not too surprising given the fact that ExoS inactivates proteins involved in the signal transduction systems of eukaryotic cells. These signal transduction systems regulate, among other things, the production of cytokines and chemokines. ExoS has a third activity. Whereas the C-terminal portion of the protein mediates the ADP-ribosylation reaction, the N-terminal portion of the protein causes tissue culture cells to round up. Rounding up of cultured cells is an indication that the cytoskeleton of the cell has been altered in some way. Investigations

have shown that the N-terminal segment actually stimulates the GTPase activity of some of the same signal transduction proteins the C terminus was inactivating. Although this may sound like two contradictory activities, with the C-terminal portion inactivating and the N-terminal portion activating the target signal transduction protein, the net effect of the bifunctional action of the intact ExoS would be to short-circuit the signal transduction system of the cell. In the case of PMNs, the effect of the toxin would be to render them unable to migrate toward the bacteria or to ingest them. Not much is known about the regulation of ExoS production. Production is maximal if bacteria are grown at 30 to 32°C (rather than 37°C) in highly aerated medium. It is not clear if the requirement for aeration simply reflects a stimulation of enzyme production as a general feature of stimulated protein synthesis under conditions that maximize energy production by the bacteria.

ExoU has not been studied nearly as intensively as ExoS. ExoU is toxic for macrophages but not for PMNs, which seem to be the main targets of ExoS. How ExoU kills macrophages remains to be determined.

Exotoxin A

P. aeruginosa produces an exotoxin, **exotoxin A,** that has the same mechanism of action as diphtheria toxin (see chapter 9). It ADP-ribosylates **elongation factor-2,** an important player in protein synthesis. However, the two proteins differ sufficiently that antibodies to diphtheria toxin do not react with exotoxin A and vice versa. Also, the receptor for exotoxin A on host cells is a 300-kDa glycoprotein, which is not the same as the receptor for diphtheria toxin. After binding to the host cell receptor, the enzymatic portion of exotoxin A is internalized by endocytosis. Proteolytic nicking and reduction of a disulfide bond activate the enzymatic portion. Another similarity to diphtheria toxin is that exotoxin A synthesis is regulated by iron, with maximal expression seen when iron levels are low. Rather than being regulated directly by a Fur-like repressor, as iron acquisition genes are regulated in many bacteria, the exotoxin A gene (*toxA*) is regulated by a transcriptional activator (**RegA**), which is in turn controlled by the *P. aeruginosa* analog of **Fur,** the iron-regulated repressor. Most clinical isolates of *P. aeruginosa* produce exotoxin A, and mutants that are deficient in exotoxin A production exhibit reduced virulence in animal models. Thus, exotoxin A appears to have a direct role in virulence, possibly acting to cause tissue damage and to diminish the activity of phagocytes.

Elastolytic Activity

Elastin is a protein that accounts for nearly 30% of the protein in lung tissue. Its name arises from the fact that it allows tissues to have elastic properties needed for an organ like the lung, in which intake and expulsion of air require expansion and contraction of alveoli. Elastin is also an important component of blood vessel walls and is responsible for their resilience. *P. aeruginosa* has elastolytic activity which appears to be due to the concerted activity of two enzymes, LasA and LasB. Originally, **LasB** (called **elastase**) was thought to be responsible for the elastolytic activity of *P. aeruginosa*. However, LasB is not, strictly speaking, an elastase (i.e., an enzyme that has substrate specificity for elastin) but is a zinc metalloprotease that cleaves a number of proteins, including elastin. Elastin is not the best substrate for LasB; purified LasB has a much lower elastolytic activity than the culture fluid of *P. aeruginosa*. This finding suggests that LasB does not act alone. It now appears likely that a second enzyme, LasA, acts synergistically with LasB to degrade elastin. **LasA is a serine-type protease** that nicks elastin but does not degrade it. Nicking elastin probably denatures it so that it is more easily attacked by LasB.

LasA and LasB are detectable in the lungs of cystic fibrosis patients, and people with *P. aeruginosa* infections produce antibodies against these two proteins. Thus, LasA and LasB are produced during an infection. Animal model studies further support an important role for LasA and LasB in virulence. Nonetheless, there is still some uncertainty as to what that role is. Elastolytic activity of *P. aeruginosa* may be a cause of direct damage to the lung in the initial phases of infection but may not have this role in chronic infections because of the presence of antielastolytic antibodies. Also, it is important to recall that, despite the name "elastase," elastin is by no means the only protein degraded by the LasA-LasB combination. LasA and LasB may also aid in initial establishment of the infection, because they can degrade antibodies, complement components, and α_1-proteinase inhibitor (which prevents damage of tissue by PMN proteases). In chronic infections, high levels of antibodies to LasA and LasB may cause immune complex formation and deposition that leads to complement activation and attraction of PMNs. PMNs produce an elastase of their own which is far more active than LasA and LasB. Small quantities of LasA might enhance degradation of lung elastin due to PMN elastase just as it enhances elastin breakdown by LasB. Breakdown of elastin in blood vessel walls could explain the hemorrhages often seen in patients with *P. aeruginosa* lung infections.

Production of LasA and LasB is affected by a number of factors, including the concentration of iron and zinc in the medium. Iron and zinc probably act at a post-transcriptional level. Zinc is needed for activation of LasB (a zinc metalloprotease). LasA and LasB are reg-

ulated at the transcriptional level by a transcriptional activator, **LasR** (Figure 16–5). LasR responds to an autoinducer, synthesized by **LasI**. The autoinducer is a **3-oxo-decanoate (C12) homoserine lactone (3-oxo-C12-HSL,** formerly called **PAI-1),** which is similar in structure to autoinducers produced by other gram-negative bacteria. In contrast to previously characterized autoinducers, this one does not diffuse freely through the bacterial membranes. Instead, it is externalized by a special efflux pump, which spans both membranes. The efflux pump is encoded by *mexA*, *mexB*, and *oprM* and is produced constitutively. How the autoinducer gets back into the cell to interact with LasR is not known. Whatever the mechanism, it is very widespread, since the autoinducer can enter *E. coli*.

The LasR–3-oxo-C12-HSL combination (activated LasR) activates a number of genes. One of them is *lasI*, which encodes the synthesizer of the autoinducer. Thus, there is a burst of further autoinducer production and more activation of LasR. This feedback loop makes it possible for the bacteria to respond quickly by producing lots of the virulence factors controlled by LasR (Figure 16–5). The genes whose expression is upregulated by activated LasR include the genes that encode LasA and LasB (*lasA*, *lasB*), a gene that encodes an alkaline protease (*aprA*; see next section), the gene that encodes

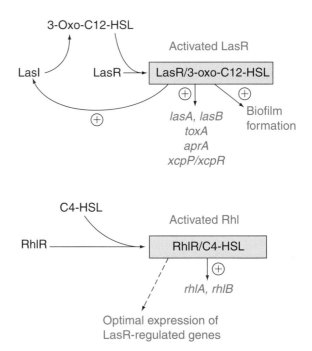

Figure 16–5 Quorum-sensing systems of *P. aeruginosa*. The autoinducers (3-oxo-C12-HSL and C4-HSL) bind to a regulatory protein (LasR or RhlR), activating it to the form that stimulates gene expression. LasI synthesizes the autoinducer. *rhlA* and *rhlB* encode the enzymes that synthesize rhamnolipid.

exotoxin A (*toxA*), and genes encoding two components of the excretion system that exports these exoproteins (**xcpP, xcpR**). Activated LasR is also essential for biofilm formation.

LasR is clearly important for virulence. There are two other autoinducers produced by *P. aeruginosa* whose role in virulence is not so well established. One is another homoserine lactone autoinducer, except with a butyryl group (C4) rather than a 3-oxo-C12 group. It is called **C4-homoserine lactone** (**C4-HSL**; formerly **PAI-2**). C4-HSL activates a protein called **RhlR** by binding it. Activated RhlR in turn activates expression of two genes (**rhlA, rhlB**) that encode enzymes involved in synthesis of a rhamnose-containing glycolipid (**rhamnolipid**). The rhamnolipid may be involved in cell damage (see next section). RhlR is also needed for optimal expression of the genes controlled by LasR, but the mechanism of this interaction remains to be worked out. There are clearly interactions between the LasR and RhlR systems that are currently under investigation. The third autoinducer was discovered because it affected *lasB* expression. In contrast to the homoserine lactone-type autoinducers, this one proved to be a **2-heptyl-3-hydroxy-4-quinolone** compound. This is the first quinolone autoinducer to be identified.

Other Extracellular Factors

P. aeruginosa produces a number of extracellular enzymes, in addition to ExoS and LasA and LasB. The roles of these enzymes are still uncertain, but they could contribute to tissue damage in lung and eye infections. The enzymes include an alkaline protease and a **phospholipase C (Plc)**. There is also an excreted nonenzyme glycolipid, rhamnolipid (Rhl), that solubilizes phospholipids. The possible significance of this can be inferred from a feature of the physiology of the lung. In the lung, the alveoli and the rest of the airway are coated with a liquid consisting of water and a phospholipid surfactant. The surfactant reduces the surface tension of the water so that the alveoli do not collapse completely when air leaves them during breathing. If they did, it would be very difficult to reinflate them. In fact, infants with a defect in surfactant production have difficulty breathing. In sections from the lungs of a cystic fibrosis patient, many collapsed alveoli are seen. This could be explained by a combination of rhamnolipid and Plc action. The rhamnolipid solubilizes the surfactant, making it easier for the Plc to degrade the surfactant (Figure 16–6). It is not clear how this would benefit the bacteria, but it could explain, at least in part, the progressive worsening of lung function in cystic fibrosis patients with recurring *P. aeruginosa* infections.

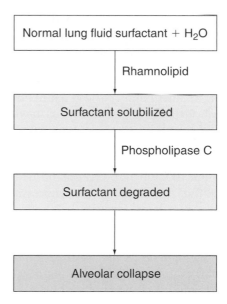

Figure 16–6 Synergistic action of rhamnolipid and phospholipase C.

Alginate Production

An interesting and unique virulence property of *P. aeruginosa*, which is unquestionably important for lung infections but may also contribute to wound and burn infections, is production of an acetylated form of the polysaccharide alginate. **Alginate** is a polymer of mannuronic and guluronic acid that forms a viscous gel around the bacteria. Alginate production is frequently referred to as mucoidy because colonies producing alginate have a wet glistening (mucoid) appearance, which is very different from that of colonies not producing alginate. Polymers like alginate allow marine bacteria to form biofilms on surfaces (rocks, aquatic plants). The ability to form biofilms appears to be important for their survival in the marine environment. *P. aeruginosa* has adapted this trait to aid its survival when it colonizes the human lung.

Alginate production is highly regulated, and bacteria rapidly lose this trait when they are grown on rich laboratory media. When nonmucoid isolates are introduced into the lung of a rat, they rapidly convert to the mucoid (alginate-producing) phenotype. This indicates there is a strong selection for alginate production in the lung. Bacteria isolated initially from the lungs of cystic fibrosis patients are not mucoid but become alginate producers over time. Thus, there seems to be a selection pressure in the human lung that causes the bacteria to begin to produce alginate. Recently, scientists uncovered a clue as to what might be controlling the switch from nonmucoid (smooth) colonies to mucoid colonies. A biofilm formed by the smooth form of the bacteria was exposed to low levels of peroxide, such as might be released by PMNs in the lung. Mucoid variants were observed. Thus, peroxide or some other reactive form of oxygen may be responsible, at least in part, for the switch from smooth to mucoid form that occurs in the lung during an infection. A curious feature of these mucoid variants is that they had mutations in *mucA*, a gene that encodes an inhibitor of *alg* gene expression. The same mutation had been seen previously in mucoid colonies isolated directly from the lungs of cystic fibrosis patients. Thus, the switch could be at the level of genetic mutation rather than activation or repression of transcription of a regulatory protein that controls alginate synthesis.

Although alginate clearly plays a role in the virulence of *P. aeruginosa*, its precise function is not completely clear. Alginate production is not essential for biofilm formation, at least in vitro, but in the lung the bacteria are embedded in a copious slime layer. One possible function for alginate in the lung is to act as an adhesin, preventing the bacteria from being expelled from the lung. A second possibility is that the alginate slime layer makes it more difficult for phagocytes to ingest and kill the bacteria, just by acting as a physical barrier.

Most of the genes that encode alginate biosynthetic enzymes are clustered in one region of the chromosome in an operon. The first gene in this cluster, *algD*, encodes **GDP mannose dehydrogenase,** the first committed step in alginate biosynthesis. Regulatory genes are located in two areas of the chromosome far removed from the biosynthetic genes, with one exception. A biosynthetic gene, *algC* (which encodes **phosphomannomutase**), is located within one of the regulatory gene clusters (Figure 16–7) but is evidently coregulated with the other biosynthetic genes.

Production of alginate is an energy-consuming activity for the bacteria. Thus, it is not surprising that expression of alginate biosynthetic genes is tightly regulated and is regulated at multiple levels. The signals for expression of alginate synthetic genes include high osmolarity and low nitrogen concentrations. Some of the regulatory proteins identified to date are listed in Table 16–2. This is certainly not a complete list, but it gives an indication of how complex the regulation of alginate production is and how different types of environmental signals might affect alginate production. Regulation occurs on at least three levels. There is a genetic switch (*algS, algT*) which allows the bacteria to switch from mucoid to nonmucoid (**phase variation**). This switch must be on for alginate production to proceed. In strains with the switch in the "on" position, alginate synthesis is further regulated at the transcriptional level by a com-

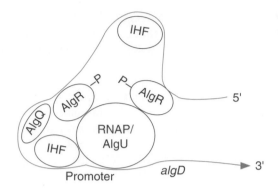

Figure 16–7 Proposed model for the complex that activates transcription of the *alg* gene cluster in which *algD* is the first gene. RNAP, RNA polymerase. (Adapted from S. Roychoudhury, N. A. Zielinski, A. J. Ninfa, N. E. Allen, L. N. Jungheim, T. I. Nicas, and A. M. Chakrabarty. 1993. Inhibitors of two-component signal transduction systems: inhibition of alginate gene activation in *Pseudomonas aeruginosa. Proc. Natl. Acad. Sci. USA* **90:**965–969, with permission of the publisher.)

plex containing **AlgP,** activated **AlgR,** and some other regulatory proteins. Formation of this complex is essential for expression of *algC* and *algD*.

AlgQ and AlgR constitute a two-component regulatory system, with AlgQ as the sensor component that phosphorylates AlgR, which in turn activates transcription of the *alg* genes. This two-component system probably senses osmolarity, because AlgR is similar in sequence to OmpR, a protein known to regulate expression of porin genes in response to osmolarity. A **histonelike protein** (AlgP) also participates in regulation of the *algD* cluster and may affect supercoiling of the operator region. Changes in supercoiling can cause changes in the level of gene expression. In other pathogens, histonelike proteins are associated with temperature regulation, but the signal sensed by AlgP remains to be determined. There are two strong and one weak AlgR binding sites upstream of the *algD* promoter, located far enough apart that DNA bending would be necessary for them to form a complex with RNA polymerase. Thus, the DNA bending protein **IHF** is probably needed to allow the complex to form. IHF stands for integration host factor. IHF was first found associated with the integration complex of phage lambda but has now been found to function as a DNA bending protein in many other types of complexes, including regulatory complexes.

Another protein, **AlgU,** which is essential for alginate production, has amino acid similarity to known sigma factors. Sigma factors determine the promoter-binding specificity of RNA polymerase. There is no con-

Table 16–2 Complex regulation of genes involved in alginate production

Regulatory protein	Characteristics	Effects on alginate production
AlgB	Activator half of two-component system (other half not identified); similar to NtrC	Enhances expression of *algD* (mechanism unknown); probably responds to nitrogen level
AlgP (AlgR3)	Histonelike protein	Part of complex that activates *algD* expression; signal unknown
AlgQ (AlgR2)	Sensory transduction component of two-component system; phosphorylates AlgR	Senses signal (probably osmolarity) that allows assembly of complex required for *algD* expression
AlgR (AlgR1)	Activator component of two-component system; similar to OmpR	Essential for expression of *algD*
IHF	DNA bending protein	Part of complex required for *algD* expression
AlgS,T	Controls switching from alginate production to nonproduction	Phase variation (on-off); signal not known
AlgU	Sigma factor	Required for *algD* expression

sensus σ^{70}-type promoter sequence upstream of *algD*, so it is possible that AlgU plays the role of a sigma factor in promoting the ability of RNA polymerase to recognize and bind to the promoter region of *algD*.

A third level of regulation is mediated by **AlgB.** Disruption of *algB* reduces expression of *algD* considerably but does not eliminate it. Thus, AlgB seems to be required for high-level expression of *algD*. There is some evidence that AlgB does not act directly on the algD promoter region, as does the AlgR complex. AlgB, like AlgR, appears from sequence similarity to be the activator component of a two-component system. The sensor component of this system has not been identified. AlgB is an NtrC homolog and may thus be sensing nitrogen starvation. There are conflicting reports about the role of the nitrogen starvation sigma factor σ^{54} in alginate production. Possibly, this is due to the fact that σ^{54} is involved with AlgB in indirect regulation of *algD* expression.

An intriguing feature of the nonmucoid to mucoid shift is that levels of some of the extracellular proteins, such as LasA and LasB, decrease during this transition. This change is reversed when the bacteria revert to the nonmucoid state.

LPS Variation

LPS structure also varies during the nonmucoid to mucoid transition. In nonmucoid strains, the *P. aeruginosa* LPS has long O-antigen chains and is negatively charged (B form), whereas in mucoid strains, LPS has shorter O chains and a sugar composition that makes it much more neutral (A form). The switch from B form to A form may not be tied directly to mucoidy but rather may reflect a phase transition system that, like the mucoid phase transition system, responds to some characteristic of the lung environment. The A form is more susceptible to the membrane attack complex formed by activated complement components C5b to C9, but this is probably not a problem in the lung, where complement levels are low. The advantage of this switch in LPS type may be that it makes the bacteria more resistant to antimicrobial peptides that kill microbes by making pores in their membranes. The killing action of airway surface liquid is due in part to the presence of such peptides. There is also a change in the lipid A portion of LPS; a palmitate group is added. This change too seems to increase resistance to killing by the antimicrobial peptides produced by the lung.

Antibiotic Resistance

One of the reasons *P. aeruginosa* is considered to be a particularly dangerous pathogen is that it is naturally resistant to most antibiotics. Only a few antibiotics are effective. These include fluoroquinolones, amoxicillin, gentamicin, and certain of the newer broad-spectrum β-lactam antibiotics, such as imipenem. Even these antibiotics are not effective against all strains of *P. aeruginosa*. The continuing problem of treating *P. aeruginosa* infections is serious enough in hospitalized patients with nosocomial infections but is most dramatically illustrated in cystic fibrosis patients, who eventually become infected with a strain that is so resistant it cannot be treated. The antibiotic resistance problem has led to intensive research into how *P. aeruginosa* interacts with antibiotics and how resistance to the few remaining front-line antibiotics develops.

The first step in the interaction between antibiotics and gram-negative bacteria occurs at the outer membrane. Some antibiotics enter the periplasm through porins. One such antibiotic is **imipenem,** a member of the β-lactam family. Imipenem enters the periplasmic space via a specific porin called **OprD**. Resistance to imipenem has developed rapidly among clinical isolates of *P. aeruginosa* as imipenem has been more widely used in clinical settings. The main mechanism of resistance appears to be a mutation that results in loss of OprD, rather than acquisition of β-lactamase. Other antibiotics, such as fluoroquinolones and aminoglycosides, appear to transit the outer membrane by a porin-independent method. In both cases, the antibiotics either bind directly to negatively charged LPS molecules or chelate divalent cations that stabilize LPS molecules in the outer membrane. In both cases, the result is destabilization of the outer membrane, disrupting this barrier sufficiently to allow the antibiotic to gain access to the periplasm and thus to the cytoplasmic membrane, through which it is transported into the cell cytoplasm, where its target is located. (Recall that the target of quinolones is DNA gyrase, and the target of aminoglycosides is the ribosome; see chapter 10.)

An intriguing finding from the analysis of the *P. aeruginosa* genome sequence data was that there are many genes encoding proteins with a deduced amino acid sequence similar to those of known antibiotic efflux pumps. In many bacteria, efflux pumps are effective resistance proteins, which pump antibiotics out of the cell. Some of these efflux pumps can eject more than one class of antibiotics. Although the *P. aeruginosa* efflux genes have not yet been shown to confer antibiotic resistance, the existence of numerous efflux pumps could explain why *P. aeruginosa* is resistant to so many antibiotics.

Future Directions

It would be impossible to remove *P. aeruginosa* from the environment, even the internal environment of a hospital, because it is so hardy and so metabolically versatile. It will always find niches to colonize, such as mop water or spent disinfectant solutions in a hospital. Now that more is known about the kind of conditions that predispose patients to develop *P. aeruginosa* infections, it is easier to monitor these patients closely for signs of an incipient infection. Infections are much easier to control if they are caught at an early stage.

Since *P. aeruginosa* seeks out chinks in the defense armor of the body, it can also be fought on that battleground. Artificial skin for burn patients is currently under development and could lessen their time at risk for infection. Better management of patients with urinary catheters, so that the catheters stay in place for as short a time as possible, reduces that window of opportunity. Careful monitoring of ventilators to make sure that the water aerosols are not contaminated with bacteria

should help to prevent ventilator-associated pneumonia. Another preventive strategy that shows considerable promise is scrupulous cleanliness, hand washing, and glove wearing in intensive care wards that contain highly vulnerable patients, such as low-birth-weight infants or patients with underlying conditions that predispose them to infection. Proper use of contact lenses to prevent scarring and the development of lenses that resist colonization by bacteria can help to lessen the threat of eye infections. Educating contact lens wearers about the problem is key to this type of preventive strategy. Now that the cystic fibrosis gene has been identified, genetic counseling to prevent the birth of children with this defect—and one day, hopefully, successful gene therapy to correct the cystic fibrosis genetic trait in those who already have the disease—may bring this problem under control. It is encouraging that improved strategies for monitoring and treating cystic fibrosis patients have already greatly extended their life spans. In the end, however, the need is still strong for new antibiotics that are effective against *P. aeruginosa*'s armamentarium of resistance mechanisms.

Scientists are also looking for new antibiotic targets, such as regulatory proteins that control essential virulence genes. Preventing colonization of vulnerable body sites such as the lung is critical for preventing episodes of disease. Although it sometimes appears that victory lies with the pseudomonads, we humans have not yet lost completely, and we are not giving up the struggle. Basic scientists like to justify their research projects as leading to the discovery of new drugs to combat the bacteria, but in the case of *P. aeruginosa*, the humbler tried-and-true methods of prevention and early intervention are most likely to have the greatest impact, at least in the near future.

SELECTED READINGS

Coburn, J., and D. W. Frank. 1999. Macrophages and epithelial cells respond differently to *Pseudomonas aeruginosa* type III secretion system. *Infect. Immun.* **67:**3151–3154.

Goehring, U. M., G. Schmidt, K. J. Pederson, K. Aktories, and J. T. Barbieri. 1999. The N-terminal domain of *Pseudomonas aeruginosa* exoenzyme S is a GTPase-activating protein for Rho GTPases. *J. Biol. Chem.* **274:**36369–36372.

Lyczak, J. B., C. L. Cannon, and G. B. Pier. 2000. Establishment of *Pseudomonas aeruginosa* infections: lessons from a versatile opportunist. *Microbes Infect.* **2:**1051–1060.

Mathee, K, O. Ciofu, C. Sternberg, P. W. Lindum, J. I. Campbell, P. Jensen, A. H. Johnson, M. Givskov, D. E. Ohman, S. Molin, N. Horby, and A. Kharazmi. 1999. Mucoid conversion of *Pseudomonas aeruginosa* by hydrogen peroxide: a mechanism for virulence activation in the cystic fibrosis lung. *Microbiology* **145:**1349–1357.

Pearson, J. P., C. VanDelden, and B. H. Iglewski. 1999. Active efflux and diffusion are involved in transport of *Pseudomonas aeruginosa* cell-to-cell signals. *J. Bacteriol.* **181:**1203–1210.

Pier, G. B. 2000. Peptides, *Pseudomonas aeruginosa*, polysaccharides, and lipopolysaccharides—players in the predicament of cystic fibrosis patients. *Trends Microbiol.* **8:**247–251.

Rahme, L. G., F. M. Ausubel, H. Cao, E. Drenkard, B. C. Goumnerov, G. W. Lau, S. Mahajan-Miklos, J. Plotnikova, M.-W. Tan, J. Tsongalis, C. L. Walendziewicz, and R. G. Tompkins. 2000. Plants and animals share functionally common bacterial virulence factors. *Proc. Natl. Acad. Sci. USA* **97:**8815–8821.

Van Delden, C., and B. H. Iglewski. 1998. Cell-to-cell signaling and *Pseudomonas aeruginosa* infections. *Emerg. Infect. Dis.* **4:**551–560.

Wall, D., and D. Kaiser. 1999. Type IV pili and cell motility. *Mol. Microbiol.* **32:**1–10.

Zhang, L., H. Wang, S. C. Masters, J. T. Barbieri, and H. Fu. 1999. Residues of 14-3-3 zeta required for activation of exoenzyme S of *Pseudomonas aeruginosa*. *Biochemistry* **38:**12159–12164.

SUMMARY OUTLINE

Characteristics of *P. aeruginosa*

Gram-negative rod

Respiratory metabolism (nonfermenter)

Great metabolic versatility allows it to occupy many niches

Diseases

Infections of burn patients (burn and lung)

Lung infections in cystic fibrosis patients

Nosocomial lung and wound infections

Nosocomial urinary tract infections

Eye infections associated with contact lenses

Infections of plants

Virulence factors

Adhesins
  Type 4 pili, twitching motility, asialo G_{M1} ganglioside receptor
  Nonpilus mucin-binding adhesin
  Core polysaccharide of LPS—CFTR protein receptor

Type III secretion system—injects ExoS and ExoU into eukaryotic cells

Xcp secretion system—secretes toxins and enzymes into the extracellular fluid

Toxic proteins

ExoS—affects GTP levels and activities of GTP-binding host cell proteins; activated by host 14-3-3 zeta protein

ExoU—toxic for macrophages

Exotoxin A—ADP-ribosylates elongation factor-2, stops host cell protein synthesis

LasA and LasB—degrade elastin, antibodies, and other proteins; act synergistically

Alginate

Alkaline protease

Phospholipase C and rhamnolipid—may act to destroy lung surfactant

Regulation of virulence genes

Quorum sensing—autoinducers
  3-oxo-C12-HSL
    Synthesized by LasI
    Externalized by efflux pump encoded by *mexA*, *mexB*, and *oprM*

(*continued*)

SUMMARY OUTLINE (*continued*)

        Activates LasR—activates several other genes
           lasI—leads to increased production of autoinducer
           lasA and *lasB*—encode elastase activity

    C4-HSL activates RhlR
        Activated RhlR activates expression of *rhlA* and *rhlB*—synthesis of rhamnolipid
        Activated RhlR needed for optimal expression of genes controlled by LasR

   Regulation of alginate biosynthesis genes (*algD* complex)—occurs at three levels
      Genetic switch (*algS, algT*)—phase variation
      Transcriptional regulation
         AlgQ and AlgR—two-component system; activates transcription of *alg* structural genes
         AlgP—histonelike protein
         IHF—allows RNA polymerase binding
         AlgU—sequence similar to sigma factor
      Nitrogen regulation—AlgB is part of two-component system

Antibiotic resistance

   Resistant to many antibiotics

   Variety of mechanisms

QUESTIONS

Answers to the questions can be found in Appendix 2.

1. In previous chapters, you have been introduced to bacteria that cause very specific diseases, the specialists. *Yersinia pestis* and *Borrelia burgdorferi* are examples of this type of bacteria. *P. aeruginosa* lies at the other end of the spectrum, with *Staphylococcus aureus* and *Streptococcus pyogenes*. Can you identify any traits that differentiate the specialists from the generalists?

2. In earlier chapters, we have belabored the concept that changing human practices create new niches for bacteria to occupy. To what extent and in what ways does *P. aeruginosa* illustrate this concept?

3. In the love-hate relationship between pseudomonads and plants, pseudomonads both protect and harm plants. By analogy, are there ways that they might be protective in the human body? If it were proved to have that trait, what are the limitations of using *P. aeruginosa* as a protective agent in the colon? On the skin?

4. In nature, nematodes ingest soil, which contains pseudomonads in abundance. How do you explain the fact that *P. aeruginosa* kills *C. elegans* in the laboratory?

5. Why has *P. aeruginosa* continued to be a major problem in hospitals, where the gram-positive cocci seem to have been displacing other gram-negative bacteria as the pathogens du jour? Is it true, as someone has undoubtedly said somewhere, that "ye shall have the pseudomonads with you always?"

6. *P. aeruginosa* and related pseudomonads are being developed as bioremediation agents. Are there some public health issues that ought to be taken into consideration as these bioremediation schemes are implemented?

7. In the lungs of cystic fibrosis patients, *P. aeruginosa* goes to a lot of trouble to produce alginate and alter its LPS. What are the potential benefits to the bacteria of these two strategies?

8. Would alginate be a good vaccine candidate? Why or why not?

9. Chemicals that act as antagonists of the *P. aeruginosa* autoinducer have been proposed as prospective antipseudomonad compounds. How would this work? What are some strengths and drawbacks to this approach?

10. Comment on the fact that mutant screens using the new worm and plant models for *P. aeruginosa* infection are not turning up the classical *P. aeruginosa* virulence genes such as *exoS* and *exoA*.

17

Bordetella pertussis

KEY FEATURES

Bordetella pertussis

CHARACTERISTICS
Gram-negative coccobacillus
Nutritionally fastidious

DISEASE
Whooping cough

RESERVOIR
Humans (mainly adults)

MAJOR VIRULENCE FACTORS
Adhesins, specificity for ciliated cells
Several toxins (e.g., pertussis toxin)
LPS and a peptidoglycan fragment (tracheal cytotoxin)
Antiphagocytic mechanisms

PREVENTION AND TREATMENT
Antibiotics not useful except to prevent spread
Vaccine—P of DTP (killed whole cells); aP of DTaP (subunit vaccine, toxoid, and adhesins)

Whooping Cough

Characteristics of the Disease

Whooping cough is an acute respiratory disease caused by *Bordetella pertussis*, a gram-negative coccobacillus. *B. pertussis* is a nutritionally fastidious bacterium and is normally cultivated on medium containing blood, a good source of many nutrients. *B. pertussis* is spread by aerosols or by direct contact with an infected person or an asymptomatic carrier. In the first stage of the infection, the symptoms of the disease resemble those of the common cold. In the second stage of the disease, a dry cough develops, which becomes paroxysmal and is later accompanied by excess mucus production and vomiting. As the second stage progresses, the episodes of coughing can become so severe that they cause convulsions and cyanosis. The sharp intake of

263

breath between paroxysms of coughing, as the infected person struggles for air, sounds like a whoop. This symptom gives the disease its name.

Because the early symptoms are so nonspecific, whooping cough is seldom diagnosed until the infected person begins to develop the severe paroxysmal cough that is the hallmark of the disease. At this point, antibiotic treatment is ineffective in ameliorating the patient's symptoms but is sometimes given because antibiotics reduce the chance for transmission of the disease to others. The infected person is most contagious during the initial stage of the disease before it is clearly distinguishable from a common cold, a fact that contributes to the spread of the disease. In some cases, edema, hemorrhages, and vascular plugs in the brain develop and produce irreversible neurological damage.

The severe form of whooping cough just described is seen almost exclusively in infants and children. Adults, even immunized adults, can develop a milder form of the disease. The disease in adults, characterized by a cough of more than 2 weeks' duration, has been called the "100 days cough." It has been estimated that 20 to 25% of adults who have a persistent cough are infected with *B. pertussis*. Adults colonized with *B. pertussis*, however, may not exhibit any symptoms. Adults with a persistent cough or asymptomatic carriers can transmit the disease to susceptible members of the population and are a particular danger to very young infants who have not received all of their immunizations.

The Vaccine Dilemma

For many years, whooping cough was considered to be a solved problem, at least in developed countries, because an effective vaccine was available (Box 17–1). The original whooping cough vaccine was a suspension of killed bacteria. It was administered for years as part of the trivalent vaccine known as **DTP** (D for diphtheria toxoid, T for tetanus toxoid, and P for pertussis killed cells). Unfortunately, the pertussis part of the vaccine caused side effects, as is frequently the case with vaccines consisting of whole killed bacteria. Approximately 20% of babies who received the DTP vaccine experienced mild side effects, ranging from pain in the area of the injection to a generalized discomfort that made them fussy for a couple of days after receiving the vaccine. About 0.1% of infants experienced convulsions soon after receiving the vaccine, and in a very small number of cases, severe and irreversible brain damage followed. This last presumed side effect is so rare that it is difficult to rule it in or out. Certainly, there is no

direct proof that the whooping cough vaccine causes brain damage.

Because whooping cough is a serious, sometimes fatal, disease, parents who had lived through whooping cough outbreaks tended to view the very low risk of serious side effects as an acceptable alternative to the disease itself. Yet, it would be better to have a form of the vaccine with reduced or nonexistent side effects. A solution to the side effects problem was to develop a new pertussis vaccine which, like the vaccines for diphtheria and tetanus, consisted of purified components and was thus much less likely to produce side effects. This vaccine, called **aP** for **acellular pertussis,** is composed of a toxoided toxin and an adhesin (see later section). The aP vaccine is now replacing the old form of the vaccine and seems to be very effective in preventing whooping cough. It clearly has fewer short-term side effects than the old vaccine. Since the existence of long-term neurological side effects is controversial because of the very low numbers of cases, it is impossible to know whether the new vaccine has reduced these effects, if in fact they exist.

Overview of the Infection Process

The first step in a *B. pertussis* infection is colonization of the respiratory mucosa (Figure 17–1). The portion of the airway colonized by *B. pertussis* lies between the entrance to the airway and the beginning of the lungs. Normally, bacteria that enter the airway are trapped in mucus, and then mucin blobs containing the bacteria are swept out of the airway by the ciliated cells. *B. pertussis* circumvents this host defense by binding preferentially to the ciliated cells in this region of the airway and multiplying on their surfaces (Figure 17–2). Colonization of ciliated cells ultimately results in the death of these cells due to production of toxic compounds by the bacteria. In some cases of whooping cough, *B. pertussis* may actually invade the lung and cause a form of pneumonia, but pneumonia is relatively uncommon. Similarly, the bacteria do not move into the bloodstream to cause septicemia.

Virulence Factors

Model Systems

ANIMAL MODELS. Primates exposed to aerosols of *B. pertussis* develop symptoms similar to those seen in humans, including the characteristic paroxysmal cough, but primates are not used for routine virulence testing because they are so expensive to acquire and maintain. Laboratory rodents can be infected with *B. pertussis*, but

BOX 17–1   What Happens When Parents Lose Faith in Vaccination?

Before the vaccine became available, whooping cough was a common childhood disease. Since most of today's parents have never seen a case of whooping cough, they tend to dismiss it as something that is not so bad. In fact, in the days before the vaccine, about 15% of infants who had whooping cough developed pneumonia, a very serious disease. Moreover, 0.1 to 4% developed severe neurological problems. Death was also a strong possibility. Today, in countries that do not provide the vaccine, thousands of deaths due to whooping cough occur each year. Introduction of the whole-cell pertussis vaccine in developed countries in the 1950s resulted in a dramatic decrease in the incidence of the disease.

In the 1970s, lulled into complacency by the low number of whooping cough cases seen during the past 2 decades, parents and physicians began to question whether the alleged risks of taking the vaccine were worth the benefit. Exaggerated media reports of the risks further fueled the fire of an antivaccination backlash. In Japan, where there had been few cases of the disease and no deaths, opposition to the vaccine became so strong that in the mid-1970s, physicians began to replace the DTP vaccine with the DT formulation. By 1976, only about 10% of children received the DTP formulation, down from over 80% a few years before. In 1979, an epidemic of whooping cough occurred. There were more than 13,000 cases and 41 deaths.

A similar progression of campaigns against vaccination, followed by large outbreaks of disease, occurred in Europe, the United Kingdom, and the former Soviet Union. In countries such as the United States and some of the Eastern European countries that stuck with their DTP vaccination program, no such epidemics occurred. The irony of this tragic error in judgment, which resulted in the deaths of hundreds of infants and children and irreversible neurological damage in some of the survivors, was that it was a decision made in the name of protecting children's health.

In the late 1990s, the antivaccination fanatics, who had now had 2 decades to forget the debacle of the 1970s, swung into action again and are still going strong. One hopes that these misguided people will not convince enough parents to forgo vaccinations for their children to doom another generation of children to experiencing the horror of whooping cough and, in some cases, dying from the disease.

Source: E. J. Gangarosa, A. M. Galazka, C. R. Wolfe, L. M. Phillips, R. E. Gangarosa, E. Miller, and R. T. Chen. 1998. Impact of the antivaccine movements on pertussis control: the untold story. *Lancet* **35**:356–361.

the resulting disease is not identical to that seen in humans. Rats colonized with *B. pertussis* develop a cough, but the other symptoms seen in humans are not reproduced. Mice inoculated intranasally do not develop a cough, but they do die of the infection and thus experience at least some of the toxic effects of *B. pertussis* colonization. The LD_{50} for mice is about 10^3 bacteria. The mouse model has been used for most of the animal studies of virulence factors. Rabbits infected with a closely related species, *Bordetella bronchiseptica*, have been used as a model system in some studies. *B. bronchiseptica* is similar in many ways to *B. pertussis*, except that it does not produce a toxin produced by *B. pertussis*, pertussis toxin. The recent outbreaks of whooping cough in countries where the DT vaccine was substituted for the DTP vaccine have unfortunately provided human subjects ("involunteers") for study, but only limited information can be obtained from investigation of clinical specimens obtained after the disease has reached its final stage.

CELL AND TISSUE CULTURE MODELS. To study the effects of *B. pertussis* on ciliated respiratory cells, cross-sections of the trachea of hamsters or mice (**tracheal rings**) have been used. The waving (or "beating") of the cilia in these cross-sections can be seen easily under a microscope. When *B. pertussis* binds to these ciliated cells, the cilia eventually stop moving, presumably because of the toxic effects of adherent bacteria. Recent studies of nasal mucosal biopsies from children with whooping cough have raised questions about whether a cessation of ciliary motion (as opposed to complete loss of ciliated cells) is actually seen in humans, but the tracheal ring assay at least provides a measure of some type of damage to ciliated cells.

Although *B. pertussis* exhibits a pronounced specific-

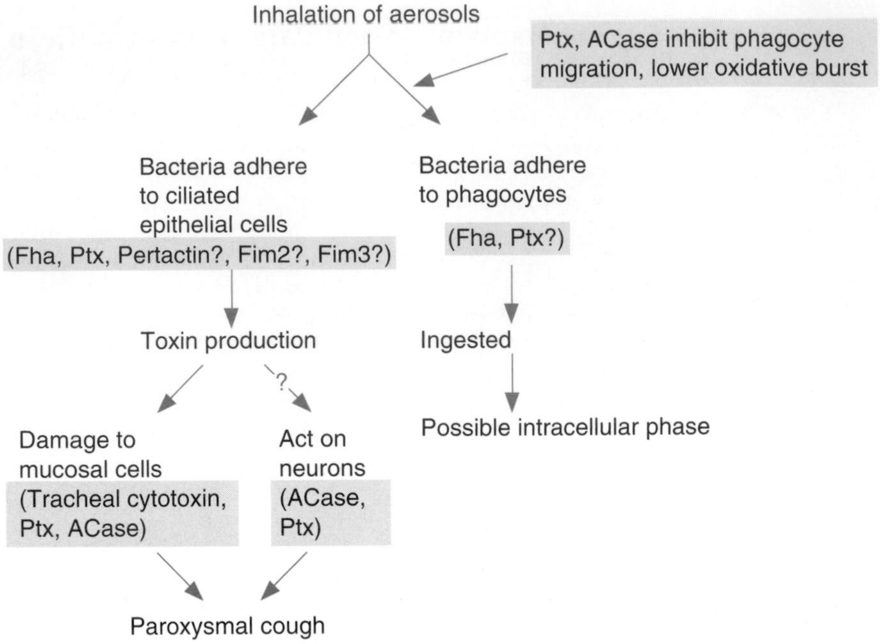

Inhalation of aerosols

Ptx, ACase inhibit phagocyte
migration, lower oxidative burst

Bacteria adhere
to ciliated
epithelial cells
(Fha, Ptx, Pertactin?, Fim2?, Fim3?)

Bacteria adhere
to phagocytes

(Fha, Ptx?)

Figure 17–1 Steps in the pathogenesis of whooping cough and associated virulence factors. Question marks indicate uncertainties about the importance of steps or virulence factors. Fha, filamentous hemagglutinin; Ptx, pertussis toxin; tracheal cytotoxin (PG fragment); ACase, invasive adenylate cyclase; Fim, pili. A question mark indicates that there is uncertainty about the role of the virulence factor in the step indicated.

Toxin production

Ingested

?

Damage to
mucosal cells
(Tracheal cytotoxin,
Ptx, ACase)

Act on
neurons
(ACase,
Ptx)

Possible intracellular phase

Paroxysmal cough

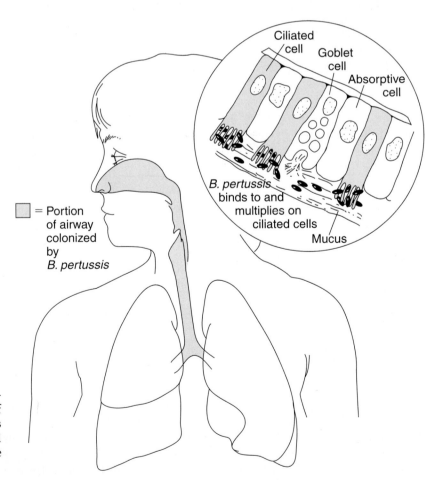

= Portion
of airway
colonized
by
B. pertussis

Ciliated
cell

Goblet
cell

Absorptive
cell

B. pertussis
binds to and
multiplies on
ciliated cells

Mucus

Figure 17–2 Colonization of the respiratory mucosa by *B. pertussis*. The portion of the airway colonized by the bacteria is shown on the left. *B. pertussis* binds to and multiplies on ciliated cells, as shown in the inset.

ity for ciliated cells when it infects the human respiratory mucosa, it will adhere to and in some cases invade a number of commonly used tissue culture cell lines (e.g., HeLa cells). The relevance of this type of binding and invasion to what goes on in the body of an infected person is questionable. Nonetheless, many investigators continue to use such model systems for evaluating *B. pertussis* virulence factors. It is only fair to point out that at least some of the virulence factors identified by this approach have actually proved to be important in assays involving animals.

Adherence

One of the unique characteristics of *B. pertussis* is its predilection for ciliated respiratory mucosal cells. Because most recent studies of *B. pertussis* and its adhesins have focused on cultured mammalian cell lines that have none of the characteristic features of ciliated cells, it is still the case that we know little about the factors that account for this remarkable host cell specificity of the bacteria. *B. pertussis* produces a number of adhesins that mediate attachment to cultured cells. The two best-studied adhesins are **filamentous hemagglutinin (Fha)** and **pertussis toxin (Ptx)**. Filamentous hemagglutinin is a large (220-kDa) protein that forms filamentous structures on the cell surface. These filaments do not have the ordered structure characteristic of pili. Fha can agglutinate red blood cells, a feature that explains the hemagglutinin part of its name.

Fha binds to galactose residues on sulfated glycolipids. A type of sulfated glycolipid called **sulfatide** is present in high levels in the membranes of ciliated cells, and this could be part of the explanation for the preferential binding of *B. pertussis* to these cells. Fha also binds a receptor, **CR3,** on PMNs. Mutants that have a disruption in the gene that encodes FhaB (*fhaB*) do not colonize the trachea of mice as well as do wild-type bacteria, but the mutants eventually kill the animal. Fha presumably plays some role in colonization, because antibodies to Fha provide protection against infection.

An unusual feature of *B. pertussis* adherence to mammalian cells is that one of its toxins, pertussis toxin, may act as an adhesin as well as a toxin. Pertussis toxin is a 105-kDa multiprotein complex consisting of subunits designated S1 to S5 (Figure 17–3). Some of the toxin molecules are released into the extracellular fluid, but the rest remain attached to the bacterial surface. Because extracellular toxins generally have a domain (the B portion) that binds eukaryotic cells, it is perhaps not surprising that toxin tethered to the bacterial cell surface might serve to attach the bacteria to the same types of cells, but precisely how the toxin exerts its adhesive effect is still not understood. Two of the toxin subunits,

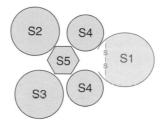 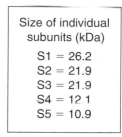

Figure 17–3 Structure of pertussis toxin. S1 is the ADP-ribosylating portion. S2 to S5 form the binding portion of the toxin.

Size of individual subunits (kDa)
S1 = 26.2
S2 = 21.9
S3 = 21.9
S4 = 12.1
S5 = 10.9

S2 and S3, appear to mediate adherence of the toxin to host cells. Although S2 and S3 have amino acid sequences that are more than 80% identical, they bind to different host cell receptors. S2 binds specifically to a glycolipid called **lactosylceramide,** which is found primarily on ciliated respiratory cells. S3 binds to a ganglioside found primarily on phagocytic cells.

Ptx is clearly an important virulence factor. Disruption of the genes encoding Ptx components increases the LD_{50} in mice by several orders of magnitude and renders the bacteria essentially avirulent. Moreover, antibodies against Ptx components prevent colonization of ciliated cells by the bacteria and give effective protection against infection. A toxoided form of Ptx has been used in some formulations of the acellular vaccine.

B. pertussis produces at least two other types of adhesins—pili and a surface protein called **pertactin.** There are two serotypes of pili, called serotype 2 (**Fim2**) and serotype 3 (**Fim3**). The importance of these adhesins in pathogenesis is not as well established as is the importance of Ptx and Fha, but they do play a role in adherence of *B. pertussis* to cultured mammalian cells.

B. pertussis can bind to receptors on PMNs. Generally, opsonization of bacteria by C3b or antibodies must occur before PMNs can ingest bacteria, but *B. pertussis* binds directly to integrin CR3 on the phagocyte's surface, via Fha, and forces its own uptake. Binding of pertussis toxin to PMNs increases the amount of CR3 on the PMN surface, so Ptx and Fha may act together to stimulate phagocytosis of *B. pertussis* by PMNs. Nonetheless, the role of this type of self-initiated phagocytosis in the disease process is still not clear. Bacteria taken up by this abnormal route may avoid phagolysosome fusion and stimulation of the oxidative burst that is normally triggered by the complement-mediated or antibody-mediated phagocytosis. Alternatively, the action of pertussis toxin and other *B. pertussis* toxins on the phagocyte (see below) could limit its killing activity.

The fact that *B. pertussis* can survive in macrophage-like cell lines and can be seen inside phagocytic cells taken from patients with whooping cough has led to the suggestion that *B. pertussis* has an intracellular phase, but this hypothesis is still unproved. Consistent with this hypothesis is the observation that cytotoxic T cells are an important part of the host defense against *B. pertussis*.

Toxins

PERTUSSIS TOXIN. Pertussis toxin, already introduced as an adhesin, appears here in the role of a protein exotoxin. Pertussis toxin consists of one enzymatic subunit and five binding subunits; the binding subunits of pertussis toxin (S2 to S5) are not identical (Figure 17–3). The binding region consists of one copy each of S2, S3, and S5 and two copies of S4. **S1,** the enzymatic portion of Ptx, ADP-ribosylates a host cell G protein, **G_i,** inactivating it. The role of G_i is to inactivate adenylate cyclase once the production of cyclic AMP (cAMP) has reached the appropriate level. Thus, ADP-ribosylation of G_i ultimately causes a rise in host cell cAMP levels (Figure 17–4). Scientists interested in mammalian G proteins have made considerable use of pertussis toxin in their studies of mammalian signal transduction. Pertussis toxin is an example of how reagents discovered by bacteriologists in the course of studying virulence factors of bacteria can be useful to scientists working in other areas.

A model for binding of pertussis toxin to a host cell and internalization of S1 is depicted in Figure 17–5. As already mentioned, S2 and S3 appear to dictate the specificity of binding. The mechanism by which the S1 subunit enters the host cell cytoplasm is still not well understood, but recent findings suggest that retrograde transport to the endoplasmic reticulum (the reverse of the process involved in production and localization of eukaryotic surface proteins) may be involved. S1 contains a disulfide bridge that must be reduced to release the active form of the enzyme. Reduction of the disulfide bond presumably occurs on the inside of the host cell membrane. ATP stimulates the internalization-reduction of S1, but the precise mechanism of stimulation is unknown.

An effect of uncontrolled cAMP production is that the cell loses the ability to control the flow of ions and other cellular processes. Pertussis toxin could thus be responsible for the increase in respiratory secretions and mucus production seen in whooping cough. Ptx probably does not contribute to the paroxysmal coughing of whooping cough, because a closely related species, *Bordetella parapertussis*, causes the same type of cough but does not produce Ptx.

INVASIVE ACASE. Not content with producing pertussis toxin, a toxin which raises host cell cAMP levels,

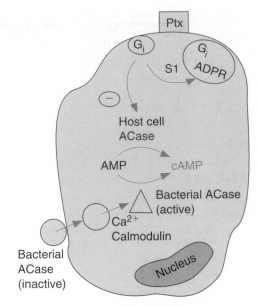

Figure 17–4 Comparison of the effects of pertussis toxin (Ptx) and invasive adenylate cyclase (ACase) on cAMP levels inside host cells. Both contribute to a rise in host cell cAMP but do so by different mechanisms. G_i normally controls the activity of the host cell ACase, but ADP-ribosylated G_i is inactive, allowing unrestricted production of cAMP by the host ACase. The invasive bacterial ACase enters the cell and is activated by Ca^{2+} and host cell calmodulin. Its activity contributes to the rise in cell cAMP levels.

B. pertussis also produces an invasive adenylate cyclase (ACase) of its own, which enters eukaryotic cells and produces cAMP directly (Figure 17–4). This toxin is a cell-associated protein when bacteria are grown in liquid media, but can be released into the extracellular fluid under some conditions. ACase appears to be important for virulence, because mutants that no longer produce ACase are avirulent in mice. They can still colonize the animals but no longer kill them. This indicates that ACase has a role in later stages of infection and may contribute to the symptoms of the disease.

The invasive ACase was originally identified as a hemolysin because it can bind to and lyse red blood cells, but it is now known to act on a variety of cell types. ACase is probably a single-chain A-B toxin (see chapter 9), because the amino-terminal portion of the ACase protein binds red blood cells and other cell types, whereas the carboxy terminus has the enzymatic activity. An interesting feature of the invasive ACase is that it is activated by calmodulin, a eukaryotic calcium-binding protein. Thus, it is only active inside a eukaryotic cell. No bacterial equivalent of calmodulin has yet been found.

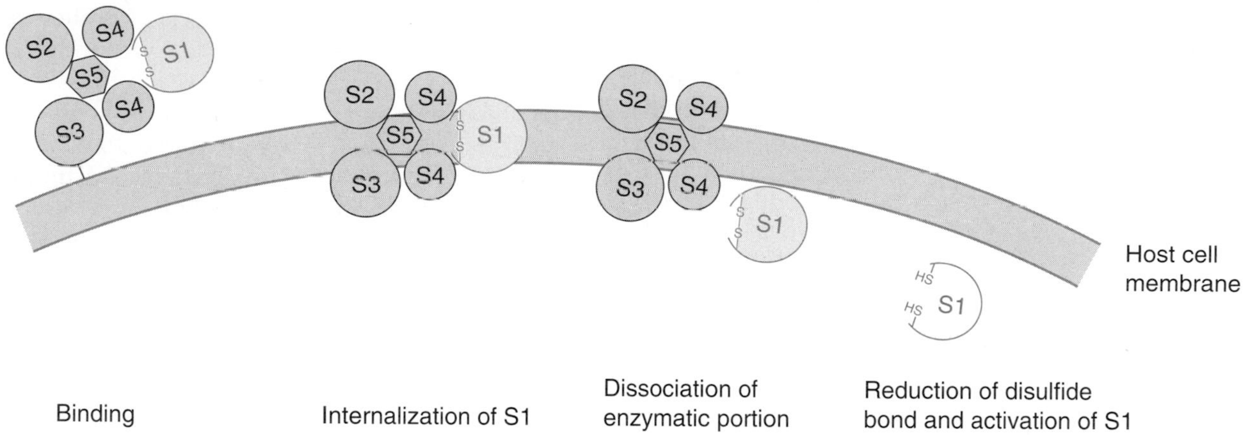

Figure 17–5   Hypothetical steps involved in the binding, internalization, and activation of pertussis toxin. Although for simplicity, the internalization process is shown here as a single step, it is probably much more complex, involving retrograde transfer through the endoplasmic reticulum.

DERMONECROTIC TOXIN (PERTUSSIS HEAT-LABILE TOXIN).   Yet another toxin produced by *B. pertussis* is dermonecrotic toxin. Dermonecrotic toxin was so named because it causes skin lesions (necrosis) when low doses are injected subcutaneously in mice. It is lethal when injected in high doses. It also appears to cause vasoconstriction. The role of this toxin in whooping cough, if any, is not known.

TRACHEAL CYTOTOXIN.   Despite its name, which suggests that the molecule is a protein exotoxin, **tracheal cytotoxin** is actually a peptidoglycan fragment: 1,6-anhydromuramic acid-*N*-acetyl-glucosamine-tetrapeptide. It is released into the extracellular fluid either as a result of bacterial lysis or as a result of natural turnover of peptidoglycan during bacterial growth. When this material is applied to hamster tracheal rings, it kills the ciliated cells, probably by inhibiting DNA synthesis. It also stimulates release of the cytokine IL-1 (which produces fever). There was initially some controversy about the significance of this compound in an actual infection, because both nonvirulent and virulent strains of *B. pertussis* produce it. However, a study using human nasal biopsy tissue showed that application of tracheal cytotoxin caused extrusion of ciliated cells from the mucosa and had cytotoxic effects on ciliated cells similar to those seen in the human form of the disease. Thus, it seems likely that tracheal cytotoxin contributes to the loss of ciliated cells that occurs in whooping cough.

LPS.   *B. pertussis* is unusual in that it produces two distinct types of LPS molecules. One has the lipid A portion seen in the *Escherichia coli*-type LPS, whereas the second LPS has a distinctive lipid portion, called **lipid X**. The two types of LPS also have different carbohydrate portions. Nonetheless, both types have the same sort of activities associated with classical *E. coli*-type LPS (e.g., activation of the alternative complement pathway and stimulation of cytokine release). No role for either type of LPS molecule in the pathogenesis of whooping cough has been established. It is possible, however, that some of the side effects of the old pertussis vaccine may have been due to LPS in the vaccine preparation. Ironically, it is also possible that LPS had a positive effect—by acting as an additional adjuvant to make DTP more effective.

B. pertussis and Phagocytic Cells

The ability of *B. pertussis* to trigger its own uptake by phagocytes has already been noted. There may be a logic in this apparently risky behavior because both pertussis toxin and ACase adversely affect phagocytes in vitro. One effect is to inhibit the migration of monocytes. In addition, these toxins lower the bactericidal oxidative response of PMNs and macrophages. Despite these in vitro effects, the ability of *B. pertussis* to survive in phagocytes, especially activated ones, during an actual infection may be marginal. The fact that *B. pertussis* does not usually succeed in infecting the lung, where lung macrophages and later PMNs are the main defense, suggests that this is the case. The interesting and important question of whether *B. pertussis* has an intracellular phase in phagocytic cells has still not been answered and deserves more scrutiny.

Is There a Type III Secretion System?

Type III secretion systems used by bacteria to inject toxic proteins directly into the cytoplasm of a host cell were introduced in chapter 9. Many bacterial pathogens have such secretion systems. *B. pertussis* is unusual in that, although it has genes that could encode a type III system, they seem not to be expressed. A closely related species, *B. bronchiseptica*, by contrast, does have a functional type III secretion system. Since *B. bronchiseptica* appears to have been the progenitor of *B. pertussis*, the question naturally arises as to why the type III system in *B. pertussis* seems not to be functional. *B. bronchiseptica* infects a broad range of four-legged mammals, but the infections are usually asymptomatic. Evidently, *B. bronchiseptica* is capable of modulating the defenses of its hosts to allow a persistent infection to develop without undue damage to the host. Type III systems often function to modulate the host response to a pathogen by affecting adversely the ability of phagocytic cells to clear the bacterium from the body. One suggested explanation for the lack of a functional type III system in *B. pertussis* is that when *B. bronchiseptica* moved from its normal animal hosts to humans and became *B. pertussis*, the type III system was deleterious in some way. In the case of *Yersinia pestis* (chapter 13), loss of certain invasion genes was associated with an increase in virulence. Since *B. pertussis* is more virulent in humans than *B. bronchiseptica* is in its normal animal hosts, loss of expression of the type III secretion system genes might be part of the reason for the increased virulence of *B. pertussis*.

Type IV Secretion System

Pertussis toxin is exported by a two-stage process. The subunits are first secreted from the cytoplasm to the periplasm by the general secretory pathway that handles secretion of most other bacterial proteins destined for the periplasm or extracellular medium. The toxin subunits are assembled in the periplasm, and the toxin is then transferred across the outer membrane by a specialized secretion system that has greatest similarity to type IV secretion systems. Initial reports on the pertussis toxin secretion system came as something of a surprise, because previously type IV secretion systems had been associated exclusively with the conjugal transfer of DNA. In retrospect, the fact that proteins not associated with DNA transfer could be exported by a type IV system should not have been surprising, because the single-stranded DNA that is transferred during conjugation is bound covalently to a protein. Thus, one could consider the conjugation apparatus to be a protein-exporting system as well as a DNA-exporting system.

There have now been several reports of protein secretion by type IV systems. Some of these will be described in the chapters on *Legionella pneumophila* (the Dot/Icm system that aids survival of the bacteria in macrophages) and *Helicobacter pylori* (export of the CagA protein, which appears to be involved in effecting cytoskeletal rearrangements in host cells).

Although the components of the pertussis toxin export system share amino acid similarity with components of conjugal transfer systems, the pertussis toxin export process differs from the conjugation process in an important way. During conjugation, the DNA protein complex is transported in a single step with no involvement of the normal secretion apparatus, whereas the export of pertussis toxin occurs in two steps, the first of which involves the general secretion apparatus of the cell. Also, conjugation transfers the DNA-protein complex directly from the cytoplasm of one bacterium to the cytoplasm of the other, whereas the type IV system responsible for the second step of pertussis toxin export simply exports the toxin into the extracellular fluid.

Regulation of Virulence Genes

Phenotypic Modulation (Transcriptional Regulation)

B. pertussis virulence genes (*fha*, *ptx*, etc.) are regulated in two ways: phenotypic modulation and phase variation. **Phenotypic modulation** is an old term indicating that genes are regulated at the transcriptional level. Expression of the *fha* and *ptx* genes is highest at 37°C and is suppressed when bacteria are grown at lower temperatures or in medium containing high levels of $MgSO_4$ or nicotinic acid. Under conditions where *fha*, *ptx*, and other genes are actively expressed, some genes, such as the genes encoding siderophore production and respiratory enzymes, are repressed. It is important to note, however, that although $MgSO_4$, nicotinic acid, and temperature modulate virulence gene expression in the laboratory, the actual signals sensed by the bacteria in the human body are unknown.

Virulence genes are scattered over the bacterial chromosome. Yet, some of them, such as the genes encoding components of pertussis toxin (*ptx* genes) and the genes required for secretion of pertussis toxin (*ptsA*, *ptsB*), are organized in operons. A locus thought to encode a central regulator of *B. pertussis* virulence genes has been identified. It contains two genes, ***bvgA*** and ***bvgS*** (*Bordetella* virulence genes), whose amino acid sequences have significant similarity to those of known two-component regulatory systems. BvgS is the histidine kinase that senses environmental signals, and BvgA is the transcriptional activator of virulence genes in the regulon. Although the deduced amino acid sequences of these two proteins suggest that they are members of a two-component regulatory system, BvgA and BvgS carry out a multistep phosphorelay system that is more complex than the simpler set of reactions catalyzed by most two-component systems. Most histidine kinases contain a single domain that is autophosphorylated and then serves as the phosphate donor for phosphorylation of the transcriptional activator (on its receiver domain), but BvgS has not only a domain of this sort but also two other domains, one of which is similar to the receiver domain on the transcriptional activator. The sequence

of phosphorylation steps is shown in Figure 17–6. BvgS ultimately transfers the phosphate to the transcriptional activator, BvgA. It is not clear why this complicated series of steps is needed, but it could allow the regulatory system to sense more complex signals or modulate responses to environmental signals more effectively.

As already mentioned, some virulence genes are activated by the Bvg system, and others are repressed. The differences between cells grown under conditions that cause the Bvg system to go into action and cells grown under conditions that turn Bvg off are sufficiently large that the two states have been termed Bvg⁺ and Bvg⁻, respectively. There is also an intermediate state, called

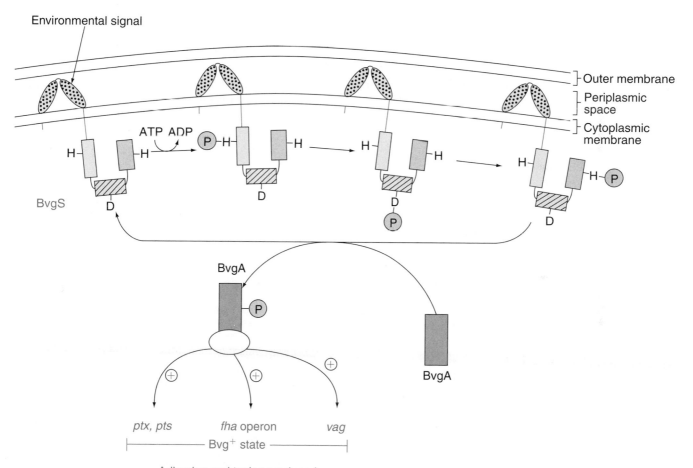

Figure 17–6 BvgS has four domains. One is exposed in the periplasmic space and presumably senses the signal. The three cytoplasmic domains (shown as rectangular boxes) contain the phosphorylation sites. The first amino acid residue to be phosphorylated is a histidine (H). Then the phosphate group is transferred to an aspartate residue (D) and finally to another histidine residue, before being transferred to BvgA to make phosphorylated BvgA, the active form of the activator. BvgA-P causes a number of genes to be expressed. When these genes are being expressed, the bacteria are said to be in the Bvg⁺ state. The state characterized by no expression of these genes is called Bvg⁻. There is an intermediate state (Bvgⁱ) in which only the BvgA-controlled adhesin genes are expressed. (Adapted from M. A. Uhl and J. F. Miller. 1996.)

Bvg^i, which occurs in the presence of intermediate levels of modulating signals. Under Bvg^i conditions, Bvg$^+$-phase adhesins are expressed but the toxins are not. Also, there are new surface proteins specific to the Bvg^i phase.

What do these phases have to do with infection of the human body? The absence in infected people of antibodies against the proteins produced by Bvg$^-$ cells suggests that the Bvg$^-$ state is not achieved in the human body. Since antibodies are made against the proteins produced by Bvg$^+$ cells, this phase is clearly achieved in the human body. Thus, in the human body, either the cells are always in the Bvg$^+$ phase or at most switch from Bvg$^+$ to Bvg^i. Bvg^i might even be involved in survival during transmission and colonization of the nasopharynx.

But what about the Bvg$^-$ state? Scientists tend to assume that bacteria do not maintain genes that are never used. Possibly, the Bvg$^-$ state was important for the ancestral *Bordetella* species that gave rise to the modern species, some of which live outside the animal body. In this case, one would have to posit that the rise of different species has occurred too recently for the Bvg$^-$ traits to be lost. A more intriguing possibility is that *B. pertussis* has a niche outside the human body. Such traits as flagella, biosynthetic enzymes, and respiratory enzymes, which are associated with the Bvg$^-$ state, could well be needed for survival outside the human body. Conventional wisdom has it that *B. pertussis* does not have such a niche outside the human body, but have scientists really looked hard enough to make sure that this is the case?

Phase Variation

A second type of regulation seen in *B. pertussis* is called **phase variation.** Nonvirulent mutants of *B. pertussis* can be obtained from virulent strains at frequencies of about 10^{-6}. Virulent revertants arise from the nonvirulent mutants at a similar frequency. These shifts are caused by frameshifts in the *bvgS* gene. Phase variation is not simply a laboratory artifact. Nonvirulent phase variants of *B. pertussis* are frequently isolated from children who are recovering from a case of whooping cough, whereas the initially infecting strain was fully virulent.

Prevention and Treatment

Although *B. pertussis* is susceptible in the laboratory to erythromycin, chloramphenicol, and some other antibiotics, antibiotic therapy of a child with the disease does not lessen the duration of symptoms. Nonetheless, antibiotics are often given to children with whooping cough because it lessens their infectivity and helps to prevent further spread of the disease. Convalescent or asymptomatic carriers can be a significant source of infection in an outbreak of whooping cough. For this reason, it is advisable to treat adults who have an asymptomatic infection, especially if they come into regular contact with an infant. Unfortunately, the way at least some adult cases of asymptomatic carriage are diagnosed is that an infant in the household gets whooping cough. Antibiotics are being used to treat adults with the "100 days cough." There is controversy, however, as to how effective this treatment is.

The development of a vaccine that prevented whooping cough virtually eliminated this disease in developed countries. A new, more defined formulation, which usually contains toxoided Ptx and Fha, is now on the market as part of the DTaP vaccine. This vaccine is given in five separate injections over the first 7 years of life to obtain maximum immunity. When the new vaccine was first administered, it was only used for the fourth and fifth injection, with the old vaccine being used for injections one through three. This was done because of concern about the possibility that use of the new vaccine for all injections might not confer immunity as effective as that achieved with the original vaccine. Clinical trials have now cleared the acellular vaccine, aP, for use in all five immunizations. Attempts are currently under way to refine the vaccine still further by replacing pertussis toxoid with portions of the S2 and S3 subunits.

SELECTED READINGS

Bassinet, L., P. Gueirard, B. Maitre, B. Housset, P. Gounon, and N. Guiso. 2000. Role of adhesins and toxins in invasion of human tracheal epithelial cells by *Bordetella pertussis*. *Infect. Immun.* **68:**1934–1941.

Belcher, C. E., J. Drenkow, B. Kehoe, T. R. Gingeras, N. McNamara, N. Lemjabbar, C. Basbaum, and D. Relman. 2000. The transcriptional responses of respiratory epithelial cells to *Bordetella pertussis* reveal host defensive and pathogen counter-defensive strategies. *Proc. Natl. Acad. Sci. USA* **97:**13847–13852.

Christie, P. J., and J. P. Vogel. 2000. Bacterial type IV secretion: conjugation systems adapted to deliver effector molecules to host cells. *Trends Microbiol.* **8:**354–360.

Cotter, P. A., and J. F. Miller. 1998. *In vivo* and *ex vivo* regulation of bacterial virulence gene expression. *Curr. Opin. Microbiol.* **1:**17–26.

Heveker, N., and D. Ladant. 1997. Characterization of mutant *Bordetella pertussis* adenylate cyclase toxins with reduced affinity for calmodulin. Implications for the mechanism of toxin entry into target cells. *Eur. J. Biochem.* **243:**643–649.

Kinnear, S. M., R. R. Marques, and N. H. Carbonetti. 2001.

Differential regulation of Bvg-activated virulence factors plays a role in *Bordetella pertussis* pathogenicity. *Infect. Immun.* **69:**1983–1993.

Ladant, D., and A. Ullmann. 1999. *Bordetella pertussis* adenylate cyclase: a toxin with multiple talents. *Trends Microbiol.* **7:**172–176.

Senzilet, L. D., S. A. Halperin, J. S. Spika, M. Alagaratnam, A. Morris, and B. Smith. 2001. Pertussis is a frequent cause of prolonged cough illness in adults and adolescents. *Clin. Infect. Dis.* **32:**1691–1697.

Uhl, M. A., and J. F. Miller. 1996. Integration of multiple domains in a two-component sensor protein: the *Bordetella pertussis* BvgAS phosphorelay. *EMBO J.* **15:**1028–1036.

Yuk, M. H., E. T. Harvill, and J. F. Miller. 1998. The BvgAS virulence control system regulates type III secretion in *Bordetella bronchiseptica. Mol. Microbiol.* **28:**945–960.

SUMMARY OUTLINE

Characteristics of whooping cough

Caused by *B. pertussis*
- Small gram-negative coccobacillus
- Fastidious, grown on media containing blood

Spread by aerosols or direct contact

First stage—resembles the common cold

Second stage
- Dry cough—paroxysmal
- Excess mucus production and vomiting
- Convulsions and cyanosis may occur

Infection process

Colonization of respiratory mucosa

Bacteria bind ciliated cells, multiply there

Bacteria rarely enter lung and cause pneumonia

Virulence factors

Model systems
- Animal models—rodents, rabbits
- Cell and tissue culture
  - Tracheal rings
  - HeLa cells

Adherence
- Filamentous hemagglutinin (Fha)
  - Binds galactose residues on sulfated glycolipids—common on ciliated cells
  - Binds CR3 on PMNs
  - Antibodies against Fha protect against infection
- Pertussis toxin (Ptx)
  - B domain (S2 and S3 subunits) may provide attachment to host cells
  - S2 binds lactosylceramide
  - S3 bind a ganglioside on phagocytes
  - Antibodies against Ptx prevent colonization
- Pili (Fim2, Fim3)—importance not established
- Pertactin—surface proteins

(continued)

Toxins
    Pertussis toxin
        Four non-identical binding subunits—S2, S3, S5, and two copies of S4
        One enzymatic subunit—S1
            ADP-ribosylates a G protein—G_i
            Increases cAMP production by host cell
    Invasive ACase
        Probably a single-chain A-B toxin
        Activated by calmodulin
        Produces cAMP directly
    Dermonecrotic toxin
        Causes skin lesions and death in mice
        Role in whooping cough unknown
    Tracheal cytotoxin
        Peptidoglycan fragment
        Kills ciliated cells
        Stimulates release of IL-1
    LPS—two types
        Typical *E. coli* type containing lipid A
        Unusual type containing lipid X
        May have been responsible for side effects in whole-cell vaccine

Interaction with phagocytes
    Fha binding to CR3 stimulates uptake of bacteria
    Ptx binding to PMNs increases CR3 receptors on PMNs
    Ptx and ACase inhibit migration of monocytes
    Bacteria can survive in macrophagelike cell lines
    Bacteria lower oxidative response of PMNs and macrophages
    May have an intracellular phase

Type III secretion system
    B. pertussis has genes that could encode a type III system
    Genes apparently not expressed

Type IV secretion system
    Subunits assembled in periplasm and then transported across outer membrane by type IV-like
        system
    Components of system have amino acid similarity with components of conjugal transfer
        system
    Major difference from typical type IV system—Ptx subunits secreted from cytoplasm to peri-
        plasm by general secretory pathway

Regulation of virulence genes

Phenotypic modulation—transcriptional regulation
    fha and *ptx* expression greatest at 37°C; suppressed at low temperature and high Mg^{2+} and
        nicotinamide concentrations
    Some genes form an operon (*ptx, ptsA,* and *ptsB*)
    Two-component regulatory system (BvgA and BvgS)
    Some virulence genes activated, others repressed by Bvg
    Control occurs in a regulatory cascade

(*continued*)

SUMMARY OUTLINE (*continued*)

    Two states of Bvg activation—Bvg$^+$, Bvg$^-$
        Also intermediate-state Bvg^i
        In humans only Bvg$^+$ (possibly Bvg^i) state occurs

    Phase variation
        Arises from frameshift in *bvgS* genes
        Nonvirulent strains appear late in infection

Prevention and treatment

    Antibiotics (e.g., erythromycin and chloramphenicol)
        Do not lessen duration of symptoms
        May prevent further spread
    Vaccine
        Old type contained whole killed cells
            Almost eliminated disease from developed countries
            Some side effects
            Stimulated antivaccine movements
        New acellular vaccine
            Contains toxoided Ptx and Fha
            Now used exclusively in the United States

QUESTIONS

Answers to the questions can be found in Appendix 2.

1. How many of the symptoms of whooping cough can be explained by the known virulence factors?

2. Whooping cough is generally considered a disease of children, but now it appears that adults are the main reservoir for persistence and transmission of the disease. How can this apparent contradiction be explained?

3. Pertussis toxin is thought to function as an adhesin as well as a toxin. How could a toxin function as an adhesin?

4. What would be the advantage to *B. pertussis* of producing two toxins that affect host cell cAMP levels?

5. "Tracheal cytotoxin" turned out to be a peptidoglycan fragment, not an exotoxin. Suggest a possible mechanism of action for tracheal cytotoxin.

6. How would you tell the difference experimentally between phase variation and phenotypic modulation? What different type of role does each play in adapting to the host?

7. Bvg-mediated regulation of *B. pertussis* is quite complex. How does the BvgSA regulatory system differ from most two-component regulatory systems? Make an educated guess as to why this system is so complex.

8. How does the type IV secretion system of *B. pertussis* differ from a type III system?

18

Streptococcus pneumoniae

KEY FEATURES

Streptococcus pneumoniae

CHARACTERISTICS
Gram-positive diplococci
Capsule, many different serotypes
Alpha-hemolytic on blood agar plates
Natural transformation system

DISEASES
Pneumonia, meningitis, septicemia
Ear infections in children

RESERVOIR
Human mouth and throat

MAJOR VIRULENCE FACTORS
Antiphagocytic polysaccharide capsule
Adhesins
Pneumolysin—pore-forming toxin
LTA

PREVENTION AND TREATMENT
Vaccines, some still in development
Antibiotics—resistance rising

Pneumococcal Disease

For those who think the ultimate goal of pathogenesis research should be finding ways to save lives and alleviate suffering caused by infectious diseases, *Streptococcus pneumoniae* (also called the pneumococcus) has to be at the top of the priority list. *S. pneumoniae* is the main cause of bacterial pneumonia, one of the leading causes of infectious disease deaths in the United States. More people in the United States die of pneumococcal pneumonia than of AIDS, but since pneumonia is an old disease that has not captured the attention of the media, the public is largely unaware of this fact. At present, although pneumococcal infections can strike all age groups, they are most commonly seen among the very old and the very young. As the baby boomers continue to age, we may see more attention paid to an illness that targets senior citizens. In addition to pneumonia, *S. pneumoniae* also causes meningitis, especially in infants, and bacteremia in people who develop pneumonia. The CDC has estimated that in the United States alone, 500,000 cases of pneumonia and 50,000 cases of bacteremia are caused each year by *S. pneumoniae*. Worldwide, the toll is far higher.

A more common but much less serious disease caused by *S. pneumoniae* is otitis media (earache). In the United States, hardly any child who reaches the age of 5 years fails to contract a pneumococcal ear infection. Although the vast majority of ear infections in children are self-limiting, the fact that these infections are so frequently—and unnecessarily—treated with antibiotics raises a potentially serious problem. Are we creating a generation of children who are colonized with antibiotic-resistant strains of *S. pneumoniae* that will later come back to hurt them in the form of incurable pneumonia and sepsis?

One of the first successes of the antibiotic era was the demonstration that pneumococcal pneumonia could be cured with penicillin. Physicians who witnessed patients seemingly at death's door recover within days to full health thought the new cure was little short of miraculous. This led to the coining of the term "miracle drugs" to describe antibiotics. Today, physicians and scientists watch with concern the gradual erosion of the effectiveness of antibiotics in treating pneumococcal pneumonia and meningitis, as the pneumococci become more and more resistant to antibiotics. In the preantibiotic era, the death rate in adults with untreated pneumococcal pneumonia was 30 to 35%. In infants with meningitis, the death rate was far higher. Loss of the ability to control *S. pneumoniae* infections would be a major public health disaster.

Despite the great importance of pneumococcal infections, support for research in this area from the funding agencies lagged badly until the 1990s. Until recently, the field was also hampered by the lack of sophisticated genetic tools. Against great odds, a few laboratories have worked miracles in recent years to bring research in this area to a point where it has moved to the forefront of modern pathogenesis research. Unfortunately, however, there are still far too few basic research laboratories working in this area.

A tragic result of the not-so-benign neglect of research on *S. pneumoniae* was the missed opportunity to develop early an effective vaccine against this serious disease. The existing vaccine is notorious for its relative lack of efficacy in the most at-risk groups—infants and the elderly. The reason for this problem will be described in later sections. Today, pharmaceutical companies and health agencies are scrambling to develop a more effective vaccine, but that effort comes too late for many. It would be possible to calculate the number of lives such an improved vaccine could have saved if the project had been given a high priority during the 1960 to 1990 period, but the exercise would be too depressing. Today, motivated by the powerful threat of increasingly antibiotic-resistant strains of *S. pneumoniae*, no one doubts the importance of a more effective vaccine.

Characteristics of *S. pneumoniae*

S. pneumoniae is a gram-positive diplococcus (Figure 18–1). In fact, the pneumococcus was originally called *Diplococcus pneumoniae*. This morphological trait can be useful for rapid diagnosis of pneumococcal infections. Demonstration of gram-positive diplococci in properly collected sputum specimens is a rapid method for preliminary diagnosis of pneumococcal pneumonia. Similarly, demonstration of gram-positive diplococci in spinal fluid is an early clue suggesting pneumococcal meningitis. In the past, a definitive diagnosis of pneumococcal pneumonia could only be accomplished by cultivating the bacteria and subjecting them to a battery of phenotypic tests. One of these tests was cultivation of the bacteria on blood agar plates. Colonies of *S. pneumoniae* produce greenish haloes (alpha-hemolysis). Classification using such phenotypic traits, however, is

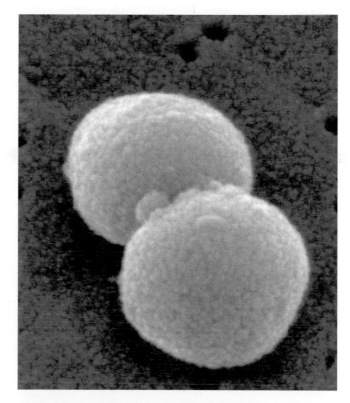

Figure 18–1 Scanning electron micrograph of *S. pneumoniae*. (Courtesy of Janice Carr, CDC.)

time-consuming and is hampered by the fact that it is not always possible to cultivate bacteria seen in sputum specimens.

To speed diagnosis, a DNA probe test has been developed for use on sputum specimens. Use of this test has revealed another problem with the classical method of diagnosing pneumococcal pneumonia: misidentification of some strains. One of the standard phenotypic tests used to identify *S. pneumoniae* has been **bile solubility.** Pneumococci produce enzymes called **autolysins** that digest peptidoglycan. The bile acid deoxycholic acid activates the autolysins of most strains. Thus, most *S. pneumoniae* strains lyse rapidly when suspended in a bile acid solution. In the past, a strain that did not lyse when exposed to bile acid would not have been classified as *S. pneumoniae*. The DNA probe test identified some strains as *S. pneumoniae* that were bile resistant. The bile resistance of these "atypical" *S. pneumoniae* strains was due to autolysins that are not activated (in fact, are actually inhibited) by bile. These atypical strains are clinically important because they are frequently associated with more invasive types of disease (e.g., meningitis). Thus, the failure of classical phenotypic tests to accurately identify these strains was a rather serious matter.

S. pneumoniae has a thick polysaccharide capsule that covers the peptidoglycan cell wall. There are over 80 distinct capsular serotypes, but most cases of pneumococcal pneumonia are caused by only 23 of these serotypes. Mixing a specimen containing *S. pneumoniae* with antibody to capsular antigens causes the capsule to appear to swell when the bacteria are viewed by phase-contrast microscopy. This **quellung** (German for "swelling") test has been used as a quick test for identification of serotypes of *S. pneumoniae*.

Although sophisticated genetic tools were slow to develop in this area, *S. pneumoniae* actually ushered in the era of DNA technology. The discovery of DNA, a discovery that launched the molecular revolution, was made using *S. pneumoniae*. *S. pneumoniae* takes up DNA from the environment naturally (natural transformation). Scientists noted that addition of a substance (which later proved to be DNA) to a culture of *S. pneumoniae* caused a nonencapsulated strain to produce a capsule and to become virulent in mice. It was decades before scientists figured out how to bludgeon *Escherichia coli*, which is not naturally transformable, to take up DNA from the environment, a discovery that helped to set the cloning revolution in motion.

Progression of Pneumococcal Disease

S. pneumoniae infections begin with colonization of the nasopharynx by the bacteria. At some time or other,

about one-third of all people will have their respiratory tracts colonized by *S. pneumoniae*. Once established in this site, *S. pneumoniae* has access to the eustachian tube of the inner ear and to the lung (Figure 18–2). If the bacteria enter the eustachian tube and begin multiplying there, they trigger an intense inflammatory response, which causes the pain and fever associated with earache.

Normally, the defenses of the upper airway keep *S. pneumoniae* from entering the lung. A case of influenza can impair these defenses, however. Influenza virus rarely causes pneumonia itself, except in years when especially virulent strains are circulating, but it can kill the ciliated cells that protect the upper airway. If pneumococci in the throat of a person with influenza manage to evade the ciliated cell defense and reach the lung, their polysaccharide capsule allows them to evade phagocytosis and killing by the alveolar macrophages and then begin to divide. Some bacteria lyse, and bacterial fragments trigger a local inflammatory response that continues to grow as more and more phagocytes and lymphoid cells are attracted to the area where phagocytes are trying unsuccessfully to kill the bacteria.

Damage to the lung, caused by inflammation, results in a breakdown of the gas exchange mechanism that is the principal function of the lung, and the patient becomes **cyanotic** because of the lack of oxygen. The classical form of pneumococcal pneumonia is rapid onset of symptoms, high temperature, shaking chills, a productive cough (cough with sputum), and blood in the sputum. Not all people with pneumococcal pneumonia

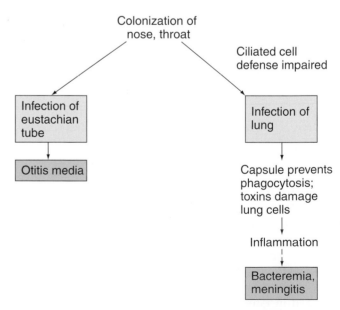

Figure 18–2   Progression of two pneumococcal diseases, earache and pneumonia.

exhibit these classical symptoms, however, a fact that complicates the diagnosis of the disease. This is most often true of people with underlying conditions, such as old age, chronic bronchitis, emphysema, heart failure, and alcoholism. In 15 to 30% of patients with pneumonia, the bacteria enter the bloodstream, where lysis of bacteria frees cell wall components that trigger cytokine release, resulting in fever and shock.

Meningitis occurs when the bacteria in the bloodstream attach to the **meninges,** a set of membranes that cover the brain and spinal column, protecting these important areas from harmful substances in blood (**blood-brain barrier**). How the bacteria get from the throat to the meninges is still unclear; the bacteria could get into the bloodstream directly from the throat or through the lungs via the bloodstream, although pneumonia is usually not a precursor of meningitis. Normally, only glucose and electrolytes can cross the blood-brain barrier, but local inflammation caused by the bacteria breaches the blood-brain barrier and admits bacteria and phagocytes to the brain and spinal fluid. Damage to the brain can lead to hearing loss, blindness, learning disabilities, paralysis, and death. Pneumococcal meningitis is characterized by fever, irritability, and drowsiness in early stages, and seizures and coma in later stages. Since early symptoms are nonspecific, it is often difficult to diagnose meningitis until the disease has advanced to a stage where the patient is in serious danger. One symptom that often signals meningitis is stiffness of the neck, but this is not seen in all cases.

The spleen is important for preventing and limiting the severity of *S. pneumoniae* infections. The importance of the spleen as a filtration organ for removing streptococci from the bloodstream can be seen from the fact that people with splenectomies or with splenic dysfunction (e.g., in sickle-cell disease) seem to be particularly prone to septic bacteremia following pneumonia. Such people can die within 12 to 18 h of the initial lung infection. The rapid progress of the disease in these individuals makes it very difficult to diagnose them in time to treat them effectively.

Virulence Factors of *S. pneumoniae*

Animal and Cell Culture Models

Although *S. pneumoniae* is normally a human pathogen, it can kill mice if it is injected peritoneally or administered intranasally in large doses. Mouse model systems are widely used to assess virulence factors of *S. pneumoniae* and to test the effectiveness of different types of vaccines. A model that has been used to study ear infections is the chinchilla model. Human PMNs and

macrophages or macrophagelike cell lines are used to test the ability of *S. pneumoniae* to resist phagocytosis. Human umbilical vein endothelial cells (HUVEC) and rat alveolar cells are used as in vitro systems for studying effects of the bacteria on endothelium (HUVEC) and lung (rat alveolar cells).

Colonization of the Nose and Throat and Entry into the Lung

The first step in the development of pneumonia is colonization of the nasopharynx by *S. pneumoniae* (Figure 18–2). A hypothesis concerning the factors involved in colonization of the nose and throat has been proposed (Figure 18–3). On agar plates, *S. pneumoniae* makes two different colony types, a transparent colony type and an opaque colony type. Most of the strains isolated from the nose and throat and most strains obtained from the lung of infected patients form transparent colonies, although they can later shift to the opaque colony type. Presumably, the different appearance of the colonies reflects differences in surface proteins or surface carbohydrate molecules that might mediate adherence. Oral epithelial cells have a disaccharide, *N*-acetylglucosamine, linked by a β1–3 bond to a galactose residue (**GlcNAc β1–3 Gal**) on their surfaces. Strains with the **transparent colony type** bind much more tightly to

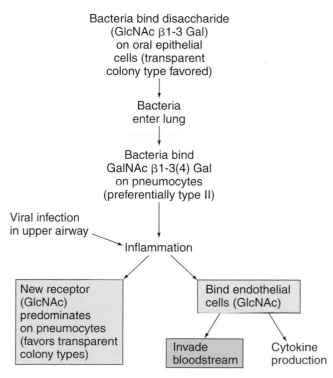

Figure 18–3 Model for progression of pneumococcal pneumonia at the molecular level.

these cells than strains with the **opaque colony type.** This tends to select for the transparent colony types.

In the lung, the walls of the alveoli are lined with cells called **pneumocytes.** These come in two types, **type I,** which has a flat appearance, and **type II,** which has a cuboidal appearance. *S. pneumoniae* seems to prefer type II pneumocytes. Type II pneumocytes have two kinds of disaccharide on their surfaces, which could be the receptors for the pneumococcal adhesin: *N*-acetylgalactosamine linked by either a β1–3 or a β1–4 bond to a galactose residue (**GalNAc β1–3 Gal** and **GalNAc β1–4 Gal**). Both colony types bind equally to these receptors, but since the transparent type starts with an advantage, it probably predominates at this stage. Pneumococci also bind to these same receptors on endothelial cells, a fact that may help them move from the lung into the bloodstream.

The advantage of the transparent phenotype increases as the infection process moves to the next stage. Inflammation caused by the infection activates pneumocytes and endothelial cells. One effect of this is a change of surface carbohydrate antigens whereby the normal antigens give way to the GlcNAc moiety on the receptor for **platelet-activating factor (PAF).** Pneumococci can also attach to this receptor, and here again, the transparent types have an advantage. Virus infection of the upper airway, a step that often precedes the development of bacterial pneumonia because it temporarily destroys the ciliated cells that guard the airway, has the same effect of causing an upshift in production of such PAF receptors on lung and endothelial cells. The ability of pneumococci to adhere to the PAF receptor increases the chances of the bacteria attaching to pneumocytes and endothelial cells, thus helping them infect the lung.

Other products of *S. pneumoniae* cause damage to cells both in the upper airway and in the lung. One is a cytotoxic protein called **pneumolysin** (Figure 18–4). Scientists now agree that this is an important virulence factor, and pneumolysin is being considered as a candidate for inclusion in an improved antipneumococcal vaccine. Pneumolysin shares amino acid homology with similar cytotoxins (hemolysins) that are produced by *Streptococcus pyogenes* (streptolysin O [SLO]) and *Listeria monocytogenes* (listeriolysin O [LLO]). Pneumolysin, unlike SLO and LLO, is a cytoplasmic protein rather than a secreted protein. It is presumably released as a result of lysis of some of the invading bacteria. Consistent with this idea, a protein called **LytA,** which is responsible for autolysis of pneumococci, has been identified as a virulence factor. Disrupting the *lytA* gene reduced the virulence of the mutant strain in an animal model. However, antibodies against LytA did not affect the course of the disease. One interpretation of these results is that LytA does not act directly but is important because it causes the release of pneumolysin from the cells.

Pneumolysin binds cholesterol in host cell membranes and disrupts them by forming pores. It might damage host mucosal cells and could aid colonization of the airway by adversely affecting ciliated mucosal cells, thus impairing the ability of the host to clear bacteria trapped in mucus. A mutant deficient in pneumolysin production had reduced virulence in mice. Also, antibodies to pneumolysin conferred partial protection in intranasally inoculated mice. Antibody titers to pneumolysin rise in humans with pneumonia, indicating that the protein is being produced by bacteria growing in the host. Thus, pneumolysin appears to be a virulence factor, although it is not nearly as important as the capsule or inflammatory cell wall components. A bewildering variety of activities have been ascribed to pneumolysin. Some of these are listed in Table 18–1.

Pneumococci have a number of surface proteins that could contribute to virulence, possibly as adhesins (Table 18–2). Unfortunately, some of them have extremely confusing names that appear at first to be almost indistinguishable. These are **pneumococcal surface protein A (PspA), pneumococcal surface adhesin A (PsaA),** and *S. pneumoniae* **surface protein A (SpsA).** The function of PspA is not known, but antibodies against it are protective. PspA is thus a possible vaccine candidate, although it is antigenically variable. SpsA has an unusual trait: it binds the secretory component of sIgA. In mucin, sIgA bound to surface antigens of microbes interacts through its Fc portion with mucin, thus trapping the bacteria. A protein that binds sIgA so that it cannot interact with mucin would reduce the chance that the bacteria would be trapped in mucin. PsaA may be an adhesin because disruption of the gene reduces binding to pneumocytes in vitro. The mutant was also rendered avirulent in mice. PsaA is another protein being considered as a candidate for a vaccine. A fourth protein of interest is **choline binding protein A (CbpA).** This is a cell surface protein that attaches to choline residues on LTA. Because LTA is anchored in the bacterial membrane, binding to this molecule would tether CbpA to the cell. The function of CbpA is still unknown, but since it is a surface protein it might be a vaccine candidate.

Survival in the Lung

Bacteria that manage to evade the ciliated cell clearance mechanism, reach the lung, and start to multiply there, encounter a very effective host defense, alveolar macrophages. Virulent pneumococci have an antiphago-

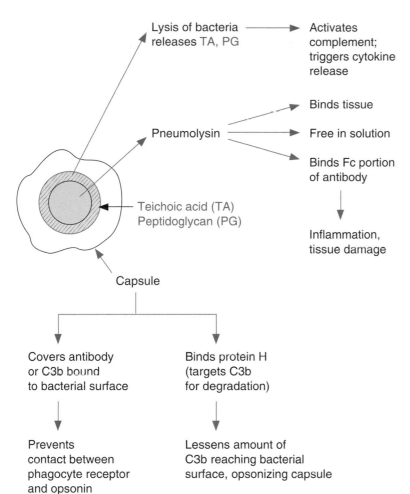

Lysis of bacteria releases TA, PG ⟶ Activates complement; triggers cytokine release

Pneumolysin ⟶ Binds tissue

⟶ Free in solution

⟶ Binds Fc portion of antibody ⟶ Inflammation, tissue damage

Teichoic acid (TA)
Peptidoglycan (PG)

Capsule

Covers antibody or C3b bound to bacterial surface ⟶ Prevents contact between phagocyte receptor and opsonin

Binds protein H (targets C3b for degradation) ⟶ Lessens amount of C3b reaching bacterial surface, opsonizing capsule

Figure 18–4 Interaction of *S. pneumoniae* virulence factors with the host. C3b and other components of the complement system are described in chapter 5.

Table 18–1 Some of the activities attributed to pneumolysin

Inhibits activity of ciliated cells

Cytotoxic for alveolar and endothelial cells

Activates classical complement pathway by binding to Fc portion of an antibody

Causes inflammation in the lung

Decreases the effectiveness of PMNs

Stimulates monocytes to produce cytokines

Table 18–2 Surface proteins of *S. pneumoniae* that are possible vaccine candidates

Surface protein	Characteristics
Pneumococcal surface protein A (PspA)	Function unknown; antibodies protective; antigenically variable
Pneumococcal surface adhesin A (PsaA)	Adhesin that mediates binding to pneumocytes; important for virulence
S. pneumoniae protein A (SpsA)	Binds the secretory component of sIgA; may prevent trapping of bacteria in mucin
Choline binding protein A (CbpA)	Tethered to LTA on cell surface

cytic capsule and are not engulfed either by macrophages or by PMNs because they are not opsonized by C3b. Bacteria that lack the polysaccharide capsule are avirulent, and antibodies against capsular components are protective in humans and in mice. The *S. pneumoniae* capsule is a complex polymer that contains sugar alcohols, amino sugars, choline, and neutral sugars, to list only a portion of the components. Different capsular types confer different levels of virulence. Strains with equally thick capsules but different capsular se-rotypes can vary considerably in virulence. An extreme example is the difference between serotype 3, one of the most virulent serotypes, and serotype 37, which is avir-ulent.

The connection between capsular composition and virulence is not understood. One indication of how composition of the capsule might affect virulence comes from serotypes that have choline residues in their capsules. A host **acute-phase protein,** called **C-reactive protein,** binds to choline residues. Although this does not appear to opsonize the bacteria (at least in vitro), C-reactive protein has been known to provide partial pro-tection against pneumococcal bacteremia in mice and might somehow aid phagocytosis in vivo.

Pneumolysin, which was mentioned previously as a possible contributor to colonization, also affects human PMNs and monocytes in vitro. Its main effect is to de-crease the oxidative burst and thus limit the killing ef-fect of phagocytes on ingested bacteria. This activity of pneumolysin may not be important in vivo, however, because unencapsulated bacteria, which still produce it, are readily killed by the phagocytes; i.e., the anti-phagocytic action of pneumolysin during an actual in-fection is not sufficient to protect the bacteria if the cap-sule has been eliminated.

Ability To Evoke an Inflammatory Response

INFLAMMATORY CELL WALL COMPONENTS. An impor-tant virulence factor of *S. pneumoniae* is the ability of cell wall constituents to provoke inflammation (Figure 18–4). Many of the symptoms of bacterial pneumonia (fever, lung damage) can be explained by the intense and largely unrestrained inflammatory response to bac-teria growing in the lung. Damage to endothelial cells allows blood to enter the lung and produces a common symptom of pneumonia, bloody sputum. Peptidogly-can fragments activate the alternative complement pathway and elicit IL-1 production by macrophages. Teichoic acid in the bacterial cell wall is also quite ef-fective in activating the alternative pathway and elic-iting cytokine production.

For some reason, most people with active pneumo-nia produce antibodies to bacterial cell wall antigens but not to capsular antigens, possibly because the cap-sular antigens are less immunogenic. Antibodies to cell wall antigens can diffuse through the porous matrix of the capsule to the bacterial surface, where they bind and activate complement by the classical pathway. This con-tributes further C5a, the PMN chemotactic factor, and C3b but does not aid phagocytic uptake of bacteria, be-cause C3b bound to the cell wall cannot make contact with phagocyte receptors owing to the physical barrier of the capsule and is targeted for degradation by protein

H bound to the capsule (see chapter 5). The net result is a continually expanding inflammatory response that causes considerable tissue damage but does not clear the bacteria. The fluid that accumulates in the lungs as pneumonia develops is due to leakage from blood ves-sels as PMNs move through vessel walls and from ac-tivated complement components that increase vascular permeability. Damage to the area also disrupts gas ex-change so that the patient literally suffocates.

PNEUMOLYSIN—AGAIN. Pneumolysin may contrib-ute to inflammation through two of its activities. First, pneumolysin by itself can activate the classical comple-ment pathway. Pneumolysin newly released from dy-ing cells by autolysis could activate complement near the surfaces of host cells, leading to further damage of host cells by the inflammatory response. A second contribution of pneumolysin to inflammation arises from the ability of pneumolysin to bind at or near the Fc portion of antibodies. Pneumolysin binding to the Fc portion of antibodies results in a conformational change in the antibody that causes activation of the clas-sical pathway. Thus, binding of pneumolysin to any an-tibodies in the area would increase complement acti-vation. Given the various ways pneumococci have of triggering the complement cascade, it is not surprising that one sign of pneumonia is depletion of complement components in the area of the infection.

Evidence supporting a role for pneumolysin in lung damage comes from the observation that purified pneu-molysin, injected into a ligated rat lung segment, pro-duced all of the histological symptoms seen in animals infected with *S. pneumoniae.* Pneumolysin has also been reported to damage endothelial cells in culture and could contribute to lung damage by damaging blood vessels. It may also help bacteria to enter the blood-stream. However, serotype 3, a highly virulent sero-type of *S. pneumoniae,* produces much lower levels of pneumolysin than other serotypes, once again raising questions about the actual function of this protein in virulence. Cell wall components can also damage en-dothelial cells and elicit a cytokine (especially TNF-α response, which would damage lung tissue). Thus, it is difficult to sort out which factors are responsible for lung damage.

Bacteria that enter the bloodstream are protected from phagocytes by their capsules. The blood also con-tains lysozyme, and levels of lysozyme rise in an area where inflammation is occurring. The *S. pneumoniae* cell wall is resistant to lysozyme, but lysozyme accelerates autolysin action, at least in vitro. Lysozyme could thus contribute to lysis of the bacteria in blood and spinal fluid, increasing the release of inflammatory cell wall components. Strains with the most active autolysins are the ones most commonly associated with the most severe disease, presumably because they are more likely to lyse and release inflammatory cell wall components. Does this mean that suicide, due to the action of *S. pneumoniae* autolysins on its own cell wall, should be considered a virulence factor?

Interaction with the Blood-Brain Barrier

The blood-brain barrier normally excludes large molecules and particulate material from the spinal fluid and brain. How, then, do pneumococci gain access to cerebrospinal fluid? The answer may lie in the ability of the bacteria to interact with endothelial cells. The blood-brain barrier contains endothelial cells. The endothelial cells are an important mediator of inflammation. Among other things, endothelial cells release a factor that helps activate the coagulation cascade (**procoagulant factor**). This factor is produced in response to LPS. Pneumococcal cell wall fragments are as effective as LPS in stimulating this activity in vitro. Teichoic acid, particularly the form with a phosphocholine moiety, may make the main contribution to this activity. Pneumococci attach to cultured endothelial cells (e.g., HUVEC). The adhesin responsible has not been identified, but cell wall fragments inhibit attachment. After attachment of the bacteria to a HUVEC monolayer, the cells of the monolayer begin to separate and eventually die. Pneumolysin is not responsible for the cytopathic effect associated with attachment because heat-killed bacteria also attached and caused the same cytopathic effects. There is a precedent for cytopathic effects being caused by peptidoglycan fragments; a peptidoglycan fragment from *Bordetella pertussis* has been shown to damage ciliated cells (see chapter 17). In the body, attachment of pneumococci to blood vessel walls of the brain and spinal column could cause breaches in the vessel walls, which lead to disruption of the blood-brain barrier and entry of bacteria and phagocytes into cerebrospinal fluid.

Signature-Tagged Mutagenesis

In the search for new insights on virulence, signature-tagged mutagenesis has been used to find new virulence genes. Recall that in signature-tagged mutagenesis (see chapter 3), a mixture of transposon variants, each tagged with a different sequence, is used to mutagenize the bacteria. The bacteria are then introduced into an animal. Bacteria that survive are screened to find which members of the original mixture of mutants did not survive in the animal. In the case of *S. pneumoniae*, this screen turned up some genes that have been described previously as virulence genes. These included a gene encoding a hyaluronidase and a gene encoding an sIgA protease. The role of these genes in virulence is

somewhat controversial, but at least there is some link to virulence. However, none of the genes with a well-established role in virulence, such as genes encoding capsule biosynthetic enzymes, pneumolysin, and surface adhesins, were identified in this screen. As usual, the screen found a plethora of housekeeping genes, including genes encoding amino acid biosynthetic enzymes and genes encoding transport proteins. It is hard to know what to make of these findings. Certainly, loss of the ability to make or take up some essential nutrient would be expected to impair the functioning of the bacteria in an animal, but it is difficult to come up with a convincing rationale for why such genes would make a specific contribution to virulence. No one questions that such general screens for genes involved in pathogenicity are needed, but how to interpret the results is still problematic. Perhaps the message is that the most important bacterial characteristic in vivo is growth rate, and anything that impacts growth rate will have a deleterious effect on the ability of the bacteria to cause infection. Certainly, we have learned this same lesson from the success of antibiotics, which drastically curtail bacterial growth rates in the body.

Antibiotic Resistance

RESISTANCE. When the penicillin-resistant pneumococci first appeared, some scientists assumed this was yet another example of resistance due to inactivation of the drug by β-lactamase. In most cases, however, as had been found with other gram-positive pathogens, mutant penicillin-binding proteins mediate resistance much more frequently than β-lactamases. To explain why this discovery was so discouraging, it is necessary to review the heartening progress that had been made in the previous decade in dealing with β-lactamase-producing bacteria. The idea was simple but effective. By combining an old β-lactam antibiotic that had been rendered obsolete by bacterial β-lactamases with a β-lactamase inhibitor, the old antibiotic became magically effective once again.

Enter the gram-positive bacteria "stage left" with a new strategy: mutated enzymes that are essential for peptidoglycan biosynthesis, enzymes that no longer bind β-lactam antibiotics. The new β-lactamase inhibitors were useless to combat this type of resistance. Bacteria were once again proving to be wily and inventive opponents, but microbiologists are tough folks too. The gram-positive cocci (those blue beach balls from hell) have a temporary advantage, but stay tuned. The only disturbing thing about this story is that microbiologists, and even more important, microbiologists who understand the physiology of gram-positive pathogens, are very thin on the ground. In military terms, we are threatened with a major attack, and all we have to counter it is a small number of—admittedly dedicated, but exhausted—defenders.

There is still more bad news to come. Physicians were so confident that pneumococci would always be treatable by penicillin and other β-lactam antibiotics that they paid little attention to the appearance of resistance to other types of antibiotics, such as erythromycin or chloramphenicol, that would have been fallback options if penicillin resistance developed. Genes encoding resistance to these antibiotics have been moving among the gram-positive bacteria on conjugative transposons (see chapter 11). The origin of these conjugative transposons is still unclear, but they are increasingly widespread. Chloramphenicol resistance is due to inactivation of the antibiotic, but the gram-positive tetracycline and erythromycin resistance genes alter the target of the antibiotic—the ribosome—so that the antibiotic no longer binds. A troubling feature of these types of resistance genes is that they often confer resistance to more than one type of antibiotic. In the case of the erythromycin resistance genes, the genes can confer resistance to three classes of antibiotics (macrolides, streptogramins, and lincosamides) (see chapter 11). No one knows why it took so long for penicillin resistance to enter the picture, but it is clear that in the interval, pneumococci have become increasingly resistant to other antibiotics as well.

Antibiotic tolerance. Just when you thought things had hit bottom, more bad news has come along in the form of **antibiotic tolerance.** Bacteria that are resistant to an antibiotic can continue to grow when the antibiotic is present. But in a patient being treated with an antibiotic, especially a patient with an impaired immune system, all the antibiotic-sensitive bacteria need to do is to shut down metabolically and survive until the end of the antibiotic therapy. This is called antibiotic tolerance. The bacteria cannot continue to multiply when the antibiotic is present, but they can survive until the antibiotic goes away. Tolerance of β-lactam antibiotics and—more worrisome—of vancomycin has been described recently. Tolerance of β-lactam antibiotics occurs in two steps. In the first step, starvation leads to depletion of autolysins. In the second step, the structure of the cell wall changes so as to make it resistant to autolysin action. Thus, any remaining autolysin is rendered ineffective. These changes allow the cells to survive exposure to the antibiotic, even though they cannot divide. If the immune system of the person being treated is in good condition, cessation of division may be sufficient to allow the host defenses to mop up the invaders. But if all of the bacteria are not cleared by the time therapy comes to an end, the bacteria will be able to make a comeback.

In the case of vancomycin tolerance, the bacteria use another pathway. Analysis of mutants that had become tolerant to vancomycin revealed that they had mutations in a gene *vncS,* which encodes a component of a two-component regulatory system. What this regulatory system controls and why such mutations cause bacteria to become vancomycin tolerant remains to be discovered. In an animal model for meningitis, an infection caused by one of these mutants was not controlled by vancomycin therapy. Thus, vancomycin tolerance may have clinical significance.

Natural Transformation

The ability of pneumococci to take up DNA from the external environment (natural transformation) is usually not listed as a virulence factor, but perhaps it should be considered one. The transformation system of pneumococci allows the bacteria to take up DNA from *S. pneumoniae* and closely related *Streptococcus* species. Double-stranded segments of DNA are bound to the cell surface, a single-stranded nick is made, and one strand is digested away. Membrane proteins of the transformation system take up the resulting single-stranded DNA. The internalized DNA can then be made double stranded and introduced into the chromosome by homologous recombination. The fact that the bacteria preferentially take up DNA from closely related strains makes it more likely that there will be enough sequence similarity to allow homologous recombination to occur.

Two possible effects of this process have been identified in connection with virulence and antibiotic resistance. Some scientists have suggested that the enormous strain-to-strain variability of the capsular polysaccharides may have resulted from events in which DNA from a strain with one capsular serotype enters a strain with another serotype. In the case of penicillin resistance, the mutant penicillin-binding proteins have a mosaic structure that may have occurred because of sequential acquisition of parts of penicillin-binding proteins from different sources.

An intriguing feature of the transformation process is that there is only a narrow window of time during which the bacteria are capable of DNA uptake (**competence**). This period of active DNA uptake occurs in mid-exponential phase and can be as short as 20 min. It is important to point out, however, that this window of opportunity may be short only in the case of bacteria growing rapidly in laboratory medium. This phase of growth could be prolonged in vivo because of nutrient limitation or other factors that limit growth. The regulation of competence has become an area of recent interest. A model for regulation of competence has been proposed (Figure 18–5). The signal is a peptide that stimulates a two-component regulatory system to activate expression of genes needed for natural transformation. A mysterious aspect of this regulation is that just as competence is triggered suddenly in mid-exponential phase, it is turned off a short time later. How this downregulation works and why the bacteria would want such a narrow window of competence are fascinating subjects for future research.

Prevention and Treatment

Antibiotic Therapy

Antibiotics have been the treatment of choice for various diseases caused by *S. pneumoniae*, but the use of antibiotics has not been completely straightforward. Not only has resistance to antibiotics muddied the waters, making treatment choices difficult in some cases, but the consequences of lysing bacteria releasing inflammatory molecules can be problematic (Box 18–1). There is also a psychological component to treatment. No one questions the use of antibiotics to treat life-threatening diseases such as pneumonia, sepsis, or meningitis, but treatment of otitis media in children is

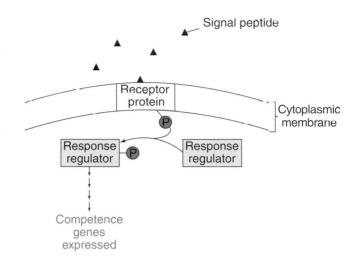

Figure 18–5 Model showing the signaling pathway leading to the development of competence in *S. pneumoniae*. A small peptide (triangles) interacts with a receptor (a transmembrane histidine kinase), causing it to become phosphorylated. The phosphorylated receptor activates a response regulator by transferring the phosphate group to it. The response regulator is a DNA binding protein. The activated response regulator in a series of unknown steps leads to expression of competence genes.

BOX 18–1   Pneumococcus Bites Back: the Meningitis Treatment Dilemma

Most strains of *S. pneumoniae* are still susceptible to β-lactam antibiotics. Thus, pneumococcal pneumonia and pneumococcal meningitis are readily curable with antibiotics in the sense that β-lactam antibiotics will rapidly kill all the bacteria in the body. Yet, until recently, many patients with pneumococcal meningitis did not survive the treatment. About 30% of children with meningitis died despite antibiotic therapy, and many survivors sustained permanent brain damage. This outcome was better than the nearly 100% mortality of untreated meningitis but was unacceptable to physicians and patients. The reason for the high death rate in antibiotic-treated patients was that β-lactam antibiotics caused the bacteria to lyse. Especially in children, pneumococci reach high levels in cerebrospinal fluid before the symptoms begin to appear. Treating such patients with β-lactam antibiotics causes a sudden release of the very cell wall fragments that were responsible for the damage seen

in cases of untreated meningitis. This leads to further inflammation, accompanied by a dangerously high level of intracranial pressure, which causes irreversible damage to the brain. The solution has been to administer the drug **dexamethasone,** an anti-inflammatory steroid, along with the β-lactam antibiotics. This therapeutic regimen has cut the death rate from 30% to less than 5%. A second treatment problem posed by meningitis is the difficulty in getting antibiotics across the blood-brain barrier. β-Lactam antibiotics do not normally reach cerebrospinal fluid. Inflammation breaches this barrier and allows some antibiotic molecules to leak through, but it would be desirable to devise some way to make the blood-brain barrier temporarily more permeable to antibiotics. Solving this problem is currently a hot area of infectious disease research.

Source: E. Tuomanen. 1993. Breaching the blood-brain barrier. *Sci. Am.* **268:**80–84.

another matter. The rationale for treating earache in children with antibiotics is less compelling because the vast majority of cases resolve spontaneously, and only in a tiny minority of cases does the child develop a more serious infection that impairs hearing. Because of this, the current recommendation for managing earache in children is to wait 24 to 48 h and then treat only if the infection is not resolving.

Yet physicians still routinely treat earache in children with antibiotics. The reason is that parents demand antibiotics. Parents may be motivated not just by their own desire to have the child become symptom free as quickly as possible, but also by the fact that some day care centers require a child with an ear infection to be taking an antibiotic before the child can return to day care. Opponents of day care like to portray parents who place children in day care as selfish adults who value their own professional commitments, income, and advancement over the well-being of their children. The more accurate image is of a desperate parent (often a single mother, who can barely afford day care) who is facing the loss of a job that supports herself and her child. It is not easy for a physician to withstand that kind of pressure.

Vaccines

The possibility that antibiotics might prove ineffective in treating pneumococcal pneumonia at some point in the future has increased the importance of having an effective vaccine. In the earlier years of vaccine development, scientists gave a high priority to developing an effective antipneumococcal vaccine, but inexperience, and in some cases incompetence, delayed the development of the vaccine that finally emerged (Box 18–2). The first successful, now widely used, vaccine consisted of the 23 most common capsular serotypes. It protected against most (but not all) virulent strains. This leaves open the possibility that outbreaks due to one of the other 57 serotypes not represented in the vaccine could occur.

Another problem with the current vaccine is that it is a polysaccharide vaccine. Since polysaccharides are less immunogenic than proteins, this vaccine does not produce a good antibody response, especially in high-risk groups such as infants (who do not respond to T-cell-independent antigens) or the elderly (whose ability to mount an antibody response is lessened). The efficacy of the currently available capsular vaccine is controversial, even in the case of adults. Clearly, it is not 100% protective, but levels of protection as high as 60% have been reported for elderly populations. In retrospect, this relatively low level of efficacy (compared with other vaccines) is not surprising.

The antipneumococcal vaccine is by far the most complex subunit vaccine ever administered to humans. Whereas most subunit vaccines consist of one or a few proteins, the pneumococcal vaccine contains 23 capsu-

---

BOX 18–2 Gold Digging and the Pneumococcal Vaccine

The search for an effective antipneumococcal vaccine goes back all the way to the 1880s. At that time, gold had recently been discovered in South Africa, and tremendous efforts were being made to mine it as fast and efficiently as possible. This required labor, which was supplied by native African miners. Unfortunately, many Africans had never been exposed to *S. pneumoniae* and were thus highly susceptible to pneumococcal infections. As the death toll rose, there was increasing political pressure to close the mines, which were under British control.

To counter this movement, the mining industry brought in microbiologists to try to prevent the spread of infection. The first scientist to make the attempt, Almroth Wright, failed not so much because the vaccine did not work, but because his data were sloppy and did not convince the skeptics. The next to try was Spencer Lister. Lister also struck out because of bad study design. He vaccinated all of the miners in one compound and used miners from a different compound as an unvaccinated control. Since, however, the attack rates were known to be different in different compounds, this was not a good enough control to establish unequivocally that the vaccine worked. It was not until 1945 that a vaccine against pneumococcal infections, the currently used mixed-polysaccharide vaccine, was conclusively proved to have some beneficial effects.

Source: R. Austrian. 1999. The pneumococcus at the millennium: not down, not out. *J. Infect. Dis.* **179**(Suppl. 2):S338–S341.

lar serotypes. Consider the statistics. If one serotype is 90% effective against infections caused by that particular serotype, how effective would four serotypes be? Try $0.9 \times 0.9 \times 0.9 \times 0.9 = 0.66$, or 66% effective against all four serotypes. Despite the relatively low level of protection, the vaccine is still recommended for high-risk groups such as the elderly on the basis that some protection is better than none at all.

More recently, scientists working on vaccine development have been attempting to reduce the complexity of the vaccine and to replace carbohydrate antigens with more immunogenic molecules. The first important development was a conjugate vaccine consisting of polysaccharide antigens covalently attached to proteins to make the vaccine more immunogenic. Such a vaccine, primarily aimed at preventing ear infections, has entered the market. It covers seven capsular serotypes.

Currently, efforts are under way to develop protein-based subunit vaccines using surface proteins such as PspA, pneumolysin, and some of the other antigens that elicit a protective antibody response and are effective against more than one capsular serotype. Moreover, since these are proteins, they should be more immunogenic in high-risk groups such as infants and the elderly. Such protein vaccines are currently being tested. The major issue has been the antigenic variability of the proteins. The ideal vaccine would consist of one or two highly conserved proteins that are exposed on the surface of the capsule and elicit a protective antibody response. The recent availability of the complete genome sequence of *S. pneumoniae* will make it easier to identify such proteins. A DNA vaccine consisting of the gene for PspA is being developed.

The increasing resistance of *S. pneumoniae* strains to antibiotics, coupled to the fact that coverage by the conjugate vaccine is incomplete, has caused scientists to take another look at an older treatment strategy—passive immunization. There is no question that opsonizing antibodies against capsular antigens are protective; the problem is that in some people the capsular polysaccharide vaccine does not elicit an effective enough antibody response. A solution to this problem is to inject antibodies against capsular antigens to give the patient's body help in clearing the bacteria from the lung or bloodstream. This type of treatment can have side effects, especially if the antibodies come from nonhuman animals. But since the death rate in untreated cases of pneumonia is so high, the potential benefits to a patient with pneumonia clearly outweigh the risks.

SELECTED READINGS

Aronin, S. I., and V. J. Quagliarello. 2001. New perspectives on pneumococcal meningitis. *Hosp. Pract.* **36**:43–51.

Briles, D. E., R. C. Tart, E. Swiatlo, J. P. Dillard, P. Smith, K. A. Benton, B. A. Ralph, A. Brooks-Walter, M. J. Crain, S. K. Hollingshead, and L. S. McDaniel. 1998. Pneumococcal diversity: consideration for new vaccine strategies with emphasis on pneumococcal surface protein A (PspA). *Clin. Microbiol. Rev.* **11**:645–657.

Coffey, T. J., M. C. Enright, M. Daniels, J. K. Morona, R. Morona, W. Hryniewicz, J. C. Paton, and B. G. Spratt. 1998. Recombinational exchanges at the capsular polysaccharide biosynthetic locus lead to frequent serotype changes among natural isolates of *Streptococcus pneumoniae*. *Mol. Microbiol.* **27**:73–83.

Cundell, D., H. R. Masure, and E. I. Tuomanen. 1995. The molecular basis of pneumococcal infection: a hypothesis. *Clin. Infect. Dis.* **21**(Suppl. 3):S204–S212.

Håvarstein, L. S. 1998. Identification of a competence regulon in *Streptococcus pneumoniae* by genomic analysis. *Trends Microbiol.* **6**:297–299.

Jedrzejas, M. J. 2001. Pneumococcal virulence factors: structure and function. *Microbiol. Mol. Biol. Rev.* **65**: 187–207.

Mitchell, T. J., and P. W. Andrew. 1997. Biological properties of pneumolysin. *Microb. Drug Resist.* **1**:19–26.

Novak, R., B. Henriques, E. Charpentier, S. Normark, and E. Tuomanen. 1999. Emergence of vancomycin tolerance in *Streptococcus pneumoniae*. *Nature* **399**:590–593.

Paton, J. C., A. M. Berry, and R. A. Lock. 1997. Molecular analysis of putative pneumococcal virulence factors. *Microb. Drug Resist.* **1**:1–10.

Polissi, A., A. Pontiggia, G. Feger, M. Altieri, H. Mottl, L. Ferrari, and D. Simon. 1998. Large-scale identification of virulence genes from *Streptococcus pneumoniae*. *Infect. Immun.* **66**:620–629.

Tomasz, A. 2000. *Streptococcus pneumoniae: Molecular Biology and Mechanisms of Disease.* Mary Ann Liebert, Inc., New York, N.Y.

Tong, H. H., L. M. Fisher, B. M. Kosunick, and T. F. DeMaria. 2000. Effect of adenovirus type 1 and influenza A virus on *Streptococcus pneumoniae* nasopharyngeal colonization and otitis media in the chinchilla. *Ann. Otol. Rhinol. Laryngol.* **109**:1021–1027.

Tuomanen, E., and A. Tomasz. 1990. Mechanism of phenotypic tolerance of nongrowing pneumococci to beta-lactam antibiotics. *Scand. J. Infect. Dis.* **74**:102–112.

SUMMARY OUTLINE

Diseases caused by *S. pneumoniae*

Ear infections in children
Very common
Usually self-limited

Pneumonia
Main cause
High death rate if untreated
Sepsis can develop

Meningitis
Especially in infants
Even if treated successfully, long-term effects may result

Characteristics

Gram-positive diplococci

Bile solubility—most strains

Polysaccharide capsule
80 + serotypes
23 most commonly involved in infections
Quellung reaction—swelling of capsule by antibodies that react with the capsule

Naturally transformable (take up DNA from the medium naturally)
Permitted discovery of DNA

Progression

Colonization of the nose and throat gives the opportunity for access to the middle ear or lung

Damage to ciliated cells (e.g., by viral infection) allows bacteria to enter lung

Antiphagocytic capsule prevents lung macrophages from acting

Inflammatory response and bacterial toxins cause tissue damage

Bacteria enter bloodstream, causing sepsis, meningitis

Virulence factors

Animal models
Mouse—pneumonia
Chinchilla—ear infections

Molecular model of progression
Changing pattern of host cell receptors
Inflammation leads to further change in receptors that aid adherence

Protein virulence factors
Pneumolysin
Binds cholesterol
Forms pores
Many activities—may impair phagocytes, contribute to lung damage
Putative adhesins—also vaccine candidates
PspA—function unknown
SpsA—binds secretory chain of sIgA
PsaA—adherence to pneumocytes
CbpA—binds choline

(*continued*)

SUMMARY OUTLINE (*continued*)

Capsule
- Polysaccharide
- At least 80 serotypes, 23 responsible for most disease
- Antiphagocytic
- Major virulence factor

Cell wall components—inflammation
- LTA
- Peptidoglycan fragments

Interaction with meninges—inflammation

Antibiotic resistance
- Mutant penicillin-binding proteins
- Multidrug-resistant strains more common; resistance genes on mobile elements, such as conjugative transposons
- Tolerance for β-lactam antibiotics and vancomycin

Transformation system
- Takes up DNA from closely related streptococci
- May contribute to variability in penicillin-binding proteins, capsular types

Prevention and treatment
- Antibiotics
- Vaccine
  - Capsular vaccine
    - Most complex vaccine available
    - 23 serotypes of capsular polysaccharides
    - Not immunogenic in infants
    - Poorly immunogenic in the elderly
  - New vaccine—protein conjugated to capsular serotypes
  - Future vaccines—mixture of surface proteins, pneumolysin; PspA DNA vaccine
  - Passive immunization—injection of anticapsular antibodies from another source

QUESTIONS

Answers to the questions can be found in Appendix 2.

1. What factors make a DNA-based test preferable to conventional methods of isolation and identification? How would you design a PCR test to detect *S. pneumoniae,* and how would you check its accuracy?

2. What host defenses must be overcome by *S. pneumoniae* in causing an infection?

3. Why does pneumolysin have so many activities in vitro? Is there any way to figure out which, if any, of these activities is actually important in vivo?

4. Should autolysins be considered a virulence factor?

5. What virulence factors are responsible for the symptoms of meningitis? Why is it necessary to give steroids along with antibiotics?

6. Would pneumococcal cell walls make a good vaccine?

7. What is the rationale for developing a vaccine based on pneumolysin or one of the surface adhesins? Would these proteins have to be modified in any way to make them vaccine components?

8. Even during the period when penicillin was still effective against most strains of *S. pneumoniae,* the use of broad-spectrum antibiotics other than penicillin to treat pneumonia had become increasingly popular with clinicians. Why?

9. It is recommended that patients in nursing homes receive the pneumococcal vaccine. In addition, it is recommended that staff members receive not only this vaccine but the flu vaccine as well. What is the rationale for this second recommendation?

10. During natural transformation, the double-stranded DNA is made single stranded before it enters the cell, then made double stranded again inside the cell. Why would bacteria do this?

19

Tuberculosis

KEY FEATURES

Mycobacterium tuberculosis

CHARACTERISTICS
Gram-positive type cell wall with unusually high lipid content; rod shape
Special stain required (acid-fast stain)
Aerobic metabolism, very slow growth in culture
Capable of long-term survival in the human body (persistence)

DISEASE
Tuberculosis (TB)

RESERVOIR
Humans, especially those with latent TB

MAJOR VIRULENCE FACTORS
Ability to survive in lung macrophages
Avoidance of activated macrophage response
Cell wall components that elicit damage to tissue
Ability to survive for decades in walled-off lesions

PREVENTION AND TREATMENT
Diagnostic techniques: skin test, acid-fast stain
Vaccine, but not effective in all populations (especially the elderly and infants)
Special anti-TB therapy requires multiple drugs taken for many months

---

A Disease of the Past Returns To Haunt the Future

As late as the 1800s, tuberculosis (TB) was still an epidemic disease in the United States, Europe, and England, and the annual death toll was nearly 1% of the population in some cities. To put this in context, consider that in a city the size of New York City, this would correspond to over 100,000 deaths per year, a patient load that would swamp the hospital capacity of even the most advanced of today's modern medical centers. As living conditions began to improve, however, the incidence of TB began to decline, at least in developed countries. Unfortunately, a similar decline did not occur in developing countries, and TB remains today one of the top three killers (with malaria and HIV) of people worldwide.

291

The discovery of a cure for TB in the 1950s, together with the development of inexpensive screening tests to detect infected people (skin test, chest X rays), made it possible for the first time to think that TB might be eradicated in the developed countries. In the United States, England, and Europe, public health programs aimed at eliminating TB were initiated and aggressively pursued. Widespread screening of the population identified people with the disease. A person with diagnosed TB was required by law to accept treatment and could be incarcerated if treatment was refused. Health care workers were hired to check that TB patients being treated on an outpatient basis were taking their medication regularly over the full period prescribed. This was very important, because the treatment regimen required the patient to take three or more pills several days a week for 6 months.

These measures were successful in decreasing the number of new TB cases to an all-time low. But, although TB was fast disappearing in developed countries, it remained a major cause of death in developing countries. Nearly 2 billion people are currently infected with the organism that causes tuberculosis, and about 8,000,000 new cases occur each year, making TB one of the most common infectious diseases worldwide. In developing countries, TB is the cause of 6% of all infant deaths, nearly 20% of adult deaths, and 26% of avoidable deaths.

Nothing Fails Like Success

Ironically, the success of anti-TB public health programs in the United States and Europe proved to be their undoing. In the early 1970s, most of these anti-TB programs were dismantled, and funds previously allotted to them were redirected to what appeared at the time to be more urgent health care needs. For the next decade, TB cases continued to decline, but suddenly beginning in the mid-1980s, some countries began to notice an increase in new cases. The number of new cases continued to increase until public concern made new action imperative. One factor contributing to this increase was immigration. Immigrants from countries where TB is endemic account for about one-fourth of the new TB cases in the United States.

Another important factor contributing to the resurgence of TB was the crowded conditions seen in many homeless shelters and prisons and the presence in these settings of people who were substance abusers or had HIV infections, two factors that increase susceptibility to TB. New cases of TB were not limited to residents of homeless shelters and prisons. People staffing such institutions and health care workers caring for people with active TB also acquired the disease and in some

cases spread the disease further before they were diagnosed and treated.

Drug Resistance—a Worrisome New Development

A resurgence of TB is cause enough for concern, but many of the new outbreaks had a frightening difference from earlier outbreaks of the disease. Strains of *Mycobacterium tuberculosis*, the cause of TB, were increasingly likely to be resistant to one or more of the drugs used to treat TB, and some strains were effectively untreatable, except by experimental drugs or surgery to remove part of the lung. Since the fatality rate of untreated TB is 50%, the appearance of untreatable strains caused a panic among public health workers. The rise of drug-resistant strains could have been predicted (and was predicted) to occur under conditions seen with increasing frequency in decaying inner cities. Yet, physicians and public health officials were caught in a state of complete unpreparedness.

With the dismantling of anti-TB programs a decade earlier, TB had been largely forgotten by the medical community. In many hospitals, young doctors were not being trained to diagnose and treat TB or were given only a cursory introduction to the disease. The ability of clinical laboratories to diagnose TB was also diminished. Research on TB had been drastically curtailed, and little effort had been expended to develop an effective vaccine. To make matters worse, the pharmaceutical companies, assured by the medical community that TB was a disease of the past in developed countries, and not considering developing countries a sufficiently lucrative market, had discontinued efforts to find new anti-TB drugs and had even stopped making some well-established anti-TB drugs, such as streptomycin. Thus, in contrast to other bacterial diseases in which the development of resistant strains can be offset by new antibiotics entering the marketplace, there were no new anti-TB drugs under development. This is a serious problem, because it can take 20 years to bring a new drug from the discovery stage to the market.

So Soon We Forget

Despite the state of unpreparedness of the health care infrastructure, an effective mobilization of resources was achieved, and the resurgence of TB was once again brought under control. The costs of reestablishing control were high. It has been estimated that New York City alone spent nearly a billion dollars to clean up a TB outbreak in that city, an outbreak caused in part by drug-resistant strains. And this outbreak only involved a few thousand cases, not the millions of cases seen in some parts of the world. Why is TB control so expensive? For one thing, patients with active TB have to be isolated in specially constructed rooms where the flow of air is monitored to make sure that air from the room is not flowing outward into nearby hospital wards. For another, control efforts—from monitoring the long-term therapy of patients to special precautions taken to protect hospital personnel from infection—are very labor-intensive.

Did we learn anything from this frightening experience? Not really. The minute the genie appeared to be back in its bottle, the medical community once more reverted to its stance of benign neglect. What infrastructure had been assembled has already started to decay.

What is very wrong with this picture is that there are thousands of people walking around in large U.S. cities today with dormant multidrug-resistant bacteria in their lungs. At least some of these people will develop active disease in the future, a form of TB called reactivation TB. Moreover, TB and HIV infection appear to be synergistic, so more HIV means more TB. From Russia comes an alarming warning. TB is spreading like wildfire in Russian prisons, creating an increasingly large reservoir of infected people. The Russian government cannot afford to treat all these people, now that their economy is in a state of collapse. Every day, airplanes from all over the world, including the TB hot spots, are landing in U.S. and European airports. Fortunately, there is no reason to panic and no reason to limit immigration or travel out of fear of TB. In fact, the most pressing problem is not immigrants but us, the citizens of developed countries. We are the ones who created the drug-resistant TB strains, which we are now exporting to the rest of the world. The best remedy is to maintain a state of preparedness so that the TB problem, when it arises again, is not allowed to get out of hand, as it very nearly did in the 1990s.

Spread and Progression of Tuberculosis

Symptoms and Mode of Spread

Tuberculosis is caused by *M. tuberculosis,* an obligately aerobic rod-shaped bacterium with a gram-positive-type cell wall that has an unusually high lipid content. The disease is spread from person to person by aerosols. An earlier view of how TB is spread is described in Box 19–1. Aerosol-spread diseases such as TB are particularly insidious because the tiny droplets generated by coughing not only bypass the defenses of the upper airway but stay in the air much longer than larger particles. Whereas cleaning of surfaces with disinfectants

provides a cheap and effective means of eliminating bacteria that settle on these surfaces, disinfecting air requires special filters and is so expensive that it is not feasible for large-scale use.

Symptoms of TB include fever, coughing (often with bloody sputum), weight loss, and loss of energy (malaise). Progressive, irreversible lung destruction occurs, and the bacteria may escape from the lungs and enter the bloodstream. *M. tuberculosis* can infect any area of the body, including bones, joints, liver, spleen, gastrointestinal tract, and brain. The systemic form of the disease is almost always fatal. TB is not normally a fast-developing disease. Often the patient continues to decline in health for years before finally succumbing. In people with AIDS, the disease kills more rapidly, and the fatality rate is nearly 80%.

TB is a serious disease, and a highly contagious one. Transmission is most likely when there is prolonged close contact between a susceptible person and a person who has an active case of TB, but that contact does not have to be intimate. Under the right conditions a single person with active TB can infect many other people (Box 19–2). The word "infect" needs to be defined carefully. A person is considered infected with *M. tuberculosis* if he or she converts from negative to positive on a TB skin test. Conversion to positive on the skin test indicates that *M. tuberculosis* has been inhaled and has been able to survive in the lung long enough to attract the attention of the immune system (see below). Only a subset of people who become skin test positive actually develop active TB; usually this subset is only about 1% of infected people, but it can be as high as 40% if the population is stressed, malnourished, or has underlying conditions, such as HIV infection.

Progression of the Disease

An important defense of the lung is the alveolar macrophage. *M. tuberculosis* has evolved the ability to survive and multiply in unactivated alveolar macrophages. Activated macrophages can kill the bacteria, however. Thus, the ability of a person to mount a rapid and effective activated macrophage response determines whether the outcome of exposure will be symptomatic disease or not (Figure 19–1). The initial interaction between *M. tuberculosis* and macrophages elicits both a T-helper (CD4$^+$) and a cytotoxic T-cell (CD8$^+$) response. There has been some controversy over the relative importance of these two types of T cells in bringing the infection under control, but both make a contribution to host protection.

The CD4$^+$ T cells stimulate antibody production, but antibodies against *M. tuberculosis* are useless since the bacteria are serum resistant and can multiply inside

BOX 19–1   Tuberculosis and Vampires

Tuberculosis was a mysterious disease until Koch demonstrated in the late 1800s that it was caused by a bacterium that was spread by aerosols. Koch announced his discovery in 1882, but this new information about tuberculosis took many years to penetrate the public consciousness. Meanwhile, since tuberculosis was a much-feared disease, other theories of causation continued to prevail.

Perhaps the most bizarre example of such a theory was the belief that vampires caused tuberculosis. This belief appears to have been widespread in the northeastern United States during the 19th century. If a vampire was thought to be feeding off the living, as indicated by cases of TB (or "consumption" as it was known at the time), the supposed vampire's body was exhumed and inspected. Signs such as failure of the body to decompose and "blood in the heart" indicated that the person was a vampire. In such cases, the heart (and sometimes other organs) was removed and burned. The skull was removed from the spinal column and placed on the upper chest, with the leg bones crossed below it, skull and crossbones fashion. These measures were believed to kill the vampire and thus to prevent further cases of tuberculosis.

Ten documented cases of this type of "therapy" have been assembled, spanning the period from 1770 to 1892. All but one took place in Rhode Island, Connecticut, or Vermont, usually in rural communities. One example is provided by the Brown family of Exeter, R.I., which consisted of a mother, a father, and seven children. The mother died of consumption in 1883. A daughter died 6 months later. Several years later, a son developed symptoms of TB and went to Colorado for the restorative effect of the dry climate. While he was gone, a second daughter sickened of consumption and died. When the son returned home, shortly after his sister's death, his condition began to worsen.

It was decided by relatives and friends that a vampire (presumably either his dead mother or one of his dead sisters) was draining him of life. Accordingly, the graves of his mother and two sisters were opened. Two were skeletons, but the third (the daughter who had died 2 months earlier) still had "blood in her heart" (probably decomposition of heart tissue, not real blood). The heart was removed and burned. In this case, the bones were not rearranged, although placing bones in the skull-and-crossbones configuration was seen in other cases. This therapeutic intervention did not work, of course, and the brother died soon after.

Why would people of that period connect vampires with TB? Three characteristics of the disease suggest an answer. One is the gradual wasting away of the sufferer, as if his or her life energy were being drained. The second is the enhanced appetite of the sick person. Such a hunger might well persist after death, causing the dead person to hunger for the life energy of those still alive. Finally, a case of TB was often followed by other cases among people who were closely related or well known to the first person to die, as if the undead one knew well where to find its victims.

Adapted from P. S. Sledzik and N. Bellantoni. 1994. Brief communication: bioarcheological and biocultural evidence for the New England vampire folk belief. *Am. J. Physical Anthropol.* **94**:268.

Two points to ponder: How would you satisfy Koch's postulates if you were testing the vampires-cause-TB hypothesis? How would you investigate this hypothesis at the molecular level?

phagocytes. The main contribution of the CD4$^+$ T cells to controlling an incipient infection seems to be production of IFN-γ, which stimulates macrophage activation. (CD8$^+$ T cells also release IFN-γ but to a lesser extent.) IFN-γ also stimulates endothelial cells to bind T cells, thus triggering their movement out of the blood vessel and into adjacent tissue so that they can converge on the infected area. The importance of IFN-γ is evident from the fact that transgenic mice that no longer make IFN-γ are much more susceptible to *M. tuberculosis* infection than normal mice.

There is some evidence that in humans other cytokines may be needed in addition to IFN-γ to stimulate the activation of macrophages, but IFN-γ still plays an important role in human infections. CD8$^+$ T cells kill infected phagocytes that have not succeeded in

BOX 19–2   Tuberculosis Outbreak in a California Prison— and in a School Bus

In 1991, in a large California prison with 5,421 inmates and 1,500 staff members, 18 cases of active TB occurred. In previous years, even one case would have been considered unusual. Ten of the cases developed in the prison, presumably in prisoners who entered prison with the disease. In other cases, the person entered prison with symptomatic TB. One of the people who developed symptomatic TB was a staff member. Three cases were caused by strains that were resistant to at least one of the anti-TB drugs. Although 18 cases out of nearly 7,000 prisoners and staff might not sound like a lot, this incidence of disease is more than 10 times higher than the incidence of TB in the general population, a difference that reflects the effect of crowding on the emergence of the disease.

This figure also underestimates the actual spread of the bacteria. Skin test information was available for nearly 3,000 inmates. Of these, 873 were skin test positive. Many inmates were skin test positive when they entered the institution, but 324 tested positive for the first time in prison. There was no systematic information about skin test results for staff members, but two staff members aside from the one diagnosed with active TB had a record of conversion from skin test negative to skin test positive during the 2 years including the outbreak. Thus, at least 324 inmates and three staff members may have been infected during the outbreak.

This outbreak was easily manageable, because the number of active cases was small enough to allow isolation and effective treatment of people with symptomatic disease. Also, only a few cases were due to drug-resistant strains, and these strains were still susceptible to enough drugs to allow the infection to be controlled. If the number of cases had been higher, or if a multiply resistant strain had been involved, the outcome could have been much worse. What frightens public health officials is the possibility that outbreaks caused by multiply resistant strains will occur and may be almost impossible to control in a large crowded prison. Such outbreaks have become common in prisons in the former Soviet Union.

You don't have to be in prison to contract TB. A bus driver who thought he had a smoker's cough but actually had active TB infected many children on a school bus in rural New York State. Thirty-two percent of the children who rode that bus were infected, and 51 of the 81 infected children developed active TB. The length of the ride made a difference too. Only 22% of children whose ride was only 10 minutes long were infected, but 57% of the children who were on the bus for more than 40 minutes were infected. This is by no means the only school-associated outbreak, and it illustrates an important aspect of TB: TB is more contagious in infants and children than it is in adults.

Sources: Anonymous. 1992. Tuberculosis transmission in a state correctional institution—California, 1990–1991. *Morb. Mortal. Wkly. Rep.* **41**:927–929; K. A. Sepkowitz. 1996. How contagious is tuberculosis? *Clin. Infect. Dis.* **23**:954–962.

destroying the bacteria so that the bacteria can be ingested and killed by activated macrophages. The importance of CD8$^+$ T cells in the protective response can be seen from the fact that transgenic mice that lack β_2-macroglobulin and do not make functional CD8$^+$ cells are more susceptible to TB than the parental line. The argument over which type of T cell makes an important contribution to immunity is not simply an academic dispute. An effective vaccine must stimulate the right type of immune response if it is to provide long-lasting immunity to TB.

In a healthy adult exposed to relatively low numbers of bacteria, activated macrophages generally appear early enough to stop the infection before appreciable damage is done to the lung. Such people become skin test positive but do not develop symptomatic TB. In an infant, or in an adult who cannot mount a rapid and effective T-cell response, activated macrophages do not appear until much later in the disease process, and the bacteria continue to multiply in lung macrophages. Since the phagocytic cells are not clearing the infection, new T cells, PMNs, and macrophages continue to be at-

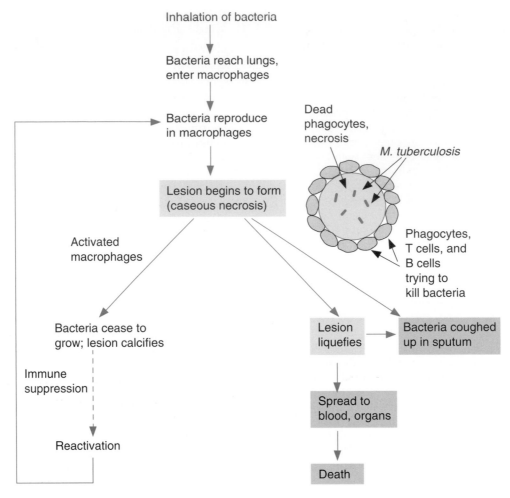

Figure 19–1   Steps in the development of tuberculosis.

tracted to the area and accumulate around the sites where bacteria are growing. Macrophages in the vicinity of the bacteria fuse to form **giant cells,** and a layer of macrophages and T cells forms around a growing focus of damaged tissue containing the bacteria.

In some cases, although the phagocytes are not able to kill the bacteria, the T cells and macrophages are successful in walling off the growing lesion with a thick fibrin coat. The walled-off lesion is called a **tubercle.** Tubercles eventually calcify, giving rise to the hard-edged lesions visible in chest radiograms. The cell-mediated (T cell plus phagocyte) response that produces tubercles is called a **granulomatous response** because the tubercles appear macroscopically as granulomas.

Phagocytes trying unsuccessfully to kill the bacteria cause considerable damage to lung tissue, both by releasing lysosomal enzymes and by producing TNF-α. TNF-α causes tissue damage and is probably also responsible for the weight loss that occurs in people with TB. An important characteristic of lesions that develop during a case of TB is the consistency of their contents. Initially, the areas where bacteria are dividing have a thick, cheeselike consistency (**caseous necrosis**). As bacteria continue to divide and phagocytes continue to enter the area, the necrotic region becomes much more liquid. Since a liquid is much more easily rendered into aerosols than the thicker caseous material, a person with liquefied lesions is much more contagious than a person whose lesions are in the caseous necrosis stage. Also, the thick consistency of a caseous lesion prevents bacterial movement out of the area. Bacteria in a liquefied lesion can escape from the lesion more readily and spread to other parts of the body, causing the disseminated form of the disease (**miliary TB**).

A person who has mounted an immune response that stops bacterial growth and prevents the development of severe symptomatic disease is not necessarily out of danger. Walled-off lesions may contain live bacteria. An unusual feature of *M. tuberculosis* is its ability to survive for decades in such lesions. Later in life, suppression of the immune system (e.g., by cancer, immunosuppressive drugs, or AIDS) may allow the bacteria to break out of the lesion and begin to multiply again. This form of the disease, called **reactivation TB** (Figure 19–1), is identical to primary TB in its infectiousness and in the damage it can cause. People infected with *M. tuberculosis* but with no other risk factor have a likelihood of 2 to 23% over a lifetime to develop reactivation TB. The spread in these estimates gives some idea of how little scientists know about what factors cause reactivation. A person who has an HIV infection has a 5 to 10% per year probability of developing reactivation TB. HIV and TB are truly the infectious disease equivalent of the one-two punch.

Latency and Persistence— Another TB Mystery

M. tuberculosis can survive for decades in an infected person's lungs before reactivating and causing an active infection. This is called **latency,** and traits that enable the bacteria to survive in the lung for a prolonged period of time are called **persistence factors.** The phenomenon of latency still mystifies scientists, who are not even sure where the bacteria are in a person with a latent infection. Most would say that the bacteria are in tubercles in the lungs or in the lung-associated lymph nodes, but some people develop a form of reactivation disease that involves organs other than the lung. This raises the possibility that latent bacteria may also hide out in other locations beside the lungs.

Another mystery is how the bacteria manage to survive for such long periods. One hypothesis is that although mycobacteria are not spore-formers, the bacteria assume a sporelike state in which they are metabolically inactive but still capable of reverting to their actively replicating form. Some indirect support for this hypothesis has come from analysis of the *M. tuberculosis* genome sequence. *M. tuberculosis* has genes that are related to genes from *Streptomyces* sp. that regulate sporulation in that spore-forming bacterium. One of these genes is *sigF*, which encodes a putative sigma factor. In *M. tuberculosis*, *sigF* is expressed in stationary phase, a characteristic that fits with the spore hypothesis. There is no sign, however, of the sporulation genes themselves. If *M. tuberculosis* has a metabolically inactive form, it is likely to differ considerably from spores of known spore-formers. An opposing hypothesis is that the bacteria are metabolically active, but only marginally so. An observation that supports this hypothesis is that antibiotic therapy reduces the likelihood of re-activation TB. Scientists assume that antibiotics only work on metabolically active bacteria.

There is an animal model for reactivation TB that was developed in the 1950s. Mice are very susceptible to *M. tuberculosis* and develop lung lesions similar to those seen in humans. The mice are inoculated with *M. tuberculosis* and then treated with anti-TB drugs for 12 weeks. Then treatment is terminated. At 4 weeks into the no-treatment period, the mice appear to have been cured. Bacteria are not seen in their organs, although PCR can detect the presence of bacterial DNA. After another 8 weeks with no treatment, about one-third of the animals develop reactivation TB and die.

The latency (or reactivation) model has been used to identify two genes in addition to *sigF* that appear to be important for persistence of bacteria in the animal. One of these genes is *acr*, a gene that encodes a protein called α-**crystallin.** This gene is expressed primarily in stationary phase and encodes a chaperone. Disruption of *acr* reduces persistence of the bacteria.

Another possible persistence gene comes as something of a surprise: **isocitrate lyase,** an enzyme of the **glyoxylate cycle** (Figure 19–2). Disruption of the isocitrate lyase gene leads to loss of the persistence phenotype in the animal model. An explanation is suggested by the fact that although mycobacteria grow on carbohydrates in laboratory medium, their real substrates in vivo may well be fatty acids. Metabolism of fatty acids requires a β-oxidation pathway, which breaks down fatty acids linked to S-coenzyme A (S-CoA) to acetyl-S-CoA. The acetyl-S-CoA is fed into the first steps of the

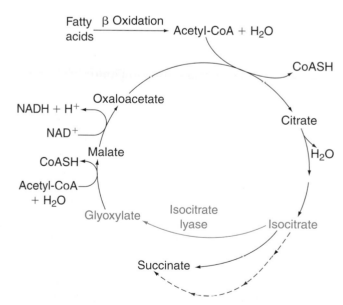

Figure 19–2   The glyoxylate cycle. Dotted arrows represent the steps in the TCA cycle that are bypassed by the glyoxylate cycle.

tricarboxylic acid (TCA) cycle and thence into the gly-oxylate pathway (Figure 19–2). The role of the glyoxylate pathway is to produce succinate, which can be used to make more microbial biomass, instead of oxidizing acetyl-S-CoA all the way to carbon dioxide, which becomes carbon lost to the cell. If fatty acids are important substrates for bacteria in the latent or persistent state, such enzymes would be critical for persistence. Efforts are now under way to determine whether isocitrate lyase would make a good target for antimycobacterial drugs. An encouraging fact is that humans lack isocitrate lyase, so drugs targeting this enzyme would be likely to have minimal side effects.

Mycobacterium tuberculosis and Its Unusual Cell Wall—a Case of Fat Making for Lean and Mean

Unlike cell walls of other gram-positive bacteria, the cell wall of *Mycobacterium* species consists not only of peptidoglycan but also of a number of unusual glycolipids that make mycobacteria impervious to mild staining procedures such as the Gram stain. To stain mycobacteria, a harsh procedure called **acid-fast staining** must be used. In this procedure, bacteria are boiled in an acid-alcohol solution with a red dye (**fuchsin**). Mycobacteria are the only bacteria that take up and retain the stain effectively when exposed to such drastic conditions. A few other genera of bacteria (e.g., *Nocardia*) stain weakly with the acid-fast staining procedure, but such bacteria are uncommon causes of human disease. Accordingly, the presence of red rods in an acid-fast-stained clinical specimen is a strong indication that a *Mycobacterium* species is responsible for the disease.

A schematic view of some of the constituents of the mycobacterial cell wall is shown in Figure 19–3. In addition to peptidoglycan, the mycobacterial cell wall contains glycolipids such as the **arabinogalactan-lipid** complex and **mycolic acids,** a type of lipid found only in the cell walls of *Mycobacterium* and *Corynebacterium* species. Lipid accounts for over 10% of the total weight of mycobacteria, a much higher percentage than in other bacteria. The complex, lipid-rich cell wall of mycobacteria protects the bacteria from the effects of toxic phagolysosomal components and is probably the reason why mycobacteria are not killed by normal, unactivated macrophages. The complex cell wall has also protected mycobacteria from researchers. Mycobacteria are much more difficult than most bacteria to disrupt, and cell wall constituents interfere with many procedures commonly used for isolation of DNA and RNA, a fact that considerably slowed the application of molecular biology techniques to the study of mycobacteria.

Mycobacterial cell wall components are highly stimulatory to the mammalian immune system. The ability of the lipid portion of the mycobacterial cell wall to enhance the antibody response to protein antigens has been exploited for years by scientists in the form of an adjuvant called **Freund's adjuvant.** The active ingredient in Freund's adjuvant is mycobacterial cell walls.

Treatment of TB and the Challenge Posed by Drug-Resistant Strains

Standard Treatment Options

Most of the commonly used antibiotics (e.g., penicillins, cephalosporins, tetracyclines, and chloramphenicol) are ineffective against tuberculosis. Exceptions are rifampin and streptomycin. Resistance to streptomycin has become so widespread in other bacterial pathogens that streptomycin is hardly used anymore in developed countries. During the outbreaks of the 1990s in the United States, the government had to appeal to developing countries for streptomycin, which is still made and used widely in poor countries. Some of the new fluoroquinolones may also inhibit mycobacterial growth, although they are still under study as therapeutic agents.

The backbone of TB therapy has been a set of special antibiotics that are effective primarily against mycobacteria: **isoniazid, ethambutol,** and **pyrazinamide** (Figure 19–4). Isoniazid and ethambutol probably act by inhibiting synthesis of mycolic acids, a major component of the mycobacterial cell wall. The mechanism of pyrazinamide action is not known. The fact that as late as the 1980s there was virtually no information about how most of the anti-TB drugs work gives you an idea how thoroughly unprepared public health officials were to deal with the resurgence of the disease. This lack of information has seriously impeded the development of new forms of these old drugs that could be used to combat resistant strains.

A mechanism of action of isoniazid has now been proposed and is shown in Figure 19–5. Isoniazid is first activated to its active form (isonicotinic acyl radical) by a **catalase, KatG.** The activated form is then covalently attached to an NADH moiety in the active site of **InhA,** an **acyl-carrier protein reductase** that acts on long-chain lipids and catalyzes a step in the synthesis of mycolic acid. Isoniazid inhibits that activity of InhA (Figure 19–5). One mechanism of resistance to isoniazid has been identified—mutations that inactivate *katG*. There

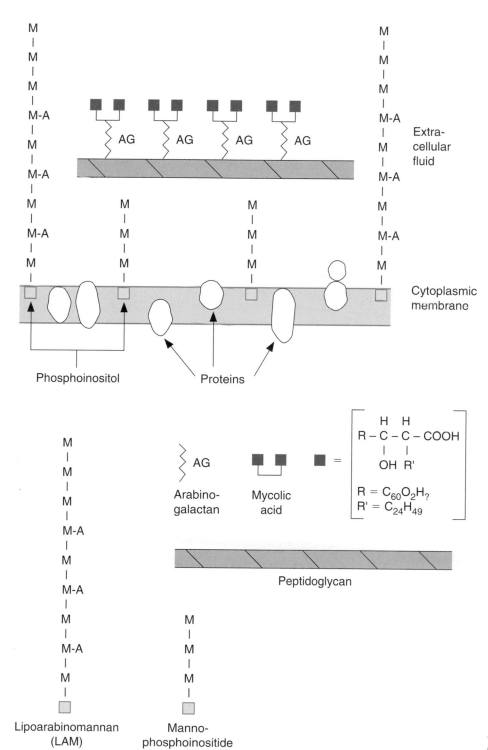

Extra-
cellular
fluid

Cytoplasmic
membrane

Phosphoinositol

Proteins

Arabino-
galactan

Mycolic
acid

$$\left[\begin{array}{c} \mathrm{H} \quad \mathrm{H} \\ \mathrm{R-C-C-COOH} \\ | \quad | \\ \mathrm{OH} \quad \mathrm{R'} \\[1em] \mathrm{R = C_{60}O_2H_?} \\ \mathrm{R' = C_{24}H_{49}} \end{array}\right]$$

Peptidoglycan

Lipoarabinomannan
(LAM)

Manno-
phosphoinositide

Figure 19–3 Schematic drawing
of the cell wall of *M. tuberculosis.*

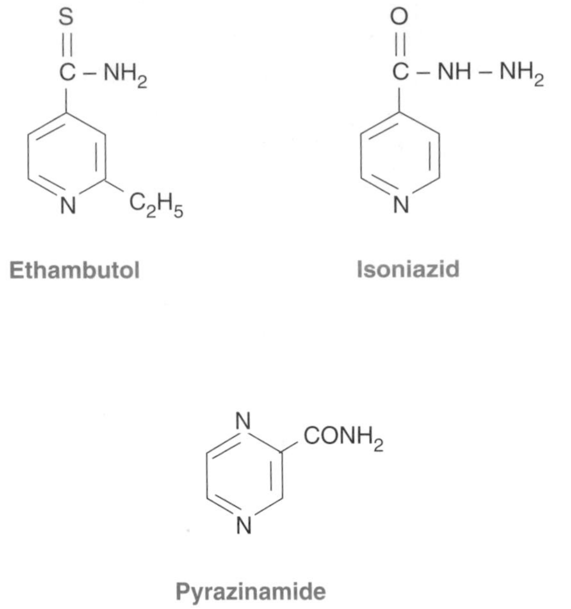

Ethambutol   Isoniazid

Pyrazinamide

Figure 19–4 Structures of ethambutol, isoniazid, and pyrazinamide.

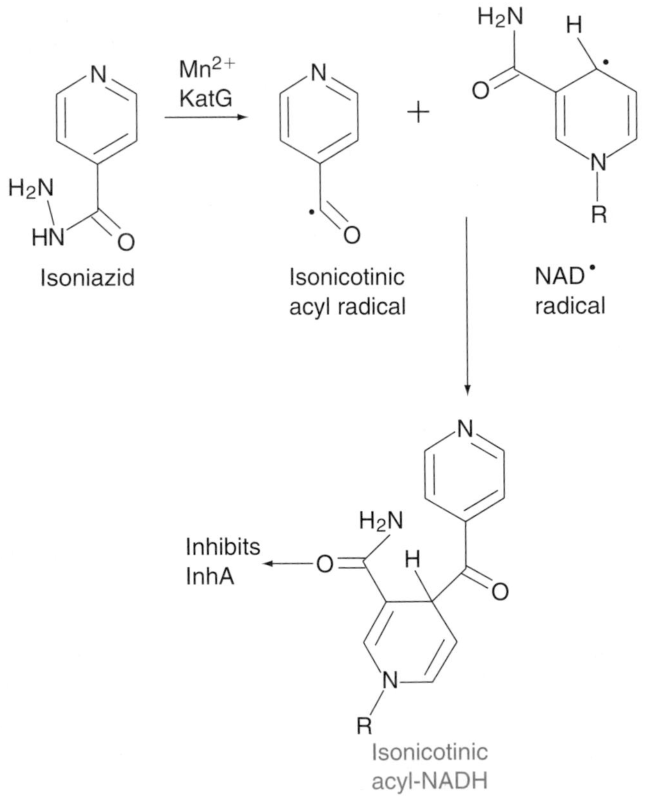

Isoniazid   Isonicotinic   NAD•
              acyl radical   radical

Inhibits
InhA

Isonicotinic
acyl-NADH

Figure 19–5 Pathway for formation of the isonicotinic acyl-NADH inhibitor of InhA. (Adapted from Rozwarski et al. [1998].)

are probably other mechanisms that remain to be discovered. Presumably, resistance to rifampin occurs in mycobacteria the same way it occurs in other bacteria; mutations in a subunit of RNA polymerase (the target of rifampin) leave the enzyme active but reduce its binding of rifampin.

The Emergence of Resistance

Resistance to isoniazid and rifampin occurs at a relatively high frequency. For this reason, and also to increase the killing efficacy of the antibiotics, combinations of drugs have been used. Isoniazid plus rifampin has been the most effective two-drug combination and is still the one most commonly used to treat TB. More than one drug reduces the risk of resistance development because the probability of a bacterium acquiring mutations that simultaneously confer resistance to both drugs is much lower than the probability of the bacterium mutating to resistance to the individual drugs. Before the emergence of drug-resistant strains, the success rate of treatment of TB with isoniazid-rifampin or other drug combinations was over 90%, even in AIDS patients. Treatment of strains that have become resistant to both isoniazid and rifampin is much less likely to be successful. In fact, the fatality rate in cases caused by such strains approaches 50% even when treatment is given (80% in the case of AIDS patients).

If combination drug therapy was effective in the past in preventing the development of drug-resistant strains, how did resistant strains emerge? Drug combinations prevent the emergence of resistance only if the drug combination is taken as directed. *M. tuberculosis* is a slow-growing bacterium and takes a long time to kill. To effect a cure, it is necessary for a person to take the prescribed drug combination daily or several times weekly for at least 6 months. Different members of this combination kill rapidly growing forms of the bacteria, and others kill slow-growing bacteria. Both are needed to sterilize the lung.

Until recently, the different anti-TB drugs were not available in a single pill form. Accordingly, patients frequently had to take at least two different (often three different) pills. Given that most people have trouble remembering to take a single pill over a long period of time, this type of complicated drug regimen made patient compliance a problem. People who are substance abusers are even less likely to take medication consistently. Also, nausea is a common side effect of some antituberculosis drugs, a factor that discourages regular taking of the medication.

It is not feasible to hospitalize people for the full term of therapy. Virtually all treatment of TB patients is done on an outpatient basis. This is the reason why earlier anti-TB programs included people hired to monitor patients closely to make sure that they were taking the prescribed drugs as directed and were completing the course of therapy. With the dismantling of these programs, doctors simply gave the patient a prescription or 2 to 3 bottles of different pills and left compliance to the patient. What happened was that many patients took the medications only intermittently—took one type of pill for a while and then another for a while, and most did not finish the full course of therapy.

In some developing countries, such as Tanzania, where aggressive anti-TB campaigns have been mounted and therapy is closely monitored, over 90% of patients finish the full course of therapy. One recent survey of compliance by patients receiving outpatient treatment from a U.S. inner city hospital found that only about 10% of patients completed a full course of therapy. This is probably a worst-case situation, but patient compliance in the United States is nowhere near 90%. With compliance numbers so low, the emergence of resistant strains was a foregone conclusion. Health workers in the United States are now monitoring patient compliance and as an incentive are giving food or clothing vouchers weekly to people who take all their medication. Better late than never.

The emergence of drug-resistant strains has complicated the treatment of tuberculosis considerably. In the case of an infection caused by a drug-resistant strain, it is necessary to tailor the therapy to the resistance profile of the strain causing the infection. Since isolation and identification of M. tuberculosis from a clinical specimen takes 2 weeks or more and since antibiotic sensitivity testing of the isolate takes at least another 2 weeks, decisions about therapy cannot await the results of clinical tests.

A patient with suspected TB is thus given a drug combination that is normally effective. Then, if the first combination seems not to be working, the combination is changed. Later in therapy, susceptibility test results will arrive to guide the choice of drugs. Such an approach requires a much higher involvement of skilled medical staff than was necessary in preresistance days. This drastically increases the cost of therapy, a critical factor for overburdened and underfunded inner city hospitals, the ones most likely to see drug-resistant TB.

Also, since the patient remains infectious until the therapy has stopped the multiplication of the bacteria, people with drug-resistant TB are more likely to spread the disease. Some patients with drug-resistant TB never respond to treatment, forcing physicians to resort to a form of treatment practiced earlier in the century: surgical removal of the infected portion of the lung. A piece of possible good news is that one of the newer fluoro-

quinolones, **sparfloxacillin,** appears to have some activity against M. tuberculosis in vitro and is actually more effective at killing M. tuberculosis in mice than isoniazid and rifampin. Unfortunately, resistance to fluoroquinolones arises as readily as resistance to rifampin and the other anti-TB drugs, so sparfloxacillin will have to be used carefully to prevent it from becoming rapidly obsolete.

The W Strain—a Taste of Things To Come?

In the 1990s, a strain of multidrug-resistant M. tuberculosis, called the W strain, emerged in New York City. It was resistant to isoniazid, rifampin, streptomycin, ethambutol, ethionamide, rifabutin, and kanamycin—in short, most of the available anti-TB drugs. It was also highly virulent and infectious. The W strain has now spread to other parts of the United States and may soon be seen in other countries. What might have become an epidemic was brought under control by a combination of measures, including isolation of patients found to be infected, surgical removal of infected lung tissue, and aggressive use of the few remaining drugs available (some of which were used on an experimental basis). Nonetheless, 74% of those infected with the W strain died. In many cases, death occurred within months, rather than the long slow progression normally seen in people with TB. In a New Jersey case, a woman was found to be infected with the W strain. She died 2 years after diagnosis, but not before she passed the strain to her two small children, who died within 6 months of diagnosis. The fact that a number of the people infected with the W strain had a concurrent HIV infection may have hastened the progression of TB, but there are indications that this strain is more virulent than previous M. tuberculosis strains.

The Search for New Drugs

Scientists at pharmaceutical companies and in academic laboratories are now working hard to find new targets for antimycobacterial drugs. One, isocitrate lyase, has already been mentioned. Another that has been proposed recently is an old player in the mycobacteria area: a protein complex called **antigen 85 complex.** This complex consists of three closely related proteins and is found on the cell surface or free in the extracellular fluid. Antigen 85 had been identified previously because it was one of the major M. tuberculosis antigens to which the human immune system responds. The activity of the complex has now been identified: it is an enzyme that transfers mycolic acid molecules onto the trehalose residues of polysaccharides in the cell wall

(Figure 19–6). Agents that inhibit this reaction have been found and are being tested.

Not only do scientists want to find new antibiotic targets; they also want to build in strategies for preventing resistance from developing. A clever and novel approach to developing antibiotics that would make it difficult for the bacteria to become resistant has been suggested on the basis of analysis of the *M. tuberculosis* genome sequence. Like other bacteria, *M. tuberculosis* produces families of proteins that share amino acid sequence similarity but have somewhat different functions. The idea is to target essential protein families, designing the antibiotic to act against a highly conserved region of the protein. Currently, all available antibiotics have a single target. Having a single antibiotic with multiple targets, which have activities essential for cell function, would make it difficult for the bacteria to mutate to resist antibiotic action.

Diagnosis of TB

Early identification of people with symptomatic TB not only allows therapy to be administered before serious lung damage occurs but also helps to prevent the spread of the bacteria to other susceptible people. Developing means for rapid identification of TB cases, especially cases caused by drug-resistant strains, has become an important goal. Acid-fast staining of **sputum** (material coughed up from the lung) has been used as a diagnostic test for years. This type of diagnostic test is complicated by the fact that other pathogenic *Mycobacterium* species also stain acid-fast, so detecting acid-fast rods does not give a definitive diagnosis of TB. Also, unless the bacteria are present in high numbers, they will not be readily found by microscopic examination. Despite these limitations, acid-fast staining has proved to be a very useful test.

A second simple diagnostic test is the TB skin test. In this test a mixture of *M. tuberculosis* protein called **purified protein derivative (PPD)**—although it is actually a crude extract containing many mycobacterial proteins—is injected intradermally. If the person being tested has or previously had tuberculosis, PPD stimulates preprimed CD4$^+$ T-helper cells at the site of the injection to secrete cytokines. These cytokines cause PMNs, then monocytes and macrophages, to be recruited to the injection site. Leakage of fluid due to migration of phagocytes through the blood vessel wall, together with the local inflammatory effect of cytokines, produces an area of redness and swelling (**erythema**). Fibrin deposition triggered by the monocytes and macrophages causes the area to harden (**induration**). The result is a raised, tough red area around the injection site (positive skin test). No reaction is seen in people who have not been sensitized by previous infection (negative skin test). The skin test must be interpreted

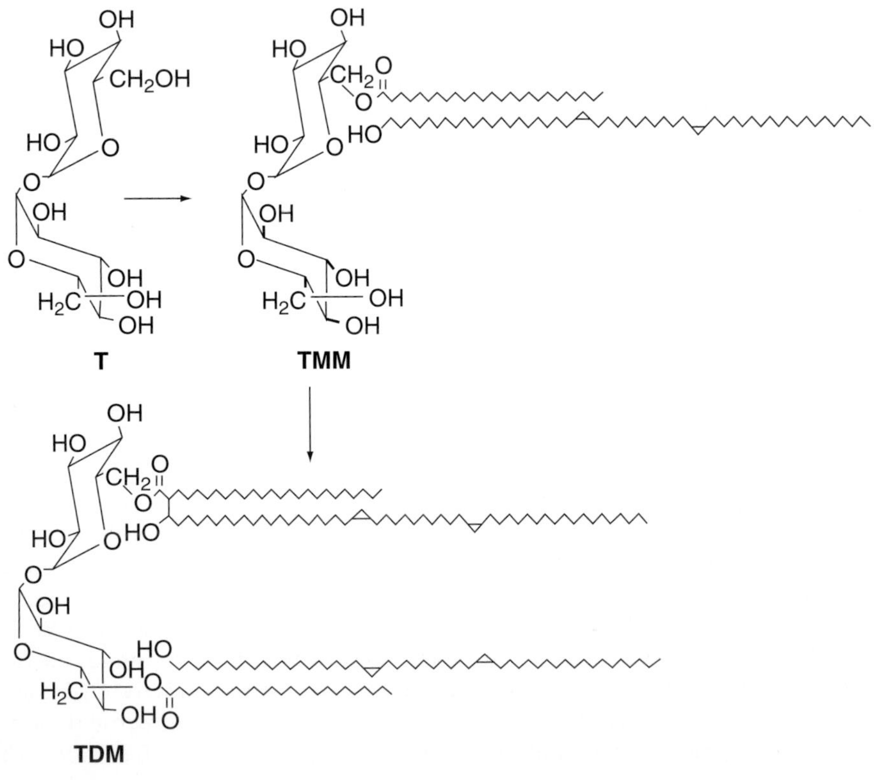

Figure 19–6 Reaction catalyzed by antigen 85 complex, which transfers mycolic acid molecules onto the trehalose residues of polysaccharides in the cell wall. T, trehalose; TMM, α-trehalose monomycolate; TDM, α,α′-trehalose dimycolate. (Adapted from D. L. Clemens. 1997. *Mycobacterium tuberculosis*: bringing down the wall. *Trends Microbiol.* **5**:383–385, with permission of the publisher.)

with care. After initial exposure to *M. tuberculosis*, it takes about 4 weeks before the person converts to skin-test-positive status. Thus, the skin test does not detect very recent infections. People who have been immunized with the anti-TB vaccine strain, **Mycobacterium bovis BCG** (see below), become skin test positive, so a positive test result gives no information about previous infection in such cases. Some people with active TB, especially disseminated TB, convert from skin test positive to skin test negative. This loss of skin test reactivity (**anergy**) in people with active TB is specific for reactivity to PPD and does not necessarily reflect a decrease in immune competence, although a general decrease in immune competence (e.g., in people with AIDS) can also cause the person to convert from skin test positive to skin test negative. The mechanism of anergy is unknown. Finally, the skin test is not absolutely specific for *M. tuberculosis*. People infected with other species of mycobacteria can become weakly positive on the TB skin test.

The skin test only indicates whether a person has been exposed to *M. tuberculosis* antigens (or has been immunized with BCG). A person with a positive skin test does not necessarily have active TB. Nonetheless, the skin test has been very useful for identifying people who may be carrying the bacteria and might thus be at risk for reactivation TB. Currently, it is recommended that people who have recently converted from skin test negative to skin test positive (not due to immunization) should take the full course of therapy for tuberculosis, even if they do not have an active case of tuberculosis at the present time, to eliminate the later risk of reactivation tuberculosis.

The need for better diagnostic tests to detect *M. tuberculosis* infections has spurred efforts to develop detection methods that do not require growth of this slow-growing organism. Using PCR to amplify 16S rRNA sequences specific to *M. tuberculosis* forms the basis for one approach. A related approach takes advantage of the fact that all *M. tuberculosis* strains identified to date carry the same insertion sequence, **IS6110**. Detection of IS6110 sequences by PCR or by DNA hybridization provides a means of demonstrating that *M. tuberculosis* is present in clinical specimens. Since PCR amplification procedures take less than 24 h from start to finish, a relatively rapid detection test for *M. tuberculosis* is possible. PCR might also be used to obtain information about the drug susceptibility of the causative strain (see below). The main drawback to the PCR diagnostic approach is the danger of cross-contamination of specimens with DNA. PCR is so sensitive that small contaminating amounts of DNA can give a positive signal.

Virulence Factors

Studying Virulence Factors

Studies of *M. tuberculosis* virulence factors have been hindered by the fact that the generation time of *M. tuberculosis* is about 18 to 24 h (which means that it takes weeks to form a visible colony on agar medium). Because *M. tuberculosis* grows so slowly, *Mycobacterium smegmatis*, a faster-growing species with a generation time of 3 h, is sometimes used as a surrogate for *M. tuberculosis*. Also, for a long time, such simple manipulations as extracting DNA from the bacteria or introducing recombinant DNA into them were very difficult, owing in part to the unusual mycobacterial cell wall. Despite these difficulties, methods for extracting clonable DNA and introduction of foreign DNA into *M. tuberculosis* have now been developed. In fact, a transposon that integrates randomly enough to be used for transposon mutagenesis has been found.

Cultured mammalian cells, especially lines of macrophagelike cells, are now being used to investigate *M. tuberculosis* virulence factors. In interpreting such studies, it is necessary to keep in mind that *M. tuberculosis* can invade many types of cultured mammalian cells, but in the human lung, monocytes and macrophages are clearly the primary targets of the bacteria. There are several animal models for studying tuberculosis. Mice, guinea pigs, rabbits, and monkeys can all be infected with *M. tuberculosis*. The disease in monkeys is closest to that seen in humans. Rabbits inoculated intranasally with *M. tuberculosis* also have symptoms similar to those seen in humans. Transgenic lines of mice that have known immune defects have already proved useful and are likely to dominate future research on host defenses against TB.

Entry into and Survival in Phagocytes

A key virulence property of *M. tuberculosis* is its ability to multiply inside monocytes and macrophages. It can also invade PMNs, but macrophages, especially the activated ones, are the key to development of the infection. Some light has now been shed on the question of how *M. tuberculosis* enters macrophages (Figure 19–7). Complement-mediated opsonization is not the answer because levels of complement in the lungs are only 1 to 3% of those in blood. Instead, *M. tuberculosis* binds directly to macrophage surface protein CR3, the normal receptor for iC3b. The bacteria also bind to other macrophage receptor proteins, such as CR4. Binding is followed by internalization of the bacteria in a vesicle. One advantage of entering a phagocyte by a pathway different from normal phagocyte-initiated phagocytosis is

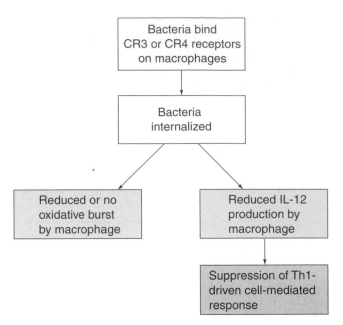

Figure 19–7 Interactions between *M. tuberculosis* and macrophages.

that the vesicle may not fuse with lysosomes. Macrophages that take up *M. tuberculosis* have a reduced ability to carry out phagolysosome fusion, because the bacteria prevent the interior of the vesicle from acidifying. Moreover, infected macrophages have a reduced oxidative burst (Figure 19–7). Another effect of the bacteria on the macrophages is to reduce their production of IL-12, a cytokine that stimulates the Th1 response. Although antibodies are useless in controlling TB, the Th1-stimulated cell-mediated response, especially the activated macrophage response, is critical. Reducing this response may give the bacteria an edge.

The ability of *M. tuberculosis* to bind to more than one surface protein on phagocytic cells may increase the ability of the bacteria to invade a variety of cells. Unstimulated macrophages have relatively little CR3 on their surfaces, but they have a moderate level of CR4. PMNs, which rush to the site in response to the infection, have more CR3 than CR4. Also, inflammation alters the amount of CR3 on the surface of phagocytic cells. Thus, the bacteria are ready for either phagocytic cell type at any stage of activation.

Whether *M. tuberculosis* multiplies in the phagosome or escapes the phagosome and enters the macrophage cytoplasm is controversial. Some studies have reported that *M. tuberculosis* inside macrophages can be seen both inside phagosomes and free in the cytoplasm, but the question arises as to whether this is true intracellular multiplication or is an artifact of the fixation process

and sectioning technique used to prepare the phagocytic cells for microscopic examination. A reason for thinking some of the bacteria might escape the phagosome and multiply in the cytoplasm is that infection with *M. tuberculosis* elicits an MHC class I-associated cytotoxic T-cell response, a response usually elicited by microorganisms growing in the cytoplasm or nucleus of the macrophage.

A careful study of the fate of the bacteria in phagocytes has now shown that there may be two stages to the invasion process. In the first stage, the bacteria are found primarily in phagosomes. Some of these are killed and degraded by the phagocyte, but others survive and divide. An interesting, but unanswered, question is what traits differentiate the ones that survive from the ones that do not. In the second stage, some of the bacteria that survived in the phagosome are seen budding off from the phagosome in vesicles whose membrane appears to be impaired. These bacteria may be escaping into the cytoplasm, although they appear to retain some vesicular membrane around them. Recently, a gene has been found in the *M. tuberculosis* genome sequence that has sequence similarity to a hemolysin that aids another gram-positive bacterium, *Listeria monocytogenes*, to escape the phagosome (see chapter 27). Thus, *M. tuberculosis* may produce a hemolysin with the same function as listerolysin, i.e., to allow bacteria to escape from a phagocytic vesicle.

Still another possible defense mechanism against phagocytic killing is that phenolic glycolipids from mycobacteria can scavenge toxic oxygen radicals in vitro. If so, the glycolipids, which are abundant in the mycobacterial cell wall, could help to protect bacteria that were exposed to the toxic forms of oxygen produced in the phagolysosome or in a region of tissue where phagocytes are active.

Avoidance of the Activated Macrophage Response

Although *M. tuberculosis* can survive inside normal, resting macrophages, the bacteria are killed by activated macrophages. Accordingly, it would be in the interest of the bacteria to produce factors that interfere with macrophage activation. IFN-γ (and possibly other cytokines as well) produced by activated T cells, especially CD4$^+$ cells, is essential for activating macrophages. In this connection, it is interesting that *M. tuberculosis* produces some compounds that (at least in vitro) interfere with T-cell activation. For example, **lipoarabinomannan,** a mycobacterial cell wall glycolipid, suppresses T-cell proliferation. It also blocks transcriptional activation of interferon-inducible genes in macrophage cell lines and might thus prevent interferon from triggering macrophage activation.

A protein complex secreted by *M. tuberculosis*, antigen 85, has already been mentioned in connection with possible new targets for antibiotics. Initially, it was reported that one of the proteins in the complex, 85A, bound fibronectin. This is now thought not to be an important activity of antigen 85, which instead catalyzes the mycolylation of cell wall polysaccharides. Antigen 85 might serve as a virulence factor in the sense that it is a powerful immunostimulant that elicits an antibody response. Excretion of antigen 85 might actually deflect the human immune system from a protective response (development of an activated macrophage defense) to a nonproductive one (antibody production).

Ability To Elicit a Destructive Inflammatory Response

Many other bacterial pathogens cause damage to host tissue by eliciting a local or systemic inflammatory response. This hypothesis is also being entertained as a possible explanation for the lung damage caused by *M. tuberculosis*, and there has been considerable interest in identifying what antigens are most important in eliciting this destructive host response. Unfortunately, most of this work has been done using skin test reactivity as an assay. The problem with this approach is that the type of cell-mediated response generated in the skin test (delayed-type hypersensitivity) overlaps but is not the same as the cell-mediated response elicited by bacteria multiplying in the lung.

A few proteins have been identified that can evoke a skin test response when administered in purified form (e.g., antigen 85B, 85C, and MPB70, a 23-kDa secreted protein of *M. bovis* BCG), but little is known about the antigens most important in provoking the destructive cell-mediated response that causes lung damage. Mycolic acids from the mycobacterial cell wall are toxic when injected into animals, and these compounds could act by stimulating the inflammatory response. Also, **muramyl dipeptide,** a cell wall component of mycobacteria, is well known for its ability to stimulate the immune system and trigger cytokine production.

One popular hypothesis is that release of TNF-α, provoked by a combination of mycobacterial cell surface components, causes most of the lung damage. Injection of TNF-α into lungs causes damage similar to that seen in tuberculosis, and antibodies to TNF-α reduce lung damage in animals infected by the bacteria without significantly affecting the growth of the bacteria themselves. Thus, bacterial products that elicit TNF-α could be important in the disease process. Release of toxic lysosomal components by macrophages trying to ingest and kill the bacteria may also contribute to lung damage.

Factors That Affect Host Susceptibility

Years ago, differences in susceptibility of different strains of laboratory mice to mycobacterial infections led scientists to posit a genetic locus called *bcg* that influenced host susceptibility. The hypothetical locus got its name from the fact that it affected the sensitivity of mice to the BCG strain of *M. bovis*. Strain BCG was isolated in the early days of mycobacterial research by two French scientists, Calmette and Guérin. This is the strain used as the current TB vaccine. The *bcg* locus has been located on mouse chromosome 1 and cloned. The gene was given the name *Nramp1* for **natural resistance-associated macrophage protein.** The fact that the gene encoded a macrophage protein made it more believable as a host susceptibility factor because macrophages are so important in the immune response to *M. tuberculosis* infections.

The importance of *Nramp1* for human susceptibility to TB has now been brought into question on the basis of two concerns. The first is that the gene had been identified on the basis of its effect on susceptibility to *M. bovis* BCG, not to *M. tuberculosis*. Of more concern was the fact that mice homozygous for the resistant allele of *Nramp1* were just as susceptible to *M. tuberculosis* as animals homozygous for the susceptible allele. It is still possible that *Nramp1* makes a small contribution to human and mouse susceptibility to TB, but its importance has probably been overstated. The demise of the *Nramp1* hypothesis is a disappointing development, but it does not mean that there are no important host susceptibility factors. Different people in a population exposed to TB respond very differently, with a range that goes from no infection at all, to latent infection, to active disease. Of course, the size of the inoculum, the length of the exposure, and the number of exposures clearly have a big effect on the outcome. Yet, the strong suspicion remains that there are genetic factors that make some people able to throw off an incipient infection and others to progress to active disease.

Understanding such genetic predispositions, if they exist, is important for two reasons. First, it would allow public health workers to identify especially susceptible members of the population and target them for first receipt of a vaccine if a good one becomes available. They would also be the focus of preventive treatment in a group of people exposed to an infected person. Second, if gene therapy ever gets off the ground, it might become possible to make susceptible people less susceptible by replacing the gene responsible for susceptibility. The hunt for the genetic factors that affect susceptibility to TB goes on.

Immunity to TB

BCG: a Widely Used but Controversial Vaccine

Since TB is a major cause of death worldwide, a vaccine that would prevent TB has long been a high-priority item. The emergence of drug-resistant strains has made the search for an effective vaccine more urgent. Even in the case of treatable TB, the cost of the therapy (not only the drugs themselves but the staff needed to monitor compliance) is so high that a vaccine provides the only realistic hope of controlling TB in rich and poor countries. An avirulent strain of *M. bovis* called BCG has been used as a TB vaccine. This strain enters macrophages and replicates briefly before being killed. It should thus elicit the types of immunity elicited by *M. tuberculosis* itself, assuming that all of the protective antigens are expressed. BCG can be administered orally and is safe enough to give to infants. Billions of doses have been administered worldwide, and the lack of toxic side effects makes this one of the safest vaccines known. The only reported problems have occurred in AIDS patients: there have been a few cases of patients developing an infection caused by the BCG strain itself. BCG is also a very cheap vaccine, costing about 10 cents per dose.

Unfortunately, the effectiveness of BCG in preventing tuberculosis is controversial. The vaccine has some efficacy in preventing tuberculosis in children but does not prevent reactivation of a preexisting infection in older people. Results of field trials of the vaccine have differed widely, some showing protection rates as high as 70 to 80%, others showing that the vaccine was completely ineffective in preventing TB. It is interesting to note that regardless of the protection rate found in different studies, all studies report that virtually all vaccinated people convert to skin test positive. This underscores the concept that skin test positivity is not correlated with a protective immune response.

Why are the field trial results with BCG so variable? One possibility is genetic differences in susceptibility of different human populations. Another is that different derivatives of BCG were used that differed in immunogenic properties. Still another possibility is suggested by an old British study, which showed that inoculation

with BCG or *Mycobacterium microti* (an avirulent species) gave protection from tuberculosis at the 70% level. Yet whereas people inoculated with BCG all became strongly skin test positive, people inoculated with *M. microti* became weakly skin test positive at best. In field trials, subjects are chosen on the basis of a negative TB skin test reaction because the skin test presumably indicates they have not had any previous contact with *M. tuberculosis*. If, however, people in some locales had been exposed to a ubiquitous, relatively nonpathogenic mycobacterium, which like *M. microti* confers some protective immunity against tuberculosis without making the person TB skin test positive, the apparent failure of BCG to give higher protection rates in inoculated people compared to control subjects might simply indicate that BCG is not capable of *increasing* the protection already conferred by the other species.

Whatever the reason for the variation in field test results, it is clear that even at its best, BCG is not the vaccine that is so desperately needed. The BCG vaccine might be improved by introducing genes from *M. tuberculosis* that encode protective antigens into the BCG strain. This approach sounds good in theory, but it will have to wait until more is known about what *M. tuberculosis* antigens elicit a protective response and how to attain the right type of response. A good vaccine must produce the sort of cell-mediated response that gives immunity, not simply elicit a useless antibody response. Intensive research is currently under way to learn how to elicit the right type of cell-mediated response with a vaccine. One thing is clear: a killed vaccine is completely ineffective. A live vaccine that replicates briefly in the body is necessary for establishing immunity.

BCG as a Carrier for Other Vaccine Antigens

Since BCG is a safe, cheap vaccine that stimulates a cell-mediated response as well as an antibody response, it is an obvious vehicle for vaccines based on protective antigens from other bacteria or viruses. Now that cloned DNA can be introduced into *M. bovis* BCG, attempts are being made to introduce genes encoding protective antigens from a variety of bacteria and viruses into the strain. The promoter of an *M. tuberculosis* heat shock gene, which is expressed at high levels when bacteria are growing in a mammalian host, is used to ensure high expression of the cloned antigen. Ideally, the strain could be made to express several antigens from different microbes. The long-term goal of these attempts is to develop a vaccine that would simultaneously immunize children against a variety of diseases, including tuberculosis.

SELECTED READINGS

Agerton, T. B., S. E. Valway, R. J. Blinkhorn, K. L. Shilkret, R. Reves, W. W. Schluter, B. Gore, C. J. Pozsik, B. B. Plikaytis, C. Woodley, and I. M. Oronato. 1999. Spread of strain W, a highly drug-resistant strain of *Mycobacterium tuberculosis*, across the United States. *Clin. Infect. Dis.* **29:**85–92.

Dussurget, O., and I. Smith. 1998. Interdependence of mycobacterial iron regulation, oxidative-stress response and isoniazid resistance. *Trends Microbiol.* **6:**354–358.

Ehlers, M. R., and M. Daffe. 1998. Interactions between *Mycobacterium tuberculosis* and host cells: are mycobacterial sugars the key? *Trends Microbiol.* **6:**328–335.

Havlir, D. V., and P. F. Barnes. 1999. Tuberculosis in patients with human immunodeficiency virus infection. *N. Engl. J. Med.* **340:**367–373.

Iseman, M. D. 1993. Treatment of multidrug-resistant tuberculosis. *N. Engl. J. Med.* **329:**784–791.

Jacobs, W. R., Jr., G. V. Kalpana, J. D. Cirillo, L. Pascopella, S. B. Snapper, R. A. Udani, W. Jones, R. G. Barletta, and B. R. Bloom. 1991. Genetic systems for mycobacteria. *Methods Enzymol.* **204:**537–555.

North, R. J., and E. Medina. 1998. How important is *Nramp1* in tuberculosis? *Trends Microbiol.* **6:**441–443.

Orme, I. M. 1998. The immunopathogenesis of tuberculosis: a new working hypothesis. *Trends Microbiol.* **6:**94–97.

Rozwarski, D. A., G. A. Grant, H. Derek, R. Barton, R. Jacobs, and J. C. Sacchettini. 1998. Modification of the NADH of the isoniazid target (InhA) from *Mycobacterium tuberculosis*. *Science* **279:**98–102.

SUMMARY OUTLINE

Historical perspective

Epidemic disease in 1800s

Incidence declined in developed countries until 1970s

In 1980s incidence in developed countries increased; drug-resistant strains emerged

Still one of the leading causes of death worldwide

Progress of tuberculosis

Caused by *M. tuberculosis*
  Obligate aerobe
  Gram-positive-type cell wall with a high lipid content

Spread by aerosols

M. tuberculosis survives and multiplies in unactivated alveolar macrophages

Activated macrophages can kill *M. tuberculosis*

Ingestion of *M. tuberculosis* by macrophages stimulates both CD4$^+$ and CD8$^+$ T cells
  CD4$^+$ T cells release IFN-γ
    Activates macrophages
    Stimulates movement of T cells from bloodstream to infected area
  CD8$^+$ T cells kill infected phagocytes that have not controlled *M. tuberculosis* growth

Tubercles may form—granulomatous response
  Bacteria, T cells, and phagocytes walled off by fibrin coat
  May calcify
  Contain live bacteria that may break out and multiply—reactivation TB

Latency
  Bacteria are not causing active infection
  M. tuberculosis most likely in tubercles or lymph nodes; possibly in other organs
  Bacteria may assume sporelike state
  M. tuberculosis may be marginally metabolically active
  Mouse model
  Disruption of *acr* (α-crystallin) reduces persistence of bacteria
  Isocitrate lyase required for bacterial persistence
    Allows bacteria to convert fatty acids to biomass and NADH
    Possible target for antimycobacterial drugs

(continued)

Bacterial cell wall

Contains peptidoglycan plus unusual glycolipids—prevents staining by Gram stain

Stained by acid-fast stain

Examples of glycolipids are arabinogalactan and mycolic acids

Protects against effects of phagolysosomal components

Hard to disrupt cells

Stimulates immune system to produce antibodies (component of Freund's adjuvant)

Treatment of tuberculosis

Most antibiotics do not work

Effective antibiotics include rifampin, isoniazid, ethambutol, and pyrazinamide

Mechanism of action not known for most of the antibiotics

Isoniazid inhibits a step in mycolic acid synthesis (catalyzed by InhA)

Antibiotics used in combination both to kill fast- and slow-growing strains and to prevent resistance

Isoniazid-rifampin most common combination

Poor patient compliance because of long-term treatment (4 to 6 months)

W strain

Multidrug-resistant strain appeared in 1990 in United States

Highly virulent and infectious

Infected patients must be isolated, aggressively treated

Infection progresses rapidly

Search for new drug targets

Isocitrate lyase

Antigen 85 complex (attaches trehalose to cell wall polysaccharides)

New antibiotics with multiple targets

Diagnosis of TB

Tentative diagnosis based on acid-fast rods in a sputum specimen

Other mycobacterial species also stain acid-fast

Need many cells in specimen to see them

PPD skin test

Indicates whether person has been infected at some time with *M. tuberculosis*

BCG vaccination causes positive test

May become negative in immunocompromised people (anergy)

New tests

PCR amplification of 16S rRNA genes

Detection of IS*6110* sequences

Virulence factors

Difficult to study

Bacteria grow slowly

Only recently amenable to genetic analysis

Animal models used

Survival in phagocytes

M. tuberculosis binds to CR3 and CR4—allows binding to a variety of phagocytic cell types

Bacteria internalized in vesicle

(*continued*)

SUMMARY OUTLINE (*continued*)

      Mycobacteria block phagolysosome fusion by preventing acidification of vesicle

      Reduced oxidative burst in infected macrophages

      Bacteria reduce macrophage production of IL-2 (less Th1 stimulation)

      M. tuberculosis may escape phagosome, enter cytoplasm (perhaps aided by hemolysin)

      Phenolic glycolipids may detoxify toxic oxygen radicals

   Avoidance of activated macrophage response

      Lipoarabinomannan from cell wall suppresses T-cell proliferation; blocks activation of genes by interferon

      Antigen 85 may deflect host response from activation of macrophages to production of antibodies—not a useful response

   Stimulation of destructive inflammatory response—some candidates

      Antigen 85

      Mycolic acids

      Muramyl dipeptide

      TNF-α elicited by bacterial cell surface components

   Factors affecting host susceptibility

      Nramp1

         Originally thought to confer resistance to tuberculosis

         Currently thought not to be very important

      Hunt for factors continues

Vaccine—BCG

   Avirulent strain of *M. bovis*

   Safe and cheap

   Efficacy highly variable

   Might be improved by adding *M. tuberculosis* genes that encode protective antigens

   Might serve as basis for multivalent vaccine effective against a variety of diseases

QUESTIONS

Answers to the questions can be found in Appendix 2.

1. Why did the incidence of TB in countries such as the United States continue to decline for several years after anti-TB programs were dismantled before beginning to increase? Now that TB incidence in developed countries is at an all-time low, is it worth the money it takes to continue to support TB programs? If you were to keep programs, which ones would they be?

2. BCG has never been administered routinely in the United States as a vaccine despite the fact that it has been widely used in Europe and many other countries. The reasons for this were as much political as scientific, but make an educated guess as to what the scientific rationale might have been for such a decision.

3. Is it possible that a vaccine can be developed that does not make the recipient positive on the TB skin test? If so, how could this be done?

4. Explain why double or triple drug therapy (if taken as prescribed) should make the development of resistant strains virtually impossible. (Assume that the frequency of spontaneous resistance is 10^{-7}, i.e., 1 in 10^7 bacteria, for each drug and that a person with TB might have 10^7 to 10^8 bacteria in their lungs.) How would failure to take medications properly allow resistant strains to emerge?

5. Why do homeless people with TB present an especially difficult problem for health care workers trying to control the spread of TB?

6. A research group reports that their candidate vaccine elicits high levels of antibodies to *M. tuberculosis* antigens when injected into healthy volunteers. Is this a good indication of the efficacy of the vaccine? Is there some reason to think that intact mycobacteria will always elicit an antibody response?

7. People who have been exposed to someone with TB are usually given isoniazid or rifampin alone rather than a two-drug combination. Explain the rationale for this.

8. How do the known virulence factors of *M. tuberculosis* resemble or differ from virulence factors of other respiratory pathogens? Given that all the respiratory bacterial pathogens face the same defenses of the lung, why should they have different virulence factors?

9. The numbers given here for the incidence of TB in developing countries were determined by estimating the number of people whose deaths were caused by TB. In Africa and some other countries, such people frequently have a concurrent HIV infection, which makes them more susceptible. Recently, for political reasons, some U.S. agencies have begun to count deaths due to TB in HIV-infected people as deaths due to HIV, thus making the number of deaths due to HIV appear to rise. Is there a justification for this change? Why would anyone want to make such a change?

20

Legionella pneumophila and Legionnaires' Disease

KEY FEATURES

Legionella pneumophila

CHARACTERISTICS

Gram-negative motile rod

Poor staining by Gram stain, but not due to high lipid content of cell wall

Complex nutritional requirements

DISEASES

Legionnaires' disease

Ventilator-associated pneumonia in hospitals

RESERVOIRS

Biofilms in water sources, including air-conditioning cooling towers

Amoebae

Ubiquitous in soil and water

MAJOR VIRULENCE FACTORS

Infect macrophages (Mip)

Survive and multiply in macrophages (Icm/Dot)

Type IV secretion system

Trigger apoptosis

Proteolytic enzymes—metalloprotease

PREVENTION AND TREATMENT

Biocides to prevent formation of biofilms in air-conditioning cooling towers

Prevent contamination of water sources that are aerosolized in hospitals

Antibiotic treatment

No vaccine yet available

The Dark Side of Modern Comforts: Air-Conditioning Turns Ugly

Legionnaires' disease is a form of bacterial pneumonia caused by *Legionella* species, most commonly by *Legionella pneumophila*. *L. pneumophila* was only recognized as a cause of pneumonia within the last 25 years, although sporadic cases of *Legionella* pneumonia probably occurred long before the disease was identified and named. The incidence of *Legionella* pneumonia has increased dramatically in recent years, owing in part to the installation of central air-conditioning systems in large buildings, such as high-rise office buildings, hospitals, and hotels. *L. pneumophila* is ubiquitous in soil and water and has proved to be particularly adept at growing in air-conditioning cooling towers. Aerosols produced by the air-conditioning machinery are inhaled, thus introducing bacteria into the lung.

Another recent technical innovation that has contributed to the rise in *L. pneumophila* infections is the use of ventilators to assist very ill patients to breathe. A tube is inserted into the patient's airway, and air is pumped into the lungs. Water is used to humidify the air so that lung tissue does not dry out. If the water in the ventilator device becomes contaminated with *L. pneumophila*, the bacteria are introduced directly into the lungs of the patient. Most ventilator patients are highly susceptible to lung infections, not only because the defenses of the upper airway have been bypassed by the ventilator tube but also because many of these patients have other predisposing conditions, such as diabetes or other forms of immunosuppression. Dust and liquid aerosols from construction sites next to hospitals and nursing homes have also been sources of *L. pneumophila* outbreaks. There was even a case in which some people contracted the disease from a spa display model in a store.

Healthy children and adults are not very susceptible to *L. pneumophila* infections. Apparently, the defenses of the healthy airway are usually sufficient to prevent *L. pneumophila* from reaching the lung and infecting it. However, people with underlying conditions that impair these defenses (heavy alcohol use, smoking, old age, and ventilator use) can be infected by *L. pneumophila*. The cluster of cases that first brought *Legionella* infections to the attention of the public occurred among a group of elderly men attending an American Legion convention (hence the designation "Legionnaires' disease"). Many of these men were smokers or heavy drinkers or both. The cooling towers of the hotel air-conditioning system were heavily contaminated with *L. pneumophila*, so the air-conditioning system was in effect spewing *L. pneumophila* into the rooms.

Legionnaires' Disease

L. pneumophila is a motile aerobic gram-negative rod with complex nutritional requirements. For example, the bacteria require high levels of cysteine and iron compounds. They use amino acids but not carbohydrates for growth. Although *Legionella* has a typical gram-negative-type cell wall, it does not stain well with Gram stain reagents. In this and other ways, *Legionella* resembles *Mycobacterium tuberculosis*, although *Legionella* does not have such a high lipid content in its cell wall.

Legionella, like *M. tuberculosis*, can survive and multiply inside phagocytic cells, especially macrophages. In the lung, it causes considerable damage unless an activated macrophage response is elicited rapidly enough to bring the infection under control.

An unusual characteristic of the disease caused by *L. pneumophila* is that, unlike most other lung infections, it appears not to be transmitted from person to person. All cases are acquired from the environment. This feature of the disease suggests that *L. pneumophila* is not very well adapted to the human body, as expected in the case of a bacterium that has only recently begun to cause human disease. *L. pneumophila* can certainly do a lot of damage to the lungs of people it infects, but the bacteria are probably in a stressed state throughout their residence in this unnatural host.

Legionnaires' disease is characterized by fever, disorientation, lethargy, and considerable lung damage, which appears on lung radiograms as patchy ("moth-eaten") regions where fluid has accumulated. Microscopic analysis of histological sections of infected lungs reveals that most of the invading bacteria are inside phagocytes, either growing inside the phagosome or filling the cytoplasm. Extensive lysis of phagocytic cells occurs where the bacteria reach high numbers. Cytoplasmic contents of lysed phagocytic cells contribute to the fluid that is found in the air sacs of infected people.

A number of *Legionella* species are capable of causing disease in humans. *L. pneumophila* is the best-studied species and accounts for about 85% of *Legionella* infections in humans. The next best studied species and next most common cause of disease is *Legionella micdadei*, the cause of a disease called Pontiac fever. Pontiac fever resembles viral flu more closely than it does Legionnaires' disease.

The Natural Host?—a Free-Living Macrophage Equivalent

In nature, *Legionella* species can often be found growing in biofilms, but another host for *Legionella* is protozoa. The protozoa ingest the bacteria with the intention of using the bacteria as food. But the protozoa are in for a nasty surprise because *Legionella* has *them* for lunch. Just as *Legionella* kills human macrophages, it also kills protozoa that ingest it. *Legionella* can infect many species of protozoa, including such environmentally ubiquitous genera as *Acanthamoeba* and *Hartmanella*. The fact that *Legionella* multiplies inside of and kills amoebae, which are similar in many ways to mammalian macrophages, may be the answer to the question, How could *Legionella* cause human disease if it is not adapted to the human body? Protozoa are not perfect equivalents of macrophages. This is evident from the fact that there are some mutations that diminish virulence in amoebae but not in mammalian cells and vice versa (Figure 20–1). Yet, there are also a number of mutations that affect the ability to kill both of these hosts, so there is clearly some overlap. Moreover, there is evidence that bacteria that were recently inside protozoa are somewhat more virulent than free-living bacteria. The difference is not very large, but its existence supports the hypothesis that growth in protozoa prepares *Legionella* to infect human macrophages.

The natural association between *Legionella* species and protozoa raises an interesting question about the evolution of bacterial pathogens, especially those that can replicate inside human cells. Is it possible that many of what we today call virulence factors evolved long before mammals appeared, as defenses against voracious protozoa? Are there other species that can do the same thing? This is an aspect of pathogenesis that has received virtually no attention.

Virulence Factors

Problems with Determining *Legionella* Virulence Factors

ANIMAL MODELS. Some characteristics of the bacteria and the disease it causes make the study of *Legionella* virulence factors particularly challenging. First, *Legionella* causes infections primarily in people with underlying conditions that impair airway defenses or in people with some form of immunosuppression. Thus, a combination of bacterial properties and host deficiencies are needed for infection to occur, and it is therefore difficult to associate single properties of the bacteria unequivocally with the ability to cause disease. The animal model most often used is the guinea pig. Intranasal or intratracheal inoculation of guinea pigs or exposure of guinea pigs to aerosols of *L. pneumophila* produces lung lesions similar to those seen in humans. However, the guinea pigs are not immunocompromised in the same way as the humans who are at highest risk for *Legionella* infection. Thus, there is some question as to whether the same types of virulence factors are important in the guinea pig as in, for example, elderly alcoholics. A strain of immunocompromised mice, A/J mice, has been used as an animal model for studies of *Legionella* virulence factors and may be a closer mimic of the situation in humans. Interestingly, this strain of mouse has a defect in a gene encoding a protein that inhibits apoptosis (**neuronal apoptosis inhibitory protein**). Since *L. pneumophila* appears to induce apoptosis of macrophages, an early development in infection of these cells,

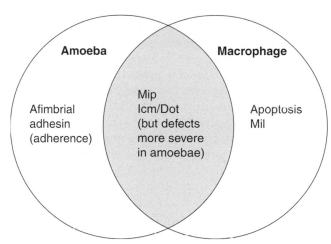

Figure 20–1   Examples of virulence factors that are important for infection of amoebae or macrophages or both. RpoS, a sigma factor that controls the stationary phase of gene expression; Mip, macrophage infectivity promoter (peptidyl prolyl isomerase that increases infective efficiency); Icm/Dot, a type IV secretion system that injects unknown effector proteins into macrophage cytoplasm; Mil, macrophage infectivity locus.

this genetic defect that makes the cells more susceptible to apoptotic killing makes sense.

CELL LINES. Murine macrophages, human macrophages, and human monocytes have been used in studies of the interaction between the bacteria and their cell target. A problem that arises in connection with these model systems is that *Legionella* strains vary in their ability to survive in macrophages. In many studies, only a small fraction of a *Legionella* inoculum survives phagocytosis. The marginality of *Legionella* survival contributes to the variability in experimental outcome. *Legionella* invades other cell types as well as phagocytic cells; cell lines such as Chinese hamster ovary cells have been used to investigate general interactions between *Legionella* and host cells. It is not clear, however, how good a model nonprofessional phagocytes are for *Legionella* invasion of alveolar macrophages.

Amoebae have been added to the list of animal models recently, and they may be very useful because of their comparative simplicity. One group has shown that the slime mold *Dictyostelium discoideum*, which has long been used as a "lab rat" by scientists who study eukaryotic development, can be infected with *Legionella*. In theory, this would be a good model because so much is known about this slime mold, and mutants with well-characterized phenotypes are available. So far, these mutants have not been particularly informative, possibly because they were isolated in studies of development and multicellular organization, not other basic cellular functions. In the long run, protozoa may prove to be more useful.

Another problem that impedes the study of *L. pneumophila* virulence factors is that it grows fairly slowly in laboratory medium. It takes about 3 days for visible colonies to form. Moreover, different research groups have tended to use different strains that vary considerably in virulence. Finally, the genetics of *Legionella* is still very primitive, although considerable progress has been made in recent years. It is now possible to obtain mutants and to introduce cloned DNA, so that virulence genes can be cloned by complementation.

Given these problems, it is impressive that the scientific community has made so much progress with *Legionella* during the past several years. When the first edition of this book was written, it was difficult to find much to say about *Legionella*, except to list the many things that were not known. Soon, given the rate of progress, the difficulty will be to keep this chapter from being too long.

Survival in Amoebae

Much has now been learned about how *L. pneumophila* infects and multiplies inside amoebae. Not surprisingly, the bacteria undergo numerous changes as they adapt to the interior of the amoeba. An **afimbrial adhesin** seems to be involved in attachment to and invasion of amoebae. This is one of the traits that are not important for infection of and survival in human phagocytic cells; it seems to be amoeba specific (Figure 20–1). In both amoebae and human macrophages, the bacteria can be internalized by an unusual mode of phagocytosis called **coiling phagocytosis** (Figure 20–2). A single pseudopod wraps around the bacterium being ingested to create a vacuole. Scientists, like most humans, are struck by visual anomalies, and this led to the initial conclusion that coiling phagocytosis had some deeper meaning. This turned out not to be the case. First, legionellae can be ingested by conventional phagocytic engulfment and the result is the same—the phagosome does not fuse, at least initially, with the lysosome. Moreover, this type of phagocytosis was not seen with all host cells or with all *Legionella* strains. What is clearly important is what happens after ingestion of *L. pneumophila*, when the bacteria somehow alter the phagosome membrane to prevent phagosome-lysosome fusion (see later section).

Some factors are important for survival of the bacteria both in amoebae and in human macrophages. These include **Mip (macrophage infectivity promoter)**, a protein that increases infection efficiency but does not affect intracellular growth. Mip is a **peptidyl prolyl isomerase.** This type of enzyme is usually found in eu-

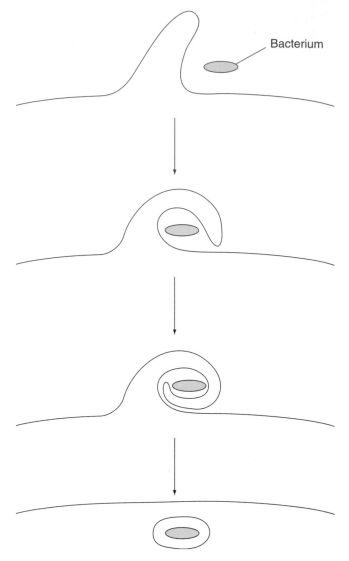

Figure 20–2 Coiling phagocytosis, a type of phagocytosis that probably plays no role in virulence but looks neat.

karyotic cells. Possibly, the bacterial version targets some important eukaryotic proteins. Another set of genes that seem to be important for survival in both amoebae and human cells are the *icm* genes (*icm* stands for **intracellular multiplication**). Some of these genes appear to encode a **type IV secretion system** (Figure 20–3 and Appendix 1). Here a fascinating mystery unfolds. Type IV secretion systems have usually been associated with conjugal transfer of DNA. Although those who study DNA transfer generally focus on the transfer of the DNA molecule, conjugation actually requires that a protein be attached to the DNA prior to transfer. So, conjugation could be viewed as the secretion and transfer of a protein to which DNA happens to be bound. A similar involvement of a type IV secretion system in the secretion of proteins without attendant DNA has been seen in *Bordetella pertussis*. It remains to be seen whether type IV secretion systems, like type III systems, are mainly responsible for the translocation of proteins from the bacterial cytoplasm to the host cell cytoplasm and have been coopted in some cases by DNA molecules. There is precedent for transfer from prokaryote to eukaryote mediated by a type IV secretion system. In the case of the plant pathogen *Agrobacterium tumefaciens*, the protein-DNA complex is transferred from a prokaryotic cell into a eukaryotic (plant) cell. It is interesting to note that *A. tumefaciens* uses gene transfer to modify the activities of plant cells so that the plant cells multiply to form a tumor that secretes opines, compounds the bacteria can use as carbon and energy sources. So the *A. tumefaciens* type IV conjugation system, like the type III and type IV systems of human bacterial pathogens, is designed to manipulate host cell physiology to the advantage of the bacteria. If the *icm*-encoded machinery is merely injecting proteins rather than a protein-DNA complex, it remains to be seen what proteins are injected and what their role is. In the case of *B. pertussis*, the purpose of the type IV secretion systems seems to be to inject proteins into phagocytic cells in order to undermine the effectiveness of these defensive host cells (see chapter 17).

Regulation of Virulence Genes

TEMPERATURE. *Legionella* exhibits both temperature- and nutrient-based control mechanisms. At 30°C, several virulence factors are preferentially expressed. These include pili, flagella, and the type IV secretion system. A mystery that remains to be explained is that, although expression of these traits in the laboratory is temperature dependent, in macrophages, where the temperature remains at 37°C, these traits are associated with late steps in the infection process, when the bacteria have filled the cell. Also, in macrophages, the type IV secretion system is produced early in infection, whereas the other traits are associated with later stages of infection. Some signals other than temperature must contribute to the control of expression of these genes. Temperature regulation is expected to be important in the transition of bacteria from amoebae, which usually experience temperatures below 30°C, to human macrophages. Given that humans are accidental hosts, what looks like temperature regulation may well be the *Legionella* equivalent of the heat shock stress response.

THYMINE LIMITATION. The vacuoles in which the *Legionella* cells find themselves are deficient in certain compounds, such as thymine and thymidine. Not surprisingly, therefore, the bacteria use a stringent response system to regulate expression of some of the same virulence factors. The **stringent response system** senses starvation for amino acids or other compounds and responds by making special compounds, such as **ppGpp**, which act as signals to activate expression of virulence genes (Figure 20–4). The virulence genes regulated by the stringent response may be more important in later rather than earlier phases of intracellular growth, because some of them, such as flagella, seem most appropriate for bacteria that are about to be released into the environment. Limitation of some important carbon and nitrogen sources could well be the

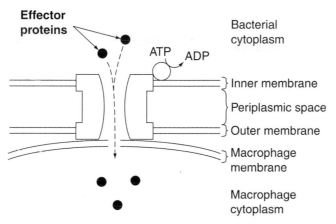

Figure 20–3 A model of the *L. pneumophila* type IV secretion system. The channel is formed by some of the proteins encoded by the *icm* and *dot* genes. Other products of these genes, the effector proteins, are injected into the macrophage cytoplasm. Unlike the classical type IV secretion system, it appears that no DNA is transferred along with the protein. (Adapted from Segal and Shuman, 1998.)

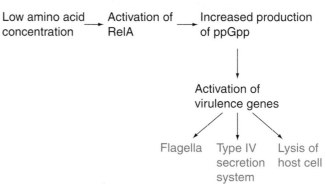

Figure 20–4 Stringent response model for *L. pneumophila* virulence regulation. When amino acids are limiting, RelA is activated. Increased concentrations of ppGpp coordinate entry into the stationary phase, with expression of virulence traits enhancing transmission to a new host. (Adapted from Swanson and Hammer, 2000.)

switch that alerts the bacteria that it is time to escape by lysing the cell in which they are multiplying and move on to more nutritionally rich pastures.

OTHER SYSTEMS.   There must be other regulatory systems, because *Legionella* goes through a rather complex life cycle (Figure 20–5). The bacteria are taken up in a vacuole. Then they start to multiply, changing the vacuole environment as they increase in numbers. As bacteria prepare to leave the cell, the stringent response kicks in, and a number of virulence genes that will help the bacteria survive outside the host cell are expressed. It is possible that the stringent response system controls all this, but it seems unlikely. Undoubtedly, other levels of regulation remain to be discovered.

Interaction with Mammalian Macrophages

For a relative newcomer to mammalian cells, *Legionella* is remarkably sophisticated in its ability to manipulate mammalian phagocytic cells. This is evident from studies of attachment and invasion and from what happens to the phagosome after invasion has occurred. *Legionella* can enter macrophages even in the absence of opsonization by C3b or antibody. This makes sense in view of the fact that the lung is deficient in complement and antibodies unless an infection is under way. Mip, the macrophage invasion protein, appears to facilitate this uptake process. How it does this is not clear. Mip is a peptidyl prolyl isomerase, a kind of peptidase. Mip may not even be involved in invasion and internalization in a direct way but might degrade lung surfactant protein. How lung surfactants might block *Legionella* invasion is not clear. Mip influences only the very early steps in invasion. Disruption of the *mip* gene reduces but does not eliminate invasion of macrophages. Mip does not seem to be required for the bacteria to survive intracellularly.

In cells that exhibit coiling phagocytosis, the vacuole is covered with endoplasmic reticulum, which is studded with ribosomes. At first, this development ap-

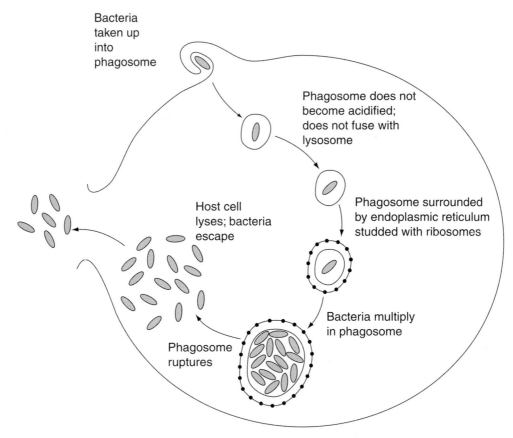

Figure 20–5   The life cycle of *L. pneumophila* in macrophages. The bacteria are taken up in a vacuole (phagosome) that does not become acidified or fuse with a lysosome. The vacuole becomes surrounded by endoplasmic reticulum. Late-stage proteins are eliminated from the membrane of the phagosome. The type IV secretion system is involved in the process. The bacteria replicate in the vacuole, escape the vacuole, and multiply in the cytoplasm. When the cytoplasm is depleted of nutrients, the macrophage lyses, and the bacteria escape and invade other phagocytes.

peared to be strange and mysterious, but then it was noted that a process called **autophagy** made the whole thing look more coherent. Apparently, in normal mammalian cells, there is a process in which components of the cytoplasm or organelles are surrounded in a similar fashion by endoplasmic reticulum. These areas contain components slated for destruction and recycling. A vacuole containing *Legionella*, especially one with its membrane proteins altered, would certainly appear to such a policing system to be aberrant and thus targeted for destruction. Nonetheless, this response of the cell is not sufficient to destroy the vacuole containing the bacteria. The answer to the question of why autophagy does not work on vacuoles that contain *Legionella* will be a fascinating one to study.

Once the bacteria are internalized inside a vacuole, a complex developmental process begins (Figure 20–5). Not only do the vacuoles not acidify to the same extent as normal phagosomes, but they also leave the normal pathway that leads to phagolysosome fusion. This outcome seems to be due to a combination of pH homeostasis and elimination of late-stage proteins from the membrane of the phagosome that indicate the maturation of the phagosome. Examples of these **late-stage proteins** of phagosomes are the **lysosomal-associated membrane proteins LAMP-1** and **LAMP-2**. They are missing from the late-stage phagosomes that contain *Legionella*. If dead or avirulent bacteria are being taken up instead of virulent ones, the phagosome contains LAMP-1, LAMP-2, and other late-stage proteins. **Icm** and **Dot** (**defect in organelle trafficking**) proteins, which comprise the type IV secretion system and the putative effector proteins this system injects into the macrophage cytoplasm, are critical for this process, but there is still no understanding of how Icm/Dot proteins actually carry out this process. Identifying the effector proteins injected by the type IV system and their function would go a long way toward explaining this interaction. There are two obvious possibilities. One is that the effector proteins are injected into the mammalian cell cytoplasm through the phagosome membrane and help to prevent phagolysosome fusion. A second possibility is that they somehow influence the flux of nutrients into the phagosome, providing nutrients for the bacteria.

However they do it, the legionellae derail the vacuole slated for assassination by phagolysosome fusion into a side road, where the vacuole becomes an incubator for bacteria. The type IV system and its effector molecules may also help to create an environment that is nutrient rich enough to support bacterial replication. What happens next is that the bacteria begin to divide (Figure 20–5). Eventually, they escape from the vacuole, continuing to replicate until they fill the cytoplasm of the macrophage. At this point, the bacteria begin to

experience nutrient deprivation and start to express traits, such as piliation, motility, and cytotoxicity, that will be useful when the current host is lysed and the bacteria are released to infect other cells (Figure 20–5). In these later stages, the starvation-induced stringent response system becomes important because, even though the Icm/Dot system may initially create a nutrient-rich vacuole, extensive bacterial replication will quickly deplete these once-abundant nutrients, signaling the bacteria to prepare to lyse the cell they have been multiplying in and prepare to look for other prey.

In contrast to the life cycle in amoebae in which the bacteria kill the cell in one stage by lysing the cells, bacteria kill lung cells by a two-stage process. The first stage is to trigger apoptosis. Much later, the bacteria produce cytolysins that actively lyse the cell. Triggering apoptosis would help to prevent normal functioning of the phagosome-lysosome pathway. In the case of mutants deficient in the ability to carry out the second step (lysis), the bacteria eventually leave the cell, although it takes longer. Either there is still some residual cytolytic activity in the mutants or the apoptotic death of the cell eventually causes the integrity of its membranes to decay to the point that the bacteria are released.

One of many questions that remain to be answered, if the foregoing description is accurate and the legionellae emerge from human macrophages ready for action, is why have there been no cases reported of human-to-human transmission? Possibly, at 37°C and in the conditions encountered in the human lung, transmission from one cell to another can occur, but the bacteria are not prepared to survive the long trip to another human lung.

Damage to the Lung

A hallmark of a *Legionella* infection is the liquid that accumulates in the alveoli. This liquid consists of lysed lung cells. The area of damage is not localized, as in most cases of typical pneumonia, but can spread throughout the lung to give the diffuse patchy densities seen in lung radiograms. The ability of *Legionella* to survive inside phagocytes contributes to lung damage because phagocytes and T cells continue to be attracted to the area and release cytokines and other toxic products without killing the bacteria.

Products of the bacteria themselves may also contribute to lung damage caused by a *Legionella* infection. *L. pneumophila* produces a number of extracellular proteases, some of which cause damage when introduced into the guinea pig lung. A particularly destructive protease is a 40-kDa zinc **metalloprotease.** The metalloprotease also has hemolysin activity. Intranasal or intratracheal administration of partially purified metalloprotease into the lungs of guinea pigs produces lesions that resemble those seen in the lungs of guinea pigs with *Legionella* infections. This metalloprotease is not, however, produced by all pathogenic *Legionella* species. *Legionella* produces other hemolysins and phospholipases (e.g., phospholipase A, phospholipase C) that could have a destructive effect on lung cells. These phospholipases can also destroy lung surfactant, the lipid that reduces the surface tension experienced by vacuolar membranes, making it easier to refill emptied air sacs. Destruction of surfactant can cause the alveoli to collapse completely when the gas they contain is released, and it can be difficult to refill them.

Prevention and Treatment

Since untreated *L. pneumophila* pneumonia can be fatal, prompt diagnosis and treatment with effective antibiotics are important. Erythromycin is currently the drug of choice for treating legionellosis, although newer macrolides, such as azithromycin, are coming into fashion. The fact that an antibiotic is effective against *Legionella* growing in laboratory medium does not mean that it will be clinically effective (see Box 20–1). The antibiotic must be able to penetrate phagocytic cells, since that is where the bacteria are replicating. An obvious way of preventing *Legionella* infections is to eliminate *Legionella* from water supplies that might produce aerosols, which would be inhaled by humans. This is difficult to accomplish in practice because of the resistance to biocides of bacteria inside amoebae. Hot water (60°C) flushed through pipes and UV light can kill *Legionella,* but these are expensive ways of treating large amounts of water, such as water stored in air-conditioning cooling towers. A renewed effort is being made to identify biocides that are safe for humans but kill *Legionella* inside amoebae. Efforts are also being made to develop a vaccine to prevent Legionnaires' disease. Since the bacteria can grow in macrophages, a protective response would require activation of macrophages and possibly recruitment of cytotoxic T cells, which can also kill macrophages infected with bacteria.

Legionella as a Paradigm for Intracellular Pathogens

As recently as several years ago, the thought of *L. pneumophila* as a model organism for studying how bacteria survive and multiply inside phagocytic cells would have generated considerable skepticism because of the difficulties encountered by scientists working with these bacteria. Compared with the other intracellular

---

BOX 20–1   Legionnaires' Disease Is Bad News

To read the descriptions of Legionnaires' disease provided by clinical microbiology texts, it might seem to be not such a big deal. But it can be a very big deal to people with a serious infection. Consider this case description of a patient with an *L. pneumophila* lung infection. A 40-year-old man was fighting for his life. His condition was so bad that he was brought to a hospital by helicopter. His initial symptoms were vague, suggesting a bout of flu. These included fever, feeling very tired, and respiratory symptoms that were not very clearly described. At first, he was treated for influenza, but as shortness of breath became a problem, the doctors knew this was serious. Bronchoscopic examination revealed fluid in the air sacs of his lungs and some inflammation of the airway. The patient was soon diagnosed by the medical team as having Legionnaires' disease. Once this diagnosis was arrived at, appropriate therapy was instituted. This story should have had a happy ending. Right diagnosis. Right antibiotic therapy. No deal. This fairly young man lingered for 9 months in a long-term-care facility before dying. The cause of death—inadequate lung function due to damage caused by *L. pneumophila*. This case shows how, even when everything is done right, including the appropriate therapy backed up by supportive therapy to maintain oxygenation of the blood, the outcome can be bad. Note also that this patient displayed none of the textbook risk factors, such as old age, alcohol abuse, smoking, or immunosuppression. The source of the infections was never determined, something that is difficult to do in an isolated case like this one. *L. pneumophila* may be new to the human lung, but it is one tough character nonetheless.

Source: P. H. Gilligan, M. L. Smiley, and D. S. Shapiro. 1997. *Cases in Medical Microbiology and Infectious Diseases,* 2nd ed., p. 61–64. ASM Press, Washington, D.C. (This is a wonderful book, crammed with descriptions of actual cases to give students an idea of what the diseases described so abstractly in most medical microbiology books really feel like at the human level.)

pathogens, with the possible exception of *Salmonella* sp., our understanding of how *Legionella* interacts with human cells has proceeded at such a fast pace that *Legionella* is now considered by many to be a model for intracellular bacterial pathogens. There is also the interesting ecological feature—its life in amoebae—to make *Legionella* even more appealing as a model organism. One could even argue that *Legionella* has caught up with and even surpassed *Salmonella* as a model intracellular pathogen. The reason is that scientists who work on *Legionella* have made themselves familiar with the pathology of Legionnaires' disease. A close intellectual connection to the pathology of the disease means that scientists who study *Legionella* are less likely to waste time on tissue culture artifacts and other distractions that have plagued scientists working in some other areas of pathogenesis.

There is one reason for concern about making *Legionella* the model intracellular pathogen. If scientists are right in thinking that humans are an accidental host, *Legionella* did not evolve as a human pathogen and could thus differ in important ways from bacteria that have. Nonetheless, the interesting question of how *Legionella* adapted so readily to cause human disease finesses this quibble. Moreover, it is unlikely that bacterial diseases will cease to emerge in the future. Insights into the traits of bacteria that can make this jump from the environment to humans without millions of years of coevolution could be very important. Also, except for *M. tuberculosis*, one could argue that competing model organisms such as *Listeria*, *Salmonella*, and *Yersinia* spp. are also accidental human pathogens whose true reservoir is some other animal or soil and water. Certainly, these bacteria have been causing human disease far longer. But has this period really been long enough to have a significant effect on the bacterium-human interaction if humans are not the main reservoir?

SELECTED READINGS

Abu Kwaik, Y. 1998. Fatal attraction of mammalian cells to *Legionella pneumophila*. *Mol. Microbiol.* **30:**689–695.

Christie, P. J., and J. P. Vogel. 2000. Bacterial type IV secretion: conjugation systems adapted to deliver effector molecules to host cells. *Trends Microbiol.* **8:**354–360.

Harb, O. S., and Y. Abu Kwaik. 2000. Characterization of a macrophage-specific infectivity locus (*milA*) of *Legionella pneumophila*. *Infect. Immun.* **68:**368–376.

Kirby, J. E., and R. R. Isberg. 1998. Legionnaires' disease: the pore macrophage and the legion of terror within. *Trends Microbiol.* **6:**256–258.

Rittig, M. G., G.-R. Burmester, and A. Krause. 1998. Coiling phagocytosis: when the zipper jams, the cup is deformed. *Trends Microbiol.* **6:**384–387.

Roy, C. R. 1999. Trafficking of the *Legionella pneumophila* phagosome. *ASM News* **65:**416–421.

Russell, D. G. 1998. What does "inhibition of phagolysosome fusion" really mean? *Trends Microbiol.* **6:**212–214.

Segal, G., and H. A. Shuman. 1998. How is the intracellular fate of the *Legionella pneumophila* phagosome determined? *Trends Microbiol.* **6:**253–255.

Solomon, J. M., and R. R. Isberg. 2000. Growth of *Legionella pneumophila* in *Dictyostelium discoideum:* a novel system for genetic analysis of host-pathogen interactions. *Trends Microbiol.* **8:**478–480.

Swanson, M. S., and S. Sturgill-Kosycki. 2000. Exploitation of macrophages as a replication niche by *Legionella pneumophila*. *Trends Microbiol.* **8:**47–50.

Swanson, M. S., and B. K. Hammer. 2000. *Legionella pneumophila* pathogenesis: a fateful journey from amoebae to macrophages. *Annu. Rev. Microbiol.* **54:**567–613.

SUMMARY OUTLINE

Legionnaires' disease

Form of pneumonia

Caused by *L. pneumophila*

First recognized in 1976

Incidence increasing

Spread by inhalation of aerosols
- Generated by air-conditioning towers
- Inhalation therapy

Most susceptible people have impaired respiratory defenses (heavy alcohol use, smoking, or old age)

Characteristics of disease
- Fever, disorientation, lethargy
- Lung damage—"moth-eaten" appearance on X rays

(continued)

    Significant fluid accumulation

    Milder self-limiting disease (Pontiac fever) caused by *L. micdadei*

    Not transmitted person to person

Characteristics of *L. pneumophila*

Motile, aerobic, gram-negative rod

Complex nutritional requirements

Does not stain well with Gram stain reagents

Lives in phagocytic cells

Normal environment
    Biofilms in nature
    Inside protozoa (*Acanthamoeba*, *Hartmanella*) and fungi (*Dictyostelium*)

Virulence factors

Problems with studying virulence factors
    Animal models
        Guinea pig can be infected by aerosols (not immunocompromised)
        A/J strain of immunocompromised mice
    Cell lines—none have been good models
    Amoebae—just beginning to be used
    Genetic studies of *L. pneumophila* not very advanced

Survival in amoebae
    Attach by afimbrial adhesin (not important in human cells)
    Coiling phagocytosis
        Pseudopods wrap around bacteria
        Probably not as important as originally thought
    Mip—macrophage infectivity promoter
        Peptidyl prolyl isomerase
        Increases efficiency of infection
    Icm—intracellular multiplication
        Type IV secretion system
        Secretes proteins attached to DNA into cytoplasm of another cell in other species
            (e.g., *Agrobacterium*)
        In *L. pneumophila* may only be injecting proteins

Regulation of virulence genes
    Temperature—important in transition of bacteria from amoebae to macrophages
    Thymine limitation
        Stringent response system
        May be more important in later stages of intracellular growth

Interaction with macrophages
    Invasion does not require opsonization
    Mip facilitates uptake
        May degrade lung surfactant
        Not required for intracellular survival
    Developmental process within a vacuole
        Phagosomes do not become acidified
        Late-stage proteins (LAMP-1 and LAMP-2) eliminated from phagosome membrane
        Effector proteins injected by Icm/Dot system involved in some way

(continued)

SUMMARY OUTLINE (*continued*)

            May prevent phagosome-lysosome fusion
            May provide nutrients to bacteria in phagosome
        Bacteria divide in vacuole, then escape to cytoplasm
        Bacterial replication continues until cytoplasm is filled
        L. pneumophila experiences loss of nutrients
            Traits such as piliation, motility, cytotoxicity expressed
            Stringent response system becomes more important
        Mammalian cell lysis requires two steps
            Bacteria trigger apoptosis
            Cytolysins later lyse cell

    Damage to lung
        Bacteria lyse lung cells
        Damage is diffuse
        Extracellular proteases contribute to damage
            Metalloprotease very destructive
            Others may destroy surfactant

Prevention and treatment

    Erythromycin current drug of choice

    Azithromycin use increasing

    Antibiotics have trouble reaching intracellular bacteria

    Prevention measures
        Eliminate bacteria from water sources—difficult
        Search for biocides to kill *L. pneumophila* in amoebae

***Legionella* as paradigm for intracellular lifestyle**

    Life in amoebae appealing as model for jump from environment to humans

    Concerns—human is accidental host; bacteria did not evolve to infect humans

    May give insights into how new diseases emerge

QUESTIONS

Answers to the questions can be found in Appendix 2.

1. Given that *Legionella* stains poorly with Gram stain reagents, how would you detect it in sputum, i.e., how would you diagnose Legionnaires' disease?

2. Although *Legionella* normally lives in water, it can only be cultivated in the laboratory on rich medium. Give a possible explanation for this observation.

3. Why might you expect that in the case of bacteria such as *Legionella*, which only infect somewhat immunocompromised people, the genetic, biochemical, and immunological approaches might yield different answers, whereas these same three approaches might give the same answer for an organism such as *M. tuberculosis* that infects healthy people?

4. It has been found that animals vaccinated with metalloprotease toxoid were protected from subsequent infection with *L. pneumophila*. This appears to conflict with the finding that a protease-minus mutant was as virulent as wild type. How can the two results be reconciled—or can they?

5. In earlier chapters, the question of whether cultured cells are good models for the bacterium-host interaction was raised. Explain why this question is even more pressing in the case of diseases like Legionnaires' disease.

6. Comment on potential problems that might arise in connection with development of a vaccine against Legionnaires' disease.

21

Mycoplasma pneumoniae and *Chlamydia pneumoniae*

KEY FEATURES

Mycoplasma pneumoniae and **Chlamydia pneumoniae**

CHARACTERISTICS

M. pneumoniae—small bacterium with a minimalist genome; no peptidoglycan; cholesterol in membrane; extracellular pathogen

C. pneumoniae—small bacterium with a minimalist genome; outer membrane but no peptidoglycan; obligately intracellular pathogen; two forms (elementary body, reticulate body)

DISEASE

Atypical pneumonia: "walking pneumonia"—*M. pneumoniae;* flulike infection—*C. pneumoniae*

Some types of heart disease (controversial): *C. pneumoniae*

RESERVOIR

Infected humans

MAJOR VIRULENCE FACTORS

M. pneumoniae: cytadherence organelle—binding to host cells; phospholipases; antigenic variation—evasion of immune system; elicit strong cytokine response

C. pneumoniae: unknown

PREVENTION AND TREATMENT

Antibiotics

Lifestyles of *Mycoplasma pneumoniae* and *Chlamydia pneumoniae*

M. pneumoniae and *C. pneumoniae* may have the same species name and cause disease in the same location—the lung—but they are very different microbes. They do share enough features, however, to be considered together in the same chapter. Both are common causes of community-acquired pneumonia in the high school and college age group. They are also a common cause of pneumonia in adults and the elderly. Both cause a type of pneumonia that has been called **atypical pneumonia.** The pneumonia is atypical in that the radiograms of infected lungs look different from those of people with "typical" pneumonia caused by bacteria such as *Streptococcus pneumoniae.* In lung radiograms of people with atypical pneumonia, the pattern of density due to inflammation is patchy and diffuse, with a "moth-eaten" appearance. In cases of typical pneumonia, the areas of density seen on lung radiograms are compact with clear edges.

M. pneumoniae causes a condition called "walking pneumonia," the bane of busy college students. The name comes from the fact that the infected person usually does not require hospitalization and, although sick enough to spend a lot of time in bed, is still capable of walking around. *C. pneumoniae* is a newly recognized cause of a flulike infection. It has also been in the news, because scientists have suggested that it may cause some types of heart disease. This hypothesis has put cardiology on its ear. If even some heart disease cases are caused by an infectious agent, what a revolution this would be for heart disease patients who might look forward to a rapid antibiotic cure! Of course it could be bad news for the pharmaceutical industry, since current heart medications that are taken daily throughout a person's life are a major source of profit.

Both mycoplasmas and chlamydiae are very small bacteria and have the smallest bacterial genomes known. This raises the question of how many genes are required for an organism to be free-living (Box 21–1). *M. pneumoniae* and a close relative called *Ureaplasma* sp. have genomes in the range of 0.5 to 0.8 Mbp. The genome of *Escherichia coli* is 8 to 10 times larger, and many bacteria have even larger genomes than that of *E. coli*. A 0.5-Mbp genome could encode about 500 genes. The essential core of genes is thought to be even smaller, possibly only 200 to 300 genes. This is not much larger than the genomes of some of the more complex viruses, which are incapable of replication independent of a host cell. By contrast, *M. pneumoniae* can grow independently of human cells if it is provided with a nutrient-rich medium. Another interesting feature of *M. pneumoniae* is that although it is clearly a bacterium (judging from 16S rRNA gene sequence data), it has some features of a eukaryotic cell: it lacks a rigid cell wall, its membrane contains cholesterol, and it has an internal protein network reminiscent of a cytoskeleton.

C. pneumoniae and other chlamydiae, such as *Chlamydia trachomatis* (chapter 31) have a somewhat larger genome (slightly over 1 Mbp in size) but are equally amazing in their capacity to squeeze maximum function out of a small number of genes. They are as small as mycoplasmas, but unlike the mycoplasmas they are obligate intracellular parasites. Despite their genomic simplicity, they undergo a two-stage developmental cycle, something scientists would have thought required a much bigger genome. The developmental cycle of *C. pneumoniae* is shown in Figure 21–1. The stage that infects human cells is a metabolically inactive form (the

BOX 21–1   New Insight into the Old Question, What Is Life?

One of the great areas of controversy in recent years has been the question, what is the minimal genome size for a free-living bacterium? This area became particularly contentious when scientists announced the discovery of "nanobacteria," bacteria only 50 nm in diameter. These nanobacteria were alleged to cause kidney stones, but there is controversy about whether they even exist, much less play a role in human health. The discoverers claimed that the nanobacteria were free-living bacteria, not obligate intracellular parasites like the viruses. Skeptics argued that a bacterium that small, approaching the size range of eukaryotic viruses, could not possibly contain enough DNA to encode the functions of a free-living microbe. This led naturally to the question of how many genes a free-living microbe really needs. *M. pneumoniae* may provide an answer.

Scientists are now making disruptions in every *Mycoplasma* gene to answer this question of the minimal genome size. *Ureaplasma urealyticum* is receiving similar attention. Scientists hope to narrow down what is the essential core group of genes that is both necessary and sufficient for a self-replicating organism. It is important to point out that although mycoplasmas and ureaplasmas replicate themselves, they do so in very close association with mammalian cells. Yet they are capable of replication in cell-free medium if given enough nutrients. Thus, their genomes could presumably carry the secret of what genes make up the minimal genome of a living organism. This approach to answering the question "What is life?" will certainly not impress philosophers, who are concerned with such concepts as intelligence and the soul, but it might reveal fundamental information about the basic biological aspects of living beings.

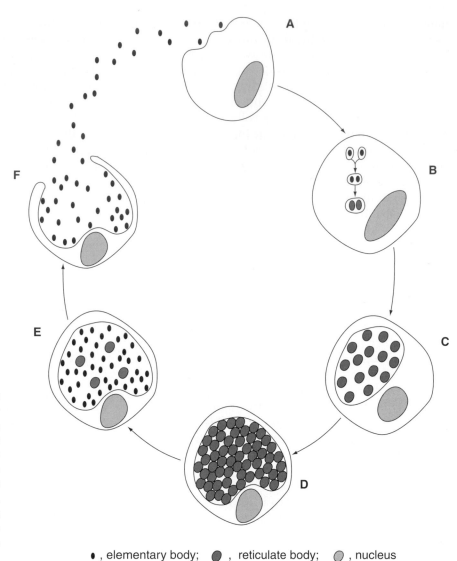

Figure 21–1 The developmental cycle of *C. pneumoniae*. The elementary body invades the host cell (**A**), where it changes into a reticulate body (**B**). The reticulate body actively replicates (**C**) until the vacuole fills most of the cytoplasm (**D**). The reticulate bodies convert into elementary bodies (**E**). The vacuolar membrane fuses with the cell membrane, and the elementary bodies are released into the environment (**F**).

●, elementary body; ●, reticulate body; ◯, nucleus

elementary body), somewhat akin to a spore, that can survive for short periods of time in the external environment and is thus able to move from cell to cell in the human body. Once inside an endosome in a human cell, *C. pneumoniae* changes into a replicating form (**reticulate body**), which begins to multiply, and as it does the vacuole becomes larger and larger, nearly filling the human cell cytoplasm. The reticulate body is larger than the elementary body and is metabolically active. As the vacuole expands in size, the reticulate bodies begin to differentiate into elementary bodies, which will be the form released to infect other cells. Thus, in addition to the genes needed for these two forms, there are undoubtedly some complicated regulatory circuits to go with the rest of the genomic package.

In contrast to some other intracellular pathogens that kill the cell they invade, chlamydiae are kinder, gentler parasites. Eventually, the vacuole in which they are rep-

licating fuses with the cytoplasmic membrane, releasing the elementary bodies into the extracellular environment with relatively little damage to the infected cell. True, the cell abandoned by all those elementary bodies probably feels about the way your mother would feel after you brought home several hundred of your closest friends for a weekend of steady eating, drinking, and laundry, but at least the parasitized cell is still alive, if spent. The tissue damage that occurs during chlamydial infections is not due to direct destruction of host cells, but to the body's inflammatory response to the bacteria.

Because of their lifestyles, neither mycoplasmas nor chlamydiae have much association with other bacteria—unless there is some part of their life cycle that has not yet been discovered. This may be the reason that resistance to antibiotics has not been a particular problem in these bacteria. The bacterial equivalent of hermits, they have little opportunity to tap into the DNA gene transfer superhighway that links so many other bacterial pathogens. Those pathogens spend at least some of their time in close contact with bacteria of the microbiota of the human body or with soil and water bacteria that may have resistance genes to pass along.

But wait! There may be more gene transfer than meets the eye. Analysis of genome sequence data revealed that both of these organisms, but especially *Chlamydia* species, have a number of eukaryotelike genes. Scientists investigating the sequencing data suggest that the bacteria may, during their long and close association with eukaryotic cells, have acquired DNA from their eukaryotic host cells. A recent discovery about chlamydiae suggests that this association may have been an even longer one than previously thought. *Chlamydia*-like bacteria have been found inside protozoa, such as *Acanthamoeba* species. A close relative of *Chlamydia* has yet another interesting association with eukaryotes (Box 21–2). Thus, chlamydiae could have

been associated with eukaryotic cells for hundreds of millions or even billions of years. The time of appearance of the first eukaryotic cell is estimated to have been at least 2.7 billion years ago.

Characteristics of *Mycoplasma* and *Chlamydia* Species

Mycoplasmas and chlamydiae do not have a peptidoglycan cell wall. Mycoplasmas have only the cytoplasmic membrane, whereas chlamydiae have a gram-negative-type cell wall with cytoplasmic and outer membranes, but neither has peptidoglycan. The outer membrane of chlamydiae has disulfide cross-linked proteins that may play the same stabilizing role as peptidoglycan in other bacteria. The cytoplasmic membrane of mycoplasmas has characteristics resembling a gram-negative outer membrane. Instead of being a phospholipid bilayer like the cytoplasmic membranes

---

BOX 21–2   And You Guys Thought Genital Herpes Was Bad!

A distant relative of the chlamydiae that lives inside the genital tissue of insects is an interesting bacterium called *Wolbachia*. *Wolbachia* species have been found in many insects, but its best-known host is the fruit fly *Drosophila melanogaster*. It has been estimated that about one-third of the *Drosophila* colonies used by scientists for research are infected with *Wolbachia*. *Wolbachia* is most closely related to the bacteria that cause the diseases typhus and Rocky Mountain spotted fever, *Rickettsia* species, which in turn are most closely related to *Chlamydia* species. *Wolbachia* is an intracellular pathogen that is not spread by sexual transmission but only by transovarial transmission. The infected eggs of an infected mother produce infected progeny. This has given rise to an unusual strategy used by the bacteria to keep themselves in an insect population.

When *Wolbachia* enters a *Drosophila* population, it spreads rapidly. The reason is that *Wolbachia* makes subtle changes, still not understood, in the testes and ovaries of the fruit flies that make a mating between an infected male and an uninfected female unlikely to produce progeny. Apparently, the infected sperm is altered in such a way as to be unable to fertilize

an uninfected egg. Yet an infected egg can "rescue" this defect and allow for numerous infected progeny. The upshot of this pattern of infection is that infected females, which can enter into productive matings with infected or uninfected males, are more likely to have progeny than uninfected females, which can mate productively only with uninfected males. This advantage in numbers of progeny is sufficient to allow the infected insects to dominate an insect population very quickly.

But the *Wolbachia* story gets even creepier as we get closer to the title of this boxed item. In some insects, *Wolbachia* uses a different strategy to ensure that transovarial transmission occurs. An infected male wood louse, for example, can be turned by a *Wolbachia* infection into a fully fertile female wood louse. In this case, the bacteria are probably affecting hormone levels sufficiently to trigger a sex change. So far, there is no known case of a *Wolbachia* infection in a vertebrate species. Still, if you know someone who works with *D. melanogaster*, watch that person very, very carefully.

Source: A. A. Salyers and D. D. Whitt. 2001. *Microbiology: Diversity, Disease, and the Environment.* Fitzgerald Science Press, Bethesda, Md.

of other bacteria, the mycoplasma membrane has the asymmetric character of the outer membrane. The inner leaflet of the bilayer is phospholipid, but the outer leaflet is composed of lipoproteins (Figure 21–2). The outer leaflet lipoproteins may be the functional equivalent of gram-negative lipopolysaccharide or gram-positive lipoteichoic acid in the sense that the lipoproteins are responsible for eliciting the inflammatory response seen during a mycoplasma infection.

The genome sequences of mycoplasmas revealed that there are few amino acid or vitamin biosynthetic genes. This was not a surprise, given that mycoplasmas require a very complex medium if they are grown away from eukaryotic cells. They also require fatty acids and sterols. Some mycoplasmas use arginine as an energy source, making ATP via the arginine dihydrolase pathway (Figure 21–3). This trait may have a role in pathogenesis, because histones, the proteins that organize and protect eukaryotic DNA, are arginine-rich proteins. Depletion of the host cell's arginine reserves could lead

to shortages in histones, and this type of shortage could explain the chromosome breakage seen in eukaryotic cells infected with mycoplasmas. Mycoplasmas may also derive nucleic acids from eukaryotic cells that have lysed in their vicinity. It is clear from the genome sequences and from metabolic studies of mycoplasmas that a major reason for their stripped-down genome is that they are obligate parasites (outside the laboratory) of eukaryotic cells.

Most of the pathogenic *Mycoplasma* species remain outside the eukaryotic cells with which they are associated, but there is variety here as well. *Mycoplasma penetrans*, an animal pathogen, can invade cultured mammalian cells. Other *Mycoplasma* species actually fuse with the membranes of the eukaryotic cells with which they associate. But the current picture of *M. pneumoniae* is that it is an external parasite that is intimately associated with mammalian cells.

Mycoplasmas have a distinctive shape (Figure 21–4), which unlike that of most bacteria is asymmetric. That is, the two ends of the cell look different and probably have different functions. The bacteria move with a gliding motility across surfaces. The leading end contains the organelle that attaches to eukaryotic cells, so one could almost imagine mycoplasmas as searching for prey with their adherence end poised to grab whatever hapless eukaryotic cell appears on their radar screen. Their movement seems to be purposeful, indicating some kind of chemotaxis. One of the several "eukaryotic" features of mycoplasmas is their histonelike proteins that may form a primitive kind of cytoskeleton. This cytoskeleton not only organizes the shape of the

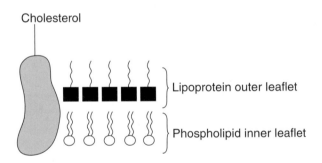

Figure 21–2 Structure of the cytoplasmic membrane of mycoplasmas. The inner leaflet consists of phospholipid, and the outer leaflet consists of lipoproteins. The membrane also contains cholesterol, a complex lipid normally associated with mammalian cells, not prokaryotes.

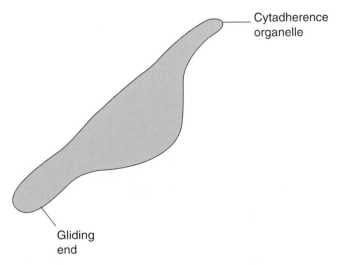

Figure 21–4 Asymmetric shape of *M. pneumoniae*. One end causes the cell to glide across surfaces. The other end contains the cytadherence organelle, which attaches to eukaryotic cells.

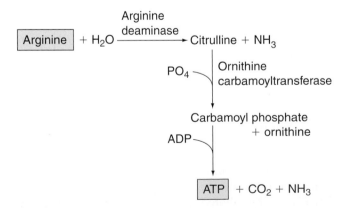

Figure 21–3 The arginine dihydrolase pathway. Some mycoplasmas use arginine as an energy source.

cell but also aids in localization of the adhesive end of the bacterial cell.

Not much will be said here about the features of *C. pneumoniae* because most of the work on the characteristics of the chlamydiae has been done with *C. trachomatis,* the subject of chapter 31. The two-stage life cycle has already been noted, as has the gram-negative structure of the cell envelope. *C. pneumoniae* was first described in the 1980s. Epidemiological studies soon revealed that it was an important cause of community-acquired pneumonia. The association of *C. pneumoniae* with coronary artery disease, the most common cause of death in developed countries, caused a veritable gold rush to assess whether this association would lead to new cures and preventive strategies. In the process, studies of the metabolic features of *C. pneumoniae* got shoved to the back of the research line. After all, there are a number of antibiotics that are still effective against *Chlamydia* species, so the argument that studying metabolism might reveal new targets for antibiotics had far less force than it does for increasingly antibiotic-resistant species. This is unfortunate because a fascinating and possibly important question about the metabolism of *C. pneumoniae* is why it colonizes the respiratory tract preferentially, whereas the other major chlamydial pathogen, *C. trachomatis,* either infects the eyes (causing a destructive disease called trachoma) or the genital tract (nongonococcal urethritis and its sequelae). Another relative, *Chlamydia psittaci,* causes systemic disease (Box 21–3).

Virulence Factors

M. pneumoniae

GENOME SEQUENCE. You might think that because of the small genome size of mycoplasmas and the availability of at least one complete genome sequence, everything must be known about how mycoplasmas cause disease, but this is not the case. Given the difficulty of working with mycoplasmas, the amount of progress made in recent years is impressive, but there is still a lot to do. One important advance is that it is now possible to introduce foreign DNA into *Mycoplasma* species. This means that directed mutations can be made to test the importance of candidate virulence genes. There is even a transposon, Tn*4001,* which can be used to mutagenize *Mycoplasma* species.

So, what has been learned from the genome sequence that might give insights into the essential features of mycoplasmas? Here the big story seems to be what genes are missing. The fact that amino acid and vitamin biosynthetic genes are missing was not all that much of a surprise, because of the rich medium needed to cul-

---

BOX 21–3   Stop! Don't Kiss That Parrot!

The *Chlamydia* species that are responsible for the most cases of human infections are *C. pneumoniae* and *C. trachomatis. C. pneumoniae,* as already noted, is a common cause of respiratory infections. *C. trachomatis* is the leading cause of a widespread sexually transmitted disease, nongonococcal urethritis (chapter 31). A much rarer cause of human infection, but one with an interesting epidemiology, is *C. psittaci. C. psittaci* is carried by many species of exotic birds. It can be transmitted by aerosols to humans who spend time in close proximity to such birds. The bacteria enter the human body and cause a disseminated febrile infection called psittacosis. At first, the symptoms resemble those of a bad case of flu, but psittacosis can be deadly. Even if the infected person survives, the disease can last for a long time. Since psittacosis is not a very common disease, doctors often misdiagnose it. This is an example of the importance of asking a patient with a mysterious complaint about the patient's occupation; the patient's history can provide useful clues to the cause of the patient's symptoms. Psittacosis is seen most commonly in veterinarians and in people who work in pet stores that sell exotic birds.

---

tivate mycoplasmas grown in the absence of mammalian cells. A more surprising feature is the apparent lack of regulatory genes. Two-component regulatory genes are missing, as are homologs of global regulatory genes, such as *crp, lrp,* and *rpoS.* It is premature to jump to the conclusion that there is no regulation of mycoplasma genes. Mycoplasmas exhibit gliding motility and chemotaxis, yet no recognizable genes of this type have been seen in the genome sequence. So the regulatory genes of mycoplasma may differ from those of other bacteria in that they do not have recognizable amino acid sequence motifs.

ADHERENCE. An important virulence factor of mycoplasmas is the ability of these bacteria to bind very specifically to the ciliated cells of the upper respiratory tract. Binding of the bacteria ultimately leads to the cessation of the "beating" of the ciliated cells, thus removing a vital defense of the upper respiratory tract. A specialized mycoplasma organelle is responsible for this **cytadherence.** It is located at only one end of the cell. The importance of this localization is not understood. The cytadherence polar tip structure has a membrane-protein surface and a core that consists of a very dense collection of proteins. Components of this cytadherence structure are beginning to be identified, but it is clear that the mechanism of adherence is probably not going to be the same as that of pili. Binding of mycoplasmas to a eukaryotic cell can depolarize the eukaryotic cell membrane, so that the cell becomes more permeable to whatever toxic substances the mycoplasmas produce. Depolarization by itself could explain the cessation of motion of ciliated cells to which mycoplasmas have bound.

TOXINS. So far, there have been no reports of protein exotoxins produced by mycoplasmas. Yet they clearly produce some toxic substances that damage eukaryotic cells. Two candidates are peroxide and other reactive forms of oxygen. This hypothesis was suggested decades ago, but not much progress has been made toward determining whether reactive forms of oxygen are really important players in eukaryotic cell damage. Given that membrane lipoproteins of mycoplasmas can elicit cytokine release and generally do most of the things done by LPS, the possibility has to be taken into account that membrane lipoproteins may be responsible for some of the toxic effects mycoplasmas have on cells.

Yet another possible virulence factor is membrane phospholipases. Mycoplasmas are so closely associated with a mammalian cell that such phospholipases could do serious damage to nearby eukaryotic cell membranes. The mycoplasma membrane is presumably protected by its asymmetric bilayer structure.

ANTIGENIC VARIATION. The lipoproteins of the mycoplasma surface appear to be a very immunogenic target for the human immune system. One of the virulence strategies suggested by recent studies of strains isolated from human infections is antigenic variation in the membrane lipoproteins. How important a role antigenic variation plays in evasion of the host defense responses remains to be established.

MANIPULATION OF PHAGOCYTIC AND IMMUNE CELLS. Phagocytes seem not to be very effective in eliminating mycoplasmas, and no one knows why. There is no shortage of hypotheses, of course. Mycoplasmas elicit a strong cytokine response. They stimulate lymphocytes such as T cells and B cells in a nonspecific manner. In fact, in their presence, B cells begin to produce in-

appropriate antibodies. This could be a diversion of the immune response. In the laboratory, given the perennial problem of mycoplasma infection of tissue culture cells, one wonders how many reports from immunology laboratories are artifacts of a mycoplasma infection giving rise to aberrant and nonspecific activation of T and B cells.

C. pneumoniae

Virtually nothing is known about the virulence factors of *C. pneumoniae.* The bacteria can adhere to and damage endothelial cells, and they elicit a strong inflammatory response. Students rejoice! This is all you need to memorize for now. The big story here, as was already mentioned, is the possible connection between *C. pneumoniae* and heart disease. But the fun doesn't stop there. *C. pneumoniae* has also been suggested to have a role in Alzheimer's disease and asthma. In the case of coronary artery disease and Alzheimer's disease, the hypothetical connection is based on the ability of *C. pneumoniae* to infect endothelial cells. Infection of endothelial cells creates a zone of inflammation that damages the blood vessel wall. Then bad things can begin to happen. In the arteries, cholesterol plaques can begin to form in the damaged regions. In the brain, protein plaques could form, and neutrophils attracted to the site could magnify the damage.

What are the reasons to think *C. pneumoniae* might cause heart disease? First, the bacteria have been detected in atherosclerotic plaques (Koch's first postulate satisfied) and have been cultivated from these lesions (Koch's second postulate satisfied). But are the bacteria simply opportunists that are colonizing preexisting lesions, or are they the cause of these lesions? Therein lies the crux of the question. Resolving this question is not as simple as it might at first appear to be. For one thing, treating middle-aged people with antibiotics to see if they have fewer heart attacks (sneaking up on Koch's third postulate) may be too little too late.

Epidemiological studies indicate that the lung disease caused by *C. pneumoniae* is primarily a disease of younger people, so the damage that precipitates plaque deposition might already have been done in earlier years. If so, treating middle-aged people with antibiotics would not be expected to work. But consider the alternative: treat adolescents or college-aged students with antibiotics, then wait decades to see how they fare. How many scientists with studies on this time scale are going to get their grants renewed? Also, there is the argument that the use of antibiotics that should have eliminated *C. pneumoniae* in people now in their heart attack years (tetracyclines, erythromycin) was widespread in the 1960s and onward, and yet the incidence of coronary artery disease seems to be increasing. But if, as proved to be the case with *Helicobacter pylori*, which causes peptic ulcers, a combination of antibiotics is required to clear the infection, this argument loses its force.

There is a rabbit model for heart disease. New Zealand White rabbits fed high-fat diets develop plaques very similar to those seen in people with heart disease. Animals infected with *C. pneumoniae* but not with *M. pneumoniae* developed atherosclerotic plaques. Investigators found that early antibiotic therapy with antichlamydia antibiotics could prevent formation of lesions in most of the rabbits, but if the disease was allowed to go on too long before treatment was started, the antibiotics were not effective. If this is a good model of human disease, the findings of such studies suggest that treating middle-aged patients with established heart disease is not the proper way to demonstrate efficacy of antibiotic treatment.

You are probably beginning to wonder if there are any chronic diseases other than ulcers that have not been claimed for *C. pneumoniae*. There are a few, but *C. pneumoniae* has certainly taken center stage in a number of areas. At the very least, a new respiratory pathogen has been added to our knowledge. In studies that have attempted to determine the cause of all of the cases of respiratory disease in the study population, scientists have often found that "unknown etiology" was one of the most common diagnoses. Knowing about *C. pneumoniae* has helped to reduce the number of "unknown etiology" diagnoses. The next few years should bring forward a lot of new information about the virulence factors of *C. pneumoniae* and perhaps some more definitive answers about the involvement of this tiny bacterium in heart disease and other chronic conditions.

SELECTED READINGS

Balin, J. J., H. C. Gerard, E. J. Arking, D. M. Appelt, P. J. Branigan, J. T. Abrams, J. A. Whittum-Hudson, and A. P. Hudson. 1998. Identification and localization of *Chlamydia pneumoniae* in the Alzheimer's brain. *Med. Microbiol. Immunol.* **187:**23–42.

Chambaud, I., H. Wroblewski, and A. Blanchard. 1999. Interactions between mycoplasma lipoproteins and the host immune system. *Trends Microbiol.* **7:**493–499.

Fong, I. W. 2000. Antibiotic effects in a rabbit model of *Chlamydia pneumoniae*-induced atherosclerosis. *J. Infect. Dis.* **181**(Suppl. 3)**:**S514–S518.

Hammerschlag, M. R. 2000. The role of chlamydia in upper respiratory tract infections. *Curr. Infect. Dis. Rep.* **2:**115–120.

Hatch, T. P. 1996. Disulfide cross-linked envelope proteins: the functional equivalent of peptidoglycan in chlamydiae? *J. Bacteriol.* **178:**1–5.

Krause, D. C. 1998. *Mycoplasma pneumoniae* cytadherence: organization and assembly of the attachment organelle. *Trends Microbiol.* **6:**15–18.

Meier, C. R., L. Derby, S. Jick, C. Vasilakis, and H. Jick. 1999. Antibiotics and risk of subsequent first-time acute myocardial infarction. *JAMA* **281:**427–431.

Micillo, E., A. Bianco, D. D'Auria, G. Mazzarella, and G. F. Abbate. 2000. Respiratory infections and asthma. *Allergy* **55**(Suppl. 61)**:**42–45.

Rosengarten, R., C. Citti, M. Glew, A. Lischewski, M. Droesse, P. Much, F. Winner, M. Brank, and J. Spergser. 2000. Host-pathogen interactions in mycoplasma pathogenesis: virulence and survival strategies of minimalist prokaryotes. *Int. J. Med. Microbiol.* **290:**15–25.

Rottem, S., and Y. Naot. 1998. Subversion and exploitation of host cells by mycoplasmas. *Trends Microbiol.* **6:**436–440.

SUMMARY OUTLINE

M. pneumoniae

Characteristics
  Very small
  Small genome (0.5 to 0.8 Mb); could encode about 500 genes
  Grows extracellularly but in intimate association with human cells
  Shares features with eukaryotic cells
    No peptidoglycan cell wall
    Cell membrane contains cholesterol
    Internal histonelike protein network similar to cytoskeleton
  Cell membrane asymmetrical
    Phospholipid inner leaflet
    Lipoprotein outer leaflet—may elicit inflammatory response

(continued)

Requires very complex media
May use arginine for energy—arginine dihydrolase pathway
Asymmetrical shape
Moves with gliding motility
Attaches with cytadherence organelle

Disease
Primary atypical pneumonia ("walking pneumonia")
Common in young adults

Virulence factors
No recognizable regulatory genes
Adherence
Bind ciliated cells
Cytadherence organelle
Depolarizes eukaryotic cell
Toxic substances
No known protein exotoxins
May produce peroxide, other reactive forms of oxygen
Phospholipases found in membrane
Antigenic variation in membrane lipoproteins
Manipulation of phagocytic and immune cells
Elicit strong cytokine response
T and B cells stimulated nonspecifically
B cells produce inappropriate antibodies

C. pneumoniae
Characteristics
Small microbes
Small genome (slightly more than 1 Mbp)
Obligate intracellular parasites
Two-stage developmental cycle
Elementary body
Infective form
Metabolically inactive
Survives in external environment
Moves cell to cell in human body
Enters via vacuole (similar to *Legionella*)
In vacuole changes to reticulate body
Reticulate body
Replicating form
Metabolically active
Multiplies and causes vacuole to fill cell
Differentiates into elementary body
Vacuole membrane fuses with cytoplasmic membrane—elementary bodies released
Have a number of eukaryotelike genes
No peptidoglycan cell wall
Gram-negative-type inner and outer membranes

(continued)

SUMMARY OUTLINE (*continued*)

Diseases
  Community-acquired pneumonia—first described in 1980s
  Coronary artery disease?
    Found in atherosclerotic plaques—cause or opportunist?
    Rabbit model
  Alzheimer's?
  Asthma?
Virulence factors
  Almost nothing known; adhere to and damage endothelial cells

QUESTIONS

Answers to the questions can be found in Appendix 2.

1. What characteristics of *M. pneumoniae* fit with the organism's small genome size? How do the bacteria make it on such a small number of genes?

2. Look up the size of some eukaryotic viral genomes. How does the size of the *M. pneumoniae* genome compare with that of the largest viral genomes?

3. Do you believe the sequencing laboratories' claims that *M. pneumoniae* has few if any regulatory genes because they found no recognizable regulatory proteins in the *M. pneumoniae* sequence? What are some possible explanations for this finding? All other sequenced microbial genomes have been littered with regulatory genes of all types.

4. How is the cytadherence organelle of *M. pneumoniae* different from pili?

5. Mycoplasmas have an asymmetric cytoplasmic membrane that is very unusual. Also, they have cholesterol in their membrane. No one knows why this membrane architecture arose in mycoplasmas. Can you come up with a hypothesis about its utility?

6. What would it take to convince you that *C. pneumoniae* causes at least some cases of heart disease and is not just an opportunist that comes along after the process has started? If this latter view were proved to be correct, would that make *C. pneumoniae* unimportant in heart disease?

7. Compare and contrast the traits of chlamydiae and mycoplasmas.

22

Bacillus anthracis, the Cause of Anthrax

KEY FEATURES

Bacillus anthracis

CHARACTERISTICS
Gram-positive rod
Sporeformer

DISEASE
Anthrax—form depends on how acquired: cutaneous, gastrointestinal, inhalation (systemic)

RESERVOIR
Infected farm animals; no human-to-human transmission

MAJOR VIRULENCE FACTORS
Survival in macrophages
Protein toxins
Capsule (poly-D-glutamate)—not very immunogenic

PREVENTION AND TREATMENT
Vaccine—designed to protect animals, but effective in humans
Antibiotics, if administered early enough

Before 1990, *Bacillus anthracis,* a gram-positive spore-forming rod, was relegated to the list of pathogenic bacteria that had not received much media attention. It had long been an important veterinary pathogen, but the number of human cases was relatively small. So, as far as the public was concerned, anthrax did not loom very large as an infectious disease issue. In the 1990s, however, this picture changed dramatically as bioterrorists began to express their interest in "weaponizing" *B. anthracis,* and anthrax was suddenly on the front page. There is still considerable controversy about how effective a biological weapon *B. anthracis* would actually be. Still, with terrorists threatening to use anthrax as a weapon of germ warfare, government officials had to take the threat seriously.

Features of the Disease

Until the germ warriors entered the picture, the people most likely to get anthrax were people who worked with wool and hides. Farm animals are the major reservoir for *B. anthracis,* and the disease has been a long-standing problem in agriculture. One of Pasteur's first coups was to develop a vaccine against anthrax that was designed to protect farm animals. People became victims of *B. anthracis* if they had cuts contaminated with spores from animal products or if they inhaled spores when working with hides or wool from infected animals. The majority of people exposed to spores of *B. anthracis* develop **cutaneous anthrax** (Figure 22–1). Spores enter a small cut or lesion and then germinate. A pustule develops with a large surrounding area of swelling (edema). After a few days, the center of the lesion becomes black owing to necrosis. This lesion is called an **eschar.** Recovery occurs in over 99% of cases if antibiotic treatment is administered. Rarely do the bacteria enter the bloodstream. **Gastrointestinal anthrax** is acquired by eating contaminated meat. This form of anthrax is rare, especially in developed countries.

The most serious form of anthrax is **inhalation (or systemic) anthrax,** which occurs when spores are inhaled and are taken up by lung macrophages. Inside the macrophage, the spore germinates and the bacteria begin to divide. There is no apparent lung disease, but since macrophages can migrate to lymph nodes, the bacteria spread beyond the lungs and into the bloodstream. Bacteria in the bloodstream cause septic shock. This is the form of anthrax that can kill a person within a few days. Antibiotic therapy, if instituted soon enough (within 24 h), can be effective, but the fatality rate is still very high. It is the sudden onset, and the difficulty in getting antibiotics to infected people fast enough if many people are infected, that makes anthrax attractive to bioterrorists. Fortunately, anthrax is not transmitted from person to person, so the risk is in the initial exposure of a population to the weaponized anthrax spores, not in continued transmission.

A vaccine is available; it consists of a crude protein preparation that contains a toxoid called **protective antigen** and is fairly effective in the short term but does not confer long-term immunity. This vaccine was originally designed to be administered to animals, not humans, and thus has not undergone the rigorous safety testing usually demanded for vaccines administered to humans. In the late 1990s, when the U.S. Department of Defense—worried about attacks by bioterrorists on U.S. troops—ordered members of the military to present themselves for vaccination, some people objected to being inoculated with a vaccine whose effects in humans were not very well documented. The people who objected were right about the vaccine not having been tested as widely in humans as the vaccines that are traditionally administered to infants and children, but there is little evidence that the vaccine has any serious

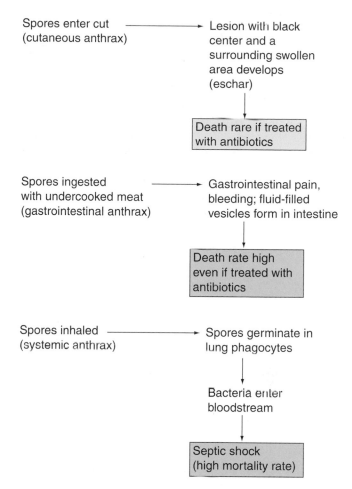

Figure 22–1   Forms of anthrax.

side effects. Finally, the military backed down and called off the vaccination program. If someone does manage to use anthrax successfully as a weapon, the tide of opinion may well turn again, especially among those military personnel in areas of the world where attacks are more likely to occur.

Virulence Factors

Ability To Germinate and Survive in Macrophages

Skin and lung macrophages and other phagocytic cells ingest spores. Not only are the spores not killed by the macrophage, but they germinate in the macrophage and begin to divide, eventually killing the macrophage. The signals that prompt the spore to germinate are not completely characterized, but they appear to be small molecules such as L-alanine. Much is known about spore production by bacteria, but the process of germination is still very poorly understood

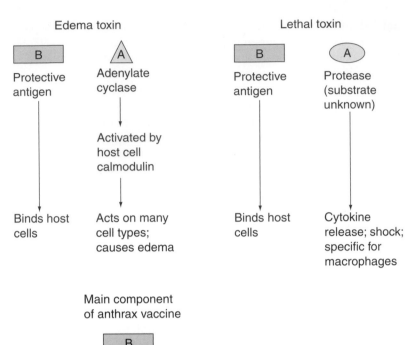

Figure 22–2 Edema toxin, lethal toxin, and the main vaccine component. A, A portion; B, B portion. The triangle represents the A portion of edema toxin; the ellipse represents the A portion of lethal toxin.

Toxins

The two main virulence factors of *B. anthracis* are both protein toxins, one that probably causes the edema seen in cutaneous anthrax (**edema toxin**) and one that is responsible for death in cases of septicemic anthrax (**lethal toxin**). An interesting and unusual feature of these toxins is that, although they are conventional A-B toxins, both have the same B (host cell binding) portion, a protein called protective antigen (Figure 22–2). The name protective antigen comes from the observation that antibodies to this protein are protective, presumably because they prevent binding of either toxin to human cells. As already mentioned, protective antigen is the active component of the current formulation of the anthrax vaccine.

The A (active) portion of the edema toxin is called **edema factor.** It appears to be an adenylate cyclase similar to the one produced by *Bordetella pertussis* (chapter 17). Like the *B. pertussis* enzyme, edema factor is activated by human calmodulin after it enters the target cell and produces large amounts of cAMP. Since cAMP is an important signaling molecule, many cell functions are disrupted, including control of the flow of ions and thus the flow of water.

The A portion of lethal toxin is called **lethal factor.** Together with protective antigen, the lethal factor at-

tacks and kills macrophages. Although edema factor acts on most cell types, lethal factor seems to exert its lethal effect only on macrophages. At the amino acid sequence level, lethal factor looks like a protease, and it has been shown to cleave human proteins. The actual protein target or targets of lethal factor are still unknown. Lethal toxin probably causes shock because it induces macrophages to produce high levels of cytokines, especially IL-1. Cytokines released by the macrophages trigger the shock process. Both the edema toxin and the lethal toxin are antiphagocytic in the sense that they interfere with or destroy the ability of phagocytic cells to ingest the bacteria. Thus, although initially, residence in a phagocytic cell seems to be a good thing for *B. anthracis,* its strategy for surviving in the human body seems to be to avoid phagocytosis after the initial stages of germination and growth.

The genes encoding the toxins are found on a large plasmid, **pOX1** (Figure 22–3). Also carried on the plasmid are genes encoding the regulatory proteins **AtxA** and **AtxR,** which control expression of the genes for lethal factor (*lef*), edema factor (*cya*), and protective antigen (*pag*). The Atx proteins respond to carbon dioxide concentration and temperature. There are a number of pOX1 genes whose functions are unknown. Since there are at least some virulence factors encoded by this plas-

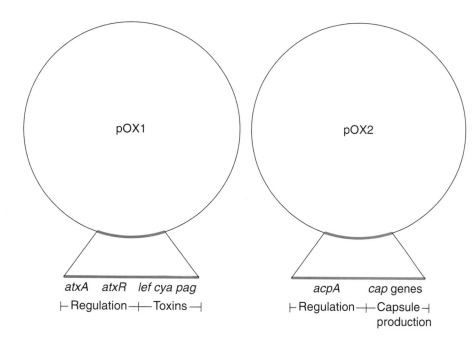

Figure 22–3 Virulence plasmids.

mid, other genes on the plasmid could be involved in virulence.

Antiphagocytic Capsule

B. anthracis not only has unusual toxins that share a common B portion, but it also has an unusual capsule. Unlike other capsules, which are composed of polysaccharides, the capsule of *B. anthracis* is composed of D-**glutamate** residues. You might expect that a poly-D-glutamate capsule would make a great vaccine candidate. After all, in the case of the gram-positive cocci that cause disease, scientists are chasing after surface proteins as possible vaccine candidates. But here again, *B. anthracis* has a surprise in store. For some reason, an immune response to the capsular protein is not protective. The genes encoding the protein capsule (*cap* genes) are located on a second large plasmid, **pOX2.** Also on this plasmid is a regulatory gene (*acpA*), whose product, AcpA, controls expression of the *cap* genes. Surprisingly, AcpA synthesis is controlled by AtxA, which is encoded by a gene carried on the other plasmid, pOX1, so there is cross talk between the plasmids. The poly-D-glutamate capsule may not be a good vaccine candidate, but it appears to be very important for virulence, at least as important as the toxins. A strain of *B. anthracis* that has been cured of pOX1, so that it no longer produces the toxins but still carries pOX2, is nearly as virulent in animal models as the wild-type parent. This observation raises the question of whether there may be toxins other than lethal toxin and edema toxin that remain to be discovered. For another interesting story featuring the virulence plasmids, see Box 22–1.

Prevention of Anthrax

The anthrax vaccine was one of the first vaccines developed because anthrax was such a problem for farmers. *B. anthracis* infects and kills many types of animals. In many countries, anthrax in animals has been virtually eradicated by using a combination of vaccination to prevent animals from getting the disease and ruthlessly culling herds found to contain infected animals. Not only does an anthrax-free herd protect the animals, but it also lessens the risk of human exposure. Most of the human cases of anthrax in the past occurred in people who worked in meat processing plants or worked with animal hides or wool. In fact, inhalation anthrax has been called "wool-sorter's disease." As always, prevention is the preferred solution. Anthrax provides an excellent example of how effective a prevention campaign can be. It is unlikely that anthrax will ever be eradicated, as smallpox was and polio may soon be, because there is a wild animal reservoir for the disease. But anthrax can be kept at bay by a consistently administered and aggressive program to keep the disease out of domestic animals.

BOX 22–1 Peas in a Pod

B. anthracis has long been viewed as one of the few villains in a genus that has many beneficial members. One widely used beneficial member is *B. thuringiensis*, a natural pesticide. Spores of *B. thuringiensis* have long been used by organic farmers as a safe and effective way to control insects. *B. thuringiensis* kills certain insect pests because it produces an insecticidal toxin that is fatal to insects that ingest it. The beauty of this toxin is that outside of a few species of insects, it does not have toxic effects on any other creatures. Thus, in contrast to chemical pesticides, it is safe for humans and leaves beneficial insects, such as ladybugs, alone. *B. anthracis* is not the only pathogen in the genus *Bacillus*; *Bacillus cereus*, a common soil bacterium, occasionally causes a form of food-borne disease that is unpleasant but not lethal. But *B. anthracis* has been the number one *Bacillus* bad boy.

Imagine the consternation when the genome sequencers began to compare the sequences of these three species and found that all three are virtually identical, clearly—despite their names—strains of the same species. Only *B. anthracis* had pOX1 and pOX2, however, so these plasmids seem to account for its ability to cause disease. This finding raises the question of whether *B. anthracis* was created by gene transfer events that introduced pOX1 and pOX2 into one of the less pathogenic, or even beneficial, species. If so, where did these plasmids come from? More important, could *B. cereus* or *B. thuringiensis* acquire pOX1 and/or pOX2 at any time by horizontal gene transfer? Such transfers must not happen very easily, because turning *B. thuringiensis* into *B. anthracis* is not occurring often enough to make *B. thuringiensis* dangerous, but such a transfer seems to have happened at least once.

Source: E. Helgason, O. Okstad, D. Caugant, H. Johansen, A. Fouet, M. Mock, I. Hegna, and I. Kolsto. 2000. *Bacillus anthracis, Bacillus cereus,* and *Bacillus thuringiensis*—one species on the basis of genetic evidence. *Appl. Environ. Microbiol.* **66:**2627–2630.

SELECTED READINGS

Bossier, F., M. Levy-Wever, M. Mock, and J. Sirard. 2000. Role of toxin functional domains in anthrax pathogenesis. *Infect. Immun.* **68:**1781–1786.

Centers for Disease Control and Prevention. 2000. Surveillance for adverse effects associated with anthrax vaccination—U.S. Department of Defense, 1998–2000. *JAMA* **283:**2648–2649.

Hanna, P., and J. Ireland. 1999. Understanding *Bacillus anthracis* pathogenesis. *Trends Microbiol.* **7:**180–182.

Little, S. F., and B. E. Ivins. 1999. Molecular pathogenesis of *Bacillus anthracis* infection. *Microbes Infect.* **1:**131–139.

Marshall, E. 2000. Bioterrorism. DOD retreats on plan for anthrax vaccine. *Science* **289:**382–383.

Smith, H. 2000. Discovery of anthrax toxin: the beginning of in vivo studies on pathogenic bacteria. *Trends Microbiol.* **8:**199–200.

SUMMARY OUTLINE

Characteristics of *B. anthracis*

Gram-positive rod

Sporeformer

Infects many animal species

Disease

Cutaneous form
  Spores enter through cuts in skin
  Characterized by pustule surrounded by edema
  Usually curable by antibiotics

Gastrointestinal form
  Acquired by ingestion of contaminated meat
  Rare in developed countries

Systemic disease
  Spores inhaled, taken up by lung macrophages
  Spores germinate, bacteria divide in macrophages
  Bacteria enter bloodstream where they cause septic shock
  Very high fatality rate

Virulence factors

Germination and survival in macrophages
  Germination prompted by small molecules, e.g., L-alanine
  Eventually kill macrophages

Toxins
  Edema toxin
    Causes edema in cutaneous anthrax
    A-B toxin
      B portion (protective antigen) same as in lethal toxin
      A portion (edema factor) is adenylate cyclase
        Activated by calmodulin
        Stimulates production of cAMP
    Attacks most cell types
    Antiphagocytic
  Lethal toxin
    A portion (lethal factor) probably acts as protease
    Targets and kills macrophages
    Induces macrophages to produce high levels of cytokines (IL-1); triggers shock
    Antiphagocytic
    Genes on plasmid pOX1
      Genes for regulatory proteins AtxA and AtxR
      AtxA and AtxR control expression of toxin genes
        lef (lethal factor)
        cya (edema factor)
        pag (protective antigen)
      Atx proteins respond to CO_2 concentration and temperature

Prevention

Vaccine
  Consists of protective antigen and other proteins
  Effective but short-term protection

Immunizing and culling infected domestic farm animals

QUESTIONS

Answers to the questions can be found in Appendix 2.

1. Why is protective antigen a better choice for a vaccine than edema factor or lethal factor, the active portion of the two toxins?

2. Why might you expect the protein capsule of *B. anthracis* to be a poor vaccine candidate, even though it is a protein?

3. Reportedly, several attempts have been made by bioterrorists to spray anthrax spores in crowded areas, such as subway stations. Nothing happened. Why is this not so surprising?

4. There were dire reports in the media at one point alleging that former Russian scientists were genetically engineering *B. anthracis* to become resistant to antibiotics. How much of a threat would this be if it were true?

5. The finding that *B. anthracis* and the benign *Bacillus* species are virtually identical at the DNA sequence level except for the virulence plasmids of *B. anthracis* is interesting, but how concerned should we be that *Bacillus thuringiensis,* used widely by organic gardeners, will someday go wild and turn into a raging pathogen because it has acquired the virulence plasmids from *B. anthracis*? What are some arguments that this is a virtually nonexistent threat?

Helicobacter pylori, a Resourceful Gastric Pathogen

KEY FEATURES

Helicobacter pylori

CHARACTERISTICS
Gram-negative curved rod
Motile due to a polar tuft of flagella (four to seven)
Microaerophile, obligately respiratory metabolism

DISEASE
Gastric and duodenal ulcers
Ulcers associated with development of gastric cancer

RESERVOIR
Human stomach

MAIN VIRULENCE FACTORS
Flagella
Urease—helps neutralize acidic pH of the stomach
Adhesins
Vacuolating toxin
LPS resembles human Lewis antigens (immune mimicry)

PREVENTION AND TREATMENT
Antibiotics cure disease and prevent ulcer recurrence
No vaccine yet

A Revolution in Gastroenterology

Good News—You're Infected!

Bacterial diseases are generally considered to be bad things, because they can cause suffering and death. Looked at from another perspective, however, a bacterial disease is a good thing. If you have to have a disease, you'd better hope it is caused by bacteria, because if it is, there is a good chance it can be cured by a course of antibiotic therapy. The success rate for curing viral, fungal, and parasitic diseases is not nearly so good. And the therapy for diseases such as cancer seems to many to be almost as bad as the disease itself. Finally, there are diseases, such as rheumatoid arthritis and heart disease, which can be controlled to some extent by medications and changes in living habits but not cured. Imagine then, the excitement generated when a disease that had long been on the incurable list is found to be caused by a bacterium. This happened in gastroenterology in the late 1980s, when scientists discovered that most gastric and duodenal ulcers are caused by the bacterium *Helicobacter pylori*. Moreover, gastric adenocarcinoma, currently the 14th leading cause of death worldwide, was strongly associated with a history of *H. pylori* infection. Thus, successful eradication of *H. pylori* from a patient's stomach could conceivably prevent gastric cancer as well as eliminate ulcers.

The discovery that a bacterium could colonize the human stomach also created something of a stir among medical microbiologists and physicians for another reason; for years, conventional wisdom had been that the environment of the stomach is too harsh to support microbial life. If those who believed this had been more familiar with environmental microbiology, they would have realized that there are plenty of bacteria capable of thriving in a low-pH environment, but the dogma that the human stomach is a sterile site had become ingrained in medical teaching. As it turned out, a bacteria-free stomach is the exception rather than the rule. In developing countries, nearly everyone is colonized with *H. pylori*. Colonization occurs early in life, and the bacteria persist in the stomach for decades. In people living in developed countries, colonization occurs much later, for reasons that are not entirely clear, but by the age of 50 years about half of adults have *H. pylori* in their stomachs. The incidence of colonization in developed countries has been dropping steadily in recent years. This is probably due in part to widespread antibiotic treatment of ulcer patients, but there may be other factors involved as well.

Before the discovery that most ulcers are caused by *H. pylori*, the standard treatment for ulcers was to administer drugs that reduced gastric acidity and to prescribe a diet that reduced irritation of the stomach lining. The idea behind this approach was that since stomach acid, and possibly some types of food, might be causing the lesions, reducing stomach acid production and eliminating diet-associated irritation of the gastric mucosa would prevent ulcer formation. Although this therapeutic approach seemed reasonable and often worked in the short run to heal the existing ulcer, it did not prevent the recurrence of ulcers. Moreover, this therapeutic regimen significantly reduced the patient's quality of life. "No more beer and extra hot salsa, doctor? How can I continue to live?" The expense of the medications also caused hardship. Ulcer medications cost thousands of dollars a year and had to be taken for life. Moreover, surgical intervention was sometimes necessary to eliminate the inflamed area.

The Long Road to Acceptance

The discovery that stomach and duodenal ulcers could be caused by a bacterium raised the possibility that a short, relatively cheap course of antibiotics could cure the condition and prevent recurrences. Naturally, the hypothesis that *H. pylori* is the cause of ulcers met with considerable skepticism, much of it justified. The basis for the skepticism was that the cause-and-effect connection between the bacteria and the ulcer is not nearly as clear-cut as it is in diseases such as cholera or dysentery. A major sticking point was that many people who had *H. pylori* in their stomachs never developed ulcers. Another impediment to convincing people that *H. pylori* causes ulcers was the initial lack of an animal model. Suitable animal models have now been found, but for a long time Koch's third postulate had not been satisfied. Scientists who believed that *H. pylori* causes ulcers were understandably frustrated by their inability to satisfy Koch's third postulate and in one case were driven to extreme measures (Box 23–1). A final source of skepticism was the failure of early attempts to cure ulcers with antibiotics. Scientists have now found several combinations of antibiotics that eliminate the bacteria and prevent recurrences. Although *H. pylori* is currently thought to be the cause of about 90% of gastric and duodenal ulcers, not all ulcers are associated with *H. pylori* infection. Other causes include nonsteroidal anti-inflammatory drugs (e.g., aspirin) and autoimmune disease.

The *H. pylori*-Inspired "Gold Rush"

It wasn't long before the implications of the discovery that ulcers are caused by bacteria began to dawn on those outside the gastroenterology community. What if there were other diseases currently on the manageable but incurable list that are caused by microbes? This intriguing question was given further force by some other infectious disease examples that were discovered at about the same time. Periodontal disease was discovered to be a bacterial disease, caused by a shift in the microbiota of the gums. Dentists began to think about replacing periodontal surgery with antibiotics as a treatment to stop periodontitis. Virologists showed that some viruses, such as hepatitis B virus and human papilloma virus, could cause cancer. This led to measures to prevent the infection from persisting long enough to proceed to cancer. One of these was a vaccine against hepatitis B virus that prevents hepatitis and, in turn,

BOX 23–1   Koch's Postulates Are Not Just Words on Paper

How much do you care about proving a theory you believe in but cannot get others to accept? Barry Marshall, a young Australian internist working with J. R. Warren, the discoverer of *H. pylori*, did not exactly put his life on the line to do so, but he placed himself at risk for a very unpleasant condition. Marshall was an early proponent of the hypothesis that many gastric and duodenal ulcers are caused by bacteria. The idea that bacteria and not stress are the cause of ulcers flew in the face of well-established medical dogma. Given this, it is not surprising that Marshall and others who advanced this outrageous notion were not at first taken seriously by others working in the field. The skeptics were on firm ground in the beginning because all that had been proved was that *H. pylori* was associated with ulcer lesions and could be isolated in pure culture from these lesions (Koch's postulates 1 and 2). Critics of Marshall's theory insisted that Koch's third postulate must be satisfied as well, i.e., that the bacteria isolated from ulcers could cause ulcers in animals or humans. At the time, Marshall had been trying unsuccessfully to get the bacteria to infect various laboratory animals. Frustrated by this, he turned to the obvious alternative: human subjects. But who would volunteer to be inoculated with a bacterium that might cause ulcers? Keep in mind that this was before a successful antibiotic regimen had been developed. And even if volunteers could be found, approval for the experiment would be denied by any committee overseeing the use of human subjects. Marshall thus turned to his most faithful and reliable supporter: himself. He first had his stomach checked by endoscopic examination to make sure that the stomach mucosa was healthy. Then he drank a turbid culture of a strain of *H. pylori*, which had been recently isolated from the lesions of a patient with peptic ulcers. Within a few hours, his stomach began to growl. A week later, he became nauseated and vomited. During this period, he felt unusually hungry and tired. Near the end of the second week, he underwent a second endoscopic examination of his stomach, and a biopsy was taken. A portion of Marshall's stomach had an inflamed appearance, and *H. pylori* was found in the mucin layer over the lesion. The bacteria Marshall had ingested were clearly capable of causing disease. Fortunately for Marshall, the infection healed spontaneously, but Marshall's point was proved.

According to an article in the *New Yorker*, which describes Marshall's experiment and its aftermath in detail, the initial event of taking the bacterial dose (a potentially momentous occasion in the history of gastroenterology) was a disappointingly undramatic affair. A fellow worker in the lab who knew what Marshall was about to do said "You're crazy." Marshall said "Here goes," drank the culture, then remarked that it tasted like swamp water. Apparently, Marshall had spent too much time thinking about the experiment he planned to do to bother providing himself with a suitably memorable statement to commemorate the occasion.

Source: T. Monmaney. 1993. Marshall's hunch. *New Yorker*, Sept. 20, 1993, p. 64–72.

---

prevents a type of liver cancer associated with a history of hepatitis B virus infection. Discovery of the connection between human papilloma virus and cervical cancer also suggested an effective preventive strategy: cauterization of cervical warts to eliminate the virus from the cervix, thus preventing cervical cancer.

These examples triggered a "gold rush" mentality in which scientists interested in curing diseases for which there was previously no cure began to reassess the possibility that the diseases they studied were caused by microorganisms. Some infectious disease experts went so far as to suggest that any disease thought previously to be an autoimmune disease should be investigated particularly closely because such diseases are triggered by the immune system and the immune system was designed to respond to—guess what!—microbial infections. The optimistic search for microbial—especially bacterial—causes of chronic diseases continues unabated. Some of the diseases that are currently being reinvestigated in the hopes of finding a microbial cause are listed in Table 23–1 along with organisms currently on the list of suspects. A few of these diseases, such as psoriasis and rheumatoid arthritis, were already being treated with antibiotics by some doctors, although this

Table 23–1 Examples of diseases that might be caused by bacteria and examples of bacteria that have been suggested as a possible cause

Disease	Suspected microbe(s)
Coronary artery disease	*Chlamydia pneumoniae*
	Helicobacter pylori
Inflammatory bowel disease (e.g., Crohn's disease)	*Mycobacterium paratuberculosis*
	Bacteroides species
Alzheimer's disease	*C. pneumoniae*
Rheumatoid arthritis	????[a]
Autism	????
Psoriasis	????

[a]????, no candidates have been identified, but antibiotics seem to help.

A

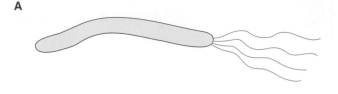

B

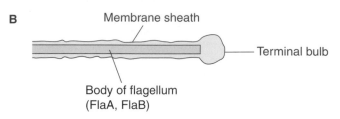

Figure 23–1 Shape of *H. pylori* (**A**) and a close-up of the structure of its unusual flagellum (**B**).

therapy was not based on data from controlled clinical trials.

Characteristics of *H. pylori*

Morphology and Metabolism

FLAGELLA. *H. pylori* is a gram-negative, curved rod, with a tuft of four to seven polar flagella (Figure 23–1A). The bacteria are actively motile, even in very viscous solutions. This is important because *H. pylori* burrows into the mucin lining the epithelial mucosa of the stomach, and mucin is a very viscous material. Many bacteria that are highly motile in low-viscosity liquids are unable to move in viscous liquids. The curved shape of *H. pylori* also contributes to its ability to move through viscous fluids because the bacteria move with a corkscrew-type motion that is characteristic of bacteria that can handle high-viscosity liquids. Moreover, *H. pylori* produces a **mucinase,** an enzyme that degrades mucus. The mucinase may help to reduce the viscosity of the mucus through which the bacteria are trying to move.

The flagella of *H. pylori* are unusual in several ways. First, they are composed of two protein subunits, **FlaA** and **FlaB.** In all other motile bacteria so far examined, the body of the flagellum is composed of a single protein subunit. The flagella of *H. pylori* have FlaA as the major component and FlaB as the minor component, but both are important. Disruption of the *flaA* gene does not completely eliminate motility but decreases it significantly. In this mutant, the flagella are short and motility is reduced, but the bacteria are still able to move. Disruption of the *flaB* gene does not affect the appear-

ance or length of the flagella but does reduce motility somewhat. Both mutants are severely impaired in their ability to colonize the stomachs of gnotobiotic piglets.

A second unusual feature of *flaA* and *flaB* is that these genes are not only located in different parts of the chromosome but are under different control. Transcription of *flaA* requires **sigma factor** σ^{28}, whose function is not known, whereas transcription of *flaB* requires **sigma factor** σ^{54}, the sigma factor associated with expression of genes needed during nitrogen starvation. The fact that the two flagellar genes are responding to different signals suggests that under different sets of conditions, *H. pylori* can vary the relative concentrations of FlaA and FlaB in its flagella. It will be interesting to learn if this is true and, if so, whether these variations are important for adaptation of the bacteria to different stages in the infection-persistence process.

A third unusual feature of *H. pylori* flagella is that the protein shaft of the flagellum is encased in a membranous sheath (Figure 23–1B). This membranous covering could help protect the flagellum from proteases in stomach secretions. Or it may have some completely different function that is not yet understood. The membrane covering is tightly associated with the flagellum along its length, but at the end, the membrane forms a terminal bulb (Figure 23–1B). The function of this bulb is not known.

Like most flagella, the *H. pylori* flagellum has a hook structure that connects the flagellar motor in the cytoplasmic membrane with the part of the flagellum that protrudes from the cell surface. The gene for the **hook protein,** *flgE*, has been cloned and characterized. Cells in which this gene is disrupted have no flagella and are completely nonmotile, although FlaA and FlaB are still produced and can be found in the cell cytoplasm. This finding indicates that the hook protein is important for assembly of the flagellum as well as for connecting the flagellum to the flagellar motor.

ENERGY METABOLISM. *H. pylori* is a microaerophile that has an obligately respiratory metabolism. Consistent with this, the genome sequence of *H. pylori* contains sequences of genes that encode enzymes of various glucose-oxidizing pathways and enzymes of the TCA cycle. The number of nutrients *H. pylori* can use as a carbon and energy source is fairly limited. Carbon sources include glucose, amino acids, and some organic acids. The bacteria can produce most of the amino acids, nucleic acids, and vitamins. The internal pH of the *H. pylori* cytoplasm is 7.0 to 7.3. Maintaining this internal pH is difficult for bacteria that find themselves in a very acidic environment because it is difficult to prevent incoming protons from acidifying the cytoplasm. A solution to this problem is that the bacteria move to and colonize the gastric mucin layer, where the pH is close to neutral.

Genomics

The first genome sequence ever to be completed was that of *H. pylori*. This came as something of a surprise to many scientists because they had naturally assumed that one of the more advanced bacterial model systems, such as *Escherichia coli* or *Salmonella enterica* serovar Typhimurium, would have this distinction. As it turned out, there is a good argument that *H. pylori* may not have this distinction after all. Almost immediately after the completion of the genome sequence was announced, the sequence data were sold to a company and thus were not released to the scientific community. There was a great deal of debate at the time about the ethics of keeping the first complete genome sequence in private hands, when the technology had been developed using public funds. One way scientists had of retaliating was to decide to ignore the *H. pylori* genome sequence and award the distinction of first genome sequence to *Haemophilus influenzae* type b. Since this unfortunate incident, there has been considerable emphasis on immediate public release of genome sequence data. The outrage and controversy over the handling of the first complete genome sequence, which after all was a scientific and symbolic milestone, clearly contributed to the current conviction that rapid public disclosure of genome sequence data, especially that generated with public funds, is the right way to proceed.

Since the first *H. pylori* sequence data disappeared

immediately into the bowels of a private company, it became necessary to obtain the genome sequence of a second strain of *H. pylori*. In retrospect, this had some important consequences. For one thing, *H. pylori* had the distinction of becoming the first microbe for which two genome sequences from different strains were determined. This distinction was earned because the company that had acquired the genome sequence data from the first strain decided belatedly to release its data to the scientific community. This made it possible for the first time to do a comparison of sequences between two strains of the same species. The results of this comparison showed that although the sequences were very similar to each other, 7% of the genes were unique to one strain or the other. About half of these unique genes were clustered together on the chromosome and may thus have come into the strain from some outside source. The results of this analysis show that even strains that are very closely related can have islands of difference. Subsequently, comparisons of genome sequences from different strains of other species were made, and these comparisons are changing the way we think about genetic variation within a species.

The *H. pylori* genome is very small, about 1.7 Mbp. *H. pylori* seems not only to have a stripped-down metabolism but also a paucity of regulatory genes. So far, only about four possible regulatory genes have been identified, far fewer than the number found in microbes with larger genomes. Analysis of the genome sequence of *H. pylori* has highlighted some problems with interpreting sequence data by using similarity to known genes as the guide for guessing the possible function of the gene. For example, the claim that *H. pylori* has a TCA cycle fits with the obligately respiratory metabolism revealed by biochemical studies. But not all the TCA cycle genes were found in the sequence. Possibly the genes encoding the "missing" functions differ at the sequence level enough not to be recognized. The problems encountered in getting the sequence data to match known metabolic functions has made it clear that sequence data are unlikely to prove anything; they are best used to generate hypotheses that can be subsequently tested with biochemical and genetic approaches.

Virulence Factors

Animal Models

Since Koch's third postulate was such a bone of contention in the early days of the debate about whether *H. pylori* causes ulcers, finding a good animal model for ulcer formation had a high priority. One of the first models was ferrets. Unfortunately, a *Helicobacter* species other than *H. pylori* (*H. mustelae*) had to be used, a fact that caused some skepticism as to how similar the two bacterial species actually are. Nonetheless, *H. mustelae* did cause ulcers in ferrets. Other animal models for ulcers that used *H. pylori* as the bacterial cause soon surfaced. They included mice and gnotobiotic piglets. A new model is beagle dogs. An advantage of beagles is that specimens can be obtained from their stomachs more easily because they are larger than rodents. This allows scientists to follow the disease over time because it is not necessary to kill the animals to obtain specimens. A recent addition to the list of animal models is the Mongolian gerbil. In this case, *H. pylori* causes a disease that closely resembles human gastric cancer.

Colonization of the Stomach Mucosa

MOTILITY. The current view of how *H. pylori* colonizes the stomach and causes an ulcer is shown in Figure 23–2. *H. pylori* is actually quite sensitive to low pH in laboratory medium. For this reason, *H. pylori* does not colonize the lumen of the stomach but rather colonizes the mucin layer that covers the gastric mucosa. Mucus resists diffusion of protons from stomach acid because it is composed largely of negatively charged, sulfated polysaccharides. Thus, mucus acts as a buffer

to maintain a slightly alkaline pH at the mucosal surface. Its role is to protect mucosal cells, which are also sensitive to acid; *H. pylori* takes advantage of this property of mucus. Since *H. pylori* must reach the mucin layer in order to survive, it is not surprising that motility is one of its most important virulence factors. *H. pylori* is not only highly motile but exhibits chemotaxis. It responds to carbonate and urea, two compounds that are secreted into the stomach by cells of the gastric mucosa.

UREASE, TEMPORARY PROTECTION FROM STOMACH ACID. Regardless of how fast the bacteria move, it takes some time to reach the mucin layer. During this rush for the border, *H. pylori* must be able to survive the acid pH of the stomach long enough to reach its destination. It does this by producing an enzyme, urease. **Urease** hydrolyzes the urea secreted by gastric cells to produce ammonia and CO_2. In effect, the bacterium surrounds itself with a layer of ammonia, which neutralizes stomach acid in its immediate vicinity. The importance of urease in the initial stages of colonization can be seen from animal model studies; a urease-negative mutant was unable to colonize and did not produce ulcers. In other experiments, urease inhibitors administered along with the bacteria also prevented infection.

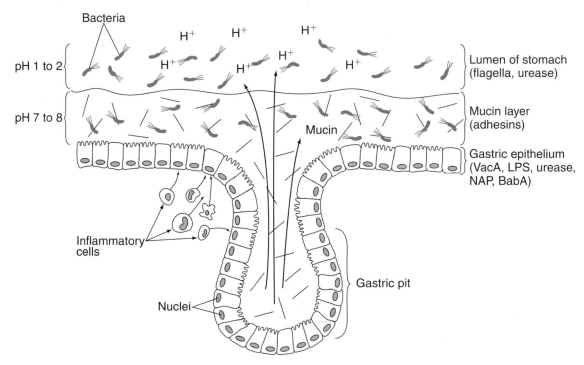

Figure 23–2 Proposed mechanism of ulcer formation by *H. pylori*. *H. pylori* uses urease to protect it from stomach acid during transit of the stomach to the mucin layer. It colonizes the mucin layer and may adhere to the gastric mucosa. Products of the bacteria provoke an inflammatory response that ultimately damages the mucosa. Virulence factors thought to be involved at each stage are indicated in parentheses.

There is still controversy over the cellular location of urease. Clearly, urease would be most effective if it were located on the cell surface or in the periplasm, but the enzyme appears to be intracellular. Either the bacteria take up urea and then export ammonia very efficiently, or urease from lysed bacteria coats surviving bacteria.

Once the bacteria are established in the mucin layer, urease inhibitors have no detectable effect on colonization or ulcer formation, suggesting that the main contribution of urease to the infection process is to protect the bacteria until they can reach the mucin layer. This does not mean that urease production by bacteria in the mucin layer makes no contribution to the pathology of the disease. Ammonia is toxic to eukaryotic cells, and the enzyme itself has an inflammatory effect on the gastric mucosa. The fact that people with ulcers produce serum antibodies against urease indicates that it is being produced by bacteria colonizing the stomach lining and is penetrating to underlying tissue. Since inhibitors of urease activity have no effect on the inflammatory properties of the protein itself, the failure of urease inhibitors to prevent ulcer formation when administered after colonization has occurred does not rule out this type of action by urease.

Urease is also important as a diagnostic tool for assessing bacterial colonization of the stomach. To assess colonization by cultivating the bacteria, it is necessary to use invasive techniques to obtain biopsy specimens. Recent studies have indicated that testing the breath for ammonia, especially when combined with testing of blood samples for antiurease antibodies, provides as good an indication of the colonization status of an individual as culturing biopsy specimens. Although cultivation of the bacteria will probably continue to be used in clinical trials of antibiotic regimens because it is the "gold standard" for assessing infection, the **ammonia breath test** is also proving to be a useful rapid test for physicians who want to monitor the success of antibiotic treatment regimens. Serological tests for antiurease antibodies and other antibodies against *H. pylori* antigens are not yet reliable enough for routine diagnostic use but are good enough to use in epidemiological studies to assess the infection rate in different human populations.

PERSISTENCE IN THE MUCIN LAYER. Flagella remain important for virulence even after the bacteria reach the mucin layer. Mucus is constantly being produced and sloughed into the lumen of the stomach. Presumably, the bacteria need to be able to burrow into new mucin as it is formed and secreted by mucosal cells. In specimens taken from an infected person or animal, most of the bacteria are located in the mucin layer, not adherent to mucosal cells. Thus, it is not surprising that *H. pylori*

possesses an adhesin that binds sulfated mucin sugars. What is more confusing is that *H. pylori* also produces adhesins that allow the bacteria to attach to epithelial cells. The best-characterized adhesin of this type is **BabA,** which recognizes the **Lewis b antigen,** a carbohydrate antigen found on the surfaces of epithelial cells. Possibly, although most of the bacteria do not attach to epithelial cells in vivo, the few that do are the ones that do the most to elicit the inflammatory response that causes the ulcer to form. In contrast to urease and flagella, which are found on all *H. pylori* strains, BabA is found only on some strains. Variation in virulence of different strains is of considerable interest, because if some strains are more virulent than others, this variation might explain why only some people colonized with *H. pylori* develop ulcers or gastric cancer. Since developing ulcers does not necessarily mean that the person will develop gastric cancer, and since cancer can develop in people who do not have a history of ulcers, there may be several different virulence types with different disease-producing capabilities.

Eliciting an Inflammatory Response

In virtually all people colonized with *H. pylori,* some inflammation of the stomach lining is seen (**gastritis**), but only in some people does the inflammation become serious enough to cause an ulcer to form. The presence of inflammation in the gastric linings of infected people has led to the proposal that inflammation somehow benefits the bacteria. Recall that *H. pylori* is not very versatile in terms of substrates it can use and that it requires amino acids as well as an energy source such as glucose. Destruction of epithelial cells could release nutrients needed by the bacteria for carbon and energy. The host's diet could also be a source of nutrients, however.

Inflammation of the gastric epithelium is the result of the infiltration of PMNs and other immune cells (B and T cells) into the submucosal tissue. As the ulcer progresses, the number of phagocytes and immune cells increases considerably. As already mentioned, urease itself could be part of the explanation for this inflammatory response because it elicits inflammation by some mechanism independent of the hydrolysis of urea. Two other possible inflammatory molecules are a cytotoxin, the **vacuolating cytotoxin (VacA),** and a **neutrophil activation protein (NAP)** that activates neutrophils. The vacuolating cytotoxin gets its name from its ability to produce numerous large vacuoles in cultured mammalian cells. These vacuoles are acidified, presumably by vacuolar H^+/ATPase. Influx of cations into the vacuoles causes them to swell. Whether the large size attained by the vacuoles is toxic to the cells or whether the cytotoxin has some other toxic activity, the result of toxin action is cell death. Death of gastric mucosal cells could contribute to the inflammatory response, which then causes further damage. Some VacA is secreted, and some is retained on the cell surface. The secreted form exists as an oligomer, which needs to be activated by exposure to pH 2 in order to become active. The form that is associated with the bacterial surface does not need exposure to acid for activation. Since protons do not penetrate very efficiently into the mucin layer, the surface-bound VacA may be the form of VacA most important for virulence.

Whatever the mechanisms by which the bacteria elicit an inflammatory reaction, they do so very effectively. Cross-sections of the mucin layer in an infected person show many bacteria, but they appear to be relatively isolated from each other. That is, microcolonies are not a common feature. This suggests that a relatively small number of bacteria per area of mucosal surface can cause an intense inflammatory response.

LPS—Immune Mimicry

Normally, LPS is responsible for eliciting an inflammatory response, but as usual, *H. pylori* does things differently. The LPS of *H. pylori* has low toxicity when injected into animals, an indication that it is not particularly good at eliciting an inflammatory response or triggering septic shock. In fact, LPS may help the bacteria evade the host's protective responses by making the bacteria look like "self." The *H. pylori* LPS O antigen of some strains contains carbohydrate moieties that are identical to human **Lewis antigens x** and **y** (**Le^x** and **Le^y**), both of which are found on the surfaces of gastric epithelial cells. This **immune mimicry** could help prevent the host from mounting an effective immune response. It could also have another effect. If the host did respond by recognizing the Le antigen portions of the LPS molecule as foreign, the antibodies would cross-react with gastric mucosal cells. This may explain why patients with symptomatic disease often have antibodies that cross-react with antigens on gastric mucosal tissue. Such cross-reacting antibodies could contribute to inflammation by activating complement or stimulating the phagocytic cells to attack gastric epithelial cells.

Type IV Secretion System

Some strains of *H. pylori* have a 40-kbp pathogenicity island, the *cag* **island,** which contains 31 genes that direct the production and assembly of a **type IV secretion system.** Strains that have the *cag* pathogenicity island are more virulent in animal models than strains that lack it. Also, *cag*-positive strains are more likely to be associated with human infections that result in ulcers or gastric cancer. What the type IV secretion system is doing for *H. pylori* is still a mystery. In many bacteria, type IV systems are associated with conjugal transfer of DNA, i.e., excretion of a protein-DNA complex as part of the process of conjugal DNA transfer. In one case, however, the type IV system mediates excretion of a toxin—the pertussis toxin of *Bordetella pertussis* (see chapter 17 and Appendix 1). So the type IV system of *H. pylori* could be mediating the secretion of a toxin.

Although the *cag* pathogenicity island is associated with virulence, things are not so simple. In people infected with *H. pylori,* it is not uncommon to find a mixture of *cag*-positive and *cag*-negative strains, which are otherwise identical to each other. The fact that the strains are otherwise identical indicates that some *cag*-positive bacteria lost their *cag* islands. This is not too surprising since there are repeat sequences at the ends of the *cag* island that would allow the island to loop out and be lost due to recombination (Figure 23–3). What is surprising is that the *cag*-negative bacteria are obviously competing successfully with the *cag*-positive bacteria in the human stomach. The apparent contradiction between this observation and others that link the *cag* island with virulence is resolved if the *cag* island is important for the initial colonization of the gastric mucosa but becomes dispensable or even detrimental once the bacteria have established an infection and have entered the persistence phase.

Prevention and Treatment

Early attempts at treating *H. pylori* infections with a single antibiotic were successful in eliminating the ulcer, but infection and ulcer production recurred in many cases after the antibiotic therapy was stopped. Since the antibiotics tested for efficacy were known to kill *H. pylori* in laboratory medium and were clearly reducing the numbers of *H. pylori* in the patients, scientists concluded that the failure to completely clear the patient of bacteria might be due to the fact that bacteria colonizing the mucin layer or inflamed site were not very accessible to antibiotics and/or the immune system. Successful therapeutic regimens which eradicate the colonization have now been developed. Some of these are listed in Table 23–2.

The first treatment regimens consisted of two antibiotics plus bismuth. Bismuth has some antibacterial activity, but it is still not clear why adding bismuth to the antibiotic combinations made such a difference in clearance of the bacteria from the gastric and duodenal

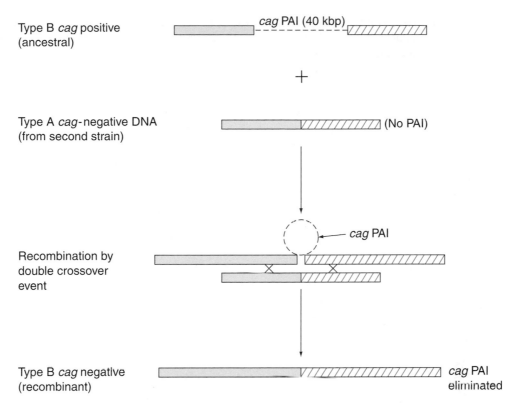

Figure 23–3 Hypothesis to explain the elimination of the *cag* pathogenicity island (PAI) in some strains by recombination with DNA lacking the *cag* PAI. The ancestral type B strain carried the *cag* PAI. The patient was colonized with a second *H. pylori* strain (type A) that did not harbor the *cag* PAI. Strain B obtained a DNA fragment from strain A (whether by transformation or conjugation is unclear). The type A DNA fragment contained sequences homologous to those flanking the sequences adjacent to the *cag* PAI segment in strain B. This allowed *cag* PAI to loop out and be lost during a double crossover event. The recombinant type B chromosome became *cag* negative. (Adapted from Suerbaum and Achtman, 1999.)

Table 23–2   Examples of drug regimens used to treat ulcer patients

Drug combination	Duration of treatment (days)
Bismuth, amoxicillin, metronidazole	7
Bismuth, tetracycline, tinidazole	4
Omeprazole, clarithromycin, metronidazole	7
Lanoprazole, clarithromycin, metronidazole	7
Omeprazole, amoxicillin, metronidazole	14

mucosa. Bismuth also acts on the inflamed gastric mucosa and may thus have an effect on the host as well as the bacteria. The obligatory requirement for bismuth in the first successful antibiotic regimens was seized on by skeptics of the *H. pylori*-causes-ulcers hypothesis to argue that the antibiotics were not really curing the condition, i.e., although *H. pylori* might exacerbate an ulcer already under way, it was not the causative agent. Now, there are regimens that include only antibiotics. Ultimately, the evidence that really convinced the skeptics that *H. pylori* was an important player came from studies comparing a conventional antiulcer drug with the antibiotic regimen. In both cases, the current ulcer was cured, but only in the group receiving antibiotics was the incidence of recurrent infection reduced significantly. Today the antibiotic treatment period usually lasts only 1 or 2 weeks. This is a big improvement over the first treatment regimens, which lasted in some cases for months. The longer oral antibiotics are taken, the more likely the patient is to experience side effects, such as diarrhea, that arise from disruptions of the normal microbiota of the colon.

A predictable development has been the appearance of *H. pylori* strains resistant to the antibiotics used in therapy. This has already given rise to clinical failures. Fortunately, there are multiple therapies, so resistance has not had as serious a clinical impact as it would if there were only one or two regimens. At least not yet. A troubling aspect of resistance to some antibiotics by *H. pylori* is a phenomenon that has been given the name **heteroresistance.** Usually, in testing for resistance, only a single colony of the isolate being studied is tested for its susceptibility to various antibiotics. Scientists have now found that if 10 colonies of a strain isolated from an ulcer patient are tested for resistance, they vary widely with respect to susceptibility. Some are resistant and some are susceptible. This raises the possibility that the appearance of resistance is simply due to selection of the resistant subpopulation within the larger population of mostly susceptible bacteria. This phenomenon has been seen so far only with resistance to metronidazole, but it raises the troubling question of how

much potential there is for strains of *H. pylori* to become resistant to antibiotics very rapidly. Now that ulcer patients and their physicians have become accustomed to being able to cure ulcers, it would be very troubling, both physically and psychologically, to have that cure taken away. It is bad enough to have failed to cure a disease, as has been the case with HIV infections, but to have found a cure, experienced the euphoria, then watched the cure lose its efficacy, is something very different. This is the kind of thing that brings villagers trooping to the town square brandishing torches and pitchforks.

Scientists who work on *H. pylori* are now more optimistic than ever about the development of a vaccine that would prevent colonization of the human stomach with *H. pylori*. There has been success in animal models of the infection, and it is likely that human clinical trials will be undertaken in the not-too-distant future. Although at first, the possibility of preventing ulcers and gastric cancer using a vaccine seems very attractive, however, there are reasons to take a more cautious approach (Box 23–2).

BOX 23–2   A Vaccine—Is This a Good Idea?

There are two reasons for proceeding with caution in the development and administration of a vaccine against *H. pylori*. The first is that *H. pylori* infections often elicit the production of antibodies that cross-react with human gastric tissue. This could be due to the Lewis x and y antigens in the LPS molecules of some strains, but it could be due to other, as yet unidentified components of the bacteria. It is very important to know exactly which *H. pylori* antigens are involved in eliciting the autoantibodies. If these antibodies cross-react with tissue other than gastric mucosal tissue, there could be some very unpleasant sequelae to administration of the vaccine, especially if it is administered systemically.

This first objection is not as serious as it sounds because scientists who develop vaccines are very well aware of how important it is to prevent elicitation of autoantibodies, and they have a lot of experience dealing with this problem. The second potential objection is not so obvious but reflects an emerging view of the effect of infectious disease pressure on human evolution. The nearly universal carriage of *H. pylori* by people in developing countries indicates that *H. pylori* has long been a resident of

the human body. Moreover, the low level of gastric and duodenal ulcers in people in developing countries suggests that early colonization may actually protect people from ulcers. (Gastric cancer, which is found more commonly in developing countries, is a different story.) People in developing countries also experience a significantly lower incidence of such diseases as asthma and inflammatory bowel disease than people in the developed world. Some scientists are beginning to wonder if the increased incidence of such diseases in the developed world might be due to loss of early stimulation of the immune system by microbial infections. A recent study found that children in day care centers, where infectious diseases are rife, had a significantly lower incidence of asthma than children raised at home, and this has reignited the debate over "How clean is too clean?" It is worth considering whether subtracting yet another widely carried human microbe, which the human body has evolved over millions of years to tolerate, is a good idea.

Source: The overactive imaginations of the authors, stimulated by an article by M. Blaser, the dean of *Helicobacter* studies (Blaser, 1998).

H. pylori Mysteries

Studies of *H. pylori* have generated many new insights into how bacteria cause human disease, but they have also raised some perplexing questions that remain to be resolved. The first of these is the question of how *H. pylori* is transmitted. Most people buy into the hypothesis that transmission from parent to child is the primary route of transmission. Yet, if daily close contact spreads the disease, why is it that spouses seem not to transmit the bacteria to each other?

The hypothesis that *H. pylori* can be spread by food or water has been entertained from time to time but never proved. But if this mode of transmission is not a common one, why has cleaning up the food and water supply in developed countries been associated with decreased carriage of *H. pylori*? The key word here is "association," which is not the same as "cause and effect," but the question of why carriage is decreasing despite continued intimacy of parents and children needs to be answered. Patterns of antibiotic use could be part of the answer, although it took combinations of antibiotics not normally used to treat other types of infections to eliminate *H. pylori* from the human stomach. The combinations were designed for quick elimination, and it is possible that antibiotics singly, while they might not rapidly eliminate the bacteria, could over the long haul make the bacteria less able to persist. The question of how *H. pylori* is transmitted is an important one. Only when this issue is finally resolved will it become possible to control the spread of this bacterium, or make it ubiquitous again as it is in developing countries—if this proves to be the best health option. This brings us to the ultimate *H. pylori* mystery: is it a good thing or a bad thing to have *H. pylori* in your stomach? Ulcers are uncommon in countries where children are colonized at a very early age, but gastric cancer is rife in some—but not all—of these same countries. Do important cofactors, such as diet or other practices, influence the progression from colonization with *H. pylori* to ulcers or cancer? Why do ulcers predominate in developed countries, whereas gastric cancer is more common in developing countries, especially in Asia? Finding the answers to these questions may well lead us to novel insights into the coexistence and coevolution of the human body and its resident bacteria.

SELECTED READINGS

Berg, D., P. Hoffman, B. Appelmelk, and J. Kusters. 1997. The *Helicobacter pylori* genome sequence: genetic factors for long life in the gastric mucosa. *Trends Microbiol.* **5:**468–474.

Blaser, M. 1998. Helicobacters are indigenous to the human stomach: duodenal ulceration is due to changes in gastric microecology in the modern era. *Gut* **43:**721–727.

Covacci, A., J. Telford, G. Del Giudice, J. Parsonnet, and R. Rappuoli. 1999. *Helicobacter pylori* virulence and genetic geography. *Science* **284:**1328–1333.

Cover, T., and M. Blaser. 1995. *Helicobacter pylori*: a bacterial cause of gastritis, peptic ulcer disease, and gastric cancer. *ASM News* **61:**21–26.

Del Giudice, G., A. Covacci, J. L. Telford, C. Montecucco, and R. Rappuoli. 2001. The design of vaccines against *Helicobacter pylori* and their development. *Annu. Rev. Immunol.* **19:**523–563.

Dore, M., M. Osato, D. Kwon, D. Graham, and F. El-Zaatari. 1998. Demonstration of unexpected antibiotic resistance of genotypically identical *Helicobacter pylori* isolates. *Clin. Infect. Dis.* **27:**84–89.

Dorrell, N., J. Crabtree, and B. Wren. 1998. Host-bacterial interactions and the pathogenesis of *Helicobacter pylori* infection. *Trends Microbiol.* **6:**379–382.

Megraud, F., and H. Doermann. 1998. Clinical relevance of resistant strains of *Helicobacter pylori*: a review of current data. *Gut* **43**(Suppl. 1)**:**S61–S65.

Parsonnet, J. (ed.). 1999. *Microbes and Malignancy: Infection as a Cause of Human Cancers.* Oxford University Press, New York, N.Y.

Sherburne, R., and D. Taylor. 1995. *Helicobacter pylori* expresses a complex surface carbohydrate, Lewis X. *Infect. Immun.* **63:**4564–4568.

Suerbaum, S. 1995. The complex flagella of gastric *Helicobacter* species. *Trends Microbiol.* **3:**168–171.

Suerbaum, S., and M. Achtman. 1999. Evolution of *Helicobacter pylori*: the role of recombination. *Trends Microbiol.* **7:**182–184.

SUMMARY OUTLINE

Characteristics of *H. pylori*

Gram-negative curved rod

Highly motile with four to seven polar flagella
- Shaft composed of FlaA and FlaB
- *flaA* and *flaB* at different sites of chromosome; regulated differently
  - *flaA* regulated by σ^{28}
  - *flaB* regulated by σ^{54}
- Shaft encased in membranous sheath with terminal bulb
- Hook protein involved in assembly of flagella

Microaerophile; respiratory metabolism only
- Uses glucose, amino acids, organic acids as carbon source
- Produces most amino acids, nucleic acids, and vitamins
- Internal pH 7.0 to 7.3

Genomics
- Small, ~1.7 Mbp
- *H. pylori* genome first one sequenced
- Comparison of sequences of two strains revealed 7% of genes unique to one strain

Virulence factors

All strains
- Urease—survival in stomach lumen, later role in inflammation (?)
- Motility—reaching the mucin layer and persisting there
- Neutrophil activation protein (NAP)—surface protein that helps to elicit the inflammatory response
- LPS—low toxicity compared to other LPS molecules; could contribute to inflammation
- VacA—vacuolating toxin, may contribute to tissue damage, inflammatory response

Some strains
- LPS capable of immune mimicry due to carbohydrate residues identical to human Lewis x and Lewis y antigens
- BabA—putative adhesin that mediates binding to epithelial cells
- *cag* pathogenicity island—contains genes for type IV secretion system; function unknown

Prevention and Treatment

Several drug combinations effective

Vaccine seems likely

QUESTIONS

Answers to the questions can be found in Appendix 2.

1. Argue for and against the statement that *H. pylori* has been conclusively shown to be the cause of ulcers.

2. Urease appears to be an important virulence factor. Would a urease inhibitor be a good therapeutic agent? Explain.

3. One perplexing question that needs to be answered is why many people who are colonized with *H. pylori* never develop the disease. What types of characteristics might explain why only a small percentage of people who are colonized by *H. pylori* ever develop ulcers?

4. An advocate of the hypothesis that *H. pylori* causes ulcers could counter the argument that many people are colonized but few develop ulcers by pointing out that *Neisseria meningitidis,* one of the leading causes of adult meningitis, colonizes at least as high a proportion of the population (during an outbreak), and a much smaller percentage of these people develop meningitis than de-velop ulcers. Is this a good argument? To what extent are the two examples similar?

5. How does the LPS of *H. pylori* differ in function from the LPS of most other disease-causing bacteria?

6. Is it appropriate to use serum antibodies to *H. pylori* as an indication of active infection at the time the serum was taken, as was done in the gastric cancer studies? Why didn't the study examine whether people with gastric cancer were currently infected with *H. pylori*?

7. Why might combinations of antibiotics be necessary to clear *H. pylori* colonization?

8. In clinical trials, conventional ulcer medications were as effective as antibiotics in curing the patients' ulcers. Given this, what is the benefit of antibiotics over conventional therapy?

9. Can you make a case for studying *H. pylori* as a paradigm organism? For what would it be a paradigm, and how does it differ from pathogens studied in more depth?

24

Clostridium difficile and Pseudomembranous Colitis

KEY FEATURES

Clostridium difficile

CHARACTERISTICS

Gram-positive rod

Sporeformer

Obligate anaerobe

DISEASE

Diarrhea

Pseudomembranous colitis (severe ulceration of the colon mucosa)

RESERVOIR

Human colon (only about 5% of the population)

MAJOR VIRULENCE FACTORS

Ability to overgrow in the colon if predominant colonic anaerobes decimated by antibiotics

Toxins A and B

PREVENTION AND TREATMENT

Avoid use of antibiotics that reduce numbers of predominant colonic anaerobes

Monitor patients receiving antibiotics known to have such an effect

Treat patients who develop symptoms with anticlostridial antibiotics

---

Pseudomembranous Colitis—a Disease Caused by Antibiotics

Emergence of Pseudomembranous Colitis

The discovery of antibiotics revolutionized medicine by providing cures for many infectious diseases that had previously caused untold suffering and death. Understandably, antibiotics were viewed as miracle drugs, and because of this it was difficult at first for physicians and the public at large to accept the fact that antibiotic use might have some negative aspects. The fact that antibiotics can sometimes have toxic side effects was recognized early on. The connection between overuse of antibiotics and the emergence of resistant strains was made much later and is still not taken seriously by a segment of the medical community. Even harder to accept was the idea that antibiotics being used successfully to treat one type of bacterial infection might actually cause another type of bacterial disease in the same patient. This happens when the antibiotics depress the resident microbiota of various body sites, thus allowing pathogens that had been kept in check by the microbiota to overgrow. Pseudomembranous colitis, one example of this type of disease, is probably the best documented. Another example is yeast vaginitis, a disease that develops in some women who take antibiotics that affect the normal vaginal microbiota.

Pseudomembranous colitis, a disease characterized by severe ulceration of the colon, was first described nearly a century ago, before the advent of antibiotics. It was a rare disease until around 1970, when outbreaks began to occur in hospitals, particularly among elderly patients. Because pseudomembranous colitis is often fatal and can kill within a few days, these outbreaks caused alarm. The reason for the sudden increase in pseudomembranous colitis cases turned out to be the widespread use of antibiotics such as clindamycin, cephalosporins, and ampicillin, which inhibit the growth of the numerically predominant genera of colonic bacteria. This gave *Clostridium difficile*, a species that is normally present in very low numbers, the chance to overgrow and cause disease. Some antitumor drugs have the same effect, although the reason for this is not clear since antitumor drugs are not overtly antibacterial. Once again, changes in human practices created a niche that a microbe could exploit.

At first, clindamycin was the antibiotic most frequently associated with the disease. Certainly, clindamycin causes more cases per amount of antibiotic used than any other antibiotic, but other antibiotics, such as ampicillin and cephalosporins, cause more cases of the disease in toto because they are used much more widely than clindamycin.

Characteristics of *C. difficile*

The bacterium that causes pseudomembranous colitis is *C. difficile*, a gram-positive, obligately anaerobic, rod-shaped bacterium. Like other clostridia, *C. difficile* is a sporeformer and is notable for its ability to produce exotoxins. *C. difficile* causes a spectrum of disease, which extends from mild diarrhea to pseudomembranous colitis. Now that diagnostic tests for detecting clostridial toxins in feces are available and the types of patients who are at highest risk for pseudomembranous colitis have been identified, early aggressive treatment of patients who show signs of developing full-blown disease

has lessened the incidence of the disease. Also, restrictions on the use of antibiotics known to cause pseudomembranous colitis have helped to reduce the incidence of the disease even further.

An interesting feature of pseudomembranous colitis is that many strains of *C. difficile* are susceptible to the antibiotics that precipitate episodes of pseudomembranous colitis. How, then, could *C. difficile* overgrow if the antibiotic is present? The reason seems to be that as antibiotic treatment comes to an end and levels of antibiotic in the intestine fall, *C. difficile* is able to resume growth faster than most other colonic bacteria and repopulates the colon before the normal microbiota can be reestablished. Also, although many strains of *C. difficile* are technically susceptible, as defined by inability to grow in concentrations of the antibiotic achievable in the colon during therapy, they are less susceptible than many of the major groups of colon bacteria. A small difference in antibiotic susceptibility could give bacteria a big edge in the colon.

It is important to note that even in people who are colonized with *C. difficile* and who are treated with the antibiotics associated with pseudomembranous colitis, only a subset develops the disease. One explanation is that the line between overgrowth by the clostridia and restoration of the normal microbiota following therapy is such a fine one that whether disease results or not is a crapshoot, with the dice weighted against the clostridial overgrowth. It is also possible, however, that some people are more likely to develop pseudomembranous colitis because of differences in the composition of their colonic microbiota or even because they are physiologically more susceptible to the effects of the clostridial toxins that mediate the disease.

Development and Ecology of the Disease

The steps in development of pseudomembranous colitis are outlined in Figure 24–1. When antibiotics or other drugs cause a reduction in concentrations of bacterial genera that normally predominate in the colon, they eliminate an important protective barrier to colonization of the site by pathogens. *C. difficile*, if present, is poised to take advantage of this opportunity. Normally, less than 1 to 5% of people in the normal population harbor *C. difficile* in their intestinal tracts, but the percentage of people colonized by *C. difficile* can become as high as 20% in a hospital setting, where the bacteria are spread from one patient to another. Risk of colonization is linked directly to the length of time spent in the hospital, particularly in the case of a hospital that has experienced outbreaks of *C. difficile* disease.

C. difficile is a strict anaerobe and dies rapidly outside

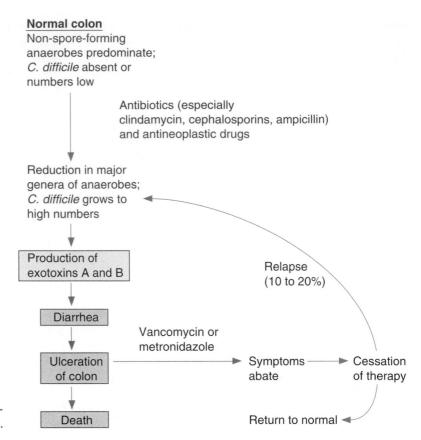

Normal colon
Non-spore-forming
anaerobes predominate;
C. difficile absent or
numbers low

Antibiotics (especially
clindamycin, cephalosporins, ampicillin)
and antineoplastic drugs

Reduction in major
genera of anaerobes;
C. difficile grows to
high numbers

Production of
exotoxins A and B

Diarrhea

Relapse
(10 to 20%)

Ulceration
of colon

Vancomycin or
metronidazole

Symptoms → Cessation
abate   of therapy

Death

Return to normal

Figure 24–1 Steps in development of pseudomembranous colitis and possible outcomes.

the colon. Thus, at first glance, it might appear unlikely that *C. difficile* would be transmissible from one patient to another. However, *C. difficile* is a sporeformer, and spores not only persist in the environment for many months, but they survive passage through the stomach if they are ingested. The spread of spores from a colonized person to the surrounding environment and then to other patients is facilitated by the fact that an early symptom of pseudomembranous colitis is diarrhea, a notorious source of aerosols. Members of the hospital staff who care for patients colonized with *C. difficile* also transmit the spores to other patients on their hands. Colonization of an otherwise healthy person with *C. difficile* causes no apparent symptoms as long as the clostridia are present in low concentrations. Only when *C. difficile* is able to attain high enough concentrations to allow appreciable amounts of toxin to be produced does symptomatic disease occur.

At first, in attempts to predict patients at highest risk for developing pseudomembranous colitis, attention was focused on patients who entered the hospital colonized with *C. difficile*. Yet, careful studies of these patients revealed that they were, if anything, less likely to develop pseudomembranous colitis than patients who acquired the bacteria in the hospital. The current model for development of *C. difficile* disease is that an unco-

lonized person enters the hospital, is exposed to antibiotics, and becomes colonized with *C. difficile*. Development of symptomatic disease now appears more likely in such cases than in previously colonized people. Why this is so is not clear. Possibly, *C. difficile* strains that survive in the hospital environment are slightly more resistant to antibiotics than strains colonizing people in the community. Or, there may be some partial immunity to *C. difficile* disease when people have carried the bacteria asymptomatically for a long time. Future research may answer these questions.

Toxins produced by *C. difficile* damage the colonic mucosa. Accumulations of fibrin, mucin, and dead host cells form a yellowish layer on the surface of the colon mucosa. Initially, numerous separate lesions appear, covered by patches of debris. Eventually, these scattered lesions coalesce, and the sheetlike layer of debris covers a larger area. This layer of debris (**pseudomembrane**) distinguishes the disease from other types of intestinal inflammation (**colitis**) and thus gives the disease its name. Untreated pseudomembranous colitis can be fatal. The symptoms are similar to those seen in cases of septic shock.

Currently, the treatment of choice for pseudomembranous colitis is to stop administering the antibiotic that precipitated the disease and begin to administer antibiotics known to be effective against *C. difficile*, such as vancomycin or metronidazole. If this treatment is successful and the patient recovers, there is still the chance of a relapse once the therapy is discontinued. Relapses occur in as many as 10 to 20% of cases, and multiple relapses in the same person are not uncommon. Presumably, relapses are due to failure to clear *C. difficile* and to restore a stable, nonpathogenic microbiota.

Virulence Factors

Toxins

PROPERTIES OF THE TOXINS. *C. difficile* produces two protein toxins that are thought to be responsible for the symptoms of pseudomembranous colitis: **toxin A** and **toxin B.** These toxins have a number of interesting properties. Toxins A and B are the largest single-molecule bacterial exotoxins known. Molecular masses reported in the literature vary considerably because of the tendency of these proteins to aggregate, but are now considered to be 308 kDa and 269 kDa, respectively, based both on biochemical data and on the DNA sequence of the genes encoding the toxins. The toxins have no recognizable signal sequence and do not appear to be activated by proteolytic nicking. They act by modifying host cell membrane G proteins that control many cellular activities, including actin polymerization. Since the discovery of the *C. difficile* toxins, other toxins with the same mechanism have been identified. Many of these were found in pathogenic *Clostridium* species, but one has also been found in pathogenic *Escherichia coli*, the cytotoxic necrotizing factor (see chapter 28). Not all of these toxins are as large as the *C. difficile* toxins, so an unusually large size is not an essential feature of toxins of this sort.

From the beginning, toxins A and B have frustrated and sometimes misled scientists working on them. As already mentioned, they were difficult to size and purify because of their tendency to aggregate. Until the genes encoding toxin A (*tcdA*) and toxin B (*tcdB*) were cloned, an added difficulty in purifying these toxins was that they have very similar properties. Another feature of these toxins that initially misled scientists was their behavior in standard toxin assays. Toxin A acted like an enterotoxin; it caused fluid release when injected into a ligated rabbit ileal loop. The fluid was not the watery type of fluid seen with enterotoxins such as cholera toxin, however, but had a more viscous, bloody appearance. This is because toxin A does not cause a fluid imbalance by disrupting ion pumps but causes fluid accumulation by damaging mucosal cells so extensively that they can no longer control water movement.

Toxin B was cytotoxic for tissue culture cells, whereas toxin A was at least a thousandfold less cytotoxic in assays of this type. Toxin B collapsed the actin cytoskeleton of the tissue culture cell, resulting in rounded-up cells, some of which still had long pointlike projections. Toxin A appeared not to have this activity. It was thus a surprise to find that both toxins not only have the same mechanism of action but are very similar in amino acid sequence (45% identity). The explanation for the apparent difference between the two toxins in mode of action proved to be that toxin B is much more active than toxin A and thus kills cells more quickly. Toxin A acts more slowly and produces milder symptoms, thus explaining the enterotoxinlike behavior in the rabbit ileal loop model.

MODE OF ACTION—MODIFICATION OF MAMMALIAN G PROTEINS. Both toxins glucosylate a threonine residue on G proteins and have more than one G protein target. Targets include **G proteins Rho, Rac,** and **Cdc42.** All of these targets are important regulatory proteins of mammalian cells, and if they malfunction, many cellular processes are affected. Among other things, they control the polymerization and depolymerization of actin. This process is normally dynamic because the actin cytoskeleton not only helps determine the shape of the cell but also allows a cell to make pseudopods for phagocytosis or to change shape, as PMNs do when they migrate between endothelial or epithelial cells. Thus, the cytoskeleton is constantly turning over. Impairment of polymerization or depolymerization or both upsets the natural balance of these processes in the cell.

G proteins cycle between a state in which they bind GDP and a state in which they bind GTP. The GTP-bound form is the form that mediates the effects of the G protein. The ratio of the GDP-bound form to the GTP-bound form is determined by the presence of signals that stimulate the phosphorylation of bound GDP to form bound GTP (Figure 24–2). Toxins A and B act preferentially on the GDP-bound form because in that form, the G protein takes on a configuration that exposes the threonine that is glucosylated by the toxins. In the GTP-bound form, the conformation of the G protein changes enough to bury the threonine residue in the protein, where it is inaccessible to toxin activity. Glucosylation does not completely inactivate the G protein, but it does reduce the GTPase activity of the protein by increasing the frequency of release of GTP from the GTP-bound form of the G protein. This creates an imbalance that disrupts the control of processes normally controlled tightly by the G protein.

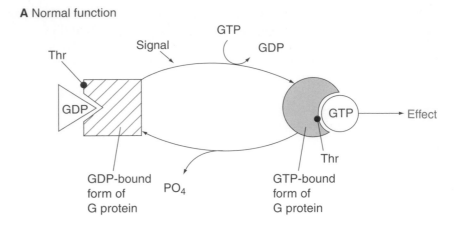

A Normal function

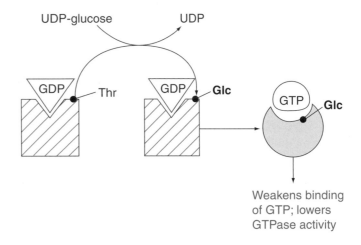

B Effects of glucosylation of G protein
   by TcdA or TcdB

Figure 24–2 Mode of action of toxins A and B. (**A**) The normal cycling of G proteins between the GDP-bound form and the GTP-bound form. The threonine (Thr) residue that will be glucosylated by the toxins is shown. It is exposed on the surface of the GDP-bound form but buried in the protein in the GTP-bound form. (**B**) Glucosylation of the threonine residue of the GDP-bound form does not prevent it from converting to the GTP-bound form, but the glucosylated GTP-bound form has a lower affinity for GTP and a lower GTPase activity. These changes disrupt the normal functions of the G protein, causing numerous changes in cell physiology.

● **Glc**, glucose bound to threonine

TOXIN STRUCTURE. The structure of the *C. difficile* toxins is illustrated in Figure 24–3 and follows the usual single chain toxin structural plan. There is a binding domain that binds to the host cell receptor, a translocation domain that mediates translocation of the enzymatic portion into the cell cytoplasm, and the enzymatic domain that glucosylates the G proteins. Since G proteins are located in the cytoplasmic membrane, the toxin need not migrate through the cytoplasm to reach its target, as do many other A-B toxins. The receptor for toxin A on human cells has been identified as **Galβ1–4GlcNAc.** This receptor is found on the surfaces of intestinal cells. The receptor of toxin B has not yet been identified but is probably also a carbohydrate antigen on mammalian cells. At one point, it was suggested that toxin B bound nonspecifically to membranes, but more

recent findings suggest that a specific receptor is involved. Differences in identity and distribution of the receptors for toxins A and B undoubtedly contribute, along with different levels of catalytic activity, to the different functions of these toxins in human disease. Not all humans are equally affected by the toxin (Box 24–1).

REGULATION OF TOXIN GENE EXPRESSION. The *tcdA* and *tcdB* genes are located on a pathogenicity island called **PaLoc** (for **pathogenicity locus**). Also in the same vicinity are the regulatory genes *tcdC* and *tcdD* (Figure 24–4). Note that all of these genes except for *tcdC* are transcribed in a single direction. Toxin levels are highest in the medium of late-exponential-phase cells. The mechanism proposed for this type of regulation starts

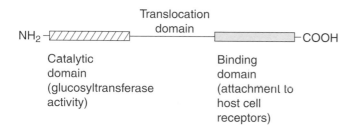

Figure 24–3 Functional domains of toxins A and B.

with the fact that *tcdD* is transcribed at highest levels in early-exponential-phase cells. The protein it encodes acts as a positive regulator of *tcdA*, *tcdB*, and *tcdE* (function unknown). As the bacteria move toward late exponential stage, the toxins begin to build up to their highest level. During this time, *tcdC*, which encodes a protein that counters the expression of *tcdD* and thus has a negative effect on toxin gene expression, is made at low levels, which are kept even lower by the antisense transcripts emanating from the other genes. As the cells enter late exponential stage, expression of *tcdC* is in-creased enough to counter the antisense effect, and TcdC begins to accumulate, shutting down synthesis of the other genes. Thus, toxin production is highest in early- and mid-exponential-stage cells; toxin concentrations increase so that, by late exponential phase, concentrations reach a maximum. That is, expression of toxin genes is not induced in late stationary phase. Rather, the rise in toxin levels is due to accumulation of toxin produced earlier in the growth curve. Of course, it is necessary to point out that the stages of the growth curve seen in laboratory medium may bear no relationship to bacterial growth patterns in nature, although the explosive overgrowth of *C. difficile* could well come close to that seen in freshly inoculated laboratory medium. Whether TcdC acts as a repressor of *tcdD* synthesis or counters the effect of TcdD in some other way is not known.

Growth phase is not the only signal sensed by the toxin regulatory genes. Stresses of various types, such as starvation for carbon and nitrogen and exposure to oxygen, also increase toxin production. These stresses may be linked, because one effect of oxygen on an ob-

BOX 24–1 Babies Are Tougher than You Think: an Unexplained "Resistance" to Toxins A and B

A curious and largely unexplained observation is that infants can harbor high concentrations of toxin-producing *C. difficile* in their colons without suffering any adverse effects. Although colonization of adults with *C. difficile* occurs in less than 5% of the population, colonization with *C. difficile* is common in infants, whose resident microbiota is still evolving. As many as 50% of infants are colonized with *C. difficile*, yet pseudomembranous colitis rarely occurs in infants, nor do the bacteria appear to cause diarrhea. In some cases, the lack of symptoms is explained by the fact that the colonizing strain is not a toxin producer, but this is not always the case. In fact, colonized infants frequently have toxin concentrations in their colons that would be fatal in an adult. An early hypothesis, now disproved, was that infants do not have toxin receptors on their colonic mucosal cells. Studies have shown that infants do have toxin A receptors. At least one of the blood group antigens that serves as a receptor for the toxin A (antigen Y) is abundant in infant mucosal tissue, and mucosal tissue from infants binds as much toxin A as adult tissue in in vitro tests. The relative immunity of infants to *C. difficile* toxins could be due to the presence of a thick undisrupted mucin layer. Moreover, the mucin of infants has a somewhat different composition than that of adults. Lack of prior mucosal damage may also be a factor. In animal studies, damage to the mucosa increased the ability of the *C. difficile* toxins to further damage the mucosa. Still another hypothesis is that infants and many adults produce toxin A-neutralizing antibodies. Such antibodies have, in fact, been detected in the feces of older infants and adults. It is good to keep in mind that only a small fraction of adults who are colonized with *C. difficile* and receive the types of antibiotics known to precipitate pseudomembranous colitis actually go on to develop the disease. Such factors as disruption of the mucin layer, damage to the mucosa, and production of toxin-neutralizing antibodies could explain not only why infants seem to be impervious to *C. difficile* toxins but also why only some adults are susceptible to the disease.

A Early exponential phase—active transcription of
TcdD; low transcription of *TcdC*

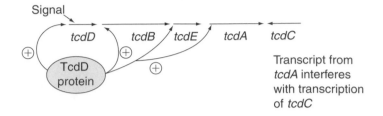

Transcript from
tcdA interferes
with transcription
of *tcdC*

B Late exponential phase—upshift in transcription
of *tcdC* overrides antisense inhibition from
tcdA transcript

Figure 24–4 Regulation of *tcdA* and *tcdB*. (**A**) In early exponential phase, *tcdD* is actively transcribed. TcdD protein activates (⊕) expression of all the genes except *tcdC*. Toxins are produced. Transcripts from *tcdA* interfere with production of *tcdC* transcripts, which are being produced at a low level. (**B**) In late exponential phase, there is an upshift in transcription of *tcdC*, which overrides the inhibitory effect of *tcdA* countertranscripts. TcdC protein somehow counteracts the effect of TcdD (⊖), shutting down synthesis of the toxin genes.

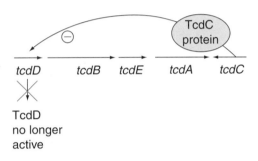

ligate anaerobe would be to reduce metabolic activities, causing a greater reliance on exogenous amino acids and other nutrients.

TOXIN ACTION AND DISEASE SYMPTOMS. A model for the contribution of toxins A and B to development of diarrhea and mucosal damage is shown in Figure 24–5. Toxin A activates neurons. It also attracts and activates PMNs, probably by stimulating intestinal mucosal cells to produce cytokines and other proinflammatory proteins. Activation of the enteric neurons affects the motility of intestinal contents and may thus contribute to diarrhea. PMNs moving into the area create an inflammatory response that damages cells, contributing to mucosal cell destruction. PMNs migrating between mucosal cells disrupt the tight junctions that normally prevent fluids from flowing across the mucosal membrane. This not only allows water to leak from tissue into the lumen of the intestine but also allows toxin B to cross the mucosal membrane by diffusion. Toxin B damages the tissue underlying the mucosal membrane, further contributing to damage of the intestinal wall. If damage becomes too extensive, LPS or bacteria from the colon can breach the intestinal wall, enter the bloodstream, and cause septic shock. Also, the extensive tissue damage caused by the toxins will elicit a strong inflammatory response that may contribute to septic shock.

Strains of *C. difficile* vary considerably in their level of toxin production; many strains produce little or no toxin. Toxigenic strains almost always produce both toxin A and toxin B, and the levels of the two toxins covary. This is not too surprising, given the fact that the toxin genes are cotranscribed. The levels of these toxins can be quite high. Under in vitro conditions that give maximum toxin production, the toxins can account for up to 5% of total protein when the bacteria are growing in pure culture, an enormous energy expenditure. The interesting question of what these toxins are doing for the bacteria remains to be answered.

Other Virulence Factors

Investigations of the virulence factors of *C. difficile* have tended to focus on toxins A and B, not only because they are clearly important factors but also because they are interesting in their own right. Little work has been done on possible adhesins of *C. difficile*. Binding to mucin or mucosal cells would bring the bacteria into close proximity to the intestinal wall, where they could do the most damage. This location might also protect them to some extent from competition with the normal microbiota of the colon, which is mostly packed in the lumen of the colon.

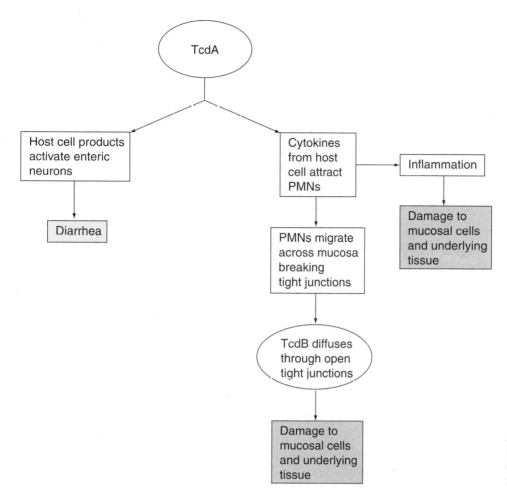

Figure 24–5 Model for how toxins A and B produce the symptoms of pseudomembranous colitis.

Another possible virulence factor, if the bacteria gain access to the underlying tissue, is LTA. LTA from lysing cells might contribute to the inflammatory response.

Prevention and Treatment

Successful treatment depends on early diagnosis. Patients receiving antibiotics known to cause pseudomembranous colitis should be watched carefully for signs of diarrhea. In many U.S. hospitals, patients with antibiotic-associated diarrhea are tested routinely for the presence of toxins A and B in their feces. If pseudomembranous colitis is suspected, the patient is given vancomycin or metronidazole, two antibiotics that are effective against *C. difficile*. Timely administration of oral vancomycin or metronidazole is usually successful in preventing the development of full-blown pseudomembranous colitis. As mentioned earlier in the chapter, relapses can occur when vancomycin therapy ceases.

One strategy, currently being tested experimentally but not used in hospitals at this point, is to aid the restoration of the resident microflora by giving the patient enemas with dilute feces taken from family members. Although an enema does not reach very high in the colon and thus might not seem to be an effective strategy for repopulating the entire colon, some studies indicate that this approach is successful in preventing relapses. Another approach, which has shown signs of success, is to feed *Saccharomyces boulardii*, a nonpathogenic yeast, to patients who are receiving antibiotic therapy. *S. boulardii* is one of several nonpathogenic yeasts and bacteria that have been embraced by the probiotics industry, based unfortunately on very little credible scientific evidence. Almost magical properties have been ascribed to these probiotic preparations, which may owe much of their perceived success to the placebo effect. Normally, it is difficult to dispute the claims for these preparations because the claims for efficacy are so diffuse. In this case, however, a very specific claim is being made—prevention of *C. difficile* disease. This claim should be easy to test. It is hard to imagine how this would work, since *S. boulardii* is not a common inhabitant of the colon. It is still too early, however, to rule out the possibility that continued ingestion of high amounts of the yeast creates an inhibitory barrier—possibly due to the physical interaction between yeast cell wall compounds and compounds in the colonic environment—to colonization by *C. difficile*, even if the yeast does not set up housekeeping in the colon.

So far, the most effective efforts to prevent pseudomembranous colitis have been restrictions on the use of the antibiotics that are most likely to cause it. At one time, some dermatologists were giving oral clindamycin to acne patients because acne is believed to be exacerbated, and possibly caused, by another anaerobe, *Propionibacterium acnes*. We now realize that giving oral clindamycin to people who are not closely supervised in a hospital setting is dangerous. Some dermatologists are still using clindamycin for acne, but they have the patient apply it to the skin as a topical preparation.

In a hospital intensive care unit, careful observation of patients taking clindamycin, cephalosporins, or ampicillin is advisable, particularly if a hospital has had a recent outbreak of pseudomembranous colitis. The fact that spores can be spread from patient to patient has increased awareness of the importance of hand washing by hospital staff caring for patients who have pseudomembranous colitis or who develop diarrhea after administration of antibiotics. The fact that carriage by people in the community (<5%) is significantly lower than carriage by hospital patients, especially in intensive care units (as high as 20%), strongly supports the hypothesis that *C. difficile* can be spread from patient to patient in the hospital environment. Careful cleaning of rooms where pseudomembranous colitis patients have stayed can reduce but not eliminate the number of spores in the environment.

There are diagnostic tests that detect *C. difficile* toxins A and B, but a completely reliable test is still not available. Recently, scientists have reported the isolation of strains that cause disease but do not produce toxin molecules detectable by the standard tests. These strains have deletions and mutations in the toxin genes that appear to have rendered the toxins inactive. Yet, the strains are still associated with disease, in some cases disease in its most severe form. Such reports raise the question of whether currently available tests that focus on detection of toxins A and B have the coverage to detect all cases of possible *C. difficile* disease. If not, this is disturbing, because once symptoms begin to develop, the attending physician does not have much time to choose the right therapy. Also, since many hospitals have been successful in reducing the incidence of pseudomembranous colitis, physicians may become less concerned about patients with diarrhea, the first sign of incipient pseudomembranous colitis. It would be a shame if the very real progress made toward prevention of infection and early detection and treatment of cases that develop should be held hostage to the lack of an adequate diagnostic test.

SELECTED READINGS

Boquet, P. 1999. The Ras superfamily of small GTP-binding proteins as targets for bacterial toxins, p. 27–44. *In* J. E. Alouf and J. M. Freer (ed.), *The Comprehensive Sourcebook of Bacterial Protein Toxins,* 2nd ed. Academic Press, Inc., New York, N.Y.

Johnson, S., and D. N. Gerding. 1998. *Clostridium difficile*-associated diarrhea. *Clin. Infect. Dis.* **26:**1027–1036.

Knoop, F., M. Owens, and I. Crocker. 1993. *Clostridium difficile:* clinical disease and diagnosis. *Clin. Microbiol. Rev.* **6:**251–265.

Mayfield, J. L., T. Leet, J. Miller, and L. M. Mundy. 2000. Environmental control to reduce transmission of *Clostridium difficile*. *Clin. Infect. Dis.* **31:**995–1000.

Mazuski, J. E, E. Grossmann, J. G. Norman, W. Denham, N. Panesar, M. J. Shapiro, R. L. Durham, D. L. Kaminski, and W. E. Longo. 2000. *Clostridium difficile* toxins influence hepatocyte protein synthesis through the interleukin 1 receptor. *Arch. Surg.* **135:**1206–1211.

Samboul, S. P., M. M. Merrigan, D. Lyerly, D. N. Gerding, and S. Johnson. 2000. Toxin gene analysis of a variant strain of *Clostridium difficile* that causes human clinical disease. *Infect. Immun.* **68:**5480–5487.

Thelestam, M., E. Chaves-Olarte, M. Moos, and C. von Eichel-Streiber. 1999. Clostridial toxins acting on the cytoskeleton, p. 147–173. *In* J. E. Alouf and J. M. Freer (ed.), *The Comprehensive Sourcebook of Bacterial Protein Toxins,* 2nd ed. Academic Press, Inc., New York, N.Y.

SUMMARY OUTLINE

Progression of the disease

Antibiotic use (clindamycin, β-lactam antibiotics) reduces concentration of normal microbiota

C. difficile overgrows, produces toxins A and B

Toxins cause diarrhea, extensive tissue damage in some people (pseudomembrane)

Can be rapidly fatal

Relapses occur

Characteristics of *C. difficile*

Gram-positive rod

Obligate anaerobe

Sporeformer

Normally found in less than 5% of people outside of hospitals

Virulence factors

Toxins A and B

    Main virulence factors—responsible for symptoms

    Properties of toxins

        Large proteins, no obvious secretion signals

        Similar amino acid sequences (45% identity)

        Same mode of action, but different effects

            Different levels of activity (toxicity)

            Different receptors

            Different efficiency of translocation of enzymatic portion

    Mode of action

        Alter actin cytoskeleton of mammalian cells

        Glucosylate G proteins that control many host cell functions

            More than one G protein glucosylated

            Glucosyl group (from UDP-glucose) added to specific threonine on G protein

            Prefer GDP-bound form of G protein (threonine exposed)

            Reduce GTP binding and GTPase activity of GTP-bound form of G protein that mediates effects of G protein on cell function

    Structure of toxin

        Binding domain—binds mammalian cell receptor

            TcdA—receptor is disaccharide

            TcdB—receptor unknown

        Translocation domain—translocation of enzymatic domain into host cell

        Enzymatic domain—catalyzes glucosylation of G protein

    Regulation of *tcdA*, *tcdB*

        tcd genes found on chromosomal pathogenicity island (PaLoc)

        TcdD—positive regulator, produced in early exponential stage

        TcdD stimulates expression of *tcdA* and *tcdB* but suppresses expression of *tcdC* (negative regulator) by antisense mechanism

        In late exponential phase, *tcdC* expression increases, TcdC suppresses *tcdD* expression

Other virulence factors—not much studied

    Adhesins

    LTA (?)

(*continued*)

SUMMARY OUTLINE (*continued*)

Prevention and treatment

Treatment

Early diagnosis vital

Withdraw drug causing the problem

Treat with vancomycin, metronidazole—drugs that kill *C. difficile* but do not affect normal microbiota adversely enough to cause the disease

Restoration of microbiota—still not very successful but important to prevent relapses

Probiotics—still controversial

Enemas with fecal slurries

Prevention

Restrict use of antibiotics that cause the problem

Rapid action in the face of a developing outbreak

Diagnostic test identifies people at risk—detects toxins A and B

Hygiene to prevent transfer of bacteria to susceptible patients

No vaccine available

QUESTIONS

Answers to the questions can be found in Appendix 2.

1. How would you satisfy Koch's postulates for *C. difficile* as a cause of pseudomembranous colitis in humans? What problems would arise?

2. Hospital staff members who care for people with pseudomembranous colitis can become colonized with *C. difficile*. Is this a cause for concern about their own health?

3. In what sense is *C. difficile* an infectious pathogen? An emerging cause of disease?

4. Many people who are colonized with *C. difficile* and who develop diarrhea after taking antibiotics do not develop pseudomembranous colitis. Propose some hypotheses to explain this observation.

5. How do two toxins with the same mode of action cause such apparently different symptoms?

6. Some hospitals have experienced multiple outbreaks of pseudomembranous colitis, whereas others have never seen a case of the disease. Assuming that the hospitals have similar levels of cleanliness and equally competent staffs, how could this be explained?

7. In some hospitals that have experienced outbreaks of pseudomembranous colitis, one procedure for ending the outbreak was not (as you might expect) to close the ward or initiate extensive decontamination procedures, but simply to move a different type of patient into the ward. Explain the rationale for this approach.

8. Would it be desirable (or possible) to develop a vaccine against *C. difficile*?

9. One way to prevent pseudomembranous colitis would be to administer metronidazole or vancomycin in combination with clindamycin or other antibiotics known to precipitate the disease. Or to give metronidazole or vancomycin prophylactically to patients found to be colonized with *C. difficile*. What are the pros and cons of this approach? (Hint: This approach has been tried and rejected as ineffective.)

25

Vibrio cholerae, the Cause of Cholera

KEY FEATURES

Vibrio cholerae

CHARACTERISTICS

Gram-negative, curved rod

Motility due to a polar flagellum

Many strains do not cause serious disease

El Tor and classical strains responsible for most epidemics

DISEASE

Cholera

RESERVOIRS

Infected humans, especially asymptomatic carriers

Marine invertebrates (e.g., copepods), algae?

MAJOR VIRULENCE FACTORS

Cholera toxin

Toxin coregulated pili (Tcp pili)—clumped at one pole of the cell

Motility (flagellum)

PREVENTION AND TREATMENT

Clean water supply, effective sewage treatment

Fluid replacement therapy

No effective vaccine available

Pathogenesis and Epidemiology of Cholera

Progression of the Disease

Cholera is a serious epidemic disease that has killed millions of people and continues to be a major health problem worldwide. Cholera is acquired by drinking water that has been contaminated with human feces or by eating food that has been washed in contaminated water. *Vibrio cholerae,* the bacterium that causes cholera, is a motile, gram-negative, curved rod with a single polar flagellum. It persists in the environment because it can survive in both fresh and brackish water. In the external environment, *V. cholerae* appears to live in close association with algae and marine invertebrates, but little is known about

363

how the bacteria spend their time between outbreaks of human disease. Recently, another invertebrate host for *V. cholerae* was identified, nonbiting aquatic midges. In this case, the bacteria infect the midges rather than living with them as beneficial symbionts.

Although its normal habitat is water, *V. cholerae* is capable of causing serious disease in humans if it is ingested in high enough numbers. In the small intestine, *V. cholerae* attaches to mucosal cells and produces an exotoxin, cholera toxin, that acts on intestinal mucosal cells. Mucosal cells have a set of ion transport pumps (for Na^+, Cl^-, HCO_3^-, and K^+) that normally maintain a tight control over ion fluxes across the intestinal mucosa. Because water can pass freely through membranes, the only way to control the flow of water into and out of tissue is to control the concentration of ions in different body compartments. Under normal conditions, the net flow of ions is from lumen to tissue (Figure 25–1), resulting in a net uptake of water from the lumen into tissues. The effect of cholera toxin on mucosal cells is to alter this balance.

Cholera toxin does not damage the mucosa nor does it invade to cause more extensive disease, but it decreases the net flow of sodium into tissue and produces a net flow of chloride (and water) out of tissue, resulting in massive diarrhea and electrolyte imbalance. A person with full-blown cholera can lose 20 liters of water per day, the equivalent of losing 50 lb! The fecal stream becomes so dilute that it looks like water in which rice has been washed, thus giving rise to the term **rice water stool** that has been used to describe diarrheal fluid from a cholera victim. The loss of skin plasticity and sunken eyes of some cholera patients are visible evidence of water loss from the tissues. A more serious result of massive water loss is collapse of the circulatory system, the cause of death in cholera victims. One beneficial effect of the copious diarrhea experienced by cholera patients is that it washes the bacteria out of the intestine. Thus, the disease is self-limiting if the infected person can survive the acute phase of the disease. This fact provides the basis for the most commonly used and effective treatment for cholera, fluid replacement therapy to prevent lethal dehydration (see below).

Although death rates can be high during a cholera epidemic, especially among infants and young children, there are also many survivors. People who recover from cholera usually acquire long-term immunity to reinfection. The fact that they are immune to reinfection in the sense that they do not develop the full-blown disease when reexposed to *V. cholerae* does not mean that they can be safely ignored as part of the overall disease picture. During an epidemic, such people may become chronic asymptomatic carriers of *V. cholerae*. They can transmit the disease to susceptible members

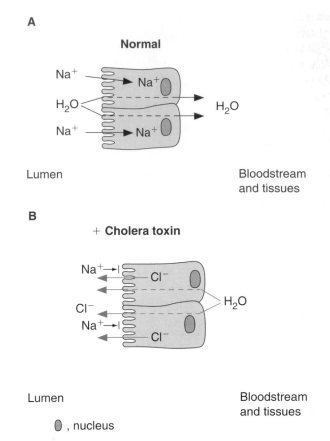

Figure 25–1 Movement of ions and water across a normal intestinal mucosa and across a mucosa affected by cholera toxin. (**A**) In the normal mucosa, the net flow of water is from the lumen to the tissues. (**B**) In the mucosa affected by cholera toxin, chloride ion secretion is increased, and absorption of sodium ions is inhibited. These effects combine to cause a rapid loss of water into the lumen, resulting in massive diarrhea.

of the population and contribute to contamination of the water supply.

History and Distribution of Cholera Outbreaks

Historically, cholera has been considered to be an Old World disease. The known pandemics of cholera and their countries of origin are listed in Table 25–1. All but one originated in the Indian subcontinent. From this location, the disease has spread widely. In some pandemics, cholera has reached the United Kingdom and the United States. After the end of the 19th century, cholera was almost unknown in the Western Hemisphere, but in the 1990s, cholera made a reappearance in this part of the world, causing a large outbreak in South America. Usually, large outbreaks of cholera are caused by a single strain of *V. cholerae*, but the identity

Table 25–1 Recorded pandemics of cholera, the source and extent of the pandemics, some associated historical events, and the strain of *V. cholerae*, where known

Pandemic	Years	Origin and extent	Associated events	Strain
First	1817–1823	Indian subcontinent; spread to Asia		
Second	1830s	Indian subcontinent; spread to Asia, United Kingdom, Canada	Lord Snow discovers that disease is water-borne	
Third	1852–1859	Indian subcontinent; reached United States	Italian physician, Filippo Pacini, describes and names the bacteria seen in human stool specimens *V. cholerae*	
Fourth	1870s	Indian subcontinent; reached United States		
Fifth	1880s	Indian subcontinent; spread to Asia, Europe	Koch isolates comma-shaped bacillus	O1 classical strain
Sixth	1889–1923	Indian subcontinent; spread to Asia		O1 classical strain
Seventh	1960–1993	Indonesia; reached South America		O1 El Tor strain
Eighth	1992–1993	Indian subcontinent; spread to Asia		O139 strain

and characteristics of the strains can change from epidemic to epidemic. Since *V. cholerae* was first isolated during the fifth pandemic, we only have information about pandemic strains since that time.

Historically, *V. cholerae* strains have been serotyped on the basis of their LPS O antigens. The fifth pandemic was caused by an O1 strain now called the **classical strain** (Table 25–1). The sixth pandemic was also caused by this strain. The seventh pandemic introduced a new O1 strain, called **El Tor,** which had somewhat different biochemical properties and phage susceptibility patterns compared with the classical strain. At that point, scientists began to believe that only O1 serotype strains caused epidemic outbreaks, whereas the so-called "non-O1" strains were responsible for smaller outbreaks and less serious disease. This notion was disproved by the eighth and most recent pandemic, which was caused by a non-O1 serotype, **O139.** This was an unpleasant surprise because it meant that simply monitoring O1 strains in the environment did not necessarily provide the early warning data that public health officials had counted on to alert them to an imminent disease outbreak. It is now clear that more information about the evolution of pandemic strains is needed if we are ever to be able to predict potential outbreaks. Scientists are beginning to probe the evolution of pan-

demic strains of *V. cholerae*, but much remains to be learned.

The history of cholera epidemics also contains some milestones in microbiology. During the second and third pandemics, a British scientist, Lord John Snow, made the connection between contaminated water and the spread of the disease. He realized that people drinking water from certain sites were the ones who contracted the disease. In the poorer areas of London and other big cities of the time, people got their water from public pumps or wells. Sewage was thrown on the streets, making it easy for a public water source to become contaminated. In a famous incident, Snow removed the pump handle from a public water source in an impoverished neighborhood in an attempt to limit the spread of the disease. Where the people who normally used the pump went to get their water is not recorded, but the incidence of cholera in the area did decrease. During the fifth pandemic, Koch isolated the "comma bacillus" we now know as *V. cholerae*.

There is an amusing sidelight to Koch's experience with the bacterium he believed to be the cause of cholera. Koch had articulated his postulates only a year earlier and was trying to satisfy them to show that cholera was caused by the bacterium he had isolated. He quickly ran into trouble, however, because he could not find an animal model to use to satisfy his third postulate. We now know that infant mice can be infected by *V. cholerae*, but Koch did not have the benefit of the experience scientists have gained during the last century in developing animal models. Frustrated by his inability to satisfy his third postulate, Koch became one of the first people to complain about his third postulate—the same postulate that bedeviled the advocates of a bacterial cause for ulcers a century later (see chapter 23). Koch declared loudly and repeatedly to all who would listen that he did not need fulfillment of his third postulate to convince him that his isolate was in truth the cause of cholera. Thus, Koch became the first victim of his own postulates (see Box 2–1).

In the seventh and eighth pandemics, death rates were much lower than in previous outbreaks, a result that can be traced directly to a massive and well-organized deployment of public health resources in the affected countries. Even poor countries can mount an effective campaign to combat a disease such as cholera if they have the will to mobilize the necessary resources. This was illustrated by the speed with which the epidemic in South America was brought under control. In the long run, however, such emergency mobilizations are not a satisfactory solution to the problem of cholera epidemics. They are expensive, divert attention and resources from other pressing public health needs, and do not save all victims of the epidemic.

Solving the Cholera Problem

An obvious solution to the cholera problem is to provide a safe water supply that is not contaminated by sewage. Doing this not only solves the cholera problem but also prevents many other types of fatal water-borne diseases. Since diarrhea is one of the main killers of children under 5 years of age, a clean water supply is an essential prerequisite for lengthening the human life span. Many countries are struggling mightily to accomplish this goal, but providing a safe water supply is an expensive proposition, especially in rural areas. It has proved to be beyond the means of many developing countries, especially those whose leaders prefer to spend money on sophisticated modern weapons rather than on public health. Even in places where a relatively safe water supply has been provided, civil strife or natural disasters can destroy in a matter of days or months the sewage treatment systems that took years to build. People in developed countries have come to take their clean water for granted, but they should not be so quick to conclude that water-borne diseases could never become a serious problem for them. Many modern cities

have aging water systems, and contamination by sewage is becoming more likely rather than less likely.

In the absence of a safe water supply in many parts of the world, the next best solution would be to develop a safe, cheap, and effective vaccine. Developing such a vaccine has long had a high priority in the world health community but has not received the sort of intensive support given to the search for vaccines against AIDS and hepatitis. This is due in part to the fact that the countries which can best afford to fund efforts to develop vaccines have come to consider themselves safe from cholera. It is true that cases of cholera are uncommon in developed countries and usually involve travelers from countries where cholera is a common disease. Nonetheless, *V. cholerae* persists in the environment in many areas of the world even where it is not currently a health problem. Thus, some future breach in sanitation facilities due to war or natural disasters such as hurricanes or floods could lead to cholera epidemics in parts of the world that have not experienced them in recent years. Unfortunately, the record of attempts by scientists to develop an effective vaccine has so far been a series of one failure after another. No one knows why.

Virulence Factors

Overview

The continuing search for an effective cholera vaccine has focused interest on the virulence factors of *V. cholerae*. Work on the molecular basis of virulence has been aided considerably by the fact that *V. cholerae* is close enough genetically to *Escherichia coli* that many of the genetic tools developed by scientists working on *E. coli* can be used in studies of *V. cholerae*. As a result, *V. cholerae* has proved to be an excellent model for studying bacterial colonization of mucosal surfaces and effects of toxin action on host cells. This is not to say that a full understanding of cholera has been achieved. In fact, if anything, recent research on how *V. cholerae* interacts with its human host has revealed how much more complex this interaction is than was previously assumed. The continued failure of efforts to develop an effective cholera vaccine that confers long-lasting immunity could be a sign that important aspects of the host-parasite interaction have been missed. In fact, recent research has tended to turn up new safety issues that have made the development of a safe vaccine seem even more elusive. An overview of virulence factors currently thought to play a role in the disease is given in Figure 25–2.

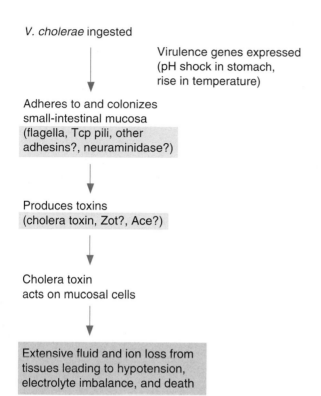

V. cholerae ingested

Virulence genes expressed
(pH shock in stomach,
rise in temperature)

Adheres to and colonizes
small-intestinal mucosa
(flagella, Tcp pili, other
adhesins?, neuraminidase?)

Produces toxins
(cholera toxin, Zot?, Ace?)

Cholera toxin
acts on mucosal cells

Extensive fluid and ion loss from
tissues leading to hypotension,
electrolyte imbalance, and death

Figure 25–2 Summary of main virulence factors thought to play a role in the pathogenesis of cholera. Virulence factors for which a role is suspected but not proven are indicated by (?).

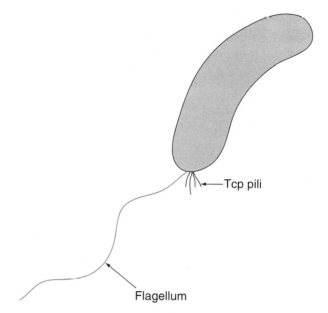

Figure 25–3 *V. cholerae* has a single flagellum and a bundle of Tcp pili (toxin-coregulated pili) located at one pole of the cell.

Colonization of the Small Intestinal Mucosa

MOTILITY AND CHEMOTAXIS. *V. cholerae* has a single polar flagellum (Figure 25–3). Evidence that flagellar motility may help *V. cholerae* reach the intestinal mucosa comes from the observation that nonmotile mutants are less virulent than wild type. The composition of the flagellum and the regulation of flagellar genes have now been analyzed in considerable detail, and some interesting features have been revealed. As was discovered previously for the flagella of *Helicobacter pylori* (chapter 23), the flagellum of *V. cholerae* is composed not of a single type of protein subunit but of multiple types of protein subunits.

The *V. cholerae* flagellum is even more complex than that of *H. pylori*. Whereas the flagellum of *H. pylori* consists of two types of protein subunits, the flagellum of *V. cholerae* consists of five protein subunit types. Granted, these subunits share high amino acid similarity, but they are encoded by different genes. Also, as was the case with the *H. pylori* flagellar genes, different *V. cholerae* flagellar genes are regulated differently. Three of them (*flaEDB*) are controlled by sigma factor σ^{28} and one (*flaA*) is controlled by sigma factor σ^{54}. Thus, as with *H. pylori,* subtle changes in relative levels of ex-

pression of the different genes could produce subtle but important changes in the properties of the flagellum. This is perhaps not surprising given that *V. cholerae* must move through both low-viscosity fluids (water) and high-viscosity fluids (mucus) at different stages in its existence in and out of the human body.

Little is known about chemotaxis or the signal(s) that guides *V. cholerae* to the mucosa. Most current research has focused instead on what happens when *V. cholerae* reaches the intestinal mucosa.

ADHERENCE. Long filamentous pili that form bundles at one end of the bacterium (Figure 25–3) make an important contribution to colonization of the intestinal mucosa. The pili have been called **Tcp pili** (for **toxin coregulated pili**) because genes encoding these pili are regulated similarly to genes encoding cholera toxin. Mutants lacking Tcp pili are avirulent in human volunteers. Not much is known about the interaction between Tcp pili and host cells; the host cell receptor for these pili has not yet been identified. Although Tcp pili are clearly an important virulence factor, purified Tcp pili do not bind to intestinal epithelial cells and thus may not mediate attachment to the mucosa. They may instead mediate bacterium-to-bacterium attachment, because bacteria producing Tcp pili aggregate.

Most research on Tcp pili has focused on the question of how pilin genes are organized and regulated and how pilin subunits are processed and assembled. Genes necessary for production of Tcp pili are organized in a cluster that contains 15 genes. One gene, *tcpA,* encodes the main pilin subunit. A second gene, *tcpB,* could encode a minor pilus structural protein, but studies of pilin binding suggest that the actual binding of the pilus to its target cell is mediated by the major pilin subunit, TcpA, and not by some minor subunit component. Three genes are involved in regulation of pilin gene expression, and at least four are involved in pilin secretion and assembly. These include *tcpC,* a gene that encodes an outer membrane protein of unknown function, and *tcpJ,* a gene that encodes a peptidase that cleaves the amino-terminal signal sequence from secreted TcpA. There is at least one gene, *tcpG,* that is located outside the gene cluster and may encode a chaperone (a protein that aids proper folding of secreted proteins). Apparently, the normal machinery for secretion and folding of most of the proteins destined for the periplasm or outer membrane is not sufficient for assembly and processing of Tcp pili, and bacteria producing these pili must provide the necessary accessory proteins as well as the basic pilin subunit proteins.

Except for *tcpG,* the *tcp* genes are clustered on what is now acknowledged to be a pathogenicity island. Also on this pathogenicity island are **accessory colonization factor** (*acf*) genes, which were earlier thought to encode an adhesin. It now appears that Acf is involved in the regulation of motility. Although the function of Acf in the infection process is still unclear, the presence of *acf* genes on the *tcp* pathogenicity island raises anew the question of whether Acf might not be more important than previously thought.

The pathogenicity island on which Tcp genes are carried is called **VPI** (*V. cholerae* pathogenicity island). This island has been shown to be the genome of yet another filamentous phage, called **VPIPhi.** TcpA turns out to be a coat protein of this virus. In addition to Tcp genes and the gene encoding a regulatory protein, ToxT (see later section), the phage also carries genes for Acf, two newly discovered regulatory proteins, **TcpP** and **TcpH,** which are activators of *toxT* expression, and **TcpI,** a negative regulatory protein. TcpP is the sensor and TcpH is the response regulator of a two-component system. The TcpP/H system is required for full expression of *tcp* genes.

Yet another interesting feature of the *tcp* pathogenicity island is that the Tcp pili have contributed to the further evolution of the virulence traits of *V. cholerae.* The Tcp pilus served as a receptor for the bacteriophage that introduced the genes encoding the subunits of cholera toxin (Box 25–1).

V. cholerae strains produce two surface proteins that agglutinate red blood cells (**hemagglutinins**). These have been named **mannose-sensitive** hemagglutinin and **mannose-fucose-resistant** hemagglutinin. The name mannose-sensitive comes from the fact that free mannose inhibits binding of the hemagglutinin to eukaryotic cells, indicating that surface molecules that contain mannose may be the receptor on the eukaryotic cell. The second hemagglutinin gets its name from the fact that neither mannose nor fucose inhibits binding. Neither of these hemagglutinins appears to have a major role in virulence, because deletions in these genes do not affect virulence of the bacteria in the infant mouse model. It is interesting that the mannose-sensitive hemagglutinin is the receptor for a filamentous bacteriophage from *V. cholerae* O139. The phage is not known to carry virulence genes, but the example of the Tcp pili and the CTX phage, which clearly had a significant effect on virulence, raises the possibility that this receptor and its phage might have some evolutionary significance, even if it is not associated with colonization of the human body.

Cholera Toxin

There is no question about the importance of cholera toxin as a virulence factor. This toxin is clearly responsible for most of the pathology seen in people with cholera. Naturally occurring strains or mutants of *V. cholerae* that do not produce cholera toxin do not cause the full-blown form of the disease, either in animals or in human volunteers. Such strains may, however, cause a milder form of diarrhea because of the presence of other toxins. Because of its importance as a virulence factor and its interesting mechanism, cholera toxin has been intensively studied at the biochemical and genetic levels, and it is currently one of the best understood of all the bacterial toxins. Cholera toxin is an A-B ADP-ribosylating toxin, which contains one A (enzymatic) subunit and five B (binding) subunits. The genes encoding the A subunit (*ctxA*) and the B subunit (*ctxB*) are part of the same operon (Figure 25–4A).

The excess of B protein over A protein is probably due to the fact that there are separate ribosome binding sites upstream of the two coding regions, and the site upstream of the B coding region is at least seven-fold stronger than the site upstream of the A coding region. Thus, *ctxB* mRNA is more actively translated than *ctxA* mRNA. The ratio of B subunits to A subunits produced during translation does not have to be precisely 5:1, because B subunit complexes (without any A portion) are excreted by the bacteria. Thus, the bacteria can rid themselves of excess B subunits. By contrast, the A subunit must be attached to five B subunits to be excreted. The 5:1 stoichiometry in the final form of the toxin is dictated by interactions between the B subunits and between the five B subunits and the A subunit, and not by relative

BOX 25–1   New Insights into the Evolution of Pathogenic *V. cholerae* Strains

Results of recent studies indicate that pandemic strains of *V. cholerae* did not develop in a gradual way but evolved by importing large chunks of DNA from an unknown source. As mentioned in the text, the first step in the evolution of the O1 strains seems to have been the acquisition by some ancestral strain of the Tcp pathogenicity island (see figure). The second step was acquisition of the cholera toxin genes via a filamentous phage, the CTX phage, which integrated into the *V. cholerae* chromosome. The finding that cholera toxin genes are located on a lysogenic phage was not particularly earthshaking, since many toxin genes have been found to be carried on lysogenic phages. What was unexpected, however, was that the Tcp pili were the receptors for this phage. Thus, importation of the cholera toxin genes via phage could only

occur after the bacteria had acquired the Tcp pathogenicity island. The O139 strain seems to have evolved by replacing a region of the genome that encoded the O1 antigen synthesis genes with a 35-kbp locus that encodes the biosynthetic genes for a different O antigen and a capsule (see text). Thus, horizontal gene transfer events involving pathogenicity islands and phages seem to be driving the evolution of epidemic strains of *V. cholerae*. This type of stepwise evolution of new strains has an ominous implication; evolution of a new strain of *V. cholerae* capable of causing cholera epidemics is easier for the bacteria than we thought.

Sources: F. Mooi and E. Bik. 1997. The evolution of epidemic *Vibrio cholerae* strains. *Trends Microbiol.* **5**:161–165; S. Richardson and D. Wozniak. 1996. An ace up the sleeve of the cholera bacterium. *Nat. Med.* **2**:853–855.

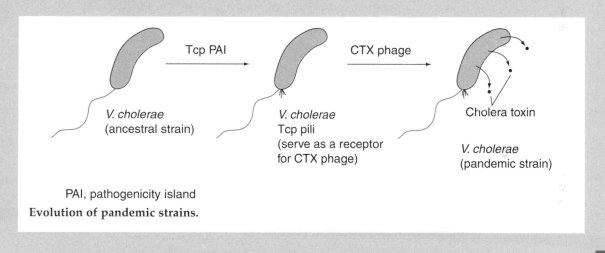

PAI, pathogenicity island

Evolution of pandemic strains.

amounts of B subunits and A subunits produced during translation (although it would obviously be wasteful for the bacterium to produce too large an excess of B subunits).

Translated A and B subunits are secreted into the periplasm, where the toxin subunits are assembled. The process by which the assembled toxin is excreted into the extracellular fluid is not well understood. An interesting finding is that excretion of the toxin requires TcpG, a chaperone that is also involved in assembly of Tcp pili. Thus, TcpG clearly has a role not only in pilus

formation but also in toxin release. Recall that the *tcpG* gene, unlike the other known *tcp* genes, is carried not on the Tcp island but on another part of the chromosome. This connection between the Tcp system, the toxin system, and a gene that is probably a *V. cholerae* housekeeping gene suggests that the Tcp pathogenicity island and the CTX phage came from a strain of *V. cholerae* or some species that is very closely related to *V. cholerae*.

Production of Tcp pili and toxin is coregulated at the transcriptional level (see below). The finding that TcpG

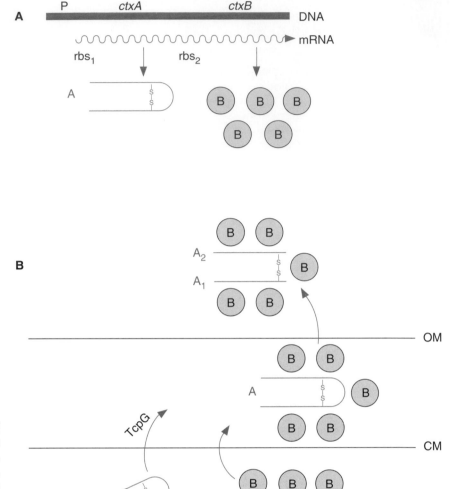

Figure 25–4 (**A**) Genetic structure of the *ctxAB* operon. *ctxA* encodes the ADP-ribosylating portion of the toxin, and *ctxB* encodes the binding subunit. (**B**) Assembly, excretion, and activation by nicking of cholera toxin. CM, cytoplasmic membrane; OM, outer membrane.

is involved in toxin excretion raises the possibility that these two processes are also linked at the posttranslational level. Intact A subunit is not enzymatically active but must be nicked to produce fragments A1 and A2, which are linked by a disulfide bond (Figure 25–4B). This nicking probably occurs after the toxin is released into the extracellular fluid.

Excreted toxin attaches to the surface of a host mucosal cell by binding to G_{M1} gangliosides. G_{M1} consists of a sialic acid-containing oligosaccharide covalently attached to a ceramide lipid (Figure 25–5). The lipid portion is embedded in the host cell membrane, and the oligosaccharide is exposed on the host cell surface. The oligosaccharide is the moiety recognized by the toxin B subunit. G_{M1} is found on the surfaces of many types of cells. Also found on many host cell surfaces are gangliosides with longer chains of sialic acid residues. *V. cholerae* secretes a **neuraminidase** (also called **sialidase**)

that removes sialic acid residues from these more complex oligosaccharides to make them structurally more similar to G_{M1}. It has been suggested that neuraminidase contributes to the virulence of *V. cholerae* by increasing the number of receptors available to bind cholera toxin. However, in animal tests, the effect of mutations affecting neuraminidase production was small (about 20% decrease in virulence associated with loss of neuraminidase).

Once cholera toxin is bound to G_{M1}, the A1 subunit is released from the toxin, presumably by reduction of the disulfide bond that links it to A2, and enters the host cell by an unknown translocation mechanism. There has been much speculation about this mechanism. One hypothesis, which was out of favor for awhile and has now resurfaced, is that the five B subunits insert themselves into the host cell membrane and form a pore through which the A1 subunit passes. This hypothesis

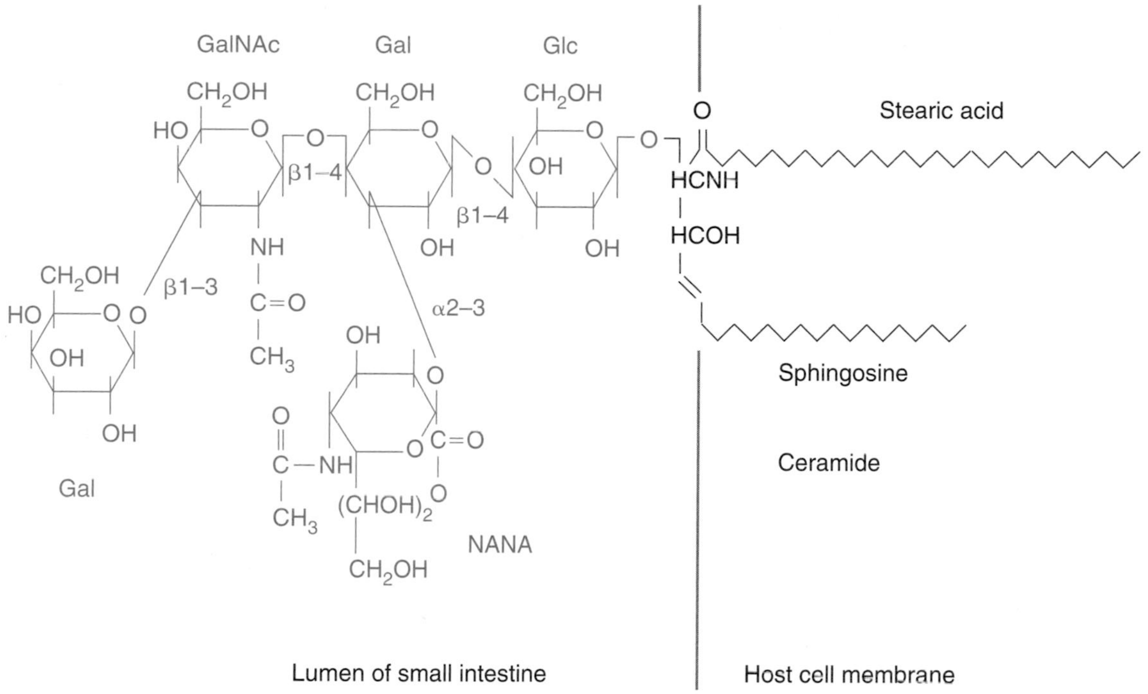

Figure 25–5 Cholera toxin binds to G_{M1} gangliosides. G_{M1} is a sialic acid residue linked to a ceramide lipid. Gal, galactose; GalNAc, *N*-acetylgalactosamine; Glc, glucose; NANA, *N*-acetylneuraminic acid (sialic acid). (From B. Spangler. 1992. Structure and function of cholera toxin and the related *Escherichia coli* heat-labile enterotoxin. *Microbiol. Rev.* **56:**622–647.)

is still controversial. Also, it is not clear whether bound cholera toxin must be taken up in endocytic vesicles for A1 to be translocated or if A1 can be translocated without endocytosis.

A great deal is known about the structure of cholera toxin; in fact, the crystal structure has been solved. This information has not yet provided much help in answering questions about how cholera toxin interacts with a host cell. Nor has it suggested any new hypotheses about translocation, although it has contributed to the revival of the B subunit pore hypothesis. The crystal structure has, however, provided an important basis for further investigations of how the A1 subunit is internalized. A challenge faced by people who solve and interpret crystal structures is how to extract from the structure of a molecule in solution clues as to how this structure alters when the molecule binds to its receptor and interacts with the hydrophobic environment of the membrane.

The A1 subunit of cholera toxin ADP-ribosylates a host cell membrane protein called G_s. A1 is capable of ADP-ribosylating other host cell proteins, but G_s appears to be the primary target. G_s is one of the family of GTP-hydrolyzing proteins (called **G proteins**) that regulate many aspects of eukaryotic cell function (Figure 25–6). G proteins are composed of three subunits ($G\alpha$, $G\beta$, and $G\gamma$). Association and disassociation of these subunits, together with hydrolysis of GTP, activate or deactivate the G protein (Figure 25–6). G_s is the G protein that regulates the activity of host cell **adenylate cyclase** in a hormone-dependent manner and thus determines the level of cAMP in host cells. The active (GTP-bound) form of G_s increases the activity of adenylate cyclase, whereas the inactive GDP-bound form renders adenylate cyclase inactive (Figure 25–6B). Normally, the active form is produced in response to hormonal stimulation and is converted to the inactive form after a short time. This on-off control ensures that cAMP (a regulatory molecule in eukaryotic cells) is produced at the levels needed to do its job but is not allowed to accumulate and thus disrupt the normal cell functions. ADP-ribosylation of G_s short-circuits this on-off control by locking G_s in the "on" form, so that cAMP levels are uncontrolled and rise to a high level. This has a variety of effects, the most important of which is that it alters the activities of sodium and chloride transporters. These alterations produce the ion imbalance that causes the water loss associated with cholera.

Early studies of cholera toxin action on mucosal cells were done with undifferentiated, nonpolarized tissue

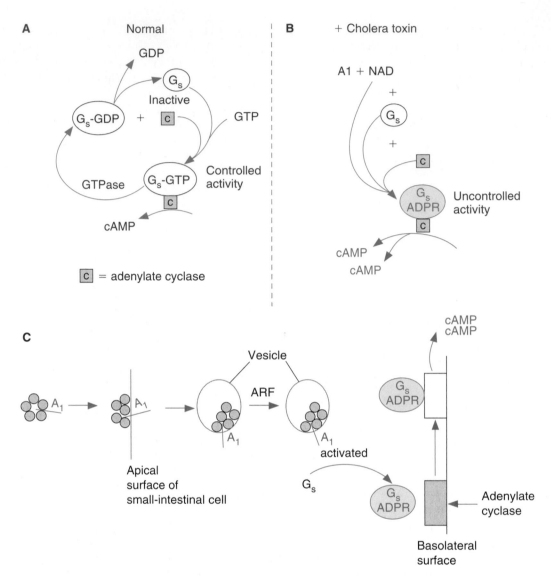

Figure 25–6 (**A**) Active and inactive forms of G proteins controlled by GTP binding and hydrolysis. (**B**) GTP-dependent G$_s$ control of adenylate cyclase by G$_s$ and effect of ADP-ribosylation of G$_s$ on adenylate cyclase activity. ADP-ribosylation (ADPR) of G$_s$ freezes adenylate cyclase in the active position so that cAMP continues to be made and levels of cAMP rise in the cell. (**C**) Model for endocytosis and transit of cholera toxin A1 subunit through the host cell. The point at which G$_s$ is ADP-ribosylated is not known, nor is it clear that the A1 subunit is actually associated with an endocytic vesicle. This model is an attempt to explain how the toxin gets from the apical surface of the host cell to its target, which is located on the basolateral surface. ADP-ribosylation factor (ARF)-mediated activation of A1 is also shown, but the point at which this happens in the host cell and its importance for A1 activity in vivo remain to be established.

culture cells. In these cells, adenylate cyclase is distributed over the entire surface of the cell. By contrast, adenylate cyclase in differentiated, polarized mucosal cells is actually located on the basolateral membrane (Figure 25–6C). Thus, cholera toxin bound to the apical surface of the mucosal cell must somehow exert its ef-

fect on a target located on the other side of the cell. A model for how this might occur is shown in Figure 25–6C. In this model, A1 is translocated through the host cell apical membrane but remains attached to an endocytic vesicle that carries it from the apical surface to the basolateral membrane where the adenylate cyclase is located. G_s is a membrane protein and is presumably found in the apical membrane, because signals are more likely to come from the apical side. If G_s is located in the apical membrane, A1 could ADP-ribosylate G_s at this point, followed by movement of ADP-ribosylated G_s through the mucosal cell to the adenylate cyclase located in the basolateral membrane. An alternative possibility is that G_s is actually located in the basolateral (not the apical) membrane and that A1, exposed on the cytoplasmic side of an endocytic vesicle, moves through the cell to contact G_s. Still another possibility is that both A1 and G_s are in an endocytic vesicle and A1 ADP-ribosylates G_s during transit of the vesicle through the cell. At this point, the only thing that is clear is that some sort of translocation must take place.

Whatever the order and cellular location of the steps that lead to the interaction of A1, G_s, and adenylate cyclase, the host cell is an active partner in the cholera toxin-host cell interaction and not simply a passive target of toxin action. That is, cholera toxin is able to exert an effect on mucosal cells only because it takes advantage of such normal host cell processes as signal transduction (G proteins) and movement of vesicles within the host cell. In other chapters, the production by bacteria of toxins and other compounds that subvert normal host cell processes to benefit the bacterium rather than the host is a recurring theme. Another way in which the hapless host cell may facilitate the action of cholera toxin was suggested recently. Eukaryotic cells produce a family of small G proteins (not to be confused with the signaling type of G proteins exemplified by G_s), which are called **ADP-ribosylation factors (ARFs)**. ARFs are thought to be involved in the traffic of proteins and membrane vesicles through the **Golgi system**. In vitro, the ADP-ribosylating activity of the A1 subunit is enhanced if it interacts with ARFs. Activation is GTP dependent and appears to result in a change in conformation of A1 that makes A1 more able to ADP-ribosylate G_s. There is no direct evidence to date for ARF activation in living cells, but the lack of evidence is unlikely to interfere with continued speculation about this very interesting possibility. Whether or not ARFs actually play a role in activating or stabilizing the A1 subunit inside the host cell, it is clear that the interaction between toxin and host cell is more complex than previously suspected.

Before we leave the subject of cholera toxin, it is worth mentioning a curious feature of mutants that do not produce cholera toxin. These mutants not only are unable to produce the symptoms of cholera but are also less able to colonize the small intestinal mucosa. Another pathogenic bacterium, *Bordetella pertussis*, which causes respiratory tract infections rather than intestinal infections, produces a toxin very similar to cholera toxin. The *B. pertussis* toxin (pertussis toxin) also appears to have a role in colonization. In fact, there is evidence that the toxin may be functioning as an adhesin as well as a toxin (see chapter 17). Virtually nothing is known about the role of cholera toxin in colonization (as opposed to production of symptoms), but it is possible that the toxin plays a role in colonization as well as in production of disease symptoms.

Other Toxins Produced by *V. cholerae*

Although cholera toxin is unquestionably the most important toxin produced by *V. cholerae*, some *V. cholerae* strains produce other toxins as well. Indications of this were first seen during early attempts to produce live vaccines by generating mutants of *V. cholerae* that produced B subunit but not active toxin. In theory, such a mutant would be a good vaccine because it contains all the desirable antigens needed to provoke a protective sIgA response against the B subunit that would prevent toxin binding to host cells. Also, such a mutant should not produce symptoms because it does not produce active cholera toxin. Yet one of the earliest toxin-negative mutants could not be used as a vaccine because it still caused diarrhea in human volunteers, although the diarrhea was much less severe than the diarrhea caused by wild type. This result indicated that the strain in which the mutation was made had another enterotoxin. Scientists hoped that the problem could be solved by making vaccine strains from strains that have no other enterotoxins, but so far no live vaccine strain has been developed that does not cause diarrhea. Obviously, there is a lot that remains to be learned about the potential of *V. cholerae* to cause diarrhea.

ZOT TOXIN. A gene has been cloned and characterized that encodes one *V. cholerae* enterotoxin. This toxin is unusual in that it affects the structure of the tight junctions (or **zonula occludens**) that bind mucosal cells together and preserve the integrity of the mucosal membrane. This was the first bacterial toxin shown to have such an effect. The tight junctions that bind mucosal cells together are so effective that even ions do not diffuse readily between mucosal cells. Thus, ion-specific pumps in mucosal cell membranes must transport ions, a feature that permits the flow of ions and water across the intestinal mucosa to be controlled and is responsible for the ability of the body to retain water. A toxin that disrupted these junctions would not only allow contents of the lumen to diffuse into underlying tissue but would also disrupt the ion balance and thereby cause diarrhea. This toxin has been called **Zot (zonula occlu-**

dens toxin). The *zot* gene lies immediately upstream of the *ctxA/B* operon on the CTX phage.

Zot may or may not play an important role in virulence, but even if Zot is not part of the disease problem, it could be part of the solution to making vaccines more effective. Zot has proved to be a powerful adjuvant for stimulating mucosal immunity. In this case, the tests involved intranasal delivery of the antigen (albumin).

ACE TOXIN. Another enterotoxin of *V. cholerae* has been named **Ace toxin (accessory cholera enterotoxin,** not to be confused with Acf). It produces fluid accumulation in the rabbit ileal loop model, a trait of many enterotoxins. This new toxin is unrelated to either cholera toxin or Zot toxin. Its role in human disease remains controversial. The *ace* gene is closely linked genetically to the *zot* gene and is part of the CTX phage.

Clearly, Zot and Ace do not make a major contribution to virulence, but at one point they were thought to be responsible for the mild diarrhea experienced by human volunteers given a vaccine strain of *V. cholerae* that had *ctxA* deleted. A strain from which this phage has been cured still caused diarrhea, however, so there must be still other toxin genes in the *V. cholerae* chromosome that are responsible for the mild diarrhea. The mild diarrhea has been a thorn in the side of scientists trying to develop a safe, effective cholera vaccine. Although adults living in cholera zones might be willing to tolerate such a side effect, the diarrhea could be a danger to infants, especially undernourished ones, who are more prone to dehydration during bouts of diarrhea.

The fact that *zot* and *ace* are located on the CTX phage raised the question of whether they might play some role in phage replication. Mutations that disrupt *zot*, *ace*, or *orfU* (another phage-encoded gene) abolished the ability of the phage to transfer to a new host. This was not true for the *ctx* genes. Scientists have long suspected that the phage-encoded genes we call toxin genes might actually be involved in the phage life cycle. The *zot* and *ace* genes seem to be the first examples of toxins that have a role in phage replication.

Gene Capture—a Role for Integrons

Scientists looking through the genome sequence of *V. cholerae* noticed a number of 123- to 126-bp direct repeats clustered in one segment of the *V. cholerae* genome. Those who work in the area of antibiotic resistance are familiar with integrons, which are elements that use a phage-type integrase to integrate circular gene cassettes into a specific site (usually less than 100 bp in length) so that an operonlike structure is created

(see chapter 11). The integron, in addition to providing an integrase and an integration site, also supplies a promoter that controls expression of the newly created operon.

The region in the *V. cholerae* genome that contains the 123- to 126-bp direct repeats looks very much like an integron that has acquired a number of genes. In this case, however, the genes were not antibiotic resistance genes but genes that might be involved in virulence. These include the gene for the mannose-fucose-resistant hemagglutinin and a gene that encodes a heat-stable enterotoxin. Neither of these genes has been proven to have a role in virulence, nor have other genes that might be part of this large operon been shown to have a function either in survival or virulence. Regardless of the true functions of the genes in this region, this discovery is important because it shows that integrons do not simply assemble antibiotic resistance genes but can assemble other genes into operons. Bacteria have many operons, but this type of genetic structure is rarely seen in archaea and eukaryotes. Is it possible that integronlike elements are responsible for the creation of many bacterial operons?

The Capsule of *V. cholerae* O139—a Difference, but Probably Not an Important One

The search for the differences between the O1 strains and the O139 strain has focused on one portion of the chromosome. This region, in the O1 strains, carries genes encoding the O1 antigen of *V. cholerae* LPS. In O139, a 22-kbp portion of this region is missing and has been replaced by a 35-kbp fragment that carries genes for synthesis of the new O antigen plus a capsule that is not found on the O1 strains. The capsule appears to be a polymer of the O139 antigen. It is doubtful that the capsule of strain O139 contributes to virulence. For one thing, O139 has the usual virulence factors of the O1 strains, such as Tcp pili and cholera toxin. For another, the DNA in this region has been found in a number of non-O1 strains, most of which appear to be nonvirulent or capable of causing only mild disease.

Antibiotic Resistance

One can question the relevance of antibiotic resistance genes in the case of *V. cholerae*. Antibiotics are usually not used to treat cases of cholera, although antibiotics can speed the resolution of the disease in some cases. Moreover, *V. cholerae*, unlike *Salmonella* species, does not cause the sort of invasive infections that become systemic and must be treated with antibiotics. Yet, the existence of antibiotic resistance genes in *V. cholerae* is of interest from an ecological point of view. Clearly, despite the absence of antibiotic selection, *V. cholerae* is acquiring antibiotic resistance genes. It would be interesting to know where these acquisition events occur.

A conjugative transposon, called the **STX element,** has been found in *V. cholerae* O139. The STX element carries genes for resistance to sulfonamide and trimethoprim, two antibiotics used widely—usually in combination—to treat a variety of human infections. There have been reports recently that some antibiotics survive wastewater treatment procedures, and that antibiotics are probably found in many freshwater and marine environments. Thus, *V. cholerae* may be experiencing its antibiotic selection pressure in the external environment rather than in the human body.

Transcriptional Regulation of Virulence Genes

Production of virulence factors by *V. cholerae* is regulated at multiple levels. These levels include duplication of the *ctxAB* region of the chromosome, regulation of virulence gene transcription, differential translation of *ctxA* and *ctxB* mRNA, activation of the A subunit by proteolytic nicking, and a possible ARF-mediated activation of A1 subunit inside the host cell. Regulation of *V. cholerae* virulence genes at the transcriptional level is the type of regulation that has received the most attention.

The ToxR/ToxS/ToxT Regulatory System

Transcription of the *ctxA/B* operon is affected by a number of environmental factors, including pH (transcription higher at pH 6 than at pH 8.5), certain amino acids, low osmolarity, and temperature (transcription higher at 30°C than at 37°C). As many as 20 other *V. cholerae* genes appear to be regulated similarly to *ctxA/B*. These include the *acf* and *tcp* genes as well as genes called ***tag*** (ToxT-activated genes) for which no function has been established. The fact that genes regulated similarly to *ctxA/B* are located in different places on the chromosome suggests that these genes are part of a regulon. Three proteins involved in controlling regulon expression are **ToxR, ToxS,** and **ToxT.** The genes encoding these proteins were cloned by taking advantage of the fact that the β-galactosidase activity of a *ctxA-lacZ* fusion was low in *E. coli*. Investigators transformed *E. coli* carrying the *ctxA-lacZ* fusion with cloned DNA fragments from the *V. cholerae* chromosome and looked for clones that increased β-galactosidase activity. The *toxR* and *toxS* genes were found as a result of this search.

ToxR is a 32-kDa protein that spans the cytoplasmic membrane. About two-thirds of the amino-terminal part of ToxR is exposed to the cytoplasm, and this portion contains the DNA-binding domain. ToxR monomers do not bind DNA and activate transcription. Only the dimer form is active; it recognizes a 7-bp repeated sequence upstream of the genes it regulates. ToxS, a 19-kDa periplasmic protein, acts to facilitate formation of ToxR dimers and stabilize them. Presumably, ToxS changes conformation in response to some sort of signal, and this change allows it to mediate dimer formation, but the precise nature of such an interaction is still undetermined. ToxR has an amino acid sequence similar to those of activator proteins from known phosphorylating-type two-component regulatory systems. Although no phosphorylation of ToxR has been detected, it is still possible that ToxR and ToxS form a standard two-component regulatory system and that the model in which ToxS activates ToxR by causing it to dimerize may not be entirely correct.

Expression of the *toxR/S* operon is itself regulated at the transcriptional level. Immediately upstream of this operon is a gene (***htpG***) that encodes a heat shock protein. Heat shock proteins are proteins produced at high levels when bacteria are exposed to high temperatures or to other forms of stress (e.g., low pH, changes in osmolarity). The *htpG* gene is transcribed divergently from *toxR/S* (Figure 25–7A), and its promoter region overlaps that of *toxR/S*. The lower level of *toxR/S* expression at 37°C could be due to increased expression of *htpG* because RNA polymerase binding and transcription from the strong *htpG* promoter would be expected to interfere with RNA polymerase transcription from the weaker *toxR/S* promoter.

A third regulatory gene has been identified on the basis of its ability to enhance expression of *ctxA-lacZ* fusions in *E. coli* in the absence of *toxR*. This gene, **toxT,** encodes a 32-kDa protein that has amino acid sequence similarity to a family of transcriptional activators. ToxT is a cytoplasmic protein. ToxR controls expression of *toxT* and the second two-component system made up of TcpP and TcpH (Figure 25–7B), and ToxT in turn activates expression of other genes, including *tcp* genes. The *toxT* gene is actually located within the *tcp* gene cluster, between *tcpF* and *tcpJ* on the Tcp pathogenicity island. This raises the possibility that ToxT originally evolved as part of the regulatory machinery for Tcp pili but was later recruited by the ToxR/ToxS system. However, the observation that some strains of *V. cholerae* that lack *ctx* genes altogether still have *toxR/S* raises the alternative possibility that ToxR/S/T originally evolved as controllers of a regulon that did not contain *ctx* and that *ctx* was recruited to become a member of this regulon. Some genes, such as the *tcp* genes and *acf* genes,

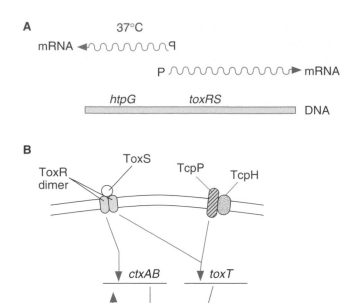

A

37°C

mRNA ◀◀◀◀◀◀◀◀ P

P ∿∿∿∿∿∿∿∿∿ ▶ mRNA

htpG   toxRS

DNA

B

ToxR
dimer
ToxS   TcpP   TcpH

ctxAB   toxT

A + B

ToxT

tcpA   Other virulence
genes

Pilin

Figure 25–7 (**A**) Regulation of *toxR/S* operon by *htpG*, a heat shock gene. Expression of *htpG* is enhanced at temperatures above 30°C and interferes with expression of the *toxR/S* operon, which is transcribed in the opposite direction from *htpG*. The promoters for *htpG* and *toxR/S* overlap. (**B**) ToxR/S, TcpP/H, and ToxT cascade of regulatory factors that control the ToxR/S regulon.

are activated directly by ToxT, but not by ToxR (i.e., ToxR does not bind to their operator regions but instead controls their synthesis indirectly by activating *toxT* expression). Other genes, such as *ctx*, are activated directly by ToxR. In the case of *ctxA/B*, ToxT participates along with ToxR in regulation of transcription, but how these two activators interact with the *ctxA/B* promoter-operator region is unknown.

Regulation in Response to Iron Levels

V. cholerae produces two types of iron-sequestering surface proteins, a siderophore binding protein and a receptor that binds hemin and hemoglobin. Not surprisingly, the genes involved in iron sequestration are regulated and are produced at highest level in low-iron medium. Other genes regulated by iron include *irgA*, a

gene of unknown function that is required for virulence of *V. cholerae* in newborn mice, and a gene that encodes a hemolysin. It is tempting to speculate that the hemolysin acts to free iron by lysing host cells and thus acts in concert with the iron-sequestering surface receptors. The iron-sequestration genes of *E. coli* are regulated in response to iron by a repressor, Fur (Fe utilization repressor). In *V. cholerae* a Fur-like repressor appears to be responsible for repressing transcription of *irgA* and the hemolysin gene and may also regulate other genes involved in iron acquisition.

Prevention and Treatment

Oral Rehydration Therapy

Because loss of water and electrolytes is what causes the death of cholera victims, replacement of fluids is an immediate goal. In people who are conscious and do not yet exhibit symptoms of extreme dehydration, oral rehydration therapy is used. The patient lies on a "cholera cot," which has a drain located under the patient's buttocks. The amount of liquid being excreted is measured, and the person is made to drink at least that same volume of liquid. This works because the small intestine and colon can still take up liquids, even though the small intestine is having trouble retaining water. The problem is that the body is losing liquid faster than it is being taken up. If enough liquid is consumed, net body water can be maintained at a sufficient level for the person to survive the disease.

Oral rehydration solution consists of a mixture of salts and glucose in water. Water alone does not work. The salts are needed for proper osmolarity, and glucose stimulates uptake of salts and water by mucosal cells. A prepackaged mixture of salts and glucose is now available but is too expensive for wide distribution in some developing countries. Accordingly, recipes have been devised that use materials found in households worldwide. A problem confronted by people creating these recipes was what to use as the measure of volume. One early solution to the problem was to use the ubiquitous Coke bottle as a standard volume.

In countries where antibiotics are readily available and affordable, antibiotics can be given to hasten the clearing of the bacteria and prevent more toxin production, but until the intestinal cells which have been attacked by cholera toxin are sloughed and replaced by healthy cells, the diarrhea will persist. Thus, oral rehydration therapy must be given even if antibiotics are being used and must be continued for days. The hardest cases of cholera to treat are those in which the disease has advanced to the point where the person is comatose and is exhibiting extreme dehydration. In such cases, rehydration by intravenous solutions is needed.

The Frustrating Search for a Safe and Effective Cholera Vaccine

The first recorded attempt to develop a vaccine against cholera took place in the late 1880s. This vaccine, which consisted of whole killed bacteria and was injected into the bloodstream, failed to elicit protective immunity. There is today a cholera vaccine, similar to this earlier vaccine, which is injected. It is not completely ineffective but confers only short-term immunity. Current understanding of the importance of an sIgA response in preventing colonization of mucosal surfaces makes a move away from an injected vaccine understandable. Also, because *V. cholerae* has a potent endotoxin, an injected vaccine could well have toxic side effects. An even more serious argument against an injected vaccine is the potential for spreading blood-borne infections such as AIDS, especially in countries where cost considerations dictate that the same needle be used to inoculate many different individuals. To obtain a good sIgA response and to avoid problems associated with injected vaccines, most recent efforts to develop a cholera vaccine have focused on oral vaccines.

Two types of oral cholera vaccine have been tested in large field trials in countries with a history of cholera epidemics. One consists of killed whole bacteria plus purified B subunit of cholera toxin. Initial protection rates were over 60%, better than those of previous vaccines. Early results of studies comparing the vaccine with and without added B subunit indicated that the vaccine might be equally effective without the added B subunit. This was good news because the purified B subunit component substantially raises the cost of the vaccine. A drawback with this particular vaccine formulation is that it gives much lower rates of protection in infants and children than in adults. Because infants and small children are the groups with the highest fatality rates, this is an undesirable property. The second type of oral vaccine is a live vaccine in which the *ctxA* gene has been inactivated by insertional mutagenesis, but the B subunit is still produced. This vaccine too has failed.

One safety concern about the more effective live vaccines has already been mentioned: they cause diarrhea that is mild in adults but might not be so innocuous in infants. Ironically, recent studies of virulence properties not only have failed to suggest any new vaccine strategies but have actually raised new safety concerns about the live cholera vaccine. First, the finding that the cholera toxin genes are carried on a lysogenic phage has raised the possibility that the vaccine strain could reacquire cholera toxin genes because of phage infection and become virulent. Eliminating the phage and its integration site would help solve this potential safety problem. A second safety issue was suggested by the finding that an integron may be recruiting new genes that might be virulence genes. This concern is less pressing since no role in virulence has been proved for any of the genes recruited by the putative integron. Yet, removing the integrase gene and thus inactivating the integron would be prudent.

The failure to find a safe, effective vaccine against cholera has been terribly frustrating to scientists dedicated to this aim. This failure is all the more galling in view of the vaccine successes in other areas that are much less highly developed, for example, the new, highly successful safe vaccine against meningitis caused by *Haemophilus influenzae*. At least the people working on the cholera vaccine have companions in misery. The search for a vaccine against *Salmonella typhimurium* and the pathogenic *E. coli* strains has been equally frustrating despite a high level of scientific development in the area and the large number of scientists working on the problem.

Future Directions

Historically, studies of *V. cholerae* have provided a wealth of new information about interactions between bacteria and mammalian cells. Scientists interested in *V. cholerae* developed the concept of a regulon. The concept of operon—genes arranged in tandem under the control of a single promoter—was well established, but work on *V. cholerae* that suggested an expansion of this concept to the notion that multiple genes and operons, in different parts of the chromosome, could be regulated by a few regulatory proteins (e.g., ToxRS, ToxT) was a new concept. The idea of the regulon—many genes controlled by central regulators—was born and has proved to be applicable to many other bacterial systems.

Cholera toxin has proved to be a valuable reagent for studies of eukaryotic cell signal transduction. Nevertheless, important questions still need to be answered. A prime question is, what is the true role of cholera toxin? It is produced optimally at temperatures lower than 37°C, indicating that it might play a role outside the human body. A relative of *V. cholerae*, *Vibrio fischeri*, can colonize a marine invertebrate, the small squid *Euprymna scolopes*. *V. fischeri* produces an ADP-ribosylating enzyme of unknown function. Could this be an analog of cholera toxin, and, if so, might cholera toxin play a role in colonization of the marine invertebrates or eukaryotic microbes with which *V. cholerae* is associated in the external environment? The larger question of what features of *V. cholerae* help it to survive in its normal setting in the environment also looms. There is a practical value to understanding better the association between *V. cholerae* and its normal hosts, the phytoplankton and marine invertebrates. People have observed, for example, that algal blooms often precede an outbreak of cholera. If this is truly a cause-and-effect relationship, knowing about it in more detail could help to predict outbreaks in time to prevent them.

Many questions remain to be answered about the interaction between *V. cholerae* and human cells. It is interesting that transcription of a heat shock protein controls transcription of *toxR/S*. The heat shock response is generally viewed as a stress response, and the fact that it is triggered when bacteria try to colonize the human body may indicate that the bacteria are none too happy in their accidental host. This raises the question of the role, if any, of the stress responses of *V. cholerae* in disease. More fundamentally, what signals is ToxR/S sensing? And how does this unusual two-component system function in response to signals? Further attempts to answer these and other questions may well usher in a new explosion of discoveries in this field.

SELECTED READINGS

Colwell, R. R. 1996. Global climate and infectious disease: the cholera paradigm. *Science* **274:**2025–2031.

Faruque, S., M. Albert, and J. Mekalanos. 1998. Epidemiology, genetics and ecology of toxigenic *Vibrio cholerae*. *Microbiol. Mol. Biol. Rev.* **62:**1301–1314.

Finkelstein, R. 2000. Personal reflections on cholera: the impact of serendipity. *ASM News* **66:**663–667. (An impressively modest historical reminiscence from the discoverer of cholera toxin.)

Jouravleva, E., G. McDonald, J. Marsh, R. Taylor, M. Boesman-Finkelstein, and R. Finkelstein. 1998. The *Vibrio cholerae* mannose-sensitive hemagglutinin is the receptor for a filamentous bacteriophage from *V. cholerae* O139. *Infect. Immun.* **66:**2535–2539.

Karaolis, D. K., S. Somara, D. Maneval, J. Johnson, and J. B. Kaper. 1999. A bacteriophage encoding a pathogenicity island, a type-IV pilus and a phage receptor in cholera bacteria. *Nature* **399:**375–379.

Klose, K., and J. Mekalanos. 1998. Differential regulation of multiple flagellins in *Vibrio cholerae*. *J. Bacteriol.* **180:** 303–316.

Manning, P., C. Clark, and T. Focareta. 1999. Gene capture in *Vibrio cholerae*. *Trends Microbiol.* **7:**93–95.

Marinaro, M., A. Di Tommaso, S. Uzzau, A. Fasano, and M. De Magistris. 1999. Zonula occludens toxin is a powerful mucosal adjuvant for intranasally delivered antigens. *Infect. Immun.* **67:**1287–1291.

Yu, R., and V. DiRita. 1999. Analysis of an autoregulatory loop controlling ToxT, cholera toxin, and toxin-coregulated pilus production in *Vibrio cholerae*. *J. Bacteriol.* **181:**2584–2592.

Thinking Out of the Box

There is an interesting beneficial relationship between a bacterium closely related to *V. cholerae*—*V. fischeri*—and a tiny squid found in the shallow water off the coast of Hawaii (*E. scolopes*). *V. fischeri* is a luminescent bacterium that lives in the light organ of the squid and protects it from predators. The surprising thing is that many of the "virulence factors" of *V. cholerae* are proving to be "colonization factors" for *V. fischeri*. For more on this interesting story, check the Internet for the primary references or turn to A. A. Salyers and D. D. Whitt. 2001. *Microbiology: Diversity, Disease, and the Environment*. Fitzgerald Science Press, Bethesda, Md.

Fiction

Infectious diseases, surprisingly, have not often inspired writers of novels to include their catastrophic consequences in a work of fiction. One exception is *The Painted Veil* by Somerset Maugham, a must-read book for cholera aficionados. In this novel, the protagonist, a microbiologist, discovers that his wife has been unfaithful and in retaliation takes her with him into the center of a cholera epidemic. The authors of this text definitely do not recommend this as a way to deal with infidelity, and cholera is the backdrop, not a major player in the novel. Yet this novel shows how microbiologists have been involved in epidemics and demonstrates the courage of microbiologists who stepped into the maelstrom of conditions that could kill them, to try to reduce human death and suffering (except that of unfaithful spouses, of course).

Characteristics of *V. cholerae*

Motile, gram-negative, curved rod

Single polar flagellum

Associated with algae and marine invertebrates in external environment

Serotyped on basis of O antigens; O1 strains most virulent until O139

Disease—cholera

Acquired by ingestion of contaminated water

Major pandemics throughout history

Characterized by prolific diarrhea

Virulence factors

Colonization of intestinal mucosa
    Polar flagellum provides motility
        Consists of five types of protein subunits
        Genes of different proteins regulated differently
    Tcp pili
        Cluster at one end of bacterium
        Coregulated with cholera toxin
        Cluster of 15 genes necessary for production of pili; make up pathogenicity island
            Two genes encode major (TcpA) and minor (TcpB) pilin proteins
            Three genes involved in regulation
            Four genes involved in pilin secretion and assembly
        Serve as receptor for bacteriophage (CTX) encoding subunits of cholera toxin

Cholera toxin
    A-B ADP-ribosylating toxin
        One A subunit; five B subunits
        Genes (*ctxA,B*) in an operon
    Subunits assembled in periplasm
    Attaches to G_{M1} gangliosides of host mucosal cells
    A subunit nicked for activity; A1 portion translocated into host cell
        A1 ADP-ribosylates G_s (membrane protein)
        A1 may interact with ARFs
        cAMP levels no longer controlled
            Activities of sodium and chloride transporters altered
            Massive fluid and electrolyte loss occurs
        Host cell actively participates in action of toxin
    May play role in colonization

Other toxins
    Zot—loosens tight junction between epithelial cells; gene located on CTX phage
    Ace—role in disease unknown; part of CTX phage

Capsule
    Present in O139 strain but not O1
    Polymer of the O139 antigen
    May not have role in virulence

Antibiotic resistance—probably not important in disease because antibiotics rarely used

(continued)

SUMMARY OUTLINE (*continued*)

Transcriptional regulation of virulence genes

ToxR/S/T regulatory system
  ToxS facilitates formation of ToxR dimers
  ToxR dimer plus ToxS may be two-component regulatory system
  toxR/S expression may be decreased because of *htpG* expression
  ToxR and TcpP plus TcpH control expression of *toxT*
  ToxT and ToxR regulate expression of *ctxA/B*

Iron regulation—Fur-like system
  Siderophores, siderophore receptor
  Receptor that binds hemin and hemoglobin
  Hemolysin

Prevention and treatment

Oral rehydration therapy—salts and glucose in water

Occasionally antibiotics used

Vaccine
  Oral vaccine is necessary
  No real success yet

QUESTIONS

Answers to the questions can be found in Appendix 2.

1. Explain why cholera epidemics are often associated with floods or typhoons. What is the significance of the fact that non-O1 strains appear capable of causing cholera?

2. *V. cholerae* dies rapidly under conditions such as those found in the human stomach (low pH, proteases). How is it able to cause infection in the small intestine?

3. Make an educated guess as to why *V. cholerae* does not cause systemic disease the way so many other diarrheal pathogens do.

4. Why does A subunit have to be cleaved by a protease in order to become active? That is, what is the advantage of having A1 connected to the rest of the toxin only by a disulfide bond and not by peptide bonds as well?

5. Why is it important that B subunits without an attached A subunit are excreted by the bacteria?

6. List the ways in which cholera toxin uses host cell molecules against the host cell.

7. Question 6 and the text of this chapter treat the host cell as the hapless victim of bacterial subversion. Can you make an argument for why interactions between host cell and toxin might actually have evolved as a form of host defense? (This seems an unlikely hypothesis, but for completeness it should be entertained.)

8. How can the fact that *ctxA/B* expression is controlled by so many apparently unlinked environmental factors be explained?

9. It was noted in the text that *toxR/toxS* is actually downregulated in response to temperature. That is, expression is *lower* at 37°C than at 30°C. How can this be explained? What are the implications of this?

10. Why would a live vaccine be expected to generate a higher degree of immunity than a vaccine consisting of killed bacteria? What are some safety criticisms that could be made of the live vaccine strain?

11. Some scientists are beginning to suspect that at least some of the so-called "virulence factors" of *V. cholerae* are actually designed to promote survival of the bacteria in the external environment. Why would this question arise in the first place, and how might some of these factors promote survival in the environment?

26

Salmonella Species

KEY FEATURES

Salmonella **Species**

CHARACTERISTICS

Gram-negative rod

Motile

DISEASES

Typhoid fever—*S. typhi*

Gastroenteritis—*S. typhimurium*

RESERVOIRS

Human carriers (especially asymptomatic carriers)—*S. typhi, S. typhimurium*

Livestock animals, reptiles—*S. typhimurium*

MAJOR VIRULENCE FACTORS

S. typhimurium: acid tolerance response; adhesins; invasion of mucosal cells (ruffling); survival in unactivated macrophages; LPS

S. typhi: capsule—Vi antigen; others not well understood

PREVENTION AND TREATMENT

S. typhimurium: proper food handling; antibiotics—cases of systemic disease; no effective vaccine

S. typhi: antibiotics; vaccine available

Salmonella Species and Serogroups

The clinical importance of *Salmonella* was recognized long before modern methods of species identification based on DNA-DNA homology or 16S rRNA sequences were developed. As a result of medical interest in this genus and the discovery of serotyping as a way to identify bacterial groups, there has been a proliferation of *Salmonella* serogroups, which until recently were all given different species names. The result was a nomenclatural nightmare. In an attempt to bring some order into this chaos, the taxonomists suggested that there should be only two species of *Salmonella*—*Salmonella enterica* and *Salmonella bongori*—and that all of the groups previously designated as disease-causing species, such as *Salmonella typhimurium* (a common cause of diarrhea) and *Salmonella typhi* (the cause of typhoid fever), should now be designated *S. enterica* serovar Typhimurium and *S. enterica* serovar Typhi. Many microbiologists who work with *Salmonella* consider this nomenclatural "cure" to be almost as bad as the original disease and have blithely ignored the new nomenclature in favor of the old one with which they are familiar—unless journal editors force them to conform. We too will use the old terminology, for the sake of simplicity and familiarity. See Box 26–1 for a description of a new species of *Salmonella*.

Salmonella strains are gram-negative, facultative, motile rods. Today, *Salmonella*, *Escherichia coli*, *Shigella* sp., and possibly *Yersinia* sp. would all be placed in the same genus. Given this, it is not surprising that the virulence factors identified by scientists working on these different organisms have proved to be very similar, despite the variety of localized and systemic infections that members of these species cause. *Salmonella* strains can cause either localized gastroenteritis or a systemic infection that leads to septic shock. *S. typhimurium* is one of the most common causes of diarrhea. Until recently, however, there were no good estimates of the total number of cases of *S. typhimurium* gastroenteritis in the United States, nor was it clear whether the rate of infection was increasing or decreasing. The CDC, an agency which has done an outstanding job of documenting and tracing large outbreaks of salmonellosis, has only recently been given the resources to track salmonellosis on a wider scale.

In the late 1990s, the CDC recruited a number of laboratories across the United States to monitor and catalog cases of salmonellosis in their areas. Of course, there are many cases that will never be brought to their attention because disease caused by *S. typhimurium* is usually self-limiting, and symptoms subside after several days. Many people with the disease do not even visit a physician, and even if they do, physicians may not bother with the paperwork needed to report the case. Nonetheless, the CDC monitoring system will provide the most accurate estimates now possible of the incidence of this very common disease.

Diseases Caused by *Salmonella* Species

S. typhimurium

S. typhimurium is transmitted by contaminated food, usually by poultry meat or eggs, although as will be explained shortly, there are other modes of transmission. Some farm practices have inadvertently increased carriage of *S. typhimurium* by farm animals. For example, the use of protein supplements in animal feed to increase weight gain has helped to increase the likelihood of *S. typhimurium* colonization of the animal's in-

---

BOX 26–1   *Salmonella* as a Reward

*S*almonella has served many purposes. It has been used as a model organism for studying bacterial metabolism and genetics and has provided many new insights into bacterial virulence. As a major source of food-borne disease, it serves as an indicator of how safe a country's food and water supplies are. It is the basis for many of the new oral vaccines. And now, believe it or not, someone has come up with a new use for *Salmonella*—as a means of honoring an admired public figure. Shortly after Michael Jordan announced his impending retirement from basketball, Stanford Shulman, chief of infectious diseases at a Chicago, Ill., hospital, announced that he was naming a new strain of *S. typhimurium* he had discovered after Michael Jordan: *Salmonella mjordan*. We will probably never know whether Michael Jordan, in his heart of hearts, felt honored by having a strain of diarrhea-causing bacteria named after him (would you?). One wonders how Mr. Jordan will represent this honor in his trophy room (if he has one). And how will the Basketball Hall of Fame handle it? Just keep it away from the snack bar, guys.

Source: USA Today, October 1993, Sports People section.

---

testinal tract. *S. typhimurium* can also be spread from one animal to another. Adult farm animals colonized with *S. typhimurium* usually do not appear to be ill, so it is difficult to identify colonized animals without resorting to expensive and time-consuming tests. During slaughter, the bacteria from the intestine of a colonized animal can easily contaminate the carcass and enter the food supply.

Eggs can be contaminated on the outside or the inside of the shell. If eggs that have been contaminated with salmonellae are left at room temperature for long periods of time, the bacteria have a chance to increase in number; this increase is not accompanied by changes in smell or appearance of the white or yolk. Anyone who likes raw eggs (e.g., in traditional Caesar salad dressing) or undercooked eggs (e.g., in egg-thickened sauces) is well advised to refrigerate eggs immediately after purchase. Farmers and the food processing industry are making every effort to reduce the level of *S. typhimurium* contamination, but there will never be a 100% guarantee of *Salmonella*-free food.

Symptoms of gastroenteritis appear within 6 to 24 h after ingestion of contaminated food or water and last as long as a week. Initial symptoms include nausea and vomiting, which subside after a few hours. These symptoms are followed by abdominal pain, diarrhea, and sometimes fever. The severity of the pain and diarrhea vary widely from one person to another, ranging from mild pain and barely detectable diarrhea to pain resembling appendicitis and severe, even bloody, diarrhea. After the symptoms subside, the infected person will continue to excrete bacteria for up to 3 months. In a small percentage of cases (1 to 3%), an infected person can continue to shed the bacteria for over a year (chronic carrier). Most cases of gastroenteritis occur in children under 10; symptoms tend to be most severe in this age group.

People commonly treat diarrhea as something of a joke—if they do not have it themselves—but *S. typhi murium* intestinal infections can turn ugly. In a small fraction of infected people, the bacteria can enter the bloodstream and cause septic shock. This is most likely to happen in immunocompromised people and the elderly, but cases of systemic disease are also seen in otherwise healthy people. The more common salmonellosis becomes, the more such serious cases will occur. Thus, preventing salmonellosis by monitoring the food supply and educating the public about proper handling of foods is clearly a good public health investment.

Although *S. typhimurium* infections have been associated primarily with chickens and chicken products, past experience has shown that infection can come from unexpected sources. During the 1950s and 1960s, when small turtles were favored pets for children, many cases of *S. typhimurium* infections were acquired by children from the turtles. Most reptiles are colonized with *S. typhimurium* or other serotypes capable of causing disease, so think twice about getting too chummy with your iguana. More recently, there have been outbreaks associated with smoked pork and even with chocolate. Is nothing sacred?

One of the largest outbreaks of salmonellosis ever documented occurred in Illinois and surrounding states in 1987. There were over 300,000 cases. This outbreak was unusual in that it was caused by contaminated milk. Pasteurization kills *S. typhimurium,* so milk seems an unlikely vehicle for the spread of salmonellosis. In this case, however, the milk was probably contaminated after it had been pasteurized; a faulty valve allowed backflow from the sewage lines into the milk that was about to be packaged for shipment. During this outbreak, some children developed systemic salmonellosis. In 1994, a smaller outbreak occurred in Minnesota and Wisconsin. This time, the cause of the outbreak was contaminated ice cream. A container truck carrying a raw egg mixture used in the preparation of the ice cream was insufficiently decontaminated before it was loaded with the pasteurized liquid ice cream mix that was destined to be frozen and whipped into the final ice cream product. Many other outbreaks of salmonellosis occurred during this same time, but these two outbreaks illustrate the fact that unexpected foods can transmit *S. typhimurium*.

An even more unusual route of transmission was responsible for a small outbreak of salmonellosis that occurred in Steubenville, Ohio, in 1981. The pattern of cases at first stumped the epidemiologist brought in to figure out what had happened. In most outbreaks, people of all ages are affected. In this case, virtually all of the cases involved young adults in the 20- to 30-year age group. Although they knew each other and occasionally socialized, there was no obvious food source that would explain the cases that had occurred. After exhausting all other possibilities, the epidemiologist finally hit on the substance responsible for the outbreak—marijuana. The epidemiologist speculated that the marijuana had probably been cut with dried cattle dung, but whatever the source of the contamination, there was a high enough concentration of *S. typhimurium* in the marijuana samples he tested to infect people who handled the drug and rolled it into cigarettes. (For a fascinating account of this bizarre case, see an article by Berton Roueche in the August 3, 1984, issue of the *New Yorker* magazine.)

S. typhi

S. typhi is a more serious pathogen than *S. typhimurium* in the sense that it is far more likely to cause life-threatening systemic infections. The disease caused by *S. typhi* is called typhoid fever. In the past, *S. typhi* caused many deaths worldwide, and it still causes many deaths in developing countries. Although many people will become very ill or die during an outbreak of typhoid fever, there are always people who become colonized with the bacteria and never experience symptoms. Or they survive the infection but remain colonized after recovery. These asymptomatic carriers are the main spreaders of typhoid fever.

The incubation period for *S. typhi* is longer than that for *S. typhimurium,* ranging from a week to as long as a month after initial ingestion of the bacteria. The bacteria multiply in spleen and liver, and large numbers of bacteria are then released into the bloodstream. This stage of the disease, which can last for 2 to 3 weeks, is characterized by a high fever, a flushed appearance, and anorexia. Chills, convulsions, and delirium can also occur. The bacteria move from the liver to the gall bladder and are shed in bile back into the intestine. Severe ulceration of the intestinal mucosa may occur at this point. An infection that proceeds to this stage is likely to be fatal.

In some people, *S. typhi* persists in the gallbladder, and these people can shed bacteria in their feces for years. Such chronic carriers are a major public health problem, especially when they are employed as food handlers. The classic case of such a chronic carrier was, of course, Typhoid Mary, a New York City cook in the early 1900s. By tracing a number of typhoid cases back to their probable source, health officials first identified Mary Mallon as the carrier who had caused several outbreaks. She was offered a gallbladder operation as a way of eliminating her carriage of the bacteria. (Antibiotics had not yet been discovered, so an operation was the only feasible solution to carrier status. Also, operations were a lot riskier because of postsurgical infections.) When she refused the operation, she was imprisoned for 3 years. She was then released, after promising not to cook for others. Apparently, she did not take the allegations about her carrier status very seriously, because she changed her name and resumed her profession as a cook. She was employed by hotels, restaurants, and even a hospital. She managed to spread typhoid fever to many more people before she was finally apprehended. After her second apprehension, she was imprisoned again, this time for the remainder of her life.

Virulence Factors

Animal Models

Although most animals that carry *S. typhimurium* do not show any signs of disease, *S. typhimurium* can cause disease in some nonhuman animals. The rhesus monkey is the animal that most closely resembles humans in its response to *S. typhimurium* infection. The guinea pig model also seems to be a close mimic of the disease in humans. Yet, these are not the models most investigators use. For reasons of convenience and cost, most investigators use mice as the animal model. The problem with mice as a model is that mice develop a fatal systemic form of the infection that is actually more similar to human typhoid fever than to gastroenteritis. In fact, the name "typhimurium" comes from the observation that the bacteria cause a *typhi*-like infection in mice.

This same objection can be raised in connection with a new animal model, the nematode *Caenorhabditis elegans*, which was first introduced by the scientists who

work on *Pseudomonas aeruginosa* and quickly taken up by those working on other bacterial pathogens. When *C. elegans* is fed *S. typhimurium*, it develops a systemic infection that is usually fatal. This is not surprising in view of the fact that the nematode does not have a mammalian-type immune system. Why *S. typhimurium* kills mice is less clear.

This is not to say that it is inappropriate to use mice or nematodes as animal models. There are many reasons for using these models. In the case of mice, a number of transgenic animals are now available that provide scientists with a highly effective way of probing the effect of specific genetic changes on the host-parasite interaction. In the case of *C. elegans*, there are also many well-characterized mutants that can be used in the same manner. Also, it is a lot cheaper and easier to maintain a nematode colony than to work with the number of mice sometimes needed to obtain statistical significance in comparisons of LD_{50} values. Moreover, increasingly onerous regulations on the care and handling of mice have forced some investigators to look elsewhere for an animal model. The regulatory situation is equally bad in the case of guinea pigs and is much worse in the case of primates.

The answer to the question of what animal model is appropriate eventually comes down to the nature of the question being asked. For most current pathogenesis research, mice are completely acceptable. Whether *C. elegans* is equally useful or just another flash in the pan remains to be seen. The nematode model will certainly be of interest in connection with the ability of the bacteria to damage eukaryotic cells when there is no immune system in the way.

S. typhi, in contrast to *S. typhimurium*, seems to be a human-specific pathogen. It does not cause disease in mice or any other nonhuman animal so far tested. This means that human volunteers have to be used for in vivo experiments. Such experiments are, for obvious reasons, complicated by a variety of regulations and ethical considerations. For the most part, human volunteers have been used primarily in trials of vaccines. Having an animal model for *S. typhi* infection would be a major step forward. For an approach to trying to get *S. typhi* to infect mice, see Box 26–2.

Overview of the Disease Process

The usual textbook description of salmonellosis states that the bacteria adhere to the ileum, that portion of the small intestinal mucosa that is nearest the ileocecal valve, and enter the body through M cells. Careful histopathological studies of the progression of disease in rhesus monkeys and guinea pigs, however, make it

BOX 26–2   Creating Chimeras as a Means of Scanning Large Chunks of a Genome for Virulence Traits

Traditionally, scientists taking a genetic approach to learning about how bacteria cause disease have looked for virulence factors by searching for individual genes or small gene clusters that are important for virulence. Even the pathogenicity islands and virulence plasmids are generally less than 100 kbp in size, a small fraction of the chromosome. In the case of a pathogen such as *Salmonella*, this approach may not work to answer some questions because the number of genes involved in virulence is so large. Results of transposon mutagenesis screens indicate that at least 4% of the *S. typhimurium* chromosome is occupied by genes needed to cause infection in mice. Although 4% may seem small at first glance, it represents hundreds of kilobase pairs in a bacterium with a chromosome size of more than 5 Mbp. Also, the genes needed for virulence are probably scattered over the chromosome. Comparisons of the genome sequences of *S. typhimurium* and *S. typhi*, for example, have so far revealed at least 50 regions of difference that are larger than an open reading frame, and these were found in many different parts of the chromosome.

Taking these findings into consideration, scientists interested in answering the question of why *S. typhi* does not infect mice decided to take a different approach. They wanted to introduce large fragments of the *S. typhimurium* chromosome into *S. typhi*, creating a *typhi-typhimurium* hybrid that was capable of infecting mice. Since the rRNA genes of *S. typhi* and *S. typhimurium* have virtually identical DNA sequences, and since several rRNA genes are scattered around the chromosome, the scientists reasoned that if a large segment of DNA containing two distant rRNA genes were introduced into the strain, the incoming DNA might be able to integrate via two crossovers, one in each of the flanking rRNA gene sequences. They created Hfr strains with an origin of transfer at an rRNA gene. This strain also carried a selectable marker located near a second rRNA gene, hundreds of kilobase pairs away from the point at which DNA transfer would begin. By selecting for *S. typhi* recipients that acquired the selectable marker, they hoped to obtain strains of *S. typhi* with a large fragment of the *S. typhimurium* chromosome integrated in them.

A problem that had to be solved was that bacteria protect themselves from imported DNA that might come from a hostile source, such as a phage, by monitoring sequence match-ups that allow homologous recombination to occur. If differences are detected, the foreign DNA is destroyed. This is called mismatch repair. The mismatch repair system of *S. typhi* had to be disrupted before the incoming DNA could be integrated and maintained stably. So far, several *typhi-typhimurium* chimeras have been created.

No chimeras have been found that infect mice the way *S. typhimurium* does, but even if the attempt to get *S. typhi* to infect mice fails, the ability to create such chimeras should prove very useful for finding other genome segments that contain widely separated virulence genes. This approach may also be applicable to creating new vaccine strains that produce antigens from other microbes.

Source: S. Maloy, and T. Zahrt. 2000. Surrogate genetics: the use of bacterial hybrids as a genetic tool. *Methods* **20**:73–79.

clear that the story is a bit more complex. In the rhesus monkey, infection occurs not only in the small intestine but also in parts of the colon, especially the distal colon (the part of the colon closest to the rectum). Limited histopathology data from humans support this same distribution of infected tissues. In the rhesus monkey and the guinea pig, the bacteria seem to be associated mainly with the villi of the enterocytes rather than M cells, and after several days the bacteria can be found inside the enterocytes. These data suggest that the main mode of infection is entry through mucosal cells into the lamina propria. It is important to keep in mind, however, that the bacteria might be entering through M cells and then infecting mucosal cells from below.

In mice, the progression of disease is somewhat simpler. Here the infection occurs primarily in the ileum. It is still the case that only about 25% of the bacteria are associated with Peyer's patches, but Peyer's patches

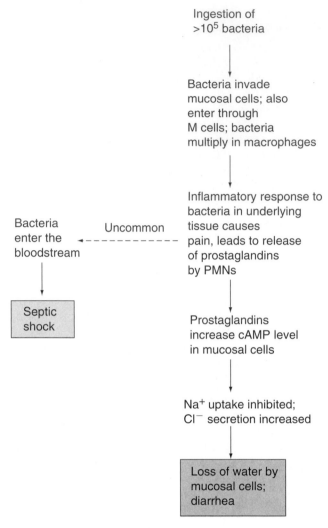

Ingestion of
>10^5 bacteria

↓

Bacteria invade
mucosal cells; also
enter through
M cells; bacteria
multiply in macrophages

↓

Inflammatory response to
bacteria in underlying
tissue causes
pain, leads to release
of prostaglandins
by PMNs

Bacteria
enter the   ◄ - - - - - - - - - - - -   Uncommon
bloodstream

↓

Septic
shock

Prostaglandins
increase cAMP level
in mucosal cells

↓

Na$^+$ uptake inhibited;
Cl$^-$ secretion increased

↓

Loss of water by
mucosal cells;
diarrhea

Figure 26–1 Steps in the progression of the disease caused by *S. typhimurium* in humans and primates.

make up such a tiny minority of mucosal cells that this amounts to a preference for the Peyer's patches. Also, in some experiments, the bacteria associated with the villi of enterocytes were not as firmly attached as those associated with Peyer's patches. If the apparent difference between mice and rhesus monkeys is real, the marked preference for Peyer's patches in mice could explain why mice are more likely to develop systemic disease. *S. typhimurium* can multiply inside unactivated macrophages. If the bacteria enter preferentially via the M cell route and are administered in high enough numbers, the bacteria might be able to multiply in mucosa-associated macrophages and enter the bloodstream before the protective activated macrophage response kicked in. In rhesus monkeys, if most of the bacteria attach to and invade through the enterocytes, their access to phagocytic cells would be more limited and the

time of transit through enterocytes might be longer, giving the activated macrophage response time to develop. Also, humans, and perhaps also rhesus monkeys, are more likely to have partial immunity because of previous contacts with low levels of the bacteria, whereas highly protected colonies of inbred mice are likely to have had little if any previous contact with the bacteria. Whatever the reason for the difference between mice and primates, humans and other primates usually control the infection within a week or so, whereas in mice the bacteria spread to the liver and spleen before the animal can mount an effective protective response.

Although the mystery of why mice respond differently than humans to *S. typhimurium* remains unsolved, another mystery—the origin of the diarrhea—seems to be unraveling (Figure 26–1). The problem was that *S. typhimurium* did not seem to produce any of the enterotoxins that have been assumed to be necessary for bacteria to cause diarrhea. This same problem arose in the case of a type of diarrheagenic *E. coli*, enteropathogenic *E. coli* (see chapter 28). At about the same time, several laboratories discovered a possible solution to this dilemma. Both *S. typhimurium* and enteropathogenic *E. coli* strains inject proteins into intestinal cells, via a type III secretion system (see chapter 13 and Appendix 1). The injected proteins disrupt host cell functions.

One consequence of metabolic disruption is that the cells produce cytokines and other signals that attract PMNs to the site. The PMNs, in turn, release prostaglandins, compounds that boost the adenylate cyclase activity in intestinal cells. Increased levels of cAMP cause an inhibition of Na$^+$ uptake and an increase in Cl$^-$ secretion by these cells, changes associated with the loss of water from tissue that is the hallmark of diarrhea. So, it is not necessary for bacteria to produce an enterotoxin to cause enterocytes to lose water.

The abdominal pain experienced by most people who have gastroenteritis is probably due to the inflammatory response and to effects of various signaling molecules on the enteric neurons. The inflammatory response is elicited directly by bacterial LPS and indirectly by cytokine release and other indirect effects of bacterial invasion of mucosal cells or macrophages.

Adherence and Invasion

ADHERENCE. *S. typhimurium* produces a number of adhesins. These include **type 1 fimbriae** (encoded by *fim* genes), **plasmid-encoded fimbriae** (*pef* genes), **long polar fimbriae** (*lpf* genes) and **thin aggregative fimbriae** (**curli**; encoded by *agf* genes). The binding specificity of the type 1 fimbriae is unknown. The plasmid-encoded fimbriae mediate binding of the bacteria to the microvilli of enterocytes. These fimbriae get their name from the fact that the *pef* genes are found on the 90-kbp plasmid, called the **virulence plasmid (pSLT),** which is found in all virulent strains of *S. typhimurium*. Loss of pSLT causes the bacteria to become avirulent, so clearly this plasmid carries important virulence genes. The *pef* genes are not among these, however, because mutants that no longer produce the plasmid-encoded fimbriae are only slightly affected in virulence. This is true of the genes that produce the other types of fimbriae. So far, the largest effect on virulence of disrupting genes encoding fimbriae is a fivefold increase in LD_{50}, a difference that is barely statistically significant. Of course, given the differences between mice and humans, these fimbriae may well play a more important role in humans than they do in mice. The long polar fimbriae mediate attachment to the Peyer's patches. Similar pili have been found in diarrheagenic strains of *E. coli*. The thin aggregative pili called curli may aid in attachment to the villi of enterocytes, but they also cause the bacteria to become attached to each other. Whether this would aid or inhibit invasion has not been determined.

A gene, *rck*, which was originally identified because it increased the resistance of *S. typhimurium* to killing by complement, encodes a surface protein. This protein also acts as an adhesin and may be involved in invasion of tissue culture cells. Its role in virulence in vivo is not known but is probably minor (see later section).

MEMBRANE RUFFLING. A number of enteric pathogens invade cultured mammalian cells by triggering actin rearrangements that ultimately result in the formation of pseudopods which engulf the bacteria. *S. typhimurium*, no exception to this rule, also forces host cells to engulf it, but the process appears somewhat different from that seen in other enteric pathogens. Binding of *S. typhimurium* to cultured cells causes a change in the appearance of the surface of the host cell that resembles the splash of a droplet of liquid hitting a solid surface (Figure 26–2). This "splash" effect, which has been called membrane **ruffling,** results in internalization of the bacteria inside an endocytic vesicle. The ruffling response has been seen in infected guinea pigs, so the tissue culture cell model accurately reflects the in vivo progression of the disease. Ruffling and internalization of the bacteria are accompanied by extensive actin rearrangements in the vicinity of the invading bacteria. After the bacteria are engulfed in a vesicle, however, the host cell surface and the actin filaments in the region return to normal (Figure 26–3).

PATHOGENICITY ISLANDS AND INVASION. SPI1 and other pathogenicity islands were identified initially by comparing the genome sequence of *S. typhimurium* with that of *E. coli* K12 (a nonvirulent *E. coli* strain) and looking for large segments of DNA found in *S. typhimurium* but not in *E. coli* K12. Other criteria for identifying a pathogenicity island included a %G+C content different from that of the rest of the chromosome and integration near a tRNA gene. Features of *S. typhimurium* pathogenicity islands identified in this way are summarized in Table 26–1.

SPI1 contains a group of genes called *inv* genes, which are responsible for the membrane ruffling associated with invasion of cells by *S. typhimurium*. The *inv* genes, together with other genes on SPI1 (*spa, prg,* and *org),* encode a type III secretion system. SPI1 also carries genes that encode the proteins that are injected into the eukaryotic cell by the type III secretion system. These genes include *sptP,* which encodes a tyrosine phosphatase. Tyrosine phosphatase is an enzyme that mimics signal transduction enzymes of eukaryotic cells and may play a role in altering the response of mucosal cells to outside stimuli, an alteration that produces diarrhea.

Other injected proteins are **SipA** and **SopE,** which are thought to be responsible for the ruffling response. One model for how *Salmonella* causes the actin rearrangements involved in ruffling is based on the finding that injected protein SopE can activate host cell G proteins such as Cdc42 and Rac, which control actin polymerization. Activation of these proteins by SopE initiates the ruffling process. Ruffling is a very localized phenomenon. Localization of the host cell's response is thought to be the role of SipA. SipA binds actin directly and inhibits depolymerization, thus increasing the amount of polymerized actin in its vicinity. For reasons that are not yet understood, the action of SipA is confined to the immediate area in which the bacteria are found, and this accounts for the localized nature of the ruffling phenomenon. In a later section, another method bacteria use to manipulate actin polymerization will be described. How these two modes of actin manipulation are coordinated remains to be determined.

SPI1 also carries genes involved in regulation of virulence genes: *hilA, invF, sirA,* and *phoPQ.* Remarkably little is known about how this cascade of regulatory genes works. The current model for regulation of SPI1-encoded genes is shown in Figure 26–4. The regulatory genes carried on SPI1 also control other virulence genes of *S. typhimurium*.

Mutations that eliminate expression of genes on SPI1 increase the LD_{50} of orally introduced bacteria by 16- to 100-fold, but they have no effect on the LD_{50} when the bacteria are introduced by intraperitoneal injections. Thus, the genes on SPI1 appear to be important in the initial phase of infection during which the bacteria

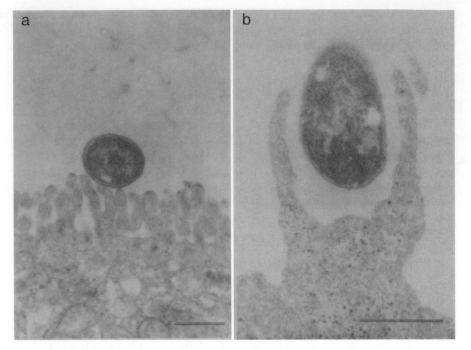

Figure 26–2 Electron micrographs showing the invasion of cultured cells by *S. typhimurium* and the membrane ruffling effect. (**a**) Bacteria adhere to the apical surface of microvilli. (**b**) Bacteria are engulfed by pseudopods creating a "splash" effect. (From B. B. Finlay, K. Y. Leung, I. Rosenshine, and F. Garcia-del Portillo. 1992. *Salmonella* interactions with the epithelial cell. *ASM News* **58:**486–490.)

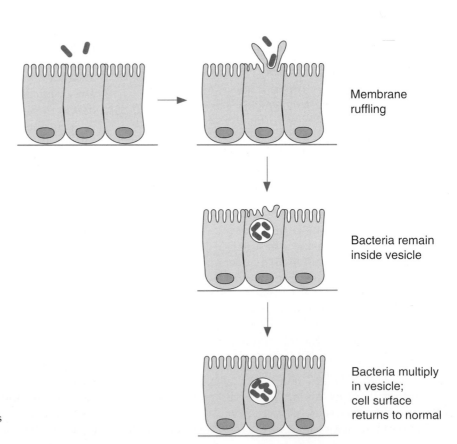

Membrane ruffling

Bacteria remain inside vesicle

Bacteria multiply in vesicle; cell surface returns to normal

Figure 26–3 Invasion of cultured cells by *S. typhimurium.*

Table 26–1   Characteristics of virulence gene clusters found so far in *S. typhimurium*

Virulence gene clusters	Virulence factors encoded in the region	Possible function of virulence factors
Pathogenicity islands		
SPI1	Type III secretion system	Involved in early stages of infection because no effect on LD_{50} due to intraperitoneal injection
	Proteins secreted by the type III system	
	Chaperones that control folding of proteins	
	Regulatory proteins (PhoPQ, HilA, InvF, SirA)	
SPI2	Type III secretion system (different from that encoded on SPI1)	Inhibition of phagosome-lysosome fusion; important during systemic phase of disease
	Proteins secreted by the type III system	
	Chaperones that control folding of proteins	
SPI3	Mg^{2+} transporter	May aid survival and growth in Mg^{2+}-poor vacuole of invaded cell
	Proteins of unknown function	
SPI4, 5	Unknown	Unknown
Lysogenic phages		
Gifsy-1, 2	Superoxide dismutase	May contribute to survival during systemic phase of infection
	Protein (GrvA) that reduces virulence	
Virulence plasmid		
pSLT	Adhesin (*pef*)	Important in all stages of virulence; Spv proteins are the most important
	Adhesin/serum resistance (*rck*)	
	Spv proteins (SpvB is a toxin that ADP-ribosylates actin)	

invade mucosal cells, rather than in later phases when the bacteria spread to liver and spleen. This is the reverse of the effect of the loss of the virulence plasmid, pSLT, which has its greatest effect on the systemic phase of the infection in mice.

Pathogenicity island **SPI2,** like SPI1, encodes a type III secretion system and the proteins it injects into eukaryotic cells. Mutations in genes carried on SPI2 have an even more dramatic effect than those in genes carried by SPI1. Eliminating expression of genes encoded on SPI2 increases the LD_{50} by 10^5-fold, regardless of whether the bacteria are introduced orally or by intraperitoneal injection. Thus, SPI2, like pSLT, seems to be involved mainly in the systemic phase of the disease. The type III secretion system encoded on SPI2 is unusual in the sense that it appears not to be used by bacteria on the surface of a host cell to inject proteins into the host cell, but rather is used by bacteria inside a phagosome to prevent phagosome-lysosome fusion. How this is accomplished remains to be discovered. A better understanding of this process could be a real breakthrough in understanding how pathogens that are internalized by mammalian cells manipulate the phagosome-lysosome fusion process.

A third pathogenicity island, **SPI3,** encodes a high-affinity Mg^{2+} transporter. This pathogenicity island may also be important for survival of the bacteria inside phagosomes. A distinguishing feature of the phagosome is that it is deficient in Mg^{2+}. Since Mg^{2+} is essential for most bacteria, this may be one way in which phagosomes reduce the metabolic activity of bacteria prior to the phagolysosome fusion.

Virtually nothing is known about two other putative pathogenicity islands, **SPI4** and **SPI5.** In addition to the pathogenicity islands so far identified, two lysogenic phages have been found that may contribute to virulence, **Gifsy-1** and **Gifsy-2.** The phages were named for a French town where the institute that housed the scientists who discovered the phages is located. So far only a few genes carried on the Gifsy phages have been characterized, but curing *S. typhimurium* of Gifsy-2 increased the LD_{50} of the strain significantly. Gifsy-2 carries a *sod* gene that encodes a superoxide dismutase. Such enzymes, which convert toxic superoxide to less toxic peroxide, may help the bacteria to survive the onslaught of the macrophage oxidative burst. One could ask how relevant this type of protection would be in the case of a bacterium that can prevent phagolysosome fusion and thus forestall the oxidative burst, but during inflammation, when PMNs and macrophages are at-

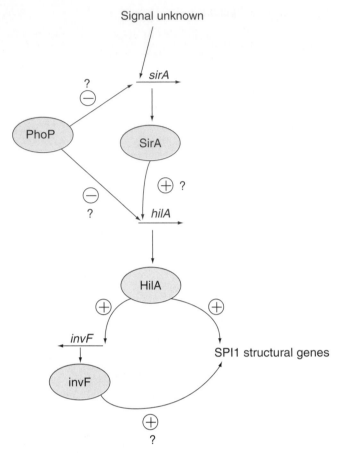

Signal unknown

Figure 26–4 Proposed cascade of SPI1 regulatory genes that control expression of structural genes on SPI1. Some of these regulators, such as PhoPQ, also control expression of genes located elsewhere in the chromosome. +, gene expression is activated; −, gene expression is repressed; ?, some uncertainty remains about the nature of the control of expression. (Adapted from Darwin and Miller [1999].)

tracted to the region where bacteria are multiplying, the bacteria could well be exposed to superoxide because of release of lysosome contents into the environment.

Also carried on Gifsy-2 is a gene designated *grvA* (for Gifsy-related virulence), a gene that has an unusual characteristic. When *grvA* is disrupted, the strain of *S. typhimurium* becomes more virulent. That is, it outcompetes the wild type in mice inoculated intraperitoneally with a mixture of wild type and mutant. (Competition assays are more sensitive than LD_{50} assays for detecting differences in virulence.) The *grvA* phenomenon is reminiscent of a phenomenon seen in *Yersinia pestis*, in which the invasin gene, *inv*, is normally inactivated. Introducing active Inv actually reduces virulence. *Y. pestis* seems to have experienced mutations that lead it in the direction of greater virulence, whereas *grvA* is still present in a form that reduces the virulence of *S. typhimurium*.

THE VIRULENCE PLASMID pSLT. Nearly 90% of *S. typhimurium* strains carry the 90-kb pSLT plasmid. This plasmid carries *pef* genes and *rck*. It also carries genes called **spv**, for *Salmonella* plasmid virulence. When **spvABCD** and **spvR** genes were cloned on a plasmid and introduced into a strain that had been cured of pSLT, full virulence was restored. This is one reason scientists now think that the *pef* and *rck* genes make only a minor contribution and that the major contribution of pSLT to virulence is the *spv* genes.

The function of the proteins encoded by the *spv* genes is still under study, but results of studies of mutants deficient in these genes suggest that the *spv* gene products are important for survival in macrophages and in steps after the initial translocation of the bacteria across the mucosa (Table 26–2). Recently, one of the *spv* genes, **spvB**, has been shown to encode an ADP-ribosylating toxin that modifies actin directly and totally disrupts the cytoskeleton of the cell. This is a new pathway for cytoskeleton modification by bacteria. In other cases, the bacteria manipulate actin polymerization by affecting the rates of polymerization or depolymerization, often indirectly by interfering with eukaryotic signal transduction pathways that affect cytoskeleton formation. In this case, actin is modified directly, a discovery that finally put *S. typhimurium* on the list of toxin-producing bacteria. For a long time it appeared that *S. typhimurium* did not produce toxins. This is still the case with respect to enterotoxins that cause diarrhea, but now it appears that *S. typhimurium* produces a cytotoxin that helps it survive in the systemic phase of the disease.

Expression of the *spv* genes is regulated by *spvR*, which in turn is regulated by the alternate sigma factor, **RpoS,** which controls many genes expressed in stationary phase. The regulatory cascade shown in Figure 26–5 is triggered by oxygen levels and nutrient starvation.

An interesting feature of pSLT was discovered recently: the plasmid is self-transmissible. Scientists examining the nucleotide sequence of this large plasmid noted the presence of transfer genes that have been found on known self-transmissible plasmids, such as F plasmid. This led them to tag pSLT with the **MudJ** transposon, which carries a gene that confers kanamycin resistance. They tested the tagged plasmid for transfer from an *S. typhimurium* donor to an *S. typhimurium* recipient. Transfer frequencies were low, but no lower than those seen with most plasmids found in natural isolates of bacteria. The fact that the virulence plasmid is self-transmissible probably explains why so many *S. typhimurium* strains now have it.

Table 26–2 Proposed order of gene expression during various stages in an *S. typhimurium* infection in mice (gene expression reflects the different environment of each site)[a]

Location of bacteria	Levels of		Genes activated or repressed
	Nutrients	Oxygen	
Lumen of intestine	High	Very low	*inv* genes expressed, *spv* genes repressed
Inside M cell or epithelial cell vacuole	Low	Low	*spv* genes induced, *inv* genes still expressed
Inside macrophages	Low	Moderate	*spv* genes still expressed, *inv* genes repressed

[a]Adapted from D. G. Guiney, S. Libby, F. C. Fang, M. Krause, and J. Fierer. 1995. Growth-phase regulation of plasmid virulence genes in *Salmonella*. *Trends Microbiol.* 3:275–279.

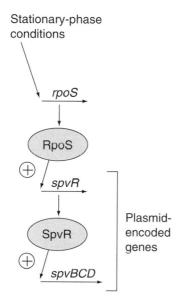

Figure 26–5 Proposed cascade of regulatory genes that control expression of plasmid-encoded *spv* genes. RpoS is encoded by a chromosomal gene; SpvR is encoded by a plasmid gene.

Table 26–3 Mutations that increase host susceptibility to *S. typhimurium* infections and other invasive pathogens

Locus	Cell type(s) affected	Effect of mutation
ity	Macrophages	Host less able to kill bacteria in spleen; increased susceptibility to infection
lps	B cells, T cells, macrophages, fibroblasts	Low responsiveness to injected LPS, failure to produce cytokines in response to LPS; decreased susceptibility to infection
xid	B cells	Decreased and delayed antibody production (IgG, IgM) in response to some antigens; increased susceptibility to infection

Host Factors That Affect Susceptibility to *Salmonella* Infections

A number of mutations in mice affect the ability of the animal to successfully resist systemic infections by *S. typhimurium* and other invasive pathogens (Table 26–3). The effect of mutations in the ***ity*** locus is controversial. Some results indicate that animals with such mutations have fewer activated macrophages and PMNs and are less able to kill bacteria. Mice with mutations at another locus, ***lps,*** do not respond normally to injections of LPS. This is reflected in the inability of murine cells to produce cytokines when the animals are injected with LPS. Animals with mutations in a gene called *xid* have altered B cells that produce antibodies (both IgG and IgM) more slowly than B cells of normal mice and seem to be less able to prevent *S. typhimurium* infections from becoming systemic.

Why Is *S. typhi* So Invasive?

S. typhi is much more invasive than the other *Salmonella* species, despite being closely related to them at the DNA level. Why is this the case? Unfortunately, there is little information on this important point. One difference between *S. typhi* and at least some other *Salmonella* serotypes is the production of **Vi antigen,** a capsular polysaccharide composed of *N*-acetylglucosamine uronic acid. This capsular antigen is produced during infection because patients recovering from typhoid fever have antibodies to Vi antigen. In some studies with human volunteers, strains of *S. typhi* that produce Vi antigen were found to be more virulent than strains that did not produce it, but the question of whether Vi antigen is a virulence factor is still somewhat controversial. Part of the problem is imagining a role for Vi antigen. Capsular polysaccharides are usually produced by bacteria to prevent phagocytosis, but *S. typhi* appears to be able to survive in phagocytes. In some other bacteria that survive inside phagocytes, surface polysaccharides appear to function as scavengers of reactive forms of oxygen. Such a function has not been proved for Vi antigen.

Help is on the way in the form of genome sequences. The genome sequences of *S. typhimurium* and *S. typhi* are now being analyzed. The genomes of these two serotypes share a 97% sequence identity, but initial genome sequence comparisons have indicated that there are differences, many of which are clustered in certain regions of the chromosome. Thus, although the two serotypes of *S. enterica* seem very similar at the DNA sequence level, certain differences may explain not only the greater virulence of *S. typhi* for humans but also the fact that, unlike *S. typhimurium*, which colonizes many animals as well as humans, *S. typhi* appears to be a human-specific pathogen.

Acid Tolerance Response

An aspect of *S. typhimurium* virulence that has received less attention than it merits is the acid tolerance response. This is the response that allows the bacteria to survive passage through the acid environment of the stomach, a necessary prerequisite for infection. *S. typhimurium* grown at neutral pH in the laboratory and shifted to lower pH conditions survive well at pH values down to about pH 4, but below that, rapid die-off of the bacteria occurs. Death presumably occurs because the bacteria can no longer pump enough protons out of the cytoplasm to maintain an intracellular pH above 5. Below that value, inactivation of important proteins occurs, and bacteria can no longer survive. *Salmonella* can survive at pH values as low as 3 if it has a chance to adapt. If *S. typhimurium* is grown at pH 6 for a generation before being exposed to lower pH conditions, it becomes able to survive at pH values as low as pH 3 for prolonged periods. A surprising and intriguing aspect of the acid tolerance response is that Fur, a protein usually associated with regulation of iron acquisition genes, appears to be a regulator of this response. Could Fur be sensing pH as well as iron? Iron binding by Fur is pH dependent, so this possibility is not completely out of the question.

More recently, an acid tolerance response to acid stress has been identified. This response is controlled by the **PhoPQ** two-component regulatory system. PhoPQ controls expression of many of the virulence genes covered in this chapter (Figures 26–4). Thus, the acid tolerance response seems to be coregulated with the modulation of genes involved in helping the bac-

teria survive and invade once they reach the intestine. This is the first time such a clear connection between the acid tolerance response and the general virulence response has been found.

Prevention and Treatment

Antibiotic Therapy

S. typhimurium infections are normally self-limiting, and there is no evidence that administration of antibiotics significantly shortens the duration of symptoms. Thus, antibiotic therapy is not appropriate for uncomplicated cases of gastroenteritis. If the disease becomes systemic, however, antibiotic therapy is necessary to clear the infection and prevent endotoxic shock from developing. Although antibiotics are usually not used to treat *S. typhimurium* infections, resistance of *S. typhimurium* to antibiotics has nonetheless become an issue.

Approximately half of all antibiotics used in developed countries are used in agriculture. A portion of this agricultural use is to treat sick animals. Most antibiotic use, however, is designed to prevent disease or to promote more rapid growth of the animal. Nontherapeutic use of antibiotics has come under fire by those who are concerned about the extent to which agricultural use of antibiotics is creating resistant strains that can cause human disease. At the center of this controversy is **S. typhimurium DT104,** a multidrug-resistant strain of *S. typhimurium* that has been causing disease outbreaks in Europe and the United States. There is little debate over the fact that agricultural use of antibiotics selects for antibiotic-resistant strains of animal intestinal bacteria. Because *S. typhimurium* is a common inhabitant of the intestines of livestock animals, it is not surprising that a multidrug-resistant strain such as DT104 should have arisen. Because virtually all cases of salmonellosis arise from contaminated food, the source of *S. typhimurium* DT104 is pretty clear: it came from an animal source.

What is controversial is the extent to which strains such as DT104 affect human health. Defenders of antibiotic use in agriculture are quick to point out that it is irrelevant whether or not *S. typhimurium* is resistant to antibiotics since antibiotics are not recommended for treatment of gastroenteritis. Those who are concerned about antibiotic use in agriculture are equally quick to point out that antibiotic resistance is very important indeed to that fraction of people infected in an *S. typhimurium* outbreak who develop the systemic form of the disease. A 1998 outbreak of *S. typhimurium* DT104 in Denmark illustrates the problem. In this case, the source of the outbreak was a smoked pork product. Smoking meat does not make the meat hot enough to kill *S. typhimurium*, so if it is consumed without further cooking, viable bacteria may be present. Apparently, quite a few people consumed the product without further cooking because there were a number of cases of *S. typhimurium* gastroenteritis. Several infected people developed the systemic form of the disease, which was treated with fluoroquinolone antibiotics. Two died.

Antibiotics are an essential part of the treatment of *S. typhi*, not only to save patients with active typhoid fever, but also to clear bacteria from carriers. Because the bacteria in carriers are localized in the liver and biliary tract, the antibiotic regimen used to clear carriers of *S. typhi* is not the same as the regimen used to treat people with typhoid fever.

Vaccines

S. typhimurium gastroenteritis can be prevented by proper handling of foods. For this reason, efforts to control *S. typhimurium* infections have focused on detecting the bacteria in foods and educating the public about proper food handling, rather than on developing a vaccine to prevent this type of food poisoning. By contrast, a considerable effort has been made to develop a vaccine against typhoid fever. Not only is the disease potentially fatal, but it is a problem in countries that are not in an economic position to provide a clean water supply for all citizens, especially those in rural areas. Three vaccines against typhoid fever are currently in use. Two are injected, and one is orally administered. The first successful injected vaccine consisted of killed whole bacteria. However, this vaccine had numerous side effects (probably due to LPS) and had to be readministered periodically. A newer injected vaccine consists of capsular material (Vi antigen). It is safer and more effective than the old injected vaccine. There is a live oral vaccine, an attenuated strain, *S. typhi* Ty21a. This strain is thought to be avirulent because of a mutation in *galE*, a gene in the galactose utilization pathway that affects O-antigen production, but there could be other mutations. In human field trials, this vaccine has proved to be safe and effective, but its efficacy has differed considerably in different trials (96% protection in Egypt, 60 to 80% protection in Chile). Although Ty21a has been used in most trials to date, there is concern about the unknown nature of the mutation in the strain and also about whether the strain is surviving long enough in the Peyer's patches to give a good immune response. Two well-characterized avirulent mutants of *S. typhi* are also being tested as potential vaccine candidates: a strain with a deletion in *crp* (which encodes the cAMP-binding protein) and a strain with a deletion in *aroA* (which encodes a protein involved in aromatic amino acid biosynthesis).

Salmonella as a Basis for Other Vaccines

An oral vaccine is easier and safer to administer than an injected vaccine. A live oral vaccine is also a cheap alternative to more expensive vaccines consisting of purified components. The current strategy for developing live oral vaccines is to take an avirulent mutant of *S. typhimurium* or *S. typhi* and introduce genes encoding various antigens into the strain. The bacteria express the desired antigen on their surfaces. *Salmonella* species are particularly desirable because they multiply in Peyer's patches and stimulate a good mucosal and humoral response.

Several candidate mutants have been evaluated as bases for oral vaccines. One is *S. typhi* Ty21a, the strain already mentioned as a vaccine against typhoid fever. This strain has the advantage that it has been proved safe and fairly effective in field trials but has the disadvantage that the genetics of *S. typhi* is considerably less developed than the genetics of *S. typhimurium*. Mutants of *S. typhimurium* that are unable to make aromatic amino acids or purines are avirulent and have been proposed as vaccine strains. Unfortunately, these mutants appear to be too crippled to elicit a good immune response. Another vaccine candidate is a strain of *S. typhimurium* that has a double mutation ($\Delta crp\Delta cya$). This mutation eliminates the cAMP receptor protein-cAMP complex global activator response. Apparently, genes controlled by this system are required for virulence because the mutants colonize but have considerably reduced virulence. Mutants that lack a functional allele of the regulatory gene, *phoP*, and mutants unable to produce diaminopimelic acid, which is essential for peptidoglycan synthesis, are also being tested as vaccine strains.

A number of vaccines based on *S. typhi* Ty21a carrying foreign antigens have been created and tested. Two examples are *S. typhi* Ty21a carrying the *Shigella* virulence plasmid and *S. typhi* Ty21a carrying a cloned O-antigen gene from *Vibrio cholerae*. The *Shigella-S. typhi* vaccine worked well in human trials, but it has proved difficult to produce effective lots of vaccine reproducibly. The *S. typhi-V. cholerae* vaccine was not as protective as expected and had some side effects. Nonetheless, the results of early attempts together with the obvious desirability of creating a single vaccine that would confer effective protection against multiple pathogens has spurred numerous attempts to create effective and safe vaccines based on the *Salmonella* carrier model. So far the *S. typhi* tetanus vaccine has only been tested in mice, but it protected mice from tetanus. *Salmonella* strains carrying genes from a hepatitis virus or the protozoal parasite that causes malaria are currently being tested as vaccines against hepatitis and malaria.

Future Directions

Given the large number of research groups that have worked on *Salmonella* pathogenesis during the past 2 decades and the early availability of advanced genetic tools, it is not surprising that the amount of information on *Salmonella* virulence has increased substantially in recent years. It is doubtless the case that there are virulence factors that remain to be discovered, but the number now known has become large enough to raise the question of what comes next. The challenge of the future will be to understand how these genes and their products interact with one another. Complicating the movement toward a more complete understanding of how the various bacterial activities work together is the lingering question of what state *Salmonella* is striving to achieve in the human body. The bias shared by many scientists in the field is still that the goal of *Salmonella* is to cause symptomatic disease in humans. Yet, the vast majority of the time spent by *Salmonella* in humans and animals is characterized by a more benign association exemplified by the carrier state. Because of this, a good case can be made for seeking colonization factors rather than virulence factors. An obvious objection to this suggestion is that it does not explain why so much of the *Salmonella* chromosome is devoted to activities that seem designed to allow the bacteria to grow in phagocytic cells.

Yet another interesting question is why some *Salmonella* serotypes (e.g., *S. typhimurium*) seem to be generalists that colonize many animal species, whereas others (e.g., *S. typhi*) seem to be specialists. What are the traits that determine host specificity? The answer to this question will likely shed as much light on differences in physiology between different animal hosts as on differences in physiology between different *Salmonella* serotypes.

SELECTED READINGS

Ahmer, B. M., M. Tran, and F. Heffron. 1999. The virulence plasmid of *Salmonella typhimurium* is self-transmissible. *J. Bacteriol.* **181:**1364–1368.

Bearson, B. L., L. Wilson, and J. W. Foster. 1998. A low pH-inducible PhoPQ dependent acid tolerance response protects *Salmonella typhimurium* against inorganic acid stress. *J. Bacteriol.* **180:**2409–2417.

Cotter, P. A., and V. J. DiRita. 2000. Bacterial virulence gene regulation: an evolutionary perspective. *Annu. Rev. Microbiol.* **54:**519–565.

Darwin, K. H., and V. L. Miller. 1999. Molecular basis of the interaction of *Salmonella* with the intestinal mucosa. *Clin. Microbiol. Rev.* **12:**405–428.

Figueroa-Bossi, N., and L. Bossi. 1999. Inducible prophages contribute to *Salmonella* virulence in mice. *Mol. Microbiol.* **33:**167–176.

Groisman, E. A., A. Blanc-Potard, and K. Uchiya. 1999. Pathogenicity islands and the evolution of *Salmonella* virulence, p. 127–150. *In* J. B. Kaper and J. Hacker (ed.), *Pathogenicity Islands and Other Mobile Virulence Elements.* ASM Press, Washington, D.C.

Hennessy, T. W., C. W. Hedberg, L. Slutsker, K. E. White, J. M. Besser-Wiek, M. E. Moen, J. Feldman, W. W. Coleman, L. M. Edmonson, K. L. MacDonald, M. T. Osterholm, and the Investigation Team. 1996. A national outbreak of *Salmonella enteritidis* infections from ice cream. *N. Engl. J. Med.* **334:**1281–1286.

Kent, T. H., S. B. Formal, and E. H. Labrec. 1966. *Salmonella* gastroenteritis in Rhesus monkeys. *Arch. Pathol.* **82:**272–279.

Takeuchi, A. 1967. Electron microscope studies of experimental *Salmonella* infection. I. Penetration into the intestinal epithelium by *Salmonella typhimurium*. *Am. J. Pathol.* **50:**109–119.

Zhou, D., M. Mooseker, and J. E. Galan. 1999. Role of the *S. typhimurium* actin-binding protein SipA in bacterial internalization. *Science* **283:**2092–2095.

Trend Alert

For those of you who like to keep current with the bar scene, you might like to know about a bar and grill located in Kankakee, Ill. (about midway between Chicago and the University of Illinois at Urbana-Champaign). The name of the bar is Sam and Ella's, pun intended. The food is nothing special, but the karma is intense, and the place is occasionally invaded by carousing microbiologists. So far, this restaurant has not attracted any adverse attention from the public health department, but you've got to admit that by giving the restaurant this particular name, the proprietors are asking for trouble.

SUMMARY OUTLINE

Characteristics of *Salmonella* strains

Gram-negative, motile rods

Facultative

Closely related to *E. coli* and *Shigella*

Can cause localized or systemic infections

Many different serotypes

S. typhimurium

Transmitted by contaminated food, especially chickens and eggs

Incubation period—6 to 24 h

Disease—salmonellosis

    Nausea and vomiting initially

    Abdominal pain and diarrhea—severity varies from patient to patient

    Rarely becomes systemic, leading to septic shock

    Progression of disease

        More severe in mice than primates

        Ingested bacteria enter enterocytes or M cells in Peyer's patches

        Bacteria grow in unactivated macrophages

    Inflammatory response leads to release of prostaglandins by PMNs

    cAMP levels rise—diarrhea results

Virulence factors

    Adherence

        Type I fimbriae (*fim*)

        Plasmid-encoded fimbriae (*pef*)—mediate attachment to enterocytes

        Long polar fimbriae (*lpf*)—mediate attachment to Peyer's patches

        Thin aggregative fimbriae (curli; *agf*)

        Surface protein encoded by *rck*

    Membrane ruffling

        Bacteria internalized in endocytic vesicle

        Accompanied by extensive but transient actin rearrangements in host cell

    Pathogenicity islands and invasion

        SPI1

            inv genes responsible for ruffling

            inv, spa, prg, and *org* encode a type III secretion system

            Contains genes for proteins injected into host cell

                sptP—tyrosine phosphatase

                SipA and SopE—involved in ruffling

                    SopE activates host cell G proteins

                    SipA binds actin, inhibits depolymerization

            Contains regulatory genes that control expression of structural genes on SPI1 and on chromosome

            Probably involved in early stages of infection

        SPI2—encodes a different type III secretion system and the proteins it injects

            Inhibit phagosome-lysosome fusion

            Important in systemic disease

(continued)

        SPI3

            Encodes Mg^{2+} transporter

            Involved in survival of bacteria in host cell vacuole

        SPI4 and SPI5—nothing known

      Lysogenic phages – Gifsy-1 and Gifsy-2

        Carry genes for superoxide dismutase and GrvA (function unknown but reduces virulence)

        May contribute to survival during systemic phase

      Virulence plasmid, pSLT

        Carries genes, *pef* and *rck*, that encode adhesins

        Also carries *spv* genes

            Encode proteins important in survival in macrophages and during translocation across membrane

            SpvB—ADP-ribosylates actin

        Regulation

            RpoS regulates *spvR*, which regulates expression of other *spv* genes

            Cascade triggered by oxygen levels and starvation

        Self-transmissible

      Acid tolerance response

        Bacteria grown at pH 6 for a generation can survive at pH 3

        Regulated by Fur

        May be coregulated with other virulence genes by PhoPQ

    Host factors affecting susceptibility

      ity mutations may affect killing by macrophages

      lps mutations reduce host response to LPS

      xid mutants produce antibodies more slowly

    Prevention and treatment

      Antibiotics used only for systemic form of disease

      S. typhimurium DT104 multidrug-resistant strain

        Resistance due to agricultural use of antibiotics

        Cannot be eliminated in systemic infections

      Prevention aimed at eliminating bacteria from foods

S. typhi

    Disease—typhoid fever

      Incubation time—1 to 4 weeks

      Bacteria multiply in spleen and liver

      Large numbers of bacteria released into bloodstream

        Lasts 2 to 3 weeks

        High fever, anorexia

      Bacteria move from liver to gall bladder, shed in bile and then into intestine

      Asymptomatic carriers are main source of bacteria

        S. typhi may persist in gallbladder for years

        Public health problem (e.g., Typhoid Mary)

    Virulence factors

      Human-specific pathogen, so factors hard to study

      Vi antigen

        Capsular polysaccharide

        Function not known

      Genome sequence may provide information about virulence factors

(*continued*)

SUMMARY OUTLINE (*continued*)

Prevention and treatment
　　Antibiotic treatment essential
　　　　Cure patients with disease
　　　　Clear bacteria from carriers
　　Vaccines—three in use
　　　　Whole killed bacteria—side effects
　　　　Injected Vi antigen
　　　　Oral vaccine
　　　　　　Attenuated *S. typhi* Ty21a
　　　　　　Ty21a also used as basis to carry foreign antigens
　　　　　　　　Shigella virulence plasmid
　　　　　　　　V. cholerae O antigen

QUESTIONS

Answers to the questions can be found in Appendix 2.

1. Why does it make sense that the incubation time for typhoid fever is longer than the incubation time for gastroenteritis caused by *S. typhimurium*?

2. In developed countries, what type of people are most likely to get typhoid fever, and how is it most likely to be spread? How would the answer differ in the case of a developing country?

3. Speculate on reasons why the disease caused by *S. typhimurium* in mice is different from the disease it causes in humans. Similarly, consider reasons for the inability of *S. typhi* to cause a lethal infection in mice.

4. Speculate on why eliminating adhesin genes seems to have a much less drastic effect on the LD_{50} than eliminating genes for invasion or type III secretion systems.

5. What was the rationale for defining pathogenicity islands by comparing the *E. coli* K12 genome with that of *S. typhimurium*? What are the advantages and disadvantages of this approach?

6. Loss of the virulence plasmid pSLT virtually eliminates virulence. Given that fact, how can some mutations in chromosomal genes also have a comparable effect on virulence even though the virulence plasmid is still present?

7. Why do investigators determine the LD_{50} both in mice to which the bacteria are administered orally and in mice to which the bacteria are administered by injection into the peritoneum?

8. How might an investigator go about establishing the order of action of regulatory genes and proteins in a cascade, such as those shown in Figures 26–4 and 26–5? How would you determine whether protein X repressed or activated the genes whose expression it controls?

9. There have been a number of alarmist reports in the media on outbreaks caused by the multidrug-resistant *S. typhimurium* strain DT104. To what extent should the public be concerned about DT104 outbreaks?

27

Listeria monocytogenes, a Doubly Motile Pathogen

KEY FEATURES

Listeria monocytogenes

CHARACTERISTICS
Gram-positive rod
Motile—flagella; actin condensation inside host cells
Ability to multiply at refrigerator temperatures

DISEASE
Listeriosis—systemic infections (immunocompromised or elderly people); infections of fetus

RESERVOIRS
Soil, water, and decaying vegetation
Many animals
Asymptomatic human carriers

MAJOR VIRULENCE FACTORS
Ability to invade host cells (internalins)
Escape from vacuole—pore-forming cytotoxin (listerolysin O); phospholipases
Movement through cell via actin condensation (ActA)
Can cross the placenta

PREVENTION AND TREATMENT
Eliminate *Listeria* from food supply
Antibiotics if diagnosed in time

Listeriosis

Characteristics of Disease Caused by *Listeria monocytogenes*

L. monocytogenes is a gram-positive, facultative, highly motile rod that causes an uncommon but potentially serious type of food-borne infection. Outside host cells, *L. monocytogenes* is motile because of its flagella. As it enters a human cell, these flagella are lost, but the bacteria are still motile because of their ability to polymerize actin into long actin tails that propel the bacteria through the cytoplasm. Another unusual feature of *L. monocytogenes* that contributes to its ability to cause disease is that it can grow at refrigerator temperatures as well as at 37°C.

L. monocytogenes is notable among the pathogens that cause food-borne infections for the high incidence of fatalities in those who develop systemic infections. Fortunately, few exposed people develop the fatal form of the disease. Most of the deaths caused by *L. monocytogenes* involve fetuses, newborns, or immunocompromised adults (Box 27–1). *L. monocytogenes* is one of the few infectious microbes that can cross the placenta. A pregnant woman who is infected may experience at worst a mild flulike infection, but if her fetus is infected, the infection is systemic and highly fatal. The tragedy of listeriosis in pregnant women is that there is no early warning; the first symptom is a severely infected newborn or a stillborn infant. In immunocompromised adults, the first sign of disease is usually fever, and the disease moves rapidly to its fatal conclusion. In immunocompromised adults, the disease most often takes the form of meningitis.

L. monocytogenes is normally found in soil, in water, in decaying vegetation, on plants, and in the intestinal tracts of many animals. It is an occasional cause of disease in cattle and sheep but usually causes no symptoms in colonized animals. *L. monocytogenes* is carried in the intestinal tracts of at least 5 to 10% of the human population without any apparent symptoms. Given its wide distribution, it is not surprising that during the past 2 decades, there have been several large outbreaks of listeriosis, all of which were associated with commercially supplied foods, especially foods containing milk. But many types of foods, ranging from fresh vegetables and coleslaw to paté and shrimp, have been implicated in outbreaks. Outbreaks have also been seen in hospitals with large concentrations of immunocompromised patients. Outbreaks involving multiple cases have received most of the public attention, but there are some indications that sporadic cases of listeriosis also occur and may be more common than has been previously appreciated.

A trait of *L. monocytogenes* that makes it very difficult to control during food processing is that it can multiply over a wide range of temperatures, including the temperatures it encounters in a refrigerator. In fact, a classical way of enriching for *Listeria* in samples that contain many other types of bacteria is to incubate the sample for prolonged periods in a refrigerator. Thus, refrigeration, a hallowed mode of protecting people from food-borne disease, is useless to prevent the multiplication of *Listeria*. One of the few pieces of good news about *L. monocytogenes* is that it is spread only by ingestion

---

BOX 27–1   Anatomy of a Listeriosis Outbreak: the Insidious Nature of the Disease

Case 1. In 1981, a listeriosis outbreak involving 41 people occurred in Canada. Thirty-four of the cases involved perinatal infections. There were nine stillbirths. Of 23 infected infants that were born alive, nearly one-third died. Two pregnant women with symptomatic listeriosis delivered live healthy infants. Of the seven nonpregnant adults who developed full symptomatic disease, nearly 30% died. The source of the outbreak was coleslaw produced by a local manufacturer. One of the farmers who supplied cabbage to the manufacturer had had two sheep die of listeriosis. Sheep manure was used to fertilize the cabbage field. This could have been the source of *Listeria* on the cabbage. Harvested cabbages were stored in a large cold storage shed until taken to the processing plant. *Listeria* is one of the few bacteria that can multiply at cold temperatures, so cold storage allowed bacteria to increase to higher numbers.

Case 2. In 1985, in California, 142 people who consumed a certain brand of soft cheese developed symptomatic listeriosis. Of these, 93 were perinatal cases and 49 were adult cases. Thirty fetuses or newborn infants died, and 18 adults died. Of the 49 adult cases, 48 occurred in people who were immunocompromised or elderly. The plant in which the cheese was produced was in compliance with safety regulations, and pasteurized milk was used to make the cheese. What appears to have happened is that on some occasions the pasteurizing equipment could not keep up with the flow of raw milk coming into the plant, and raw milk may have gotten into the final product.

Source: A. Schuchat, B. Swaminathan, and C. V. Broome. 1991. Epidemiology of human listeriosis. *Clin. Microbiol. Rev.* **4:**169–183.

of contaminated foods and not by human-to-human transmission.

One reason *L. monocytogenes* is a rather uncommon cause of human infections is that it has a high ID_{50}. It is necessary to ingest a hefty dose of bacteria to acquire even a mild infection. Anything that compromises the acid barrier of the stomach, such as antacids or H_2 blockers, can increase the likelihood of infection. Pregnancy also increases the risk of infection for unknown reasons. The incubation period is long, from 11 to 70 days (average 31 days). This long incubation period can make it difficult to trace the source of an outbreak, because people do not remember very clearly what they ate a month ago.

Listeria as a Model for Studies of the Cell-Mediated Immune Response and Cytoskeleton Formation

L. monocytogenes elicits a predominantly cell-mediated immune response during infection of mammals. This has made *L. monocytogenes* a good organism for studying the mammalian cell-mediated response; immunologists have used *L. monocytogenes* for this purpose since the 1950s. More recently, *L. monocytogenes* has also become a model organism for studies of actin polymerization, because a surface protein, **ActA,** triggers the polymerization of actin to form long filaments. This activity has become even more important recently because it turns out that many bacteria that stimulate normally nonphagocytic cells to ingest them also manipulate cytoskeleton polymerization or depolymerization to elicit the formation of the pseudopods that engulf the cell. Studies of *L. monocytogenes* were the first to alert scientists working on invasive bacterial pathogens to the fact that bacterial manipulation of host cell cytoskeleton was an important virulence factor.

Virulence Factors

Animal and Cell Culture Model Systems

L. monocytogenes causes a systemic infection in mice, and this animal model system is used to assess virulence of mutants. Pregnant mice injected intraperitoneally with *Listeria* exhibit transplacental transmission of the bacteria. If pregnant gnotobiotic mice are used, *Listeria* can be introduced by the oral route to achieve the same end, thus providing a more natural model for listeriosis. When the first edition of this book was published over 5 years ago, these models of transplacental infection were new. They seemed exciting because they opened up the possibility of investigating one of the

most important pathological features of *L. monocytogenes*—its unusual ability to cross the placenta and infect the fetus. Oddly enough, the availability of these animal models has not sparked interest in molecular studies of transplacental transfer.

L. monocytogenes readily invades intestinal cell lines (e.g., Caco-2 cells) and macrophages, and these cell lines are used for in vitro studies of invasion and actin rearrangement. *L. monocytogenes* makes **plaques** (zones of killing) in fibroblast monolayers. To make a visible clearing in the monolayer, the bacteria must be able to invade and kill many mammalian cells. Accordingly, the plaque assay is used to assess cell-to-cell spread by *L. monocytogenes*. There are now several cell-free in vitro systems, including a cell-free extract from *Xenopus* oocytes, in which *L. monocytogenes* polymerizes actin. Using the cell-free extracts allows scientists to exert more control over experimental conditions.

Genetic System

L. monocytogenes genes are generally not expressed in *Escherichia coli*, nor are *E. coli* transposons and plasmids functional in *Listeria*. Initially, the lack of genetic tools delayed the development of *L. monocytogenes* genetics. This problem has now been solved by using *Bacillus subtilis* instead of *E. coli* for cloning and expressing *Listeria* genes. Also, derivatives of the gram-positive transposon Tn*916* can be used for transposon mutagenesis. Another important development has been a method for making gene replacements.

Motility

L. monocytogenes is acquired by ingestion. If it survives passage through the stomach, it must find and adhere to the small intestinal mucosa in order to infect that site. Thus, it might seem that motility due to flagella would be an important virulence factor. In fact, although *L. monocytogenes* has flagella and is highly motile under some conditions, motility is observed only at temperatures considerably below those found in the human body (20 to 25°C). At 37°C, production of flagella is much decreased, so it is likely that motility due to flagella is not important as a virulence factor. It is possible, however, that ingested *L. monocytogenes* cells that come from a lower-temperature environment may have flagella for a period after they reach the intestine, and these flagella could help the bacteria reach the intestinal mucosa.

Invasion and Cell-to-Cell Spread

L. monocytogenes attaches to and invades tissue culture cells. Adherence and the invasion process are thought to mimic what happens during a *Listeria* infection. Steps in invasion and cell-to-cell transfer, and the virulence factors thought to be involved at each step, are summarized in Figure 27–1. Initially, the phagocytosed bacteria are contained within a vacuole that has a single membrane. They escape the vacuole by rupturing the vacuolar membrane. The bacteria then begin to polymerize actin filaments at one end, forming long actin tails that propel them through the cytoplasm. The bacteria can move by this mechanism into adjacent cells, producing long projections, which are then pinched off in the newly invaded cell. At this point, the bacteria are encased in a vacuole surrounded by a double membrane. They eventually escape from this vacuole and enter the cytoplasm of the newly invaded cell.

Adherence and invasion are mediated by membrane proteins called **internalins—InlA** and **InlB.** The importance of internalins is evident from the fact that a transposon insertion in *inlA* completely eliminates the ability of the bacteria to invade tissue culture cells. The *inlA* gene is part of an operon that contains a downstream gene, *inlB,* which encodes a protein that also appears to be involved in invasion. InlA seems to be the more important of the two internalins because providing *inlA* alone in *trans* in a mutant that does not produce InlA or InlB restores the mutant to full invasiveness.

More recently, scientists have developed an animal model to study the role of InlA in the uptake of *L. monocytogenes* by host cells. A strain of transgenic mice was created that expresses the human cell receptor E-cadherin on the surface of enterocytes. InlA binds to the E-cadherin, thus allowing *L. monocytogenes* first to invade enterocytes, then to multiply, and finally to cross the intestinal epithelium.

LLO (*hly*)

Forced phagocytosis brings *L. monocytogenes* into the host cell encased in a vesicle from which the bacteria must escape in order to enter the host cell cytoplasm. One of the proteins responsible for this escape is a hemolysin, **listeriolysin O (LLO).** LLO is responsible for the zone of beta-hemolysis seen around the bacteria when *Listeria* is grown on blood agar plates. LLO is a pore-forming cytotoxin, which has considerable amino acid sequence similarity to cytotoxins produced by two other gram-positive pathogens, *Streptococcus pyogenes* (streptolysin O) and *Streptococcus pneumoniae* (pneumolysin). The gene encoding LLO has been named ***hly,*** for "hemolysin." LLO is a major virulence factor of *L. monocytogenes.* LLO-negative mutants have an LD_{50} for mice that is 5 logs higher than that of wild type. LLO-negative mutants also do not survive in macrophages. This suggests that survival of *L. monocytogenes* in mac-

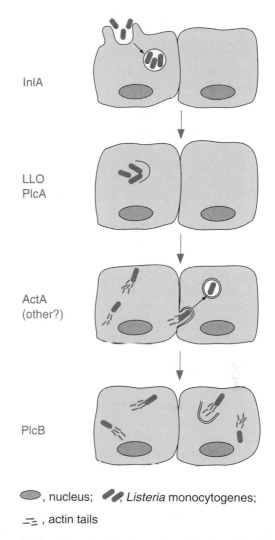

Figure 27–1 Steps in the invasion of cultured cells and intracellular spread by *L. monocytogenes.* The virulence factors thought to be involved at each step are indicated. "?" means that there is some uncertainty about the importance of the particular factor for that step. InlA is probably not necessary for ingestion of the bacteria by macrophagelike cell lines, which are naturally phagocytic, but is essential for invasion of cells, such as enterocytes, that are not normally phagocytic.

rophages could be due to its ability to escape the phagosome before phagolysosomal fusion occurs, but this has not been proved.

The importance of LLO for escape from the phagocytic vesicle was shown by an experiment in which the *L. monocytogenes hly* gene was expressed in *B. subtilis.* The *B. subtilis* strain was incubated with a macrophagelike cell line. Although wild-type *B. subtilis* remained inside the phagocytic vesicle, *B. subtilis* expressing *hly* escaped the vesicle and entered the cytoplasm of the cell.

PI-PLC (*plcA*) and PC-PLC (*plcB*)

L. monocytogenes produces at least two other hemolysins besides LLO, but these are enzymes, not pore-forming proteins. One is **phosphatidylinositol-specific phospholipase C (PI-PLC),** which hydrolyzes phosphatidylinositol. The second one is a broad-specificity **phospholipase C (PC-PLC)** that cleaves most phospholipids. The designation PC-PLC came from the initial observation that this phospholipase could cleave phosphatidylcholine. PC-PLC has now been shown to be able to cleave many other phospholipids, not just phosphocholine.

PI-PLC (*plcA*) was originally reported to be a virulence factor because a mutant with an insertional disruption in *plcA* was unable to cause listeriosis in mice. Also, this mutant formed very small plaques on a fibroblast monolayer, indicating that PI-PLC might aid intracellular spread of *Listeria*. However, a more careful analysis of this mutant revealed that the effects of the mutation were due to a polar effect of the mutation on a downstream gene, *prfA*. PrfA is a regulatory protein that appears to activate a number of genes, including *hly* and *mpl/actA/plcB* (see later section). Loss of expression of these genes has a strongly negative impact on virulence.

More recently, the role of *plcA* has been clarified. A nonpolar mutation in *plcA* had only a slight effect on virulence (about a threefold reduction in virulence). But a double mutant that lacked both PlcA (PI-PLC) and PlcB (PC-PLC) was 500-fold less virulent than wild type. Because a mutant that lacked only PlcB was only 20-fold less virulent than wild type, it is clear that the two phospholipases are acting synergistically. Judging from the ability of different mutants to escape from vacuoles, it would appear that PlcA contributes most to escape from the primary vacuole, whereas PlcB is more important for escape from the double-membrane vacuole in which the bacteria find themselves during cell-to-cell spread (Figure 27–1).

Another possible role for PI-PLC and PC-PLC is suggested by the fact that tissue culture cells infected with *L. monocytogenes* have aberrant expression of some important signal transduction molecules, such as mitogen-activated protein kinase and NF-κB. This makes sense because both PLCs release diacylglycerol from phospholipids and PC-PLC releases ceramide from sphingolipids (Figure 27–2). Molecules such as diacylglycerol and ceramide can trigger a variety of signal transduction responses in a cell. One reason to think PLCs might be doing this is that a cell line (NIH 3T3) that was stably transfected with *plcB* lost control of growth rate, a clear sign that signal transduction pathways were being aberrantly expressed. Although loss of growth control would probably not help the bacteria directly because they quickly kill the cell, it might help indirectly because dividing eukaryotic cells take up more nutrients than nondividing cells.

Metalloprotease

A gene encoding a **Zn-dependent metalloprotease (mpl)** is near *plcB* on the chromosome of *L. monocytogenes*. Transposon insertions in this locus reduce virulence. The mutants not only fail to make the metalloprotease but also fail to make active PC-PLC. However, the mutants make a protein that is somewhat larger than mature PC-PLC (33 kDa versus 29 kDa) but that still cross-reacts with antiserum to PC-PLC. The protein may be an unprocessed form of PC-PLC. If so, this result suggests that Mpl has some role in processing PC-PLC.

Actin-Based Motility

Inside the infected cell, *L. monocytogenes* uses host cell actin to move within and between host cells. Many bacterial pathogens can disrupt the host cell cytoskeleton, but only *L. monocytogenes* and a gram-negative pathogen, *Shigella* (a cause of dysentery), can organize actin filaments into long tails that propel the bacteria through the cytoplasm. The process of actin nucleation by *L. monocytogenes* requires only one protein, a surface protein called ActA. ActA appears to act by stimulating host cell proteins that normally participate in the nucleation of actin filaments to form the actin filaments. Examples of such host cell proteins are profilin and Arp proteins. These proteins normally help to make the host cell's cytoskeleton. In the presence of ActA, such proteins polymerize actin filaments at the surface of the bacterium, not in the normal location.

The bacteria polymerize actin only at one end of the cell (asymmetric polymerization). This is necessary for unidirectional movement. There is controversy as to whether asymmetric polymerization is due to asymmetric distribution of ActA on the cell surface or to some other mechanism. One group found ActA only at one end of the cell; another found ActA uniformly distributed over the surface. These different results may reflect differences in the strains used and differences in the reagents used to detect ActA. An explanation for these two apparently contradictory views comes from the observation that ActA has to be phosphorylated to become active. Possibly, ActA is distributed uniformly over the bacterial surface but only ActA molecules at one end of the cell are phosphorylated or otherwise activated.

What makes the issue of surface distribution of ActA

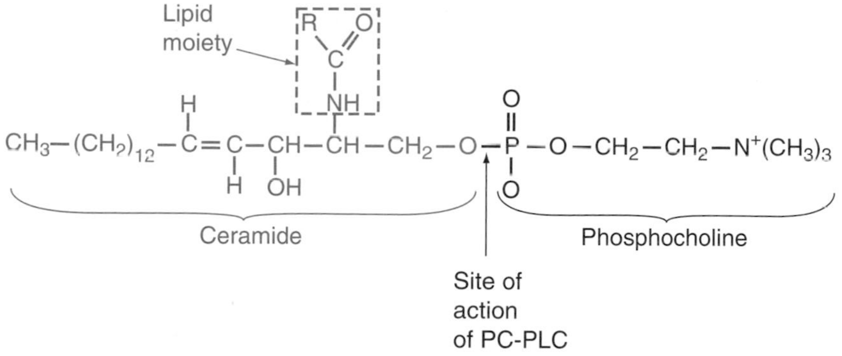

Lipid moiety

Ceramide

Site of action of PC-PLC

Phosphocholine

$$CH_3-(CH_2)_{12}-\overset{H}{\underset{H}{C}}=\overset{}{C}-\overset{\overset{NH}{|}}{CH}-\overset{\overset{|}{OH}}{CH}-CH_2-O-\overset{\overset{O}{||}}{\underset{\overset{||}{O}}{P}}-O-CH_2-CH_2-N^+(CH_3)_3$$

Figure 27–2 Site of hydrolysis of sphingolipids by PC-PLC. Ceramide, which can trigger a variety of signal transduction responses in the host cell, is released by the action of PC-PLC.

more perplexing is that some bacteria make "clouds" of actin rather than "tails." That is, they polymerize actin over the entire cell surface and do not move. The actin cloud appears to be less organized than an actin tail. This observation, taken together with the observation that bacteria can switch from cloud production to tail production, suggests that cloud formation may be an early step in the process that ultimately leads to tail formation. A model proposed to explain the cloud to tail switch is shown in Figure 27–3. Initially, the bacteria polymerize actin over their entire surface. Then, they begin to divide. Somehow the division process causes the polymerization of actin to become asymmetric, forming actin tails.

An early question that perplexed scientists was whether the tails were actually propelling the bacteria or whether the bacteria were moving by other means, leaving polymerized actin in their wake. An elegant experiment to answer this question was to incorporate a photoreactive compound in a growing actin tail. A section of the tail was then pulsed with light to activate the label, thus marking that part of the tail. By watching whether the band of light moved or remained stationary the scientists concluded that the actin tail remained stationary, and that growth of the tail by actin nucleation at the end of the bacteria propelled the bacteria through the cytoplasm. The actin tail is actually a hollow cylinder that is continuously elongated. After a period of time, the actin meshwork at the older end of the tail is depolymerized by host cell depolymerases. Thus, after the tail reaches a certain length, it appears to have a relatively constant length because actin is being depolymerized at the end of the tail as rapidly as it is being polymerized at the bacterial surface.

In the host cell cytoplasm, *L. monocytogenes* multiplies rapidly. It has been estimated that the bacteria inside a host cell divide as often as once every 50 min, a high rate of growth for an intracellular pathogen. *L. monocytogenes* also moves rapidly inside cells, at a rate of about 1.5 μm/s.

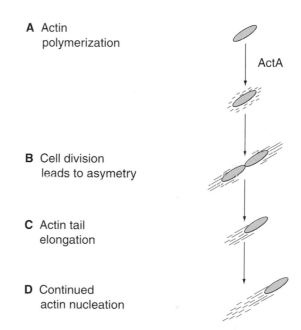

A Actin polymerization

ActA

B Cell division leads to asymetry

C Actin tail elongation

D Continued actin nucleation

Figure 27–3 A model of the steps involved in motility of *L. monocytogenes* inside host cells. (**A**) Actin polymerization is initiated by ActA, and a cloud of actin forms over the entire surface of the bacteria. (**B**) The bacteria divide, leading to what appears to be an asymmetrical distribution of actin at one end of each cell. (**C**) The actin tail elongates, and the bacteria begin to move. (**D**) Actin nucleation continues at the end of the bacteria, thus propelling them through the host cell cytoplasm. (Adapted from Smith and Portnoy, 1997.)

Systemic Spread of *L. monocytogenes*

In mice infected with *L. monocytogenes*, the bacteria first appear in macrophages, and then invade liver cells (hepatocytes). Most of their replication probably occurs in the liver. Because the bacteria are growing intracellularly in hepatocytes, a cell-mediated host response that kills infected cells is important for eliminating the bacteria. It has been shown that infection of macrophages with *L. monocytogenes* leads to presentation of bacterial antigens in a complex with MHC class I, thus stimulating the cytotoxic T-cell response. Cytotoxic T cells (and NK cells, another type of phagocytic cell that recognizes infected host cells) presumably help to kill the infected hepatocytes. Bacteria released from these lysed host cells could then be killed by activated macrophages, which, unlike resting macrophages, are able to kill *L. monocytogenes*. T-cell-deficient mice are able to survive *L. monocytogenes* infection, so although the cytotoxic T-cell response may help clear hepatocytes infected by bacteria, this response is not essential. Mice lacking the ability to produce IFN-γ are more susceptible to *L. monocytogenes* than normal mice, a fact that reflects the importance of activated macrophages as part of the host response; IFN-γ stimulates macrophage activation. A failure of the host's cell-mediated response to control *L. monocytogenes* allows the bacteria to spread systemically. The placenta is largely composed of endothelial cells. Thus the ability of *L. monocytogenes* to cross the placenta could be due to its ability to invade these cells and move from cell to cell, but this possibility remains speculative.

Organization and Regulation of Virulence Genes

Many of the *Listeria* virulence genes are clustered in the same region of the chromosome (Figure 27–4). The genes *mpl, actA, plcB,* and three open reading frames of unknown function appear to be organized in an operon. However, Northern blot analysis indicates that there may be more than one promoter in this region; in particular, there may be a promoter downstream of *mpl*. Thus, insertions in the *mpl* gene appear to be only partially polar on *actA* and other downstream genes. The *plcA* gene is part of an operon which contains *prfA*. *prfA*

encodes a positive regulatory protein that activates transcription of itself, *plcA, hly,* and the *mpl/actA/plcB* operon. There are three lines of evidence for this. First, mutations that disrupt *prfA* dramatically reduce expression of *hly* and the other genes in this region. Second, providing *prfA* on a multicopy plasmid leads to elevated expression of *hly* and the other genes in this region. Third, PrfA activates transcription of a *hly-lacZ* fusion in *B. subtilis*. Genes controlled by PrfA are thermoregulated; they are expressed at higher levels at 37°C than at lower temperatures.

Prevention and Treatment

Antibiotic treatment of pregnant women or immunocompromised people who have eaten food contaminated by *L. monocytogenes* can prevent the most serious consequences of listeriosis, but only if the infection is diagnosed in time. Usually, infections are not diagnosed early enough for antibiotics to be useful. Often, the first signs of an outbreak are stillbirths or serious infections in susceptible adults. Because cases of listeriosis are frequently associated with commercially produced foods, avoiding contamination of foods during processing would be the ideal solution. Although the food processing industry has labored mightily to prevent contamination of food by *L. monocytogenes*, contamination incidents continue to occur. Since the tests that detect contamination can take days, the food is often already on the grocery shelf before the contamination is detected. Another complication is that *Listeria* is able to grow well at low temperatures. Thus, refrigeration is not as effective in preventing growth of *Listeria* in food as it is for most other bacteria that cause foodborne disease. Add to this the fact that at least 5 to 10% of adults are asymptomatic carriers of *L. monocytogenes*,

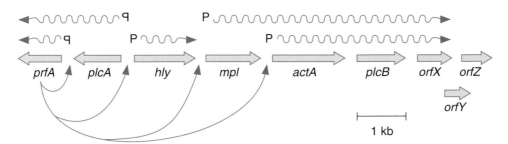

Figure 27–4　Organization and regulatory control of some *L. monocytogenes* virulence genes that are clustered on the chromosome. *prfA*, regulatory protein (activator); genes activated by PrfA are indicated by arrows: *plcA* (encodes PI-PLC); *plcB* (encodes PC-PLC); *hly* (encodes LLO); *actA* (encodes ActA, a protein involved in actin polymerization); *mpl* (encodes a protein that may be involved in processing of phosphocholine), *orfX, Y, Z* (open reading frames of unknown function), and *prfA* itself. Probable locations of promoters are indicated by "P"; wavy lines indicate mRNA transcripts.

and it is easy to see why *L. monocytogenes* is a food processor's nightmare.

For the present, the ultimate responsibility for prevention is in the hands of the consumer. Pregnant women and immunocompromised people are advised to take the following precautions. Avoid all soft cheeses, and do not consume unpasteurized milk. It is also wise to avoid coleslaw and other deli foods that are not normally heated before eating. Thoroughly heat all meats, especially processed meat products, such as cold cuts and hot dogs. Because *L. monocytogenes* grows in the refrigerator, all leftover meats should be reheated until steaming hot before they are eaten. Raw vegetables should be washed thoroughly.

A recently introduced change in the way food processors monitor food safety may help prevent the shipment of contaminated lots of food in the future. The new system is called **HACCP,** for **hazard analysis and critical control point** program. The manufacturer identifies certain critical points in the processing of the food at which contamination is most likely to occur. At each of these points, the food is monitored for contamination. By testing before the processing is completed rather than just at the end, there is more time for test results to be obtained that might prevent the shipment of the food. HACCP also identifies weak links in the safety chain. This would not only help protect consumers from infection but would prevent expensive recalls that make the food processors look bad.

SELECTED READINGS

Broome, C. V. 1993. Listeriosis: can we prevent it? *ASM News* **59:**444–446.

Kuhn, M., and W. Goebel. 1998. Host cell signaling during *Listeria monocytogenes* infection. *Trends Microbiol.* **6:**11–14.

Lecuit, M., S. Vandormael-Pournin, J. Lefort, M. Huerre, P. Gounon, C. Dupuy, C. Babinet, and P. Cossart. 2001. A transgenic model for listeriosis: role of internalin in crossing the intestinal barrier. *Science* **292:**1722–1725.

Lorber, B. 1997. Listeriosis. *Clin. Infect. Dis.* **24:**1–11.

Smith, G. A., and D. A. Portnoy. 1997. How *Listeria monocytogenes* ActA protein converts actin polymerization into a motile force. *Trends Microbiol.* **5:**272–276.

Smith, G. A., H. Marquis, S. Jones, N. Johnston, D. A. Portnoy, and H. Goldfine. 1995. Two distinct phospholipases C of *Listeria monocytogenes* have overlapping roles in escape from a vacuole and cell-to-cell spread. *Infect. Immun.* **63:**4231–4237.

Songer, J. G. 1997. Bacterial phospholipases and their role in virulence. *Trends Microbiol.* **5:**156–161.

Welch, M., J. Rosenblatt, J. Skoble, D. A. Portnoy, and T. J. Mitchison. 1998. Interaction of human Arp2/3 complex and the *Listeria monocytogenes* ActA protein in actin filament nucleation. *Science* **281:**105–108.

SUMMARY OUTLINE

Characteristics of *L. monocytogenes*

Gram-positive rod

Motile by flagella at lower temperatures

Motile inside mammalian cells because of asymmetric polymerization of actin (actin tails)

Found widely in soil, water, and intestinal tracts of animals and humans (5 to 10%)

Capable of growth over a wide range of temperatures (4 to 40°C)

Listeriosis

Acquired from contaminated foods

Large number of bacteria must be ingested

Immunocompromised people—systemic disease, meningitis

Pregnant women—transplacental transfer causes fetal infections, stillbirths

Virulence factors

Invasion of mammalian cells
Internalin A—probably most important
Internalin B

(continued)

SUMMARY OUTLINE (*continued*)

Escape from primary vacuole (single membrane)

LLO; also called hemolysin (*hly*)—pore-forming cytotoxin

PI-PLC—enzyme that removes charged head group from phospholipids (especially phosphatidylinositol)

Movement through cytoplasm, cell-to-cell spread

ActA—interacts with host cell proteins to stimulate actin polymerization

Actin tail forms at one end of cell, propels bacterium through cytoplasm

Projections from host cell surface caused by bacteria enter adjacent cells; bacteria inside double-membrane vacuole

Escape from the double-membrane vacuole

PC-PLC—phospholipase that cleaves the head group from many different kinds of lipids

Disruption of signal transduction pathways of host cell

PI-PLC

PC-PLC

Regulation of virulence factors

PrfA—positive regulator of virulence genes, may respond to temperature

Many virulence genes clustered in the same location on the chromosome

Prevention and treatment

Antibiotics usually not useful unless disease diagnosed very early

Avoid products made with unpasteurized milk

Avoid coleslaw and deli meats

Cook meat thoroughly, and reheat after refrigerator storage

QUESTIONS

Answers to the questions can be found in Appendix 2.

1. How could an actin structure such as that produced by *L. monocytogenes* cause movement of the bacteria?

2. A transposon insertion in *actA* stops tail formation by *L. monocytogenes*. Does this fact alone prove that ActA is an actin nucleator? What were some other possibilities scientists had to consider before concluding that ActA is the only bacterial protein that participates in the actin polymerization process?

3. How did scientists decide whether LLO or the phospholipases were important for escape from the primary vacuole or from the double-membrane vacuole?

4. How could you determine whether the actin polymerization factor responsible for actin tail formation was (i) produced by the bacteria as opposed to being a host cell factor and (ii) a protein?

5. Mention was made of the fact that another bacterium that forms actin tails is *Shigella*, one cause of dysentery (bloody diarrhea). The invasion and cell-to-cell spread of *Shigella* is similar to that of *Listeria* in this and other respects. Yet listeriosis is generally a systemic infection, whereas dysentery is usually localized to the intestinal mucosa and underlying tissue and does not become systemic. Speculate about why listeriosis is so different from dysentery in its symptoms and progression despite the fact that *Listeria* and *Shigella* seem to be so similar in their invasion and intracellular behavior.

6. Infection with *L. monocytogenes* produces an antibody response, but this response is not protective. Explain why this is so. Also, make an educated guess as to why most adults exhibit only mild symptoms whereas intrauterine infections or infections of immunocompromised people can be serious.

Diarrheagenic
Escherichia coli Strains

KEY FEATURES

Diarrheagenic *Escherichia coli* Strains

CHARACTERISTICS
Gram-negative rod
Motile
Facultative metabolism

DISEASES
Diarrhea
Urinary tract and other extraintestinal infections (chapter 29)

RESERVOIR
Humans
Other animals

MAIN VIRULENCE FACTORS
Vary with strain
Adhesins
Toxins (most diarrheagenic strains)

PREVENTION AND TREATMENT
Prevent fecal contamination of water supply
Proper food handling
Fluid replacement therapy
Antibiotics usually not appropriate

Different Types of Diarrheagenic
Escherichia coli Strains

Some bacteria, such as *Vibrio cholerae* (chapter 25) and *Listeria mono-cytogenes* (chapter 27), are one-disease organisms. By contrast, *E. coli* strains can cause an impressive variety of diseases. Diseases caused by *E. coli* strains include diarrhea, dysentery, hemolytic uremic syndrome (kidney failure), bladder infections, septicemia, pneumonia, and meningitis. In general, different strains are associated with different conditions. That is, a strain of *E. coli* that causes diarrhea will not cause urinary tract infections or meningitis and vice versa. The versatility of *E. coli* strains is due to the fact that different strains have acquired different sets of virulence genes. Some of these genes resemble those found in other pathogenic species and may have been acquired by lateral gene transfer, but others seem to be unique to *E. coli*. This chapter will focus on gastrointestinal infections caused by *E. coli*. Urinary tract infections and other extraintestinal diseases caused by *E. coli* will be covered in chapter 29. It should be noted that *E. coli* is by no means the only bacterium that causes a variety of infections. On the gram-positive side, *Staphylococcus aureus* (chapter 14) and *Streptococcus pyogenes* (chapter 15) certainly rival *E. coli* in pathogenic versatility. These bacteria too owe their pathogenic versatility to the acquisition of different sets of virulence genes that allow them to adapt best to conditions in certain parts of the human body.

Classification of Pathogenic *E. coli* Strains

Serogroup and Serotype

Because most strains of *E. coli* are not pathogens and because different strains cause different types of disease, it is important to be able to identify particular strains or groups of strains so that outbreaks caused by a particular type of strain can be identified. Before the advent of molecular biology and the identification of virulence factors, scientists turned to bacterial surface antigens as a convenient method for "fingerprinting" bacteria. This led to a serological classification scheme based on the reactivity of highly variable bacterial surface molecules with different antibodies (**serotyping**). Serotyping is still widely used, especially for tracing outbreaks of intestinal disease. More recently, a classification scheme based on virulence factors (which has been called **virotyping**) has been proposed. This latter approach to strain typing represents a promising new use of emerging information about virulence factors of *E. coli* strains. Its advantage is that this method of classification is more directly associated with the disease process than serotyping. Virotyping could be done using DNA hybridization or PCR, but so far no such test is in widespread clinical use. For practical reasons the serotyping approach to strain identification, a technique with which clinical microbiologists are more familiar, will continue to be widely used in the foreseeable future.

Two types of *E. coli* surface structures form the basis for the serological classification system: O antigen of LPS (**O**) and flagella (**H,** for "hauch," the German term for a flagellum). The O antigen identifies the **serogroup** of a strain, and the H antigen identifies its **serotype.** For example, two strains labeled O111:H4 and O111:H12 react with the same anti-O antibody and are thus in the same serogroup but react with different anti-H antibodies and are thus different serotypes. At least 160 different serogroups are known. There is some correlation between serogroup or serotype and virulence. For example, members of serogroup O86 are commonly found as members of the resident human microbiota and rarely cause disease, whereas members of serogroup O55 are rarely found in the resident microbiota and are almost always associated with disease. Recently, serotype O157:H7 has been associated with a type of intestinal infection that can cause kidney failure in children. The emergence of other serotypes with the same capability has somewhat blurred this picture of the lone serotype, but the ability to identify potentially dangerous strains has been a big help in preventing the dissemination of these strains through the food supply by detecting the strains before shipment of contaminated lots. Contamination of meat by *E. coli* is a common occurrence and usually does not pose any danger, so it is important to be able to identify lots that contain strains of *E. coli* that do pose a danger.

In cases where the strain has a capsule, a capsular (**K**) antigen is also used for classification. Strains classed as K1, for example, cause systemic infection in infants.

Virotype

The characteristics that form the basis for the virotyping system include patterns of bacterial attachment to host cells, effects of attachment on host cells, production of toxins, and invasiveness. A **virotype** usually contains more than one serogroup and serotype. A word of caution is in order. Although the classification scheme based on virulence-associated characteristics is a conceptually useful way of grouping *E. coli* strains, it can be somewhat misleading because it gives the impression that clear-cut distinctions can always be made on the basis of virulence factors. Some strains of *E. coli* have properties associated with more than one virotype. Also, the virotype classification scheme is based, in some cases, on incomplete information about adherence properties and toxin production and will undoubtedly need to be refined as more information becomes available. For example, the production of toxins by diarrheagenic strains of *E. coli* is so widespread that assertions that a particular virotype does not produce a toxin may simply mean that there is a toxin that has not yet been discovered. Currently, at least six *E. coli* virotypes have been identified: **enterotoxigenic *E. coli* (ETEC), enteroaggregative *E. coli* (EAggEC), diffusely adhering *E. coli* (DAEC), enteropathogenic *E. coli* (EPEC),**

enterohemorrhagic *E. coli* (EHEC), and **enteroinvasive *E. coli* (EIEC).** This chapter will focus on the best studied of these virotypes: ETEC, EAggEC, EPEC, and EHEC. Salient features of these four virotypes are summarized in Figure 28–1.

A useful test for classifying type of adherence is the HEp-2 tissue culture cell attachment assay. The strain to be typed is incubated with a monolayer of HEp-2 cells for 3 h. Then the tissue culture cells are washed with buffered saline to remove nonadherent bacteria. Formation of isolated patches of adherent cells, which are one or two bacterial cells thick, is called *localized adherence*. This pattern of adherence is typical of ETEC, EHEC, and EPEC strains. Formation of lumplike aggregates of bacteria, many cells thick, is called *aggregative adherence* and is typical of EAggEC strains. Dispersal of individual cells over the surface of the monolayer is called *diffuse adherence* and is a trait that distinguishes the most recently named virotype, DAEC. Tissue culture cells are also used to determine whether or not a strain is invasive.

A striking feature of different virotypes of *E. coli* is the extent to which virulence factors of these strains are encoded by genes carried on mobile elements. The mobile elements include plasmids (ETEC toxin genes), transposons (ETEC heat-stable toxin [ST]), pathogenicity islands (many genes of EPEC and EHEC strains), and bacteriophages (EHEC Shiga toxin [Stx]). The carriage of virulence genes on mobile elements is thought to be the reason for the variety of *E. coli* virotypes, which appear to have resulted from acquisition of particular sets of genes on mobile elements acquired from other bacteria.

EHEC strains have only recently been recognized as a cause of serious disease. A number of outbreaks of disease caused by EHEC have occurred in developed countries. Usually, pediatric diarrhea seen in developed countries is not a fatal disease. Disease caused by EHEC strains, however, can cause death because acute kidney failure (hemolytic uremic syndrome [**HUS**]) is a complication of the disease (Box 28–1). EHEC strains cause a disease that is more similar to dysentery (bloody diarrhea) caused by the gram-negative bacterium *Shigella* than to the usually uncomplicated diarrhea caused by ETEC or EPEC strains. Whereas diarrhea due to ETEC and EPEC strains is seen most commonly in developing countries, EHEC dysentery has so far been reported mainly in developed countries, such as the United States and Canada. This apparently localized distribution of EHEC diarrhea could be misleading, however, because EHEC disease has only recently been recognized and thus is only beginning to be included routinely in surveys done in developing countries. Some early reports of broader international surveys suggest that EHEC will prove to be a problem worldwide.

EIEC strains cause a bloody diarrhea similar to that caused by EHEC strains, but to date no cases of HUS

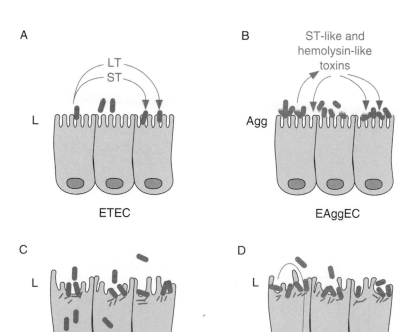

Figure 28–1 Comparison of properties of four of the virotypes of *E. coli* strains that cause intestinal disease. LT, *E. coli* heat-labile (choleralike) toxin; ST, *E. coli* heat-stable toxin; Stx, Shiga toxin; L, localized adherence; Agg, aggregative adherence.

BOX 28–1   Fast Food Furor: O157:H7 Visits the Northwestern United States

In January 1993, physicians and hospital staff members at a Seattle, Wash., hospital were overwhelmed by an unusually large number of children with acute kidney failure. All of the children had had painful bloody diarrhea prior to the onset of kidney failure. Some of the children died. Similar cases of bloody diarrhea and kidney failure occurred at the same time in Nevada, Idaho, and California. All of these cases were eventually traced to consumption of contaminated hamburgers from a single fast-food chain, and all were due to EHEC strain O157:H7. Food-borne disease outbreaks associated with fast-food chains pose a particularly serious problem because hamburger patties are made by a single, central supplier and then delivered to the various chain outlets. A single lot of contaminated hamburgers can thus end up in many widely separated locations.

What happened in response to the 1993 outbreak in different states is instructive. In Seattle, the hospital laboratory had the new tests for O157:H7 in place and was routinely testing people complaining of bloody diarrhea for O157:H7 because of the danger of HUS in children. Thus, the pathogen was rapidly identified, and contaminated hamburgers were recalled in time to prevent further cases. In Nevada, hospital laboratories were not routinely monitoring for O157:H7, and the outbreak in that state was not recognized in the early stages. In fact, it was discovered only because the parent of a child who had had bloody diarrhea read about the Washington cases of HUS in the newspaper and called the state health department. Thus, in Nevada, contaminated hamburger shipments continued to be served by fast-food outlets after they were recalled in Washington. The dangers posed by O157:H7 infections have only recently begun to be properly appreciated, and the experience of different states with this particular outbreak underscores the importance of routine testing of patients (especially children) who present with bloody diarrhea. The sooner the condition is identified, the sooner the source of the outbreak can be identified and remedied.

Another important point illustrated by this outbreak is the importance of adequately cooking meat. Fast-food chains have done an exemplary job of maintaining cleanliness in their kitchens, and, given the number of meals they serve every year, they have had a remarkably good record for safety. However, when too much emphasis is placed on the "fast" in fast foods, inadequate cooking of hamburgers and other meats can result. Properly cooked hamburgers would be safe even if contaminated by O157:H7 because thorough cooking kills *E. coli*. Emphasis on proper cooking of hamburgers is the most direct route to preventing further outbreaks of this type. Unfortunately, monitoring of ground meat for O157:H7 contamination using presently available technology is impractical, because it is difficult and often impossible to isolate the bacteria from the likely source of the outbreak. This is probably due to the fact that O157:H7 has a very low ID_{50}, similar to that of *Shigella*, so concentrations of bacteria in meat that are too low to detect easily in routine screening can still pose a hazard. New approaches to detecting low numbers of bacteria, such as the rapid enzyme-linked immunosorbent assay and a chip test now on the market, are already making routine monitoring of meat and other food products possible.

Although the first outbreaks of EHEC disease were associated with ground beef, subsequent experience has shown that many foods can become contaminated and can spread disease. A brand of apple juice, which was not pasteurized at that time, caused the death of a little girl who acquired *E. coli* O157:H7. Needless to say, the company that produced the juice is now a strong advocate of pasteurization.

A larger outbreak of EHEC disease occurred in Japan in 1996 among schoolchildren. The contaminated food was radish sprouts used in a salad included in school lunches. The seeds had come from the United States. There was much international finger-pointing as a result of this outbreak, with U.S. farmers blaming Japanese sprouting companies for the contamination and Japanese companies and government spokespeople claiming that the bacteria came to Japan on the seeds used to generate the sprouts. The limited available evidence suggests that the Japanese are right about the origin of the epidemic, but there are those who still do not consider the case proven.

Adapted from P. Knight. 1993. Hemorrhagic *E. coli*: the danger increases. *ASM News* **59**:247–250.

have been seen in people with EIEC dysentery. EIEC strains actively invade colonic cells and spread laterally to adjacent cells. A number of serogroups are included in the EIEC virotype, but three serogroups predominate. These serogroups are not seen among ETEC, EPEC, or EHEC strains.

Virulence Factors

ETEC Strains

OVERVIEW OF ETEC DIARRHEA.   ETEC strains adhere to the small intestinal mucosa and produce symptoms not by invading the mucosa but by producing toxins that act on mucosal cells to cause diarrhea. There are no apparent histological changes in host cells, except for a mild inflammatory response. ETEC diarrhea can nonetheless be fatal, especially in infants and young children. ETEC diarrhea is still a major cause of death in infants and children in many developing countries. ETEC strains also cause disease in adults, although deaths are rare. Adults in a country where ETEC strains are endemic or epidemic usually have at least partial immunity, but travelers from areas that are relatively free of ETEC strains are susceptible. For this reason, the adult version of ETEC diarrhea is commonly called **traveler's diarrhea.** ETEC strains produce two types of enterotoxin: a choleralike toxin called **heat-labile toxin (LT)** and a second diarrheal toxin called **heat-stable toxin (ST).** A number of different O serogroups and H serotypes are represented among ETEC strains.

ADHESINS.   ETEC strains produce several types of pili or fimbriae. Two types have received the most attention: **type 1 pili** and **colonization factor antigens I and II (CFA/I, CFA/II).** CFAs have also been called CS (for coli surface antigens), but to minimize confusion the CFA designation will be used here. Whereas type 1 pili are found on many *E. coli* strains, avirulent as well as virulent, CFAs are found mainly on ETEC strains. This is one of the reasons for believing that the CFAs are more important for virulence than type 1 pili.

CFAs look different from type 1 pili in that they are thinner and some are much longer. For this reason, they are called fimbriae rather than pili. The receptors for CFAs have still not been identified conclusively but are thought to be glycoproteins. The main CFAs associated with human ETEC strains are CFA/I, CFA/II, CFA/III, and CFA/IV. CFA/I is a rigid rod composed of a single protein subunit. CFA/II is not a single pilus type but is actually a group of at least two related adhesins. The predominant fimbria on CFA/II strains is a flexible fim-

bria, which is associated with CS antigen CS3, but the rigid pilus associated with CS1 and CS5 is also seen. **CFA/III** is a bundle-forming pilus, which consists of long, flexible pili that are often seen entwined around each other. CFA/III pili may be responsible for the bacterium-bacterium adherence that allows microcolonies to form. The newest ETEC adhesin to be described has been called longus. This type of pilus is found on many ETEC strains. The name longus refers to its unusual length: it extends 40 μm from the cell surface.

CFA genes are frequently (but not always) located on plasmids. Relatively little is known about regulation of CFA genes. Low-iron medium favors CFA production, but iron level is probably not the only signal controlling CFA production. CFAs are still produced in medium containing excess iron, although at a much lower level than in iron-deficient medium. In medium containing a high iron concentration, CFA production can be abolished completely by substituting acetate for glucose as the carbon source. It is not clear whether acetate itself or the slower growth rate on acetate is responsible for this effect. Interestingly, CFA production is inversely correlated with production of type 1 pili. When CFAs are produced, type 1 pili are not, and vice versa.

ENTEROTOXINS.   The diarrhea produced by adherent ETEC strains is caused by the action of either or both of two different toxins: heat-labile toxin (LT) and heat-stable toxin (ST). ("Heat stable" is defined as retention of toxin activity after incubation at 100°C for 30 min, and "heat labile" means that toxin activity is lost in 30 min under these conditions.) There are two types of LT, **LT-I** and **LT-II.** LT-I shares a high degree (ca. 75%) of amino acid identity with cholera toxin (see chapter 25). Given this, it is not surprising that LT has the same structure (five B subunits, one A subunit) and the same mechanism of action as cholera toxin. The B subunits of LT-I even interact with the same host cell receptor as cholera toxin, the host cell surface antigen G_{M1}.

The initial version of how LT causes diarrhea was fairly straightforward. The B subunits of LT bind to host cell antigen G_{M1}, and the A subunit of the toxin is internalized. Inside the cell, the A subunit ADP-ribosylates G_s, a protein which normally controls cAMP production. Inactivation of G_s causes an increase in cAMP production in intestinal cells by ADP-ribosylating protein. The rise in cAMP concentration activates **CFTR,** which, coincidentally, is the chloride channel that is mutated in people with cystic fibrosis. Chloride secretion is increased, and uptake of NaCl is inhibited. The ion imbalance causes intestinal cells to lose control of the flow of water, resulting in loss of water from tissue and diarrhea.

More recently, scientists have found that LT may have other effects. For example, LT affects the synthesis and release of prostaglandins and leukotrienes, proteins that stimulate electrolyte transport and thus could contribute to the ion imbalance. LT also has effects on the enteric nervous system, the network of neurons that surrounds the small and large intestine and controls intestinal motility and ion secretion. Inappropriate stimulation of the enteric nervous system, which controls the contractions that determine the rate of flow of contents through the intestine, could contribute to diarrhea. Finally, LT stimulates the production by intestinal epithelial cells of cytokines, a fact that could explain the mild inflammation of the mucosa that is seen in people with ETEC diarrhea. All or most of these effects could well be secondary results of the increase in cAMP production rather than primary effects of the toxin itself, but they illustrate the numerous ways in which LT affects the ion and water homeostasis of the intestinal mucosa.

The gene organization of LT-I genes is the same as for cholera toxin (i.e., the genes encoding the A and B subunits are cotranscribed in the same operon). Although the DNA and amino acid sequences of LT-I and cholera toxin are similar, the promoter regions are completely different. Thus, regulation of LT-I production is probably different from regulation of cholera toxin synthesis. Expression of genes encoding the A and B subunits of LT-I appears to be regulated rather than constitutive, because medium composition affects the amount of toxin produced. For example, certain mixtures of amino acids stimulate LT-I production by two- to threefold. The type of carbohydrate and the presence of zinc also affect LT-I production. Sublethal concentrations of the antibiotics lincomycin and tetracycline, but not of other protein synthesis inhibitors, stimulate LT-I production. Either regulation of LT-I production is highly complex, or all of these conditions have some common effect that has so far eluded investigators.

ST is not a single toxin but is rather a family of small (ca. 2 kDa) peptide toxins that fall into two subgroups: **methanol-soluble ST (STa)** and **methanol-insoluble ST (STb).** The small size of STs explains why they are not inactivated at high temperatures as rapidly as a full-length protein. High temperatures inactivate large proteins by unfolding them. A peptide as short as ST would not be affected to the same extent as a large protein. STs are excreted into the medium in a series of steps that alter the length of the peptide. In the case of STa, the precursor toxin (ca. 72 amino acids long) is first secreted to the periplasm. During secretion, 18 amino acids are removed, leaving a 54-amino-acid peptide. This peptide is excreted into the extracellular fluid, where it is cleaved to its final 17- to 19-amino-acid form by a process that is not well understood. A similar set of steps is involved in excretion of STb.

The receptor for STa is host cell guanylate cyclase, the enzyme responsible for regulating levels of intracellular cyclic GMP (cGMP) (Box 28–2). STa causes an increase in the cGMP level in the host cytoplasm, which leads to the same type of fluid loss caused by an uncontrolled rise in cAMP (Figure 28–2). **cGMP,** like cAMP, is an important signaling molecule in eukaryotic cells, and changes in cGMP affect a number of cellular processes, including activities of ion pumps. Guanylate cyclase is located in the apical membrane of the host cell, so it can act as both a receptor and a target. Binding of STa somehow activates guanylate cyclase (Figure 28–2). The activation process requires ATP, but the role of ATP is not understood, and there may be auxiliary factors involved (e.g., ATP-binding proteins).

STb appears to act by a different mechanism than STa, a fact that is not surprising since STb has a different amino acid sequence. STb has so far been found only in porcine ETEC strains, and it is questionable whether it contributes to human intestinal disease. By contrast, the role of STa in disease is well established. STa is encoded by a single gene, and its expression is regulated. Expression is controlled by cAMP, and there is a catabolite gene activator protein (CAP) binding site upstream of the promoter. CAP and cAMP control expression of a number of bacterial genes, including those involved in carbohydrate utilization.

Genes encoding LT-I and STa are carried on plasmids. These same plasmids often carry CFA genes in addition to toxin genes. This explains why production of LT-I and STa is highly correlated with production of CFAs. The plasmids carrying LT-I, STa, and CFA genes share regions of homology with each other, and these homologous regions could be insertion sequence elements (IS) associated with transposons. The variety of arrangements of STa and LT-I genes could well be due to the action of transposons and IS elements. Not only can transposons and IS elements move from replicon to replicon (see chapter 11), but some can mediate fusion of two plasmids, gene rearrangements, and gene duplication. Consistent with this hypothesis, the gene encoding STa has been shown to be carried on a transposable element.

EAggEC Strains

EAggEC strains cause a persistent form of diarrhea in children. EAggEC strains resemble ETEC strains in that they bind to small intestinal cells, are not invasive, and cause no obvious histological changes in intestinal cells to which they adhere (Figure 28–1B). They differ from

BOX 28–2   STa: a Bacterial Hormone?

For a long time, scientists working on intestinal cell physiology were intrigued by the fact that STa looked suspiciously like a peptide hormone, and they had pretty much convinced themselves that STa was exerting its effect by mimicking a naturally occurring hormone. Yet, the guanylate cyclase "receptor" that was the target for STa was not the target for any known hormone. Eventually, a hormone named guanylin was identified that is probably the hormone that normally binds guanylate cyclase. The function of guanylin is still unclear, but it causes intestinal cells to release water when it binds to guanylate cyclase. The role of the hormone could be to keep the mucin layer wet. The effect of guanylin stimulation on guanylate cyclase activity is not nearly as drastic as that of STa binding, which is consistent with the fact that ETEC-type diarrhea is not the normal state in the human body.

STa is the first example of a bacterial toxin that acts as a hormone analog. Bacteria have long been known to produce hormonelike compounds, but no pathological or ecological function had been associated with them. Using hormone analogs to alter host cell metabolism, possibly for the purpose of producing nutrients for the bacteria, may turn out to be a more common strategy for human pathogens than has been suspected. STa also stands as yet another example of how bacteria have developed ways to subvert host molecules to their own purposes, although it is still far from clear what the bacteria are getting out of this interaction. The discovery of a new hormone as a result of studying bacterial toxins illustrates the way in which studies of bacterial virulence factors have led to important discoveries in eukaryotic cell biology.

Source: M. Stroh. 1992. New hormone may lift Montezuma's vendetta. *Sci. News* **142**:5.

ETEC strains primarily in that they do not adhere uniformly over the surface of the intestinal mucosa but tend to clump in small aggregates (hence the name of the virotype). EAggEC strains produce an ST-like toxin and a hemolysin.

ADHESINS. EAggEC strains are covered with unusually thin (4 to 7 nm wide) fibrillar structures, which are presumed to be the adhesive pili of these strains. These pili have been purified and shown to be composed primarily of an 18-kDa subunit. The amino-terminal amino acid sequence of this subunit protein, GVVPQ, as well as other features of the pili are similar to those of a thin filamentous adhesin found on some strains of *Salmonella*. The name **GVVPQ fimbriae** has been proposed for this class of adhesin. It is still not clear what role, if any, these adhesins play in the disease caused by EAggEC strains. EAggEC are called aggregative because of their tendency to grow as aggregated clumps, both in vivo and in vitro. Thus, it is possible that the GVVPQ fimbriae promote adherence of bacteria to each other rather than adherence of bacteria to host cells. The GVVPQ fimbriae of EAggEC strains resemble another interesting type of pilus previously found on strains of *Salmonella typhimurium* (see chapter 26), a thin coiled pilus that has been named curli because the pili resemble curled hairs emanating from the surface of the bacteria. Curli is a virulence factor of the *E. coli* strains that produce it.

ENTEROTOXINS. The fact that EAggEC strains adhere to the intestinal mucosa without invading or causing an intense inflammatory response suggests that EAggEC strains produce some sort of diarrheal toxin, similar to ETEC strains. There was no evidence for LT production by these strains, and initially it appeared that EAggEC strains did not produce ST either. It has now been shown, however, that EAggEC strains produce an ST-like toxin called **EAST (enteroaggregative ST).** The importance of EAST as a virulence factor remains to be proved.

A second type of toxin has been associated with EAggEC strains—a 120-kDa exotoxin that is similar to a hemolysin produced by *E. coli* strains that cause urinary tract infections (see chapter 29). This toxin forms pores in host cell membranes. Binding of this toxin to HEp-2 cells causes an increase in host cell intracellular calcium levels. The increase is due to uptake of Ca^{2+} from the medium, presumably through the pore created by the toxin, and not to release of Ca^{2+} from intracellular Ca^{2+} stores. Ca^{2+} is an important signaling molecule in eukaryotic cells, and changes in Ca^{2+} levels

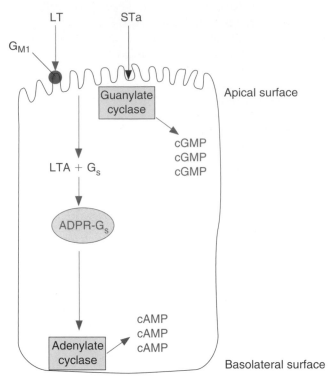

Figure 28–2 Comparison of the mechanism of action and cellular location of the targets of LT and STa. LT B subunits bind the host cell receptor G_{M1}, and the A subunit is internalized. Inside the cell, the A subunit ADP-ribosylates a G protein, G_s, that controls the activity of adenylate cyclase, an enzyme located on the basolateral surface of the host cell. This results in an increase in intracellular cAMP. STa activates guanylate cyclase, which is located on the apical surface, by binding it. The result is a rise in host cell cGMP levels.

have a number of effects on cellular function. Ca^{2+}-dependent phosphorylation of host cell proteins has been seen in HEp-2 cells to which EAggEC strains were attached, but the significance of this phosphorylation has not been established, and the identity of the target proteins is not known.

EPEC Strains

EPEC strains, like EAggEC strains, exhibit a patchy pattern of adherence to mammalian cells but do not form the same type of aggregates as EAggEC strains. Unlike ETEC and EAggEC strains, adherence of EPEC strains produces rather dramatic alterations in the ultrastructure of host mucosal cells (Figure 28–1C). Normal mucosal absorptive cells have numerous short fingerlike projections (microvilli) on their apical surfaces. Cells to which EPEC strains have adhered exhibit elongated microvilli where the bacteria are not bound and no microvilli where the bacteria are bound. This phenomenon is called **attaching and effacing.** It is the result of extensive rearrangement of host cell actin in the vicinity of the adherent bacteria, rearrangements that result in the formation of a cuplike pedestal structure under the bacteria. EPEC strains are more invasive than ETEC or EAggEC strains and elicit an even more pronounced inflammatory response. The diarrhea may be caused primarily by bacterial invasion of host cells and subversion of signal transduction systems that control ion flow rather than by production of exotoxins.

For a long time, the idea that EPEC strains were a common cause of human disease was controversial. This controversy arose from the fact that early epidemiological surveys of bacterial strains responsible for childhood diarrhea tended to focus on ETEC strains, a proven cause of diarrheal infection. As a result, there was little positive evidence in the literature for the association of EPEC strains with disease. It is now well established that EPEC strains, like ETEC strains, can cause a severe, often fatal, diarrhea in children and infants, and EPEC strains are acknowledged to be a major cause of pediatric diarrhea and death in developing countries. Interestingly, countries where pediatric diarrhea due to ETEC is a problem generally have relatively little EPEC diarrhea and vice versa. Nonimmune adults can also acquire EPEC diarrhea, and this type of diarrhea is sometimes included under the heading "traveler's diarrhea." The virotype EPEC contains a number of O serogroups. In general, serogroups associated with EPEC are limited to the EPEC virotype and are not associated with ETEC or other virotypes. One exception is serogroup O128, which is represented in both ETEC and EPEC strains, but it is a common serotype among ETEC strains and an uncommon one among EPEC strains.

EPEC diarrhea is a more complex disease than ETEC diarrhea and is thought to occur in three stages (Figure 28–3). The study of events that take place at the molecular level in the host cell after EPEC strains bind to its surface has been facilitated considerably by the discovery that attachment of EPEC strains to HEp-2 cells results in a series of changes in the HEp-2 cells that resemble histologically the changes seen in mucosal cells in the intestine of gnotobiotic piglets infected with EPEC. Thus, HEp-2 cells appear to be a good model for studying the attachment-effacement process. The first stage in association of the bacteria with the host cell is **nonintimate binding,** which is mediated by pili called **bundle-forming pili (Bfp).** In the second stage, attachment of the bacteria to the host cell triggers a signal transduction event, which is associated with activation of host cell tyrosine kinases and which results in increased host cell intracellular Ca^{2+} levels. In the third

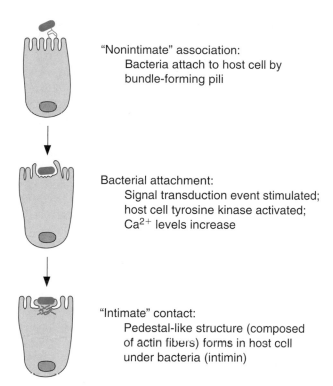

"Nonintimate" association:
Bacteria attach to host cell by bundle-forming pili

Bacterial attachment:
Signal transduction event stimulated; host cell tyrosine kinase activated; Ca^{2+} levels increase

"Intimate" contact:
Pedestal-like structure (composed of actin fibers) forms in host cell under bacteria (intimin)

Figure 28–3 Steps in the binding of EPEC strains to host cells and effect of binding on host cell functions.

stage, the bacteria associate more closely with the host cell (**intimate binding**), and extensive rearrangement of actin in the vicinity of the bacteria occurs. Histologically, the second and third stages are seen as a deformation of some microvilli and elimination of others, as well as the formation of a pedestal-like structure at locations on the host cell surface where bacteria have adhered. The pedestal-like structure is composed of a dense mat of actin fibers that causes an outpouching of the host cell membrane. The genes encoding proteins involved in the attaching-effacing process are designated *eae* for (*E. coli* attachment-effacement).

The Bfp, which mediates the first step in the interaction just described, is similar both in structure and amino acid sequence to the Tcp pili of *V. cholerae*. It is also similar but not identical to the ETEC bundle-forming pilus called longus. The importance of Bfp for virulence of EPEC strains has not yet been established, but Bfp appears to be responsible for adherence to HEp-2 cells. Given the tendency of EPEC strains to aggregate during growth, it is possible that Bfp mediates bacterium-bacterium interactions rather than (or in addition to) adherence of bacteria to host cells. EPEC strains carry a plasmid that is essential for adherence. This plasmid has been called EAF (EPEC Adherence Factor). A gene encoding the subunit of Bfp (*bfpA*) is located on this plasmid. Other virulence factors may

also turn out to be plasmid encoded, as is the case with virulence genes of ETEC strains. Some indirect evidence suggests that Bfp may not be the only EPEC adhesin involved in nonintimate attachment to host cells. First, although most EPEC strains exhibit a localized pattern of adherence to HEp-2 cells, there are some strains that exhibit a diffuse pattern of adherence. (This is a good example of the fact that virotypes are not always clear-cut.) The differences in adherence patterns suggest that some EPEC strains have adhesins that recognize receptors different from the receptor recognized by Bfp. Second, the gene for Bfp is located on a plasmid, but a transposon insertion in the chromosome has been identified that eliminates binding to HEp-2 cells. This mutation could have occurred in some gene that is necessary for Bfp secretion and assembly, but it could also have occurred in a gene encoding some other, as yet undiscovered, EPEC adhesin. This raises the daunting possibility that further study of EPEC adhesins will generate the same bewildering variety of adhesins that have been found in ETEC strains.

The intimate binding of EPEC strains to host cells is mediated by a 94-kDa outer membrane protein called **intimin.** The intimin gene has been designated *eaeA*. Mutants that lack intimin are significantly less virulent than wild type when tested in human volunteers, indicating that intimin is an important virulence factor. Intimin is also essential for the actin rearrangements that lead to formation of the pedestal-like structure in the host cell, but other proteins may also be involved in this process.

EFFECTS OF EPEC ADHERENCE ON HOST CELLS. Production of LT, ST, or other known diarrheal toxins has not been detected in EPEC strains. This raises the question of how these strains cause diarrhea. One possibility is that there is a toxin that is not detected by standard assays for diarrheal toxins, but it is also possible that diarrhea is caused by loss of the absorptive capacity of mucosal cells because of damage to the host cell surface. Mucosal cells absorb water as well as retain it. Thus, diarrhea can occur as a result of either water loss from tissue (as in the case of ETEC strains) or failure of water to be absorbed. Although the cause of diarrhea associated with EPEC strains has not been determined, the complex set of effects precipitated by binding of EPEC strains to intestinal cells and the damage done to the absorptive apical surface in the process point to the possibility that loss of absorptive power by mucosal cells could be responsible for the diarrhea. One effect of bacterial binding to HEp-2 cells is an increase in the concentration of free Ca^{2+} in the host cell cytoplasm. In contrast to the increase in intracellular Ca^{2+} concentration seen in HEp-2 cells in response to binding of

EAggEC, which is caused by influx of extracellular Ca^{2+}, the increase in intracellular Ca^{2+} caused by EPEC adherence appears to be due to release of Ca^{2+} from intracellular stores. A possible result of increased Ca^{2+} levels is activation of actin-depolymerizing enzymes, giving rise to abnormalities in cytoskeletal maintenance. Another effect of EPEC binding is phosphorylation of some host cell proteins. Phosphorylation and dephosphorylation of eukaryotic proteins is involved in signal transduction. EPEC activates a protein tyrosine kinase that might have a signal transduction role. The increase in Ca^{2+} level could also trigger phosphorylation of host cell proteins. Phosphorylation of cytoskeletal proteins following EPEC adherence has been detected in HEp-2 cells, and effects on the cytoskeleton could explain the changes that occur in microvillus structure and the abnormal assembly of the actin mat under the adherent bacteria. One consequence of deformation of the microvilli near the bacteria, at least in HEp-2 cells, is that some of the bacteria are internalized in endocytic vesicles. It is unclear whether invasion of mucosal cells actually occurs in human disease.

EHEC Strains

ADHESINS. Little is known about adhesins of EHEC strains except that they mediate the same type of binding and actin reorganization seen with EPEC strains. EHEC strains have an *eaeA* gene (encoding intimin) which is similar to the *eaeA* gene of EPEC strains and probably has the same function (i.e., to mediate tight binding of bacteria to the host cells).

TOXINS. So far, the main difference found between EPEC and EHEC strains is that EHEC strains produce a toxin that is virtually identical to **Shiga toxin (Stx),** a toxin that is probably responsible for the dysentery caused by *Shigella* species. *Shigella* species also cause HUS. There are two types of EHEC Stx—Stx1, which is most like the classical Stx from *Shigella* species, and Stx2, which is related to Stx1 but differs enough at the amino acid sequence level that there are antibodies that differentiate Stx2 from Stx1. This difference is of more than academic interest, because Stx2 is more often associated with the EHEC strains that cause HUS than Stx1.

Stx is an important virulence factor in EHEC infections. Receptors for the toxin are found on kidney cells as well as intestinal cells. Thus, dissemination of Stx to the kidney after bacterial colonization of the intestinal mucosa could be responsible for the acute kidney failure and kidney hemorrhages that are hallmarks of the fatal form of EHEC infections. The gene encoding Stx is found on a temperate bacteriophage. This fact has been invoked in connection with the controversy over whether antibiotics are helpful in the treatment of EHEC infections (Box 28–3). If Stx is a major virulence factor, its presence on a bacteriophage may allow it to convert other diarrheal strains to a more lethal form. In fact, the current view of the evolution of EHEC strains is that EHEC arose from an EPEC strain that acquired additional DNA, including the bacteriophage that carries the Stx genes. It is interesting to note that one of the surprises coming out of genome sequence comparisons is that the genome of O157:H7 contains 1 Mbp (one-fifth of the chromosome) of DNA that is not found in the K12 strain that has long been the "lab rat" in *E. coli* studies. Talk about strain-to-strain variation!

A characteristic of EHEC strains that might be considered a dissemination factor rather than a virulence factor, but which has importance for the transmission of the disease, is that O157:H7 seems to readily colonize the intestinal tracts of cattle and other farm animals. Contamination with intestinal contents during slaughter is almost certainly responsible for the initial contamination of the meat that eventually appears on supermarket shelves. Grinding of the meat for hamburger would further mix the bacteria into the meat and thus make them less likely to be killed by surface searing of the hamburger during cooking. This may explain why hamburger has been a common source in recent outbreaks. However, outbreaks associated with unpasteurized milk, apple cider, and municipal water supplies have also been reported.

Prevention and Treatment

One important mode of transmission of diarrheal infections is water contaminated with sewage. Having a water supply that is free from sewage has been one of the biggest health advantages enjoyed by people in developed countries. Constant vigilance to protect this barrier to disease is one of the most important roles of public health officials. Before dismissing the water supply from your mind as a hopelessly boring subject, take into account that in cities all over the developed world, there are rapidly aging water supply systems, with leaking pipes that can and are allowing the contents of sewage-bearing pipes to leak into tap water-bearing pipes. Also, in both urban and rural areas, heavy rains, floods, or hurricanes can overwhelm the sewage treatment facilities' barriers against premature release of sewage, and raw sewage can enter the water supply. In midstate Illinois, where this book was written, there are fairly frequent "boil orders"—announcements on the radio instructing residents of such-and-such a county to boil all

BOX 28–3   Do Antibiotics Make EHEC Disease Worse?

Normally, antibiotics are not used to treat diarrhea because the disease is self-limiting. But the disease caused by EHEC strains is so dangerous, especially to children, that physicians initially rushed to treat cases of the disease with antibiotics in the hope that antibiotics would shorten the duration of the disease and thus lessen its severity. Prompt antibiotic therapy can reduce the duration of symptoms of other types of *E. coli* diarrheal disease, such as that caused by ETEC and EPEC strains, so there was reason for optimism about the efficacy of antibiotic therapy in the case of EHEC infections. To everyone's dismay, however, certain antibiotics, such as fluoroquinolones and trimethoprim—antibiotics that have been used to treat other types of bacterial diarrhea—seemed to make the disease worse.

The explanation seems to be emerging from studies of the location of the *stx* genes, which encode the Stx toxin that is thought to be responsible for HUS and bloody diarrhea. As mentioned in the text, the *stx* genes are carried on a bacteriophage that can be induced to lytic growth. One of the stimuli that cause the phage to go from integrated to lytic phase is the SOS response. The SOS response is induced under conditions of stress, especially stress caused by

DNA damage. Some antibiotics, such as the fluoroquinolones, cause DNA damage as a side effect of their primary action. Recall that fluoroquinolones inhibit DNA synthesis by binding DNA gyrase. Apparently, the SOS system induces high-level expression of phage genes, leading to lytic growth. Not only does lytic growth provide many copies of the phage genome, but *stx* genes are induced along with phage replication genes. The combined result is the production of elevated levels of the Shiga toxin Stx. Another effect of inducing the phage to enter the lytic growth mode is that the likelihood of transfer of the phage and the genes it carries increases considerably. This has led to speculation that the use of antibiotics such as fluoroquinolones in agriculture might have inadvertently caused increased dissemination of the phages and the *stx* genes they carry, causing the emergence of EHEC strains. This last suggestion is likely to be controversial but is an interesting view of the ecology of emerging pathogens.

Source: P. T. Kimmit, C. R. Harwood, and M. R. Barer. 2000. Toxin gene expression by Shiga toxin-producing *Escherichia coli:* the role of antibiotics and the bacterial SOS response. *Emerg. Infect. Dis.* **6:**458–465.

water being used for drinking or cooking until further notice, because a breach in the water protection system has occurred. Water safety may well become a serious health issue in developed countries in the not-too-distant future.

E. coli can also be transmitted by meat products because of contamination of meat with intestinal contents during slaughter. It would be prohibitively expensive to eliminate bacteria completely from meat, especially ground meat. Irradiation would help, but public misunderstanding of this benign sterilization method has prevented its implementation. Also, irradiation would not kill the bacteria internalized in ground meat. You can protect yourself, however, by being careful to cook ground meats thoroughly. Rare steak is all right because the bacteria are on the surface of the meat and are killed during the searing of the surface, but rare hamburger is a potentially serious risk, especially for children.

Although meat is the most common vehicle for transmitting diarrheagenic *E. coli,* plants and juices can also play this role (Box 28–1). There are some precautionary measures that are effective. First, monitoring of foods likely to be contaminated for *E. coli* O157:H7 and other serotypes now known to cause EHEC disease would prevent contaminated foods normally consumed raw, such as juices and sprouts, from entering the food supply. This type of monitoring is now very expensive, but new rapid tests are in the exploratory phase and may make routine checking of produce possible in the future. Also, a rule of thumb parents can follow is never—repeat, never—give a small child any commercial drink that is unpasteurized. Unpasteurized is definitely dangerous, not healthful as many seem to think.

In the case of diarrhea caused by ETEC, EPEC, and EAggEC, fluid loss is the main problem. In groups at high risk for dehydration, such as infants and children, fluid replacement therapy is advisable. A mixture of water, salts, and glucose is administered to prevent severe dehydration. Fluid replacement therapy is discussed in chapter 25. Fluid replacement therapy can be administered orally or intravenously.

Antibiotics are not usually used to treat diarrhea, especially mild diarrhea. Nonetheless, travelers going to countries with an unsafe water supply are generally offered antibiotics if they consult a travel clinic. In cases of travelers who develop severe diarrhea, antibiotics can reduce the duration of the symptoms, but only if the antibiotic regimen is started early in the infection. Antibiotics are definitely not indicated in a suspected case of EHEC, until the question of whether they make the disease worse or not is settled. Unfortunately, in the case of EHEC infections, all that can be done is to try to compensate for possible kidney failure with dialysis and hope the patient survives the self-limited infection. This is why prevention of EHEC infections is so vitally important.

SELECTED READINGS

Kaper, J. B., J. L. Mellies, and J. P. Nataro. 1999. Pathogenicity islands and other mobile genetic elements in diarrheagenic *Escherichia coli,* p. 33–58. *In* J. B. Kaper and J. Hacker (ed.), *Pathogenicity Islands and Other Mobile Virulence Elements.* ASM Press, Washington, D.C.

Kaper, J. B., and A. D. O'Brien. 1998. *Escherichia coli O157:H7 and Other Shiga Toxin-Producing E. coli Strains.* ASM Press, Washington, D.C.

Nataro, J. P., and J. B. Kaper. 1998. Diarrheagenic *E. coli* strains. *Clin. Microbiol. Rev.* **11:**142–201. (This review is so exhaustive that it is one-stop-shopping for information on diarrheagenic *E. coli* strains.)

Fiction

If you are interested in a grim, graphic description of the meat-processing industry as well as a case of EHEC infection, you might want to read the following: Cook, R. 1998. *Toxin.* G. P. Putnam's Sons, New York, N.Y.

SUMMARY OUTLINE

Characteristics of all *E. coli* strains

    Gram-negative, motile rods

    Facultative metabolism

    Most strains nonpathogenic

    Serological classification
        Based on reactivity of surface molecules with different antibodies
        Serotype (O) based on O antigen of LPS
        Serogroup (H) dependent on flagella type
        Capsule antigen (K) also used

    Virotyping system
        Based on virulence factors of different strains
        Six virotypes known
        Genes for factors most often on mobile elements

ETEC

    Causes diarrhea, no major histological changes
        Infant diarrhea—often fatal
        Traveler's diarrhea in adults

    Virulence factors
        Adhesins
            CFAs; found only on ETEC strains
                Long thin fimbriae
                CFA/I—composed of single protein subunit
                CFA/II—consists of a group of at least two related adhesins; flexible fimbria more common than rigid pilus

(continued)

CFA/III—bundle-forming pilus
   Long, flexible pili entwined together
   Similar at amino acid level to Tcp pili of *V. cholerae*
   May be responsible for bacterium-bacterium adherence (microcolony formation)
CFA/IV—mixture of different types of fimbriae
Genes usually on plasmids
Longus—also related to Tcp of *V. cholerae*

Enterotoxins
  Heat-labile toxin
  LT-1
    75% amino acid identity with cholera toxin
    5B:1A subunits (genes in operon)
    Mechanism of A subunit same as cholera toxin—increases cAMP levels because of
     ADP-ribosylation of G_s
    B subunits bind to G_{M1} (same as cholera toxin)
    May have other effects
     Increase in leukotrienes and prostaglandins
     Affects nerves controlling intestinal motility and ion secretion
     Increases production of cytokines—mild inflammation
  Heat-stable toxin—family of small toxins
   STb (methanol insoluble)—found only in porcine strains
   STa (methanol soluble)
    Excreted into medium in series of steps; cleaved during process
    Binds to guanylate cyclase on host cells
    Causes increase in cGMP—effect same as increased cAMP
    Genes for LT-1 and STa on plasmids (often on same plasmids as CFA genes)
    Different arrangementss of LT-1 and STa genes on plasmids may be due to transposons
    STa gene on transposable element

EAggEC

Causes persistent diarrhea in children

Like ETEC binds small intestinal cells; not invasive; causes no histological changes

Clumps in aggregates on mucosa

Adhesins
  Covered with fibrillar structures (GVVPQ fimbriae)
   Role in virulence not known
   Similar to filamentous adhesin of some *Salmonella* strains

Enterotoxins
  Enteroaggregative ST—similar to ST of ETEC
  Hemolysin
   Forms pores in host cell membranes
   Similar to hemolysin produced by uropathogenic *E. coli*
  Affects Ca^{2+} levels in HEp-2 cells in culture

EPEC

Causes severe, often fatal diarrhea in infants and children (especially in developing countries)

Causes traveler's diarrhea in adults

Patchy pattern of adherence to host cells

(*continued*)

SUMMARY OUTLINE (*continued*)

Causes change in ultrastructure of host cells
   Attaching and effacing—formation of pedestal under bacteria
   Elongated microvilli in areas without bacteria
   No microvilli where bacteria are bound

More invasive than ETEC and EAggEC—causes inflammation

Effects due to damage of host cells and signal transduction systems, not exotoxins

Interaction with host cells occurs in three stages
   Nonintimate binding of bacteria to host cell—mediated by bundle-forming pili (similar to Tcp
      pili of *V. cholerae*)
   Attachment triggers signal transduction event—activates host cell tyrosine kinases (increases
      Ca^{2+} levels in host cell)
   Intimate binding—actin rearrangement occurs
   Last two steps cause pedestal formation

Adherence
   Bfp mediates nonintimate binding
      May mediate bacteria-bacteria interactions
      Gene (*bfpA*) on plasmid EAF
   Initial adherence may be due to unidentified adhesin binding different receptor from that
      of Bfp
   Intimin mediates intimate binding
      Encoded by *eaeA* gene
      Required for actin rearrangements

No exotoxin identified; diarrhea due to host cell damage and failure to absorb water

EHEC
   Adhesins
      Mediate tight binding and actin rearrangement similar to EPEC
      Encoded by *eaeA* gene

   Shiga toxin (Stx)
      Receptors on intestinal and kidney cells
      May be responsible for HUS
      Gene on temperature phage
         May allow conversion of other diarrheal strains to more lethal form

   Strain O157:H7 colonizes gastrointestinal tract of domestic animals—leads to contamination
      of meat

QUESTIONS

Answers to the questions can be found in Appendix 2.

1. If you were going to develop a new way to type *E. coli* strains based on DNA probes that recognize virulence genes, what probes would you use in your classification system?

2. There are more serotypes than virotypes. Granted that typing on the basis of virulence genes has some

appeal, what is the continued relevance of serotypes? Looking back at the early chapters of this book, what might be an even better way to categorize strains of *E. coli*, especially if the goal is to trace an outbreak?

3. Many clinicians are of the opinion that diarrhea is diarrhea and it doesn't matter what the causative agent is. In their view, expensive tests to identify the causative agent are not worthwhile. Provide arguments for and against this view.

4. Given that many virulence genes of *E. coli* are located on plasmids, phage, or other transmissible elements and could thus conceivably be transmitted to any *E. coli* strain, it seems odd that only certain small subsets of *E. coli* strains cause diarrheal disease. Speculate on why the number of *E. coli* strains that cause intestinal disease is so small, compared with the total number of *E. coli* strains known.

5. How do the virulence factors of EPEC strains differ from those of other types of pathogenic *E. coli* strains?

6. Describe different ways of eliciting the response called "diarrhea" (i.e., excessive loss of water by the body).

7. The recent outbreaks of EHEC disease have raised public concerns about safety of the food supply. One camp argues that the consumer (or food preparer in a commercial setting) is responsible for proper cooking of ground meat to ensure that all *E. coli* O157:H7 are killed. Another camp argues that the meat processors ought to be responsible for providing safe meat to the public. Argue for and against each of these views.

8. Antibiotics are usually not used to treat diarrheal disease. Explain why this is the consensus among clinicians and why traveler's diarrhea might be an exception.

29

Escherichia coli
Extraintestinal Infections

KEY FEATURES

Escherichia coli **Extraintestinal Infections**

CHARACTERISTICS

Gram-negative rod

Motile by flagella

Fermentative metabolism

DISEASES

Diarrhea, dysentery (chapter 28)

Urinary tract infections

Sepsis and meningitis

RESERVOIRS

Human distal ileum and colon

Nonhuman animal intestine

MAJOR VIRULENCE FACTORS

Urinary tract infections: adhesins; invasion of epithelial cells; LPS; toxin—alpha-hemolysin; iron acquisition

Sepsis and meningitis: capsule (K1 antigen); adhesins (S fimbriae); invasion of brain epithelial cells; toxin; LPS

PREVENTION AND TREATMENT

No vaccine available

Antibiotics

Escherichia coli strains are mostly benign and live in the human gastrointestinal tract without causing any adverse effects. Some *E. coli* strains, however, have acquired the ability to cause infections ranging from intestinal infections, such as diarrhea and dysentery (see chapter 28), to extraintestinal infections, such as urinary tract infections, meningitis, and sepsis. Strains that cause extraintestinal disease have been given the designation **ExPEC** in line with the terminology used for diarrheagenic strains. Uropathogenic strains are designated UPEC.

Epidemiology of Urinary Tract Infections

Community-Acquired Urinary Tract Infections

There are an estimated 7 million urinary tract infections in the United States each year. *E. coli* causes over 85% of the cases that occur outside hospitals (community acquired). Urinary tract infections are very unpleasant, but only rarely are they life-threatening in otherwise healthy people. Community-acquired, as opposed to hospital-acquired, urinary tract infections are most commonly caused by uropathogenic strains of *E. coli* (**UPEC** strains). *Klebsiella* and *Proteus,* two other genera of gram-negative bacteria, are the next most frequent causes of community-acquired infections. UPEC strains have a sexist agenda. Most community-acquired infections occur in females under the age of 10 or between the ages of 20 and 40. Although men have urinary tract infections, the incidence of male infections is much lower. An exception to this is older men with prostate enlargement. Thus, as the population ages, UPEC strains may become more equal-opportunity pathogens.

Why is there a difference between men and women in the incidence of urinary tract infection? One reason is that uropathogenic strains are usually harbored in the colon and must travel from the colon to the urethral opening to gain admission to the urethra and bladder. In men, the distance from the colon to the urethral opening is greater than in women, and the urethra of men is longer than that of women, forcing the bacteria to move farther to reach the bladder. Also, the urethral opening of females is close to the vaginal tract, an area more easily colonized by bacteria than the relatively dry skin of the tip of the penis. So in women, UPEC strains can stage a two-step maneuver: first colonize the colon and then the vaginal tract, where they have constant access to the urethra.

Not all girls under 10 and women between the ages of 20 and 40 are equally susceptible to urinary tract infections, and it is becoming clear that susceptibility has a genetic component. In children, infections are most likely to be seen when there are abnormalities of the urinary tract which lead to a partial obstruction that allows stagnant pools of urine to form. In women who have recurrent urinary tract infections, however, abnormalities of the urinary tract are frequently not the explanation. In this case, the colonization of the vaginal tract by uropathogenic strains provides a constant source of bacteria. One practice that has been linked to a greater risk of urinary tract infections is the use of spermicides. The hunt continues for an explanation for the age distribution of urinary tract infections in women. If predisposing factors could be identified, more effective preventive strategies could be developed.

A woman who experiences a urinary tract infection is likely to have similar infections in the future. Two hypotheses have been advanced to explain why women in the 20- to 40-year age group are prone to recurrent urinary tract infections. One hypothesis is that coloni-

zation of the colon by a UPEC strain capable of causing urinary tract infections provides a reservoir. If treatment of the initial infection does not also eliminate the bacteria from the colon, there is a chance for reinfection at a later period. Another hypothesis has been suggested by the finding that during a bladder infection, some UPEC cells invade the uroepithelial cells that line the bladder. These bacteria, hiding inside epithelial cells, may evade the action of antibiotics and persist in this location in a sort of dormant state, only to be reactivated later to cause a repeat infection. It is important to understand the cause of recurrent infections so that treatment regimens can be designed not only to clear the primary infection but to prevent recurrences.

Community-acquired urinary tract infections are almost always **ascending infections.** That is, bacteria first infect the urethra and then move to the bladder (Figure 29–1). The resulting conditions are called **urethritis** (inflammation of the urethra) and **cystitis** (inflammation of the bladder). Both conditions are associated with a burning sensation during urination. If the concentration of bacteria is high enough, the urine will become cloudy. In some cases, the infection continues to ascend, and the kidneys are infected (**pyelonephritis**). Symptoms of kidney infection include back pain and fever. Pyelonephritis is a more serious disease than cystitis or urethritis because more tissue invasion occurs and thus more inflammation. Also, since the kidney is a highly vascularized organ, there is a greater potential for bacteria to leak into the bloodstream, causing a bloodstream infection.

Hospital-Acquired (Nosocomial) Urinary Tract Infections

Hospital-acquired or nursing home-acquired urinary tract infections are most often associated with indwelling urinary catheters. Approximately 50% of all patients who have an indwelling urinary catheter in place for more than 5 days will experience bacterial colonization of the bladder. In many cases, removal of the catheter is followed by clearance of the bacteria, and a symptomatic infection does not develop. Thus, although the bacteria have gained access to the bladder and are multiplying in the bladder, they are not able to remain in the bladder once the normal flushing action of urine is restored. Some colonized individuals, however, will go on to develop a urinary tract infection. Other risk factors besides catheterization are abnormalities of the urinary tract and fecal incontinence. Infections in hospital patients or nursing home residents are particularly dangerous because they may be undetected until late in the course of the infection, when the bacteria have infected the kidney or entered the blood-

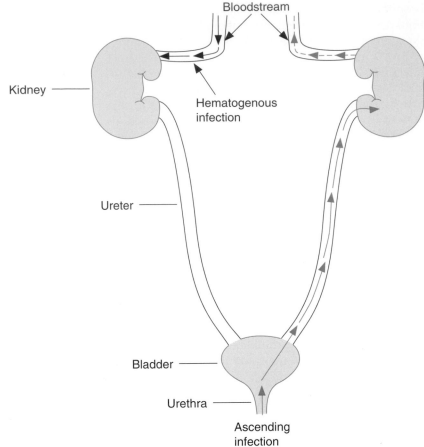

Figure 29–1 Anatomy of the urinary tract and types of urinary tract infections. Bacteria that colonize the vaginal tract can migrate up the urethra to infect the bladder. In some cases, the bacteria ascend to the kidney and cause an infection there. Rarely, the bacteria enter the bloodstream from the kidney. The kidney may also be infected directly from the bloodstream (hematogenous infection). Infection of the bladder is called cystitis. Infection of the kidney is called pyelonephritis.

stream. This is a problem in the case of comatose patients, senile patients, or patients receiving painkillers. Ascending infections that reach the kidney are a common starting point for septicemia in hospitalized patients. Once bacteria are in the bloodstream, any organ may be infected, and conditions ranging from pneumonia to meningitis can develop. In immunocompromised patients, the progression from simple urinary tract infection to systemic infection is even more likely to occur.

Urinary tract infections in a hospital or a nursing home are not always ascending infections. It is also possible for bacteria in the bloodstream (e.g., in patients with pneumonia) to seed the kidneys and cause a kidney or bladder infection. Such an infection is called a **hematogenous urinary tract infection** (Figure 29–1). Hematogenous infections almost always involve gram-positive bacteria, whereas ascending infections are most commonly caused by gram-negative bacteria. Because patients in a hospital are more likely to have impaired defenses, the spectrum of causative agents is broader than it is in community-acquired cases. Although *E. coli* is still the leading cause of urinary tract infections, other bacteria, such as *Pseudomonas aerugi-*

nosa, Klebsiella species, and *Proteus* species, are seen more often as causative agents. Even the yeast *Candida albicans*, which is a common colonizer of the human body, emerges as a significant cause of nosocomial infections.

Another group with a high risk for developing urinary tract infections caused by a variety of microbes is people with spinal cord injuries. Many such people must wear indwelling urinary catheters permanently, since they have no control over urination.

Virulence Factors of *E. coli* Strains That Cause Urinary Tract Infections

Colonization of the Colon and Vagina

Ability to colonize the colon is usually not listed as a virulence factor for UPEC strains because benign strains also have this ability, but the ability to colonize the colon is a very important first step in causing urinary tract infections. How UPEC strains get to the colon is unknown. Since there seems to be no correlation between dietary habits and urinary tract infections, the bacteria may enter the colon from the anus. Another important characteristic of UPEC strains is their ability to colonize the vaginal tract. In the vaginal tract, most of the available niches are occupied by the resident microbiota, especially lactobacilli. Thus, any disruption of the resident microbiota opens the way for colonization of the vaginal tract by *E. coli* or other potential pathogens. The association between spermicide use and higher incidence of urinary tract infections may be explained by the fact that nonoxynol-9, the active ingredient in spermicides, inhibits growth of lactobacilli and thus helps to create a favorable environment for colonization of the vagina by UPEC strains.

Adhesins

One of the main host defenses of the urinary tract is the washing action of urine. Bacteria that do not adhere will be washed out of the bladder if they cannot divide rapidly enough to keep their numbers high in the urethra or bladder. Thus, it is not surprising that the key feature of uropathogens is their ability to adhere to bladder mucosa (but see Box 29–1). Also, adherent bacteria are in close proximity to mucosal cells and are thus in a better position to provoke an inflammatory response or invade epithelial cells than bacteria growing in the lumen of the bladder. A number of adhesins of UPEC strains have been identified and studied. Rather than try to present a complete list of known adhesins, which would not only be confusing in its complexity but would probably become obsolete before this book is published, only a few of the well-studied adhesins will be described. This should give you an idea of the characteristics of adhesins that may be important for colonization of the bladder and kidney.

Type 1 pili are now thought to make an important contribution to colonization of the bladder. Earlier, the type 1 pili were dismissed as an important bladder colonization factor because most strains of *E. coli*, pathogenic and nonpathogenic strains alike, produce them. More recent findings, however, have provided a new appreciation of their importance. Type 1 pili bind mannose residues on bladder glycoproteins. This binding is followed by invasion of uroepithelial cells (see next section).

Another important adhesin, especially in strains that cause kidney infections, is **P fimbriae** (sometimes called P pili). P fimbriae are associated primarily with UPEC strains and are not found on nonpathogenic strains. The name P fimbriae comes from the fact that they are found mainly on the strains that cause pyelonephritis. The genes encoding proteins involved in synthesis and

BOX 29–1   Is Adherence Really an Essential Trait for All Uropathogens?

Many questions remain about the virulence features of UPEC strains, but one trait that seemed to be universally accepted as essential by everyone working on uropathogens is the ability of the strain to adhere to bladder mucosal cells. It is obvious why adherence should be an important trait for infection of the bladder, but sometimes it is worthwhile raising questions about such a well-accepted dogma. Someone has had the temerity to ask the question whether ability to multiply rapidly in urine could allow bacteria to remain in the bladder without adherence. Using a mathematical simulation of bladder filling and emptying, Gordon and Riley (1992) estimated that if a bacterial strain had a doubling time of about 50 min or less in urine, it could maintain itself in the normal bladder without adhering. They tested isolates from urinary tract infections and found that many of them had doubling times of 50 to 60 min in urine. Isolates from the colon or from other non-urinary tract infections tended to double much more slowly in urine. Also, the lag time before urinary tract infection isolates began to multiply (when introduced from laboratory medium to urine) was much shorter than that of other types of isolates. It is essential to keep in mind that this study only raises a theoretical possibility and does not disprove the importance of adhesins, but it is useful from time to time to consider alternative explanations for virulence. Ability to multiply rapidly in urine may well be more critical for virulence than has previously been thought. An important factor that is not taken into account by this study, or by many studies of adherence, is how the host's immune response, including the cytokines that are released into the bladder during an acute infection, affects bacterial multiplication and activities.

Source: D. M. Gordon, and M. A. Riley. 1992. A theoretical and experimental analysis of bacterial growth in the bladder. *Mol. Microbiol.* **6:**555–562.

assembly of P fimbriae are called *pap* genes, for **pyelonephritis-associated pili.** (The name fimbriae came into widespread use after these genes were named.) There are many different antigenic types of P fimbriae, but all have in common that they recognize the same receptor: α-D-Gal-(1,4)-α-D-Gal **(globobiose)** (Figure 29–2) or repeats of this disaccharide. Globobiose is bound to a **ceramide lipid** that is embedded in the host cell membrane. UPEC strains that do not produce P fimbriae produce a variety of other adhesins. Some examples of this group are the **afimbrial adhesins,** which do not have a fibrillar structure (**AFAI, AFAIII**), and the **Dr** adhesins. The receptor recognized by AFAs is not known. The Dr adhesin binds the Dr blood group antigen.

S pili are associated with strains that cause neonatal meningitis rather than with those that cause urinary tract infections. Yet they have the same binding pattern in vitro as P pili. That is, when bacteria with S pili were incubated with bladder tissue, they bound to the same areas of tissue as cells producing P fimbriae. Yet they seem not to function as virulence factors for UPEC strains. This puzzling observation was explained by the fact that binding of S pili, but not P fimbriae, was inhibited by a glycoprotein (**Tamm-Horsfall glycoprotein**) which is the most abundant protein in normal human urine. Thus, prevention of S pili binding by urine glycoproteins may play a role in excluding some potential pathogens.

Invasion of Uroepithelial Cells

A newly recognized virulence strategy of UPEC strains is invasion of bladder epithelial cells. The bladder epithelium (**uroepithelium**) is a layer of poorly differentiated, multinucleate cells called **umbrella** or **facet** cells. Several layers of epithelial cells are arranged on a base-

ment membrane. The cells of the top layer have an intriguing trait. They secrete proteins called **uroplakins** that form small hexagonal particles, arranged in a larger array that covers the surface of the top uroepithelial layer. The type 1 pili of UPEC strains bind to mannose residues attached to the uroplakins. Binding to the uroplakins causes the epithelial cells to engulf the bound *E. coli* cells. Binding by pili seems to be all that is necessary, since the bladder cells will internalize beads coated with isolated type 1 pili.

Normally, the umbrella cells do not slough very often. Cells filled with bacteria, however, are sloughed rapidly and are excreted in urine. This response to bacterial invasion may be an important defense of the bladder. The invading bacteria activate signal transduction pathways and cause modifications of cytoskeleton that are presumably recognized by the infected cell as a signal to slough. A small proportion of the invading bacteria do not have this effect. Instead they seem to become dormant and stay within cells that are not sloughed from the uroepithelium. Bacteria in the cells that remain attached are not only protected from the washing effect of urine but may also be a reservoir for future infections. The β-lactam antibiotics usually used to treat bladder infections do not enter eukaryotic cells and thus cannot get at the internalized bacteria. Also, bacteria that are not actively growing are not susceptible to β-lactam action because they are not actively synthesizing peptidoglycan. Thus, treatment will not affect most of these internalized bacteria, and they can remain in the site until some change of conditions causes them to reemerge and begin to divide actively.

The discovery of a possible latent phase of UPEC strains has suggested an answer to the question of why women so often experience repeated infections with the same strain. The party line had been that the strain lurked in the colon, where it was partially protected

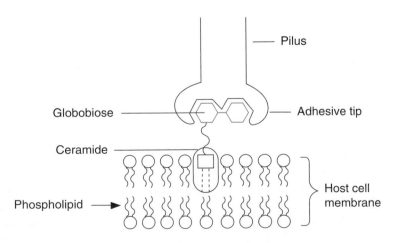

Figure 29–2 Structure of globobiose, the receptor for P fimbriae.

from antibiotic therapy directed at the bladder. Now, dormant *E. coli* inside uroepithelial cells is being considered another potential source of infection, possibly more important than intestinal and vaginal colonization. It is very important to determine which explanation for recurrent infections is the correct one, because each suggests a different therapeutic approach. If continued colonization of the colon or vagina is the most important factor in recurrent infections, then eliminating these uropathogenic strains from the colon and vagina by appropriate antibiotic therapy is of primary importance. If the bacteria inside uroepithelial cells are the main source of recurrent infections, antibiotics that either reduce invasion or act on internalized bacteria are needed.

Toxins

How does a simple colonization of the bladder lead to the strong inflammatory response that appears to be responsible for the symptoms of an acute urinary tract infection? Two possible explanations are (i) stimulation of an inflammatory response by LPS and (ii) production of exotoxins by the uropathogens. There is some evidence that LPS acts synergistically with P fimbriae to evoke the inflammatory response. Inoculation of UPEC strains into the urethra of a mouse creates an inflammatory response similar to that seen in humans. This response is characterized by movement of PMNs through the mucosa into the lumen of the bladder. The inflammatory response is also seen with P fimbriae plus LPS or LPS alone, but much less LPS was needed if P fimbriae were present. In an isogenic strain of mice that does not mount an inflammatory response to LPS (**lps nonresponder**), no inflammatory response was seen. However, these mice did not clear the infecting bacteria as the normal mice did, supporting the contention that the PMN response, though it may produce some of the unpleasant symptoms of urinary tract infections, actually has a beneficial effect. The main conclusion from these results is that binding of P fimbriae to the mucosa somehow causes LPS on the bacterial surface to be presented to the host defense system in such a way as to enhance its ability to provoke inflammation.

Evidence for production of exotoxins has also been found. Some UPEC strains secrete an extracellular protein, which was originally called a hemolysin because it lyses red blood cells but is now known to kill other cell types as well. Thus, a more appropriate name for this protein would be cytotoxin, but it is generally called **alpha-hemolysin.** The alpha-hemolysin (HlyA) belongs to a family of proteins which have been designated **RTX toxins** (for repeats in toxin) because all pro-

teins of this family contain a tandem duplication of nine amino acids.

RTX toxins act by creating pores in eukaryotic cell membranes. Binding of calcium by the toxin is necessary for pore formation. Calcium binds to the toxin in the region containing the tandem amino acid repeats that give the toxin family its name. High levels of toxin lyse cells because the pores the toxin forms allow cytoplasmic contents to leak out. At levels of toxin too low to cause lysis, a variety of effects on eukaryotic cell function have been noted. Effects that might be important in urinary tract infections are stimulation of cytokine production, stimulation of superoxide production, and depression of ATP levels in kidney cells.

E. coli strains that lack alpha-hemolysin are less virulent than wild type when injected into the peritoneal cavity of mice. In a mouse model for ascending urinary tract infections, strains producing both P fimbriae and hemolysin (P^+, H^+) colonized the bladder and kidney and killed nearly two-thirds of the mice tested. Isogenic strains that produced only P fimbriae (P^+, H^-) colonized but did not cause kidney damage or death. Strains producing neither P fimbriae nor hemolysin did not colonize. Thus, at least in this animal model, hemolysin seems to mediate kidney damage. Another line of (admittedly circumstantial) evidence implicating hemolysin in kidney damage is that a hemolysin very similar to the *E. coli* HlyA is produced by the *Proteus* sp. strains that cause kidney infections.

Another toxin produced by some UPEC strains is called **cytotoxic necrotizing factor 1 (CNF-1).** Like the alpha-hemolysin, this toxin kills epithelial cells. Its role in urinary tract infections has not been determined.

Other Virulence Factors

Iron acquisition is an important virulence factor. UPEC strains have multiple siderophore-based iron acquisition systems. These include an **enterobactin,** an **aerobactin,** and a **yersiniabactin** (like the one in *Yersinia pestis*) iron acquisition system. Capsules and serum resistance are also traits associated with many uropathogenic strains, especially those that cause kidney infections and systemic infections arising from urinary tract infections. Antiphagocytic mechanisms may help the bacteria to resist the influx of PMNs into the lumen of the bladder that occurs in response to infection. The O antigen of LPS may be important because only strains with certain O serotypes (e.g., O1, O4, O6, and O18) cause urinary tract infections. These O antigens may be linked to the serum resistance trait of uropathogens.

Finding a trait that looks as if it might be important for virulence and showing that its loss reduces virulence in an animal model are important steps toward understanding how bacteria cause an infection. But these approaches may miss important virulence factors. Recently, scientists have taken a gene fusion approach to finding genes that are expressed in bacteria growing in human urine but not in laboratory medium. The genes identified so far by this approach are some amino acid biosynthetic genes, a gene encoding a periplasmic arginine binding protein (*artJ*), a gene encoding a protein that could be involved in iron acquisition (*iron*), and a gene of unknown function. The picture that arises from these findings is very different from the one outlined in previous sections. Since the evidence for the importance of adhesins, invasion, and cytotoxins is compelling, the difference may point to biases implicit in the different approaches.

UPEC Strains—a Paradigm for Adhesin Biogenesis

Some of the most elegant work on how pili and fimbriae are assembled has come from studies of the UPEC strains. This work is important not only because it shows how bacteria can carry out the complex task of organelle construction, but also because information about pilus structure and assembly may lead to new strategies for prevention and treatment of urinary tract infections (Box 29–2). In this section, we will focus on the synthesis and assembly of P fimbriae. Considerable work has also been done on the synthesis and assembly of type 1 pili, but the same picture emerges in both cases. Production of external structures such as pili and fimbriae is an amazing exercise in construction. Not only do the proteins that make up the stalk and the tip have to pass through both the cytoplasmic membrane and the outer membrane, but they must do so in the proper order, with the tip proteins being assembled and externalized first, followed by assembly and extension of the stalk of the fimbria.

The structure of the adhesin tip has been deduced from electron micrographs of type 1 pili (Figure 29–3). The stalk of the pilus is larger in diameter than the tip. The components of the tip are **FimH** (the globobiose adhesin), **FimG,** and possibly **FimF.** The nonadhesin proteins presumably provide a structural support for the adhesin FimH.

The proposed steps in assembly of a P fimbria are illustrated in Figure 29–4, which shows the export of the tip protein PapG. Other fimbrial proteins are assumed to be externalized by the same route. The structural protein to be exported is first secreted by the **general secretory (Sec) pathway** of *E. coli*. After secretion to the periplasm, PapG is folded, a process that is

BOX 29–2   Progress toward a Vaccine To Prevent Urinary Tract Infections

Women who have had one or more urinary tract infections are understandably interested in preventing recurrences. An obvious preventive strategy is a vaccine that prevents *E. coli* from attaching to uroepithelial cells in the first place. Since most *E. coli* strains produce type 1 pili, this type of pilus was the obvious candidate for vaccine development. Scientists had identified the tip protein that mediates the binding of the pilus tip to globobiose on the epithelial cell uroplakins. This tip protein is FimH. Antibodies bound to FimH should be bulky enough to block the tight binding of FimH to globobiose that is necessary for stable attachment of the bacteria (Figure 29–2).

In 1997, a group of scientists reported that immunizing mice with FimH reduced *E. coli* colonization of the bladder by more than 99%. This was a very exciting development that may be the first step in developing an effective vaccine that would prevent urinary tract infections. One concern raised in connection with such a vaccine is that intestinal *E. coli* also produces type 1 pili. Could the vaccine interfere with colonization of the colon by *E. coli* strains that are not pathogenic? And if it did, would there be any untoward consequences? So far the answer seems to be that the vaccine does not affect colonization by benign strains of *E. coli*. It is still unclear how soon this vaccine will enter human trials.

Source: S. Langermann, S. Palaszynski, M. Barnhart, G. Auguste, J. S. Pinkner, J. Burlein, P. Barren, S. Koenig, S. Leath, C. H. Jones, and S. J. Hultgren. 1997. Prevention of mucosal *Escherichia coli* infection by FimH-adhesin-based systemic vaccination. *Science* **276:**607–611.

guided by the **chaperone** PapD. PapD then conveys the PapG protein to PapC, a protein which forms a pore in the outer membrane. The binding of PapD to the PapG protein helps to keep the PapG protein from interacting with other pilus proteins before it reaches the PapC pore.

The diameter of the interior hole in the PapC pore is about 2 nm, large enough for the folded PapG protein

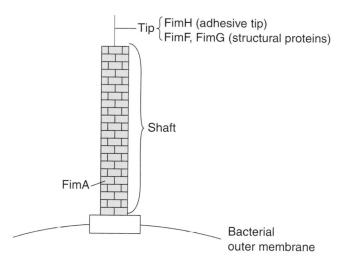

Tip { FimH (adhesive tip)
     { FimF, FimG (structural proteins)

Shaft

FimA

Bacterial
outer membrane

Figure 29–3 Structure of the type 1 pilus, as determined by electron microscopic studies. The shaft is composed of many FimA proteins. The adhesive tip has a smaller diameter and may be more flexible.

to pass through. Protein-protein interactions between pilus proteins that occur on the outer surface of the outer membrane probably play an important role in assembly of the tip and stalk structures. The PapC pore is also thought to aid in creating the proper structure by constraining the conformation of the folded pilus protein until it is ready to be assembled. Because of this activity, PapC has been called an usher. The steps illustrated in Figure 29–4 look very neat and straightforward, but a problem that probably arises rather frequently is the production of improperly folded pilus proteins, which could accumulate in the periplasmic space. Such an accumulation could well be toxic to the bacteria.

To prevent such a buildup of improperly folded proteins in the periplasm, *E. coli* has a feedback mechanism based on a two-component regulatory system consisting of **CpxA** (the sensor) and **CpxR** (the response regulator). This regulatory system is illustrated in Figure 29–4. Free, unassembled PapG and PapE, with the help of an outer membrane lipoprotein, **NlpE**, stimulate CpxA to phosphorylate CpxR. Phosphorylated CpxR activates expression of a number of genes. Among these are *dsbA*, which encodes a periplasmic protein that aids the proper folding of proteins in the periplasm, and *degP*, which encodes a protease that degrades improperly folded proteins. The combined action of these two proteins would help to get the folding and delivery of the Pap structural proteins back on track.

Another potential problem is aggregation of PapD proteins in the periplasm. This problem is solved by the fact that PapD protein contains two flexible domains. When two PapD proteins associate with each other,

these flexible domains assume a configuration that discourages dimerization. This process has been called **self-capping.** A major question that remains to be answered is how the bacteria decide when the tip structure is complete and begin to assemble the stalk, which is composed of PapA subunits. The Cpx feedback pathway suggests the possibility that a similar regulatory system exists, possibly with an outer membrane protein component that "counts" the tip proteins that are conveyed to PapC and then shuts down synthesis and/or secretion of these proteins in favor of PapA.

Results of studies of the biosynthesis and assembly of pili and fimbriae have revealed in part how this fascinating process works, but there is also a very important practical reason for knowing the structure of pili and fimbriae. Since pili and fimbriae mediate the first step in the infection process—adherence to uroepithelial cells—adhesin proteins, especially the tip proteins that mediate the actual attachment, make excellent candidates for a vaccine to protect high-risk populations from *E. coli* urinary tract infections (Box 29–2).

Organization and Regulation of Virulence Genes

GENES INVOLVED IN P FIMBRIA PRODUCTION. Production of P fimbriae occurs maximally at 37°C, but other factors, such as growth on agar medium or presence of glucose, also affect production. The temperature regulation presumably allows *E. coli* coming in from the external environment to adapt to the human body. The bacteria must also have some way of recognizing whether they are in the colon, the vaginal tract, the bladder, or the kidney, but such signals and their associated regulatory proteins have not yet been identified. In addition to allowing the bacteria to adapt to different mucosal surfaces and environments they encounter, regulation of adhesin genes may give the bacteria a way of evading host defenses. UPEC strains commonly produce multiple adhesins and can display combinations of different pilus or fimbrial types or combinations of different serotypes of the same adhesin on their surfaces. Thus, shutting down production of one type of adhesin and switching to production of another type could help the bacteria circumvent the host's sIgA response.

Genes encoding P fimbriae are clustered on the bacterial chromosome (Figure 29–5). The cluster contains genes for the major subunit (**PapA**), the adhesin tip proteins (**PapE-G**), the processing and assembly proteins (**PapC, D, H**), and some regulatory proteins (**PapB, I**). The structural genes are transcribed from a single promoter. An interesting question arises in connection with this arrangement of genes and the promoter that con-

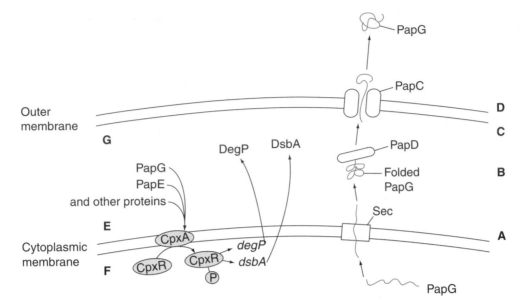

Figure 29–4 Steps in secretion and localization of pilin proteins, using PapG as an example. Also depicted is the regulatory pathway for preventing the buildup of improperly folded pilin proteins in the periplasmic space, a potentially lethal event. (**A**) PapG is synthesized in the cytoplasm and then secreted into the periplasm by Sec. (**B**) PapD assists folding of PapG. (**C**) PapD ushers folded PapG to the PapC pore. (**D**) PapG is secreted through PapC. (**E**) PapG, PapE, and possibly other proteins in the periplasm stimulate CpxA to phosphorylate CpxR. (**F**) Phosphorylated CpxR activates expression of several genes (e.g., *degP* and *dsbA*). (**G**) DegP (protease that degrades improperly folded proteins) and DsbA (protein that aids proper folding) enter periplasm and prevent buildup of improperly folded pilin proteins. (Adapted from Jones et al., 1997.)

trols their expression. Many more copies of the PapA protein are made compared with the other proteins encoded in this region. Yet the genes are all under control of a single promoter. How can this be? The answer seems to have two parts. First, degradation of mRNA from the 3′ end decreases the number of mRNA molecules that contain copies of the downstream genes. Second, the ribosome-binding site of *papA* is much stronger than those of the other genes. Working together, these features ensure that there will be many PapA proteins for every one of the other Pap proteins.

The regulation of *pap* genes at the transcriptional level has proved to be quite complex but is worth describing, both because it shows how the expression of these genes changes in response to multiple signals and because it provides another mechanism for phase variation (switching from "on" to "off" rather than modulation of expression level). Expression of *pap* genes changes in response to temperature, level of glucose in the medium, and concentrations of certain amino acids. A model for *pap* gene regulation, which explains most of the experimental results obtained to date, is illustrated schematically in Figure 29–6.

The promoter region contains two sites for **Dam-mediated methylation** of the DNA (GATC). The methylation state of these Dam sites determines whether binding of critical activators occurs and thus whether the region is in the "on" or "off" configuration. Al-

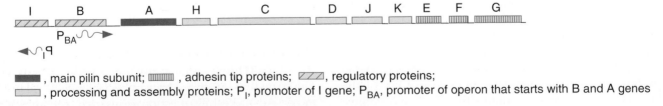

, main pilin subunit; , adhesin tip proteins; , regulatory proteins;
, processing and assembly proteins; P_I, promoter of I gene; P_{BA}, promoter of operon that starts with B and A genes

Figure 29–5 Arrangement of P fimbrial genes (*pap*) on the *E. coli* chromosome.

though Dam methylase actively methylates DNA, there should be a period shortly after DNA replication when one or both sites have not yet been methylated. **LRP (leucine response protein,** a global regulator of *E. coli* genes) binds to methylated or unmethylated sites, but only binding to methylated sites allows it to activate RNA polymerase. Methylation of the site closest to the promoter of the operon containing the *pap* genes (P_{BA}) is necessary for binding of the active form of LRP. LRP-PapI only binds to an unmethylated site. Thus, the PapI-LRP site must be unmethylated for the "on" configuration to form. Once LRP and PapI-LRP bind to the correct sites, and if conditions in the cell are such that cAMP-binding protein can bind its site, the active ("on") complex shown in Figure 29–6 can form, and the pilin genes can be transcribed from P_{BA}. Transcription from the other promoter, P_I, controls the levels of PapI. The temperature regulation of transcription may be mediated through **H-NS** (the histonelike protein), which may be needed to form the bend in the "on" configuration. Formation of the "on" complex or dissolution of the "on" complex (possibly by DNA replication through the region that would dislodge LRP-PapI long enough for the Dam site to be methylated) are infrequent events. This fits with the observation that the frequency of switching is only about 1 in 10^5. Whether the model shown in Figure 29–6 is correct in all of its details remains to be seen, but it illustrates how different signals (temperature, glucose levels, and amino acid levels) might control transcription from a single operator region.

PATHOGENICITY ISLANDS. UPEC strains have most of their virulence genes located on the chromosome. As in many other cases where an excreted toxin or pilin subunit is involved, there are auxiliary genes encoding the assembly-excretion machinery. A number of these genes are located on DNA segments called **pathogenicity islands,** which are scattered around the chromosome (Figure 29–7). Pathogenicity islands often have a %G + C content that is different from that of other genes in the chromosome, a feature which indicates that the DNA may have been acquired from another organism. Many pathogenicity islands have phagelike characteristics, such as phage integrase genes near one end of the DNA segment and small direct repeats (5 to 20 bp) at the ends, such as those created by site-specific recombination of a phage. Pathogenicity islands are so called because they carry virulence genes, sometimes large clusters of them. Sizes of the pathogenicity islands found in UPEC strains range from 25 to 100 kbp. Some of the pathogenicity islands identified in UPEC strains are listed in Table 29–1. These have been placed into four groups based on their sizes and other properties.

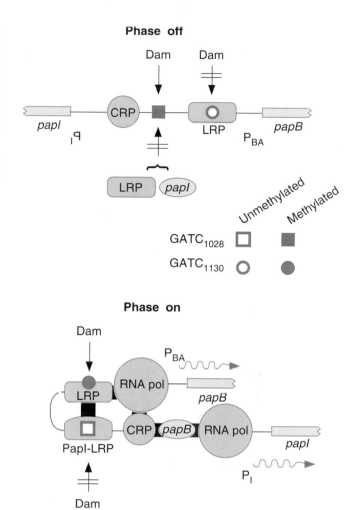

Figure 29–6 Model for control of phase variation of the *pap* genes. The formation of the "on" complex depends on the methylation state of two adjacent GATC sites. cAMP binding protein (CRP) mediates the glucose effect, and temperature regulation is presumably mediated by histonelike protein (H-NS), which may be needed to form the bend in the DNA required to form the "on" complex. H-NS is not shown in the figure because its involvement is only hypothetical at this point, but it (or some other DNA bending protein) would be needed to allow the bend to form in the "on" conformation. Leucine response protein (LRP) is a global activator whose regulation is still not well understood. LRP plays a central role in this model. (Reprinted from M. W. van der Woude et al. 1992. Evidence for global regulatory control of pilus expression in *E. coli* by LRP and DNA methylation: model building based on analysis of *pap. Mol. Microbiol.* **6:**2429–2435.)

Often a strain will contain more than one pathogenicity island. A limitation of the studies of pathogenicity islands of UPEC strains is that the pathogenicity islands have all been identified using strains that cause kidney disease, not uncomplicated cystitis. It remains to be

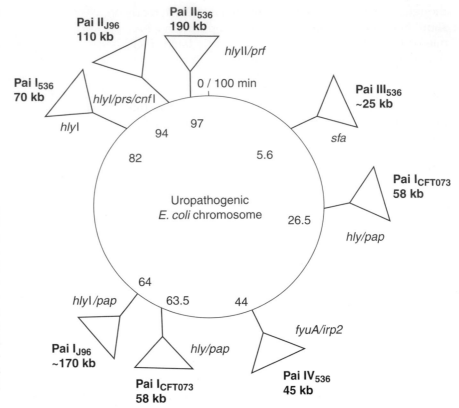

Figure 29–7 Distribution of known pathogenicity islands on the *E. coli* chromosome. The number seen in the subscripts of the Pai designations identifies the strain in which that island was located. Thus, not all of these islands are found in a single strain, although a single strain may contain more than one. The numbers inside the circle are minutes, the units used to define distances on the *E. coli* chromosome. By convention, 0 minute is the origin of replication. (Adapted from Hacker et al., 1999.)

Table 29–1 Examples of pathogenicity islands identified in uropathogenic *E. coli* strains[a]

Designation	Virulence factors encoded on the island	Size of the island (kbp)
I	Alpha-hemolysin	70
II	Alpha-hemolysin	190
	P fimbriae	
III	S fimbriae	25
IV	Yersiniabactin iron-chelating system	40
	Iron-repressible proteins of unknown function	

[a]Adapted from Hacker et al., 1999.

seen whether similar islands will be found in cystitis-causing UPEC strains.

Meningitis and Other Disseminated Infections

E. coli is now one of the leading causes of infant meningitis. This dubious distinction used to belong to *Hae-*

mophilus influenzae type b, but the conjugate vaccine that prevents *H. influenzae* b infection has knocked that cause of meningitis out of contention, one hopes forever. The bad news is that other pathogenic bacteria capable of causing meningitis in infants, such as group B streptococci and *E. coli*, remain in circulation. Fortunately, such infections are relatively uncommon, occurring about once in every 5,000 births, but unfortunately the incidence of this disease shows no sign of declining. Little is known about the factors that allow certain strains of *E. coli* to cause meningitis, although the knowledge base is increasing rapidly.

E. coli septicemia is a problem for all ages. It occurs primarily in people whose intestinal tracts have been perforated during an accident or as a result of appendicitis or surgery. People with urinary tract infections may also develop an infection that ascends to the kidney and enters the bloodstream. *E. coli* may have been displaced in hospitals as a leading nosocomial pathogen by the gram-positive cocci, but *E. coli* is definitely still around. As the nosocomial *E. coli* strains become more resistant to antibiotics, concern about these infections rises. Here too, the rate of infection is, if anything, rising because of the presence of sicker and older patients in large modern hospitals. In hospitalized patients, especially those with tubes in their airways to support breathing (ventilator patients), *E. coli* can cause lung infections that become bloodstream infections if bacteria escape from the lung.

Virulence Factors Associated with Strains That Cause Meningitis, Pneumonia, and Septicemia

CAPSULE.　A characteristic of strains that cause invasive diseases such as septicemia and meningitis is the presence of a capsule composed of a polysaccharide called **K1 antigen.** K1 capsules are antiphagocytic, a trait that would be helpful to a bacterium moving through blood and tissue. Generally, the strains that cause disseminated disease are also serum resistant, a fact that makes them resistant to killing by the membrane attack complex formed during the complement cascade. This is also a trait that would be helpful to bacteria in blood and tissue, where complement activation is bound to occur.

INVASION OF ENDOTHELIAL CELLS.　The meninges (the membranes that form the blood-brain barrier) are composed largely of endothelial cells called brain microvascular endothelial cells (BMECs). There is now a cell line of human BMECs that is being used to study invasion of endothelial cells, a trait that could have great importance in the initial steps of meningitis. Oddly enough, the BMECs of adults are invaded to about the same extent as the BMECs of infants and fetuses, so the higher susceptibility of neonates to *E. coli* meningitis is not due to differences in endothelial cell physiology (assuming that these cultured cells are good models of what happens in the human body). The reason for the higher susceptibility of infants to *E. coli* meningitis remains to be determined. Since adults are prone to septicemia caused by *E. coli* K1 strains, the difference is presumably not due to defenses of the bloodstream.

A type of adhesin called **S fimbriae** appears to make an important contribution to the ability of the K1 strains to cause meningitis and septicemia. These fimbriae (also called pili in some older literature) are found mainly on the *E. coli* strains that cause extraintestinal disease. In vitro, S fimbriae bind cellular fibronectin but not plasma fibronectin, so cellular fibronectin could be the receptor for S fimbriae in the human body.

Studies using the human BMEC model have shown that the K1 antigen is not involved in invasion, although the presence of the capsule seemed to contribute to increased survival of the bacteria after invasion occurred. The role of S fimbriae in invasion is still unclear. An *E. coli* surface protein that may play a role in invasion is an outer membrane porin called **OmpA.** The presence of OmpA increased the invasiveness of *E. coli* in the BMEC model and was associated with actin rearrangements in the endothelial cells being invaded. Thus, OmpA may be part of a system that mediates invasion by an actin rearrangement strategy similar to that seen in the diarrheal *E. coli* strains that invade intestinal cells (see chapter 28). Whether OmpA is acting directly as an adhesin or functions as part of a pathway for delivery of the actual adhesin protein remains to be established.

TOXIC COMPOUNDS.　LPS is certainly a virulence factor in disseminated infections because of its ability to elicit an inflammatory response and cause septic shock. The protein toxin cytotoxic necrotizing factor 1 (CNF-1) was mentioned earlier in this chapter as a possible contributor to urinary tract infections. This toxin is also produced by some meningitis-causing strains of *E. coli* and could be a virulence factor for these strains. This toxin activates GTPases of the Rho family, enzymes that are important regulators of cellular functions and could thus have a devastating effect on brain endothelial cells.

Prevention and Treatment

Urinary tract infections are unpleasant but usually are not life-threatening. By contrast, infant meningitis and adult septicemia are devastating diseases. In these cases, prevention is clearly superior to intervention. This is especially true in the case of meningitis and septicemia, invasive diseases that can cause lifelong damage to the nervous system (meningitis and septicemia) or to important organs such as the heart, kidneys, or lungs (septicemia) if the infected person survives. Unfortunately, the risk factors that lead to urinary tract infections and the more invasive infections caused by the K1 *E. coli* strains have still not been fully revealed.

The association between indwelling urinary catheters and urinary tract infections is the one clear clue to how to prevent infections in a subset of patients. It is still far from clear, however, why only some women have repeated urinary tract infections and why only some infants succumb to meningitis. There are surprisingly few epidemiological data on risk factors, and this is clearly an area that needs to be emphasized in the future. There has been one report that dogs are a reservoir of *E. coli* strains that cause extraintestinal infections, although the significance of this finding is not clear. Nonhuman reservoirs are more likely to be a factor in adults than in infants. In infants, vaginal colonization by K1 strains of *E. coli* would be a conceivable risk factor but has not been established as such.

Cases of extraintestinal *E. coli* infections, from urinary tract infections to meningitis, are treated with antibiotics. As already indicated, antibiotic treatment does not always prevent recurrences of urinary tract infections, and antibiotic treatment of meningitis in infants may come too late to prevent brain damage. Antibiotics are better than nothing but are clearly not the final answer to the problem presented by extraintestinal *E. coli* infections. The fact that *E. coli* strains are becoming more and more resistant to antibiotics makes antibiotics less attractive as a solution. The need to identify people who are highly susceptible to extraintestinal *E. coli* infections and to identify the risk factors that predispose people to such infections is clear. Perhaps one of these days, the funding agencies will figure this out; prevention studies may not be sexy science, but prevention beats intervention every time.

SELECTED READINGS

Buetow, L., G. Flatau, K.Chiu, P. Boquet, and P. Ghosh. 2001. Structure of the Rho-activating domain of *Escherichia coli* cytotoxic necrotizing factor 1. *Nat. Struct. Biol.* **8:**584–588.

Gonzalez, M. D., C. A. Lichtensteiger, and E. R. Vimr. 2001. Adaptation of signature-tagged mutagenesis to *Escherichia coli* K1 and the infant rat model of invasive disease. *FEMS Microbiol.* **198:** 125–128.

Hacker, J., G. Blum-Oehler, B. Janke, G. Nagy, and W. Goebel. 1999. Pathogenicity islands of extraintestinal *Escherichia coli,* p. 59–76. *In* J. Kaper and J. Hacker (ed.), *Pathogenicity Islands and Other Mobile Virulence Elements.* ASM Press, Washington, D.C.

Hoffman, J. A., C. Wass, M. F. Stins, and K. S. Kim. 1999. The capsule supports survival but not transversal of *Escherichia coli* K1 across the blood-brain barrier. *Infect. Immun.* **67:**3566–3570.

Johnson, J. R., A. L. Stell, and P. Delavari. 2001. Canine feces as a reservoir of extraintestinal pathogenic *Escherichia coli. Infect. Immun.* **69:**1306–1314.

Jones, C. H., P. N. Danese, J. S. Pinkner, T. J. Silhavy, and S. Hultgren. 1997. The chaperone-assisted membrane release and folding pathway is sensed by two signal transduction systems. *EMBO J.* **16:**6394–6406.

Jones, C. H., J. S. Pinkner, R. Roth, J. Heuser, A. V. Nicholes, S. N. Abraham, and S. Hultgren. 1995. FimH adhesin of type 1 pili is assembled into a fibrillar tip structure in the *Enterobacteriaceae. Proc. Natl. Acad. Sci. USA* **92:**2081–2085.

Kim, K. S. 2000. *E. coli* invasion of brain microvascular endothelial cells as a pathogenic basis of meningitis. *Subcell. Biochem.* **33:**47–59.

Mulvey, M. A., J. D. Schilling, J. J. Martinez, and S. J. Hultgren. 2000. Bad bugs and beleaguered bladders: interplay between uropathogenic *Escherichia coli* and innate host defenses. *Proc. Natl. Acad. Sci. USA* **97:**8829–8835.

Prasadarao, N. V., C. A. Wass, M. F. Stins, H. Shimada, and K. S. Kim. 1999. Outer membrane protein A-promoted actin condensation of brain microvascular endothelial cells is required for *Escherichia coli* invasion. *Infect. Immun.* **67:**5775–5783.

Russo, T. A., U. B. Carlino, A. Mong, and S. T. Jodush. 1999. Identification of genes in an extraintestinal isolate of *E. coli* with increased expression after exposure to human urine. *Infect. Immun.* **67:**5306–5314.

van der Woude, M., B. Braaten, and D. Low. 1996. Epigenetic phase variation of the *pap* operon in *Escherichia coli. Trends Microbiol.* **4:**5–9.

SUMMARY OUTLINE

Types of infections

 Urinary tract infections

  Community acquired—*E. coli* is the most common cause
  Hospital acquired—associated with indwelling urinary catheters
  Predisposing factors
   Age
   Sex
   Urinary catheter
   Colon colonized with uropathogenic strain
  Complications
   Kidney infection
   Bloodstream infection

 Meningitis—especially in infants

 Septicemia, lung infections—mostly nosocomial cases

(continued)

SUMMARY OUTLINE (*continued*)

Virulence factors of strains that cause urinary tract infections

Ability to colonize and persist in colon, vaginal tract

Adhesins such as type 1 pili or P fimbriae

Invasion of uroepithelial (umbrella) cells
  Attachment mediated by type 1 pili
  Most infected cells slough off
  Some infected cells persist
  Bacteria in infected cells protected from immune system, some antibiotics; may be source of recurring infections

Toxins
  LPS—inflammatory response
  Alpha-hemolysin—pore-forming protein that lyses many types of mammalian cells
  CNF-1—role in infection unknown

Other
  LPS
  Iron acquisition systems
  O-antigen serotypes—serum resistance
  K-antigen capsule—antiphagocytic

Pilin biosynthesis (P fimbriae)
  PapD
    Chaperone, aids folding of secreted Pap protein
    Conveys protein to PapC pore in outer membrane
  PapC
    Forms pore through which pilin proteins pass
    May aid in assembly of fimbrial structure
  Preventing accumulation of improperly folded proteins via a two-component regulatory system

Distribution and regulation of virulence genes
  Regulation of *pap* gene expression
    Involves methylation and demethylation of sites in promoter
    Several global regulators (e.g., Lrp, Crp) involved in control
  Characteristics and distribution of pathogenicity islands

Virulence factors of strains that cause disseminated infections

K1 antigen—antiphagocytic capsule

Serum resistance

LPS

Others?

QUESTIONS

Answers to the questions can be found in Appendix 2.

1. Why are ascending infections far more common than hematogenous infections as a cause of urinary tract infections? What factors predispose people to urinary tract infections?

2. Critique the following statement: if a bacterium can colonize the bladder, it can cause cystitis.

3. Why are some of the same virulence factors associated with both UPEC strains and strains that cause septicemia and other disseminated infections?

4. Why does each serotype of P fimbriae have its own secretion and assembly apparatus? Why not use the same apparatus for all serotypes of the same fimbriae?

5. Predict the phenotypes of mutations in each of the *pap* genes.

6. What considerations have to be kept in mind when deciding on appropriate therapy for someone with a urinary tract infection or a systemic infection?

7. If the vaccine currently being tested is successful, should this vaccine be given to anyone or only to selected portions of the population? Since there are effective antibiotic strategies already available, is this vaccine really needed?

8. What virulence factors are important for *E. coli* strains that cause extraintestinal infections, and how do they differ from factors important for urinary tract infections?

30

Neisseria Species

KEY FEATURES

Neisseria Species

CHARACTERISTICS
Gram-negative diplococci
Nonmotile

DISEASES
Gonorrhea (Neisseria gonorrhoeae)
Epidemic meningitis (Neisseria meningitidis)

RESERVOIRS
Humans

MAJOR VIRULENCE FACTORS
N. gonorrhoeae: adhesins (bundle-forming pili); hypervariable surface antigens; serum resistance; iron acquisition strategies
N. meningitidis: capsule; invasion of epithelial cells; serum resistance; iron acquisition strategies

PREVENTION AND TREATMENT
Vaccine available for some serotypes of N. meningitidis
Antibiotics

The Two Pathogenic Neisseria Species

The genus Neisseria contains two pathogenic species, which cause very different diseases. One is Neisseria gonorrhoeae, the cause of gonorrhea. The other is Neisseria meningitidis, a cause of epidemic meningitis. Members of these two species look alike. They are both gram-negative diplococci and have many similar traits, including shared virulence factors. Yet they cause diseases that seem on the surface to be radically different from each other. A closely related species, Moraxella catarrhalis, is found normally in the mouth. Originally considered to be part of the normal microbiota, it is now known to be capable of causing lung disease, especially in people whose lungs are damaged by smoking or exposure to industrial pollution. M. catarrhalis is also a common cause of otitis media. In this chapter, we will focus on the two pathogenic Neisseria species.

Types of Disease

Gonorrhea is a sexually transmitted disease that is characterized by inflammation and a purulent discharge. It is almost always localized to a mucosal surface, depending on the route of inoculation: the male urethra and the female cervix in the case of transmission by genital sex, the throat in the case of transmission by oral sex, and the anus in the case of transmission by anal sex. As with most sexually transmitted diseases, it can be transferred from mother to infant during passage of the infant through an infected birth canal. The eyes of the infant are the main sites of infection. The bacteria rarely enter the bloodstream.

By contrast, *N. meningitidis* does not cause inflammation of mucosal tissues. Rather, it enters the bloodstream and infects the meninges, the membranes that surround and protect the brain. There it causes inflammation that can disrupt the blood-brain barrier, allowing phagocytes and serum proteins to enter spinal fluid. The inflammatory process in spinal fluid increases pressure on the brain; this is the reason that meningitis is often fatal if not treated early enough with effective antibiotics. Whereas gonorrhea is a very common infectious disease, meningococcal meningitis is a relatively rare disease in most parts of the world except Africa, where it causes thousands of deaths each year. Even in places like the United States, where it is an uncommon disease, it has a great psychological impact when it strikes. Episodes of meningococcal meningitis have occurred several times in Midwestern U.S. universities over the past decades. Although the number of cases was small, the disease caused both students and parents considerable anxiety. Many universities now provide information to incoming students about meningococcal meningitis and the availability of a vaccine.

Commonalities

A closer look at these two species and the diseases they cause reveals some important similarities. For both, the asymptomatic carrier state seems to be the rule rather than the exception. Many people are infected, but few progress to symptomatic disease. When an outbreak of meningococcal meningitis is under way, the carrier rate in the highest-risk populations can be as great as 70 to 80%. Yet only a few people develop meningitis. With gonorrhea, the picture is a bit more complicated. Among women, asymptomatic carriage rates are high, but the word "asymptomatic" has to be defined with care. Asymptomatic in this context means that the women do not experience immediate symptoms of infection, such as a vaginal discharge. The bacteria may, however, be ascending to the fallopian tubes, where

they can do enough silent damage to render the woman infertile and put her at risk for ectopic pregnancy, a serious condition in which the egg is fertilized and begins to develop into a fetus in the fallopian tubes. The subsequent rupture of the fallopian tubes can be fatal. In infants and men, the asymptomatic carrier rate is much lower. Neonatal gonococcal eye infections were once a leading cause of blindness worldwide before the routine use of antibiotic eyedrops to treat newly born infants in the developed world. Gonococcal eye infections are, unfortunately, still a major cause of blindness in the developing world, where for financial reasons antibiotic drops are not routinely placed in the eyes of newborns. In men infected with *N. gonorrhoeae*, about 85 to 90% will develop a copious penile discharge, accompanied by painful urination. Still, some males are asymptomatic carriers.

Gonorrhea

Gonorrhea—Still a Major Public Health Problem

Gonorrhea rates have been declining steadily in developed countries, where effective treatment is readily available, but gonorrhea is still a significant cause of sexually transmitted disease in some countries. In the United States, about 400,000 cases a year are reported to the CDC. Some experts estimate that the actual number of cases may be as high as twice this figure. Given that gonorrhea is a treatable disease and that treatment is cheap and readily available for anyone who seeks it, why is gonorrhea still so common? People with symptomatic disease usually seek treatment immediately and are likely to be willing to suspend sexual activities until cured. Because a cure can be effected in a matter of days to weeks, this is not much of a sacrifice except to commercial sex workers. The problem is that many infected people do not have discernable symptoms. These carriers do not realize they need to be treated, unless a sexual contact reports a symptomatic infection, and they continue to spread the disease. An effective vaccine against gonorrhea would help to solve this problem, but no such vaccine is on the horizon.

A massive effort has been directed toward development of an effective vaccine against gonorrhea. In previous chapters, problems encountered by people seeking vaccines have been described, but gonorrhea surely presents one of the most difficult challenges ever faced by scientists interested in vaccine development. The reason is that *N. gonorrhoeae* has evolved an effective strategy for avoiding a successful host immune response. It constantly changes its surface antigens so that an initially effective antibody response is rendered obsolete, as *N. gonorrhoeae* assumes yet another surface complexion. In addition to constantly changing its surface antigens, *N. gonorrhoeae* also has ways of making itself appear like host tissue, thus avoiding recognition by the host's immune system in the first place.

There is one area in which public health officials can take quite justifiable pride: the virtual elimination of infant blindness due to infection of the eye by *N. gonorrhoeae*. The routine administration of antibacterial eye drops has been very effective in stopping eye infections before they start. The bad news is that the initially asymptomatic women who do not seek treatment because they do not know that they are infected are increasingly at risk for ectopic pregnancy or infertility, which is difficult if not impossible to reverse by surgical means. In the next chapter, you will learn that infertility and ectopic pregnancy are also complications of a very similar disease caused by *Chlamydia trachomatis*.

Although the incidence of gonorrhea has been declining in the United States, it is still disgracefully high, as much as 10 times higher than the incidence in other developed countries. In fact, it is higher than the incidence in some developing countries. How could this happen? Easy. The people most likely to be infected with *N. gonorrhoeae* in the United States are poor and undereducated and live in areas that are the least served by the health care system. The United States could easily eradicate gonorrhea within a few years, if the relatively modest funds needed to support the activities of inner city and rural clinics were provided. Some of the new cephalosporins (β-lactams) are relatively cheap and can be administered in the clinic in a single dose that could effect a cure, eliminating concern about patient compliance with regimens that take 1 or 2 weeks of unsupervised treatment. Also, the length of the period of infectivity is lessened. Proper use of effective drugs could stop the persistence of gonorrhea in areas where it can grow increasingly resistant to cheap antibiotics such as penicillin, which will eventually threaten even those who think gonorrhea is not their problem.

Just When We Thought We Were Seeing the Light at the End of the Tunnel, It Turned Out To Be the Headlight of an Oncoming Train

The reason so much progress has been made toward reducing the incidence of gonorrhea in developed countries is the availability of cheap and effective antibiotics for treatment of the disease. Enter the inevitable villain—multiply antibiotic-resistant strains of *N. gonorrhoeae*. Most U.S. strains of *N. gonorrhoeae* are still susceptible to β-lactam antibiotics and tetracyclines, two

classes of cheap antibiotics that have been widely used to treat gonorrhea. In other countries, especially in Asia, resistance is more widespread.

The incidence of strains resistant to tetracycline or penicillin has been increasing, and some strains are now resistant to both. These strains are still treatable using other antibiotics, but the antibiotics are more expensive than the ones which were formerly effective, a serious problem for clinics with a high case load and a low budget (two characteristics that all too often go together). The incidence of gonorrhea has been decreasing since the 1970s due largely to the facts that it can be treated on an outpatient basis with a simple drug regimen and that the same therapy works for virtually all infected people. Few clinics can afford to do a full microbiological work-up on all possible gonorrhea cases. Also, the patient may not return to learn the results of the diagnostic tests and may not abstain from sexual relations while the diagnostic tests are being run. If multiply resistant strains become common, clinics that treat sexually transmitted diseases will either have to start dispensing expensive front-line broad-spectrum antibiotics or start doing diagnostic work-ups on patients.

Two types of β-lactam resistance have been seen in *N. gonorrhoeae* strains—a chromosomal gene that encodes a mutant penicillin-binding protein that no longer binds penicillin and a plasmid-borne gene that encodes a β-lactamase. The gene for tetracycline resistance is also carried on a plasmid and encodes a ribosome protection type of resistance.

What You Don't Know Can Hurt You: Complications of Gonorrhea

In the vagina, infection is restricted to the cervix because the vaginal mucosa consists of squamous rather than columnar epithelial cells, and *N. gonorrhoeae* is unable to infect the squamous epithelial cells. In clinical specimens, gonococci are seen in pairs (diplococci), with many inside PMNs. Gram-negative cocci are uncommon in nature, a fact that has given rise to a simple presumptive test for diagnosing gonorrhea in men. A Gram stain of discharge from a man with gonorrhea contains many gram-negative diplococci, mostly inside PMNs, whereas gram-negative cocci are seen rarely, if at all, in specimens taken from an uninfected urethra.

At first, gonorrhea might seem to be a female-friendly disease. After all, women are far less likely to develop symptoms than men. This is actually a bad thing for women in the long run. Since men are more likely to develop symptoms, they are also more likely to seek treatment because of those symptoms. For an infected woman, the first signs of the disease may be the serious complications of an untreated infection, ranging from pelvic inflammatory disease to infertility. Bacteria infecting the cervix can ascend into the uterus and fallopian tubes to cause **salpingitis** or **pelvic inflammatory disease.** The main symptom of this condition is persistent pain in the abdominal area, but many women with infections of the fallopian tubes are either asymptomatic or do not have sufficient pain to cause them to seek medical attention. Pelvic inflammatory disease is a serious condition that must be diagnosed and treated as early as possible, because the inflammatory response can cause irreversible damage to the delicate fallopian tubes. One result is infertility because scarring makes the passageway through which the egg must travel too small, preventing the egg from reaching the uterus. Another potential consequence of fallopian tube scarring is ectopic pregnancy, one of the most serious complications of gonorrhea. In an ectopic pregnancy, the egg trapped in the fallopian tube is fertilized, and the fetus begins to develop there. If this is not detected and if the fetus is not surgically removed, the tube can rupture, causing the woman to go into shock.

In about 1% of infected men and women, the disease becomes systemic. A common symptom of the systemic phase of gonorrhea is arthritis, which if left untreated can destroy the affected joint. Less common but more serious complications of systemic infection are infections of the heart (endocarditis) and meninges (meningitis). *N. gonorrhoeae* can also infect the throat.

Meningococcal Meningitis

In infants, *Streptococcus pneumoniae, Escherichia coli,* and group B streptococci are now the leading causes of meningitis, but in older age groups, meningitis is more likely to be caused by *N. meningitidis.* Such meningitis cases occur most often in the winter, when people are inside in crowded locations and forced air heat dries the mucous membranes (Box 30–1).

Meningitis is a frightening disease, not just because of the damage it causes but because it can progress so rapidly. The first signs of meningitis are nonspecific—a fever, a stiff neck, a bad headache, or a rash. In an outbreak, the first few people to contract the disease are the ones most likely to die, because meningitis is not a diagnosis that would normally occur to a physician or a patient when confronted with a symptom like severe headache. Once *N. meningitidis* is known to be on the loose again, effective public education that acquaints people with the initial symptoms can be very effective in preventing further cases.

Still, communities and institutions can be confronted

BOX 30–1   A "Date" No One in the Bar Wanted To Pick Up

The University of Illinois at Urbana-Champaign, the home base of the authors of this book, has had several outbreaks of meningococcal meningitis in recent years. Most of the cases involved undergraduates. The university offers free vaccination to anyone interested, but this vaccine protects against only some serotypes of *N. meningitidis.* It is thus important to prevent the spread of disease. Epidemiologists decided to follow one of the outbreaks to find out where the disease was most likely to be acquired. Among other places, they checked campus bars frequented by undergraduates. Anyone who has been to such a place will know that these bars give the word "crowding" new meaning. One bar, in particular (dubbed "bar A" in the paper describing the study results), proved to be a hotbed of colonized people, including bar employees as well as patrons.

The association of *N. meningitidis* and campus bars makes sense. Not only are they crowded environments in which students spend hours, but in some of them, smoking is allowed, a behavior that predisposes people to become colonized. Apparently, copious consumption of alcohol does not have a protective effect. The bar in question was never named, but the word is that it has since gone out of business for other reasons.

Source: P. B. Imrey, L. A. Jackson, P. H. Ludwinski, A. C. England III, G. A. Fella, B. C. Fox, L. B. Isdale, M. W. Reeves, and J. D. Wenger. 1995. Meningococcal carriage, alcohol consumption, and campus bar patronage in a serogroup C meningococcal disease outbreak. *J. Clin. Microbiol.* **33:**3133–3137.

---

with impossible choices. During one of the first outbreaks of meningitis at the University of Illinois, university officials did nothing except issue warnings and information. This was actually the responsible thing to do in the circumstances. Irate parents soon forced the university into action, however, and students were herded together in a large room, where they were given a vaccine or prophylactic antibiotic treatment. Fortunately, the crowded setting did not set off a new round of infection, but it could have done so.

Virulence Factors

N. gonorrhoeae

ANIMAL AND CELL CULTURE MODELS. *N. gonorrhoeae* is a human-specific pathogen. Thus, in vivo studies are usually done with human volunteers. You might think that few volunteers would come forward, but the experience is actually not all that bad. Only male volunteers are used, and they are inoculated in the urethra (a painless procedure, if an uncomfortable one for many) and watched closely for several days to determine whether the strain being tested will cause disease. Once signs of the disease are evident, the volunteer is given an antibiotic that clears up the infection in short order. And, of course, human volunteers are paid or given some other reward.

N. gonorrhoeae adheres to and invades many different types of tissue culture cells. A popular cell line (because it is an epithelial cell line) is **Chang conjunctival epithelial cells,** but epithelial cell lines derived from cervical and prostate carcinomas have also been widely used. *N. gonorrhoeae* will not adhere to and invade nonhuman cell lines such as CHO (Chinese hamster ovary) cells, unless the cells have been transfected with cloned human DNA so that they are producing the receptor found on human cells. Such cell lines can be useful for testing individual receptors one at a time, whereas human cells may have multiple receptors.

PMNs and macrophagelike cell lines are used to study the fate of *N. gonorrhoeae* ingested by phagocytes. There is an animal model of sorts. Mice implanted subcutaneously with a chamber into which the bacteria are injected are used as a model for studying virulence factors associated with systemic spread. Fallopian tissue provides an organ culture model for studying effects of bacterial colonization of fallopian tubes. This type of tissue is readily available in any hospital where hysterectomies are done.

N. gonorrhoeae is naturally transformable (takes up DNA without chemical shock or electroporation), but the transformation system discriminates against foreign DNA. There are transposons that integrate in the *N. gonorrhoeae* chromosome (e.g., Tn*916* and its derivatives), but integration is not completely random. Tn*1545*del, a derivative of a conjugative transposon which is closely related to Tn*916,* has been used successfully in some transposon mutagenesis experiments but, like Tn*916,* probably does not integrate completely randomly. Gene disruption and gene replacement are possible but not as easy as with *E. coli.* The genetic tools are getting better all the time, however.

ADHERENCE AND INVASION. The picture of how gonorrhea progresses has changed significantly in recent years. *N. gonorrhoeae* was once classified as an extracellular pathogen, which was only found outside cells, except for PMNs. Today, invasion and intracellular residence are believed to be an important part of the gonococcal lifestyle. The first stage in the infection process is colonization of a mucosal surface lined by columnar epithelial cells. As a result of the inflammatory response elicited by the bacteria, the bacteria soon encounter phagocytes, especially PMNs. PMNs in the purulent discharge of a person with gonorrhea often contain numerous bacteria.

There is some uncertainty about whether the bacteria inside phagocytes are in the process of being killed or whether *N. gonorrhoeae* can survive inside PMNs. Microscopic analysis of bacteria inside PMNs indicates that many are in the process of being broken down and killed, but a fraction of the ingested bacteria appear to remain viable. Whatever the intracellular fate of *N. gonorrhoeae* inside PMNs, it appears that *N. gonorrhoeae,* like many of the bacteria described in previous chapters, can also bind to human epithelial cells and stimulate these cells to phagocytose them by a process that involves actin rearrangement. A major gonococcal adhesin is **type 4 pili;** its pilin subunits are processed by a type II secretion system (see Appendix 1). The first amino acid in the mature protein is a modified phenylalanine. This is the same type of pilus found on a number of human and plant pathogens. The receptor for the *N. gonorrhoeae* pilus is a human cell surface protein called CD46. CD46 is normally involved in regulation of the complement cascade.

The gonococci produce a number of variants of the type 4 pili. Some variants form bundles, and these **bundle-forming pili** appear to attach more efficiently to host cells than pili that do not form bundles. The reason some pili form bundles has not been established with certainty, but pilin proteins are glycosylated. One explanation is that lack of glycosylation makes the pili more able to stick together, forming the bundles. This introduces a theme that is seen repeatedly in gonococcal virulence factors: the variability of surface antigens. The finding that bacterial proteins could be glycosylated was a surprise. Prior to this discovery, the dogma had been that eukaryotic cells glycosylated proteins but prokaryotic cells did not.

After adhering to the surface of cervical or urethral epithelial cells, the bacteria are ingested by the epithelial cell and transcytose through the cell to the basolateral surface, where they exit into the space below the cells. This signals the body to mount the pronounced inflammatory response that is responsible for most of the symptoms of gonorrhea. This progression can be demonstrated in cervical tissue samples (ex vivo organ culture). There is some controversy as to whether binding via pili is sufficient to induce phagocytosis of the bacteria or whether some other intermediate is required. Gonococcal outer membrane porin proteins (called **PorA** and **PorB**) may have a role in triggering phagocytosis. First, both PorA and PorB proteins can nucleate actin. Thus, they could contribute to the actin rearrangements that contribute to formation of the pseudopods that engulf the bacteria. Second, PorA and PorB proteins can enter the cytoplasmic membranes of eukaryotic cells, causing transient changes in membrane potential. This could be a signal that sets off the signal transduction cascade that leads to ingestion of the bacteria.

Another type of surface protein, which was originally thought to have a role in adherence to the host cell but may actually have another role in virulence, is **Opa proteins.** Opa proteins are a family of gonococcal outer membrane proteins. The name Opa stands for opacity; bacteria with Opa proteins on their surfaces form colonies that have a more opaque-looking surface than those not expressing the protein. This easily visible phenotype has been used to identify mutants that express aberrant levels of Opas. The reason Opa proteins were once thought to be adhesins was that bacteria producing Opa but not pili were taken up by tissue culture cells. Two findings have raised questions about the involvement of Opa proteins in the early steps of infection. First, bacteria that produce pili but not Opa proteins are taken up by epithelial cells in organ cultures and transcytose similarly to wild-type bacteria. Thus, Opa proteins are not essential for uptake. A second problem is that the receptors for Opa proteins are located on the basolateral surface of properly polarized cells. Opa proteins seem to be important for virulence, because mutants lacking them are less virulent in human volunteers than wild-type bacteria, but their precise role in the progression of infection is still uncertain. Some of them mediate opsonin-independent uptake of the bacteria by PMNs. If the bacteria are able to survive in PMNs, a characteristic that is still in dispute, Opa proteins might be aimed more at PMNs than at epithelial cells.

How *N. gonorrhoeae* Evades the Host Defense Responses

HYPERVARIABLE SURFACE ANTIGENS.   People infected with *N. gonorrhoeae* mount a vigorous antibody response to bacterial surface proteins. Why, then, does the person not become immune to reinfection? The main reason is that *N. gonorrhoeae* varies its surface antigens, especially pilin antigens, so the original sIgA response rapidly becomes obsolete. The bacteria have an anti-

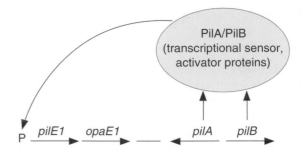

Figure 30–1   Regulation of expression of *pilE*.

genic repertoire that may be large enough to produce 1 million different antigenic variants.

Figure 30–1 illustrates some of the mechanisms of phase variation of pilin genes. *N. gonorrhoeae* controls both the amount of pilin subunit produced and the amino acid composition of the subunits. Phase variation refers to the on/off expression of genes, whereas antigenic variation (also mentioned in this chapter) refers to changes in the gene sequence leading to changes in amino acid composition of the gene product. Expression of ***pilE***, the gene that encodes the pilin subunit, is controlled at the level of transcription by a two-component regulatory system (**PilA, PilB**). PilA is the transcriptional activator and PilB is the sensor component that phosphorylates PilA. The signal recognized by PilB is still unknown. Whether pili are assembled on the cell surface (Pil$^+$) or not (Pil$^-$) is controlled at several levels. Switching between the Pil$^+$ and Pil$^-$ state is called **phase variation.** One type of phase variation arises from the fact that there are two possible processing sites on the newly translated protein, P$^+$ and P^s. PilE nicked at P$^+$ assembles into pili (Pil$^+$ phenotype), whereas PilE nicked at P^s lacks the hydrophobic region

Figure 30–2   Structure of *pilE* (**A**) and recombination exchanges of DNA between *pilS* and *pilE* (**B** and **C**). P$^+$ is the processing site that produces a mature protein that can be assembled into pili (Pil$^+$). Cleavage at the other processing site, P^s, results in release of pilin subunit from the bacteria (S stands for soluble pilin) to give a Pil$^-$ phenotype. Regions labeled "mc" (minicassette) vary from one copy of the gene to another. Mc2 is the most variable and occurs between two cysteine residues that form a disulfide linkage. Regions at the amino terminus and between mc regions are highly conserved. These conserved areas are the sites where homologous recombination can replace a section of *pilE* with a section of *pilS*. Because of the presence of repetitive sequences within *pilE* or *pilS*, recombination events can also produce copies of PilE that are larger than normal (L-pilin).

A Structure of pilin protein

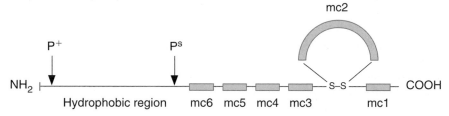

——, segment highly conserved in different copies of the gene; ▨, variable segment

B Antigenic variation in PilE

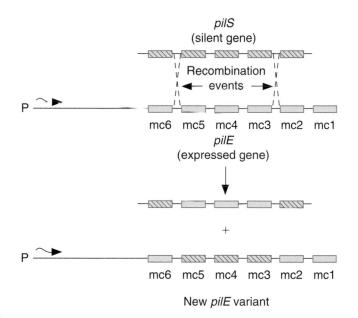

New *pilE* variant

C Origin of L-pili

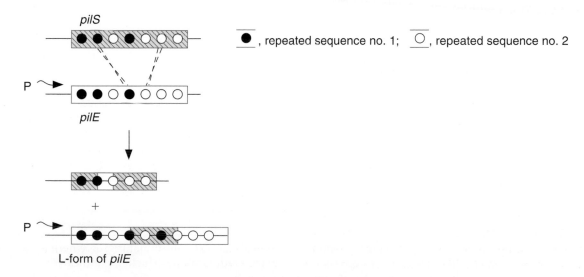

●, repeated sequence no. 1; ○, repeated sequence no. 2

L-form of *pilE*

needed for assembly. Protein processed at P^s is secreted and released from the cell rather than assembled into pili, so pili are not made.

A second type of transition also arises from production of an aberrant form of PilE that is not assembled into pili. To understand how this type of phase variation works, it is first important to know that, although there are multiple copies of the pilin gene scattered around the chromosome, there is usually only one copy (occasionally two) that has a promoter and is expressed (Figure 30–2B). This expressed copy is called *pilE* (E stands for expression), whereas the other nonexpressed copies are called *pilS* (S stands for silent). *pilE* and *pilS* contain internal repeated DNA sequences. Homologous recombination events can occur between *pilS* and *pilE*. Such events result in exchanges of the interior portions of the genes (antigenic variation, see below). However, homologous recombination between different copies of the genes sometimes results in uneven exchange of DNA because of the internal repeated DNA sequences in *pilE* and *pilS* (Figure 30–2C). The result is a form of PilE that is much larger than normal. This form is not processed and assembled into pili.

A third mechanism of phase variation involves another pilin gene, *pilC*. **PilC** protein is necessary for proper assembly and maturation of pili. Early in the *pilC*-coding region, there is a long run of G residues (Figure 30–3). During DNA replication of regions containing highly repetitive DNA sequences, a process called **slipped-strand mispairing** (Figure 30–4) changes the number of repeated bases in a run of repeats. If this occurs within the coding region of a gene, a frameshift results. In the case of *pilC*, the number of G residues in a run of G's near the beginning of the coding region determines whether the protein is prematurely terminated (out of frame) or whether intact protein is made. Frameshift mutations give a PilC$^-$ and thus a Pil$^-$ phenotype.

Changes in the DNA sequence of *pilE* that cause changes in amino acid composition of the protein are called **antigenic variation.** Antigenic variation allows the bacteria to still produce pili but avoid the immune response to them by changing the amino acid sequence of the pili so the antibodies no longer bind. The main

mechanism of antigenic variation is recombination between different versions of the *pilS* and *pilE*. As seen in Figure 30–2, *pil* genes contain variable regions (mc1 to mc6), the most variable of which is mc2, and highly conserved regions (amino terminus and between mc segments). Homologous recombination events involving conserved regions of *pilS* and *pilE* replace the variable regions between crossover points with new variable regions.

The DNA involved in crossover events could come from elsewhere in the chromosome of the same cell or it could come from DNA taken up by transformation. *N. gonorrhoeae* is naturally transformable. If homologous crossover events occurred between *pilS* and *pilE* on the same chromosome, the result would be a reciprocal exchange of DNA that would alter both *pilE* and the copy of *pilS* involved in the exchange (Figure 30–5). However, examination of antigenic variants of a strain of *N. gonorrhoeae* has shown that although *pilE* is altered, copies of *pilS* in the same strain are not changed. This is the pattern one would expect to see if DNA from lysed bacteria were taken up from the environment and used in the crossover. Because the short DNA fragments taken up from the medium would not be replicated during cell division, the altered form of pilS would be lost, and only the altered chromosomal *pilE* would be recovered. Support for this hypothesis came from the observation that transformation-deficient mutants had a much-decreased ability to produce new PilE variants. Also, antigenic variation was much reduced if DNase was included in the medium.

Phase variation and antigenic variation usually occur in only a fraction of the population (frequencies, 10^{-2} to 10^{-4}). But even if the original form of pilin is being expressed by most members of the population, a new variant that is not recognized by host antibodies will soon be selected and become the dominant form in the population. The strategy of *N. gonorrhoeae* is to produce a population of different variants (Pil$^+$, Pil$^-$, different antigenic variants), at least one of which is sure to survive.

LOS. LOS (**lipo-oligosaccharide**) is the neisserial equivalent of LPS. It is called LOS because its O antigen

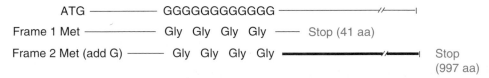

Figure 30–3 Structure of *pilC* gene showing repeats in amino-terminal region where slipped-strand synthesis can occur and change the reading frame. Thick line indicates amino acid differences between frame 1 and frame 2.

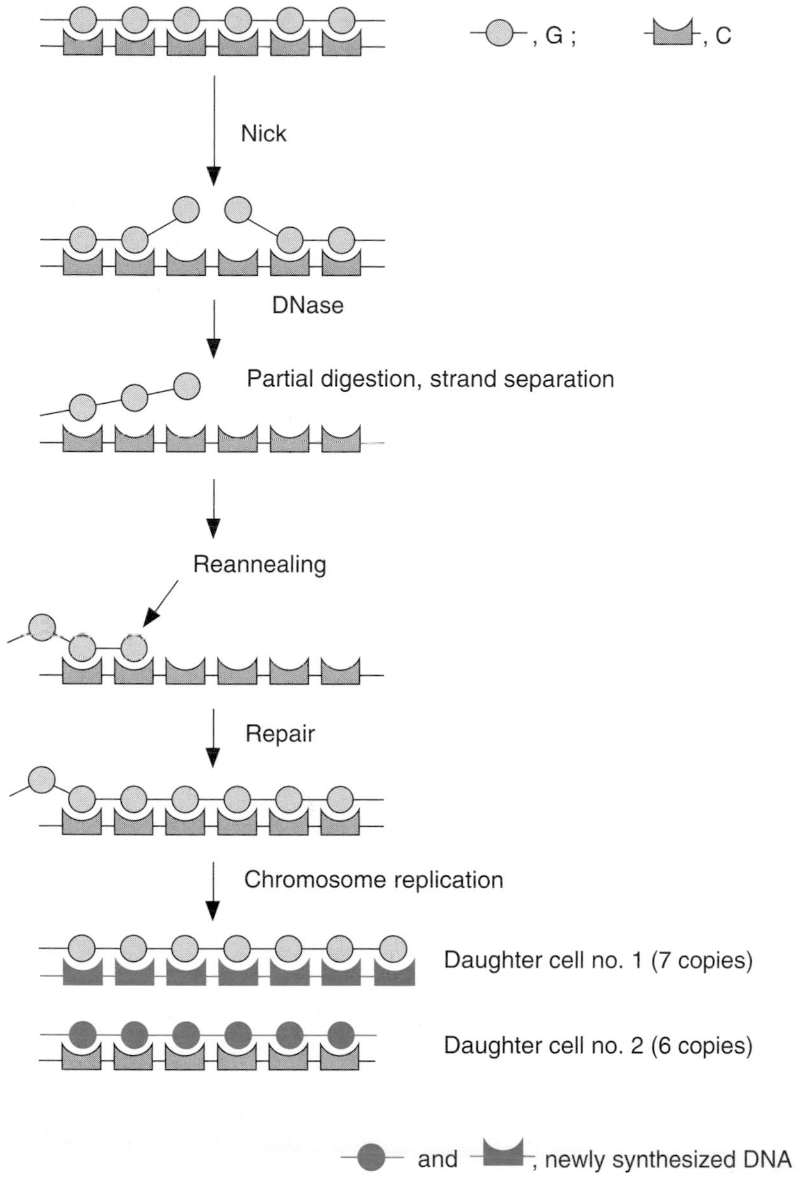

Figure 30–4 Example of how slipped-strand DNA synthesis could alter the number of G repeats. Slipped-strand synthesis can delete, as well as add, repeats.

consists only of a simple oligosaccharide and is thus less complex than that of LPS. LOS is probably responsible for most of the symptoms of gonorrhea because it triggers an inflammatory response. Activation of complement and the influx of phagocytes contribute to the purulent response and to tissue damage. Local production of TNF-α is thought to be the cause of damage to fallopian tubes.

LOS also contributes to serum resistance, the ability of the bacteria to resist the killing action of the membrane attack complex of complement. Serum resistance appears to be an important trait for strains that cause systemic infection. Serum resistance may play a local role, too, because complement activation occurs in tissue as well as blood. The importance of late-acting com-

plement components as a host defense against systemic disease can be seen from the fact that people with a genetic defect in late-acting complement components are more prone than normal people to develop disseminated *Neisseria* infections.

Some *N. gonorrhoeae* strains take *N*-acetylneuraminic (sialic) acid from human blood (CMP-*N*-acetylneuraminic acid) and attach it to galactose residues on LOS. Bacteria with sialylated LOS become serum resistant, both because sialic acid is a ubiquitous host molecule and thus does not activate complement and because the membrane attack complex does not form productively around the altered LOS. Also, sialylation of LOS prevents access of bactericidal antibodies to Por1 and other surface proteins.

A Reciprocal exchange between *pilS* and *pilE* on the same chromosome

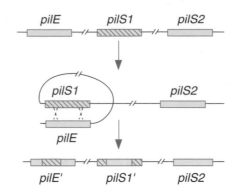

B Transformation

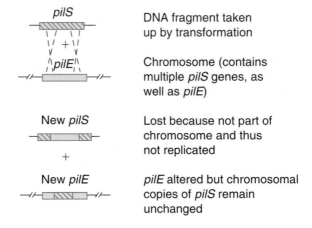

C Recombination between two copies of the chromosome in the same bacterial cell

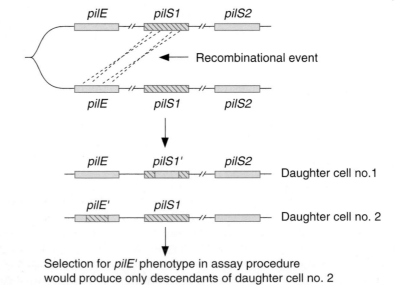

Figure 30–5 (**A**) Recombination of *pilS* and *pilE* on the same chromosome, resulting in reciprocal exchange. (**B** and **C**) Two possible origins of nonreciprocal exchanges between a copy of *pilS* and *pilE*.

BLOCKING ANTIBODIES. Some antibodies elicited by the gonococci during an infection actually block the binding of other antibodies to the bacterial surface. A surface protein called **Rmp** elicits such an antibody response. Antibodies to Rmp block the binding of antibodies to LOS and Por, two types of antibodies that are bactericidal because they elicit complement-mediated killing of the bacteria.

IRON ACQUISITION. *N. gonorrhoeae* can acquire iron in two ways. It has surface receptors that allow it to use the siderophores produced by other bacteria. This type of iron acquisition strategy is more likely to be of use to bacteria growing in the vaginal tract, where there is a dense population of bacteria, than it is to bacteria growing in the male urethra, which is normally sterile. *N. gonorrhoeae* can also use the human iron-binding proteins transferrin and lactoferrin as sources of iron. The gonococcal transferrin receptor is specific for human transferrin and does not bind transferrin from other animals, yet another reason why *N. gonorrhoeae* is a human-specific pathogen. The ability to acquire iron from transferrin appears to be important for virulence, because mutants unable to do this are avirulent. Mutants unable to strip iron from lactoferrin, however, are still virulent. Also, most clinical isolates of *N. gonorrhoeae* do not have the lactoferrin-binding receptor. A model for how transferrin-bound iron might be removed from the molecule by a bacterial surface protein called transferrin-binding protein (**TbpA**) is shown in Figure 30–6. Binding of the two parts of transferrin to different sites on TbpA results in a conformational change in the transferrin molecule that reduces the affinity of transferrin for iron and allows the bacteria to capture the iron molecule. *N. gonorrhoeae* can also acquire iron from heme and hemoglobin, but little is known about the proteins that mediate this type of acquisition.

N. meningitidis

Much less is known about the virulence factors of *N. meningitidis*, although *N. meningitidis* seems to possess many of the same virulence factors as *N. gonorrhoeae*. These factors include the ability to bind to and invade epithelial cells, serum resistance, and mechanisms of iron sequestration. A fascinating question is why two species that are as closely related as are *N. gonorrhoeae* and *N. meningitidis* cause such different diseases. For starters, when *N. meningitidis* colonizes the human nose and throat, why does it not cause the type of inflammation seen when *N. gonorrhoeae* colonizes the urethra or cervix? One suggestion has been that *N. gonorrhoeae* in the male urethra or female fallopian tube is

in an area that is normally sterile, and the body may react differently to bacteria in such sites than to bacteria in sites where many types of bacteria are normally found. This suggestion does not explain, however, why *N. gonorrhoeae* causes an inflammatory response when it colonizes the cervix.

A difference between *N. meningitidis* and *N. gonorrhoeae* is that *N. meningitidis* has a polysaccharide capsule. This capsule has a number of antigenic variants. The most important are A, B, C, Y, and W135. Not only does the capsule prevent uptake and killing of the bacteria by phagocytes, but it contributes to the serum resistance of meningococci. Serum resistance due to the polysaccharide capsule, sialylated LOS, and the outer membrane porin Por is important for protecting the bacteria from complement-mediated killing when they enter the bloodstream. How the bacteria enter the bloodstream is unknown. There are M cells in the tonsils, and this could be one route of entry. Direct invasion through epithelial surfaces has not been ruled out.

New insights into the differences between gonococci and meningococci may be revealed by comparisons of the genome sequences of the two species. In a recent comparison by subtractive hybridization, eight regions of difference ranging from 2 to 40 kbp were identified. The proteins encoded in such regions may help to explain the differences in the diseases caused by these very closely related bacterial species.

Prevention and Treatment

Gonorrhea

The treatment for gonorrhea was once straightforward, and it still is in some parts of the world, where the prevailing strains have not become resistant to antibiotics. For a long time, penicillin was effective against gonorrhea, but the incidence of penicillin-resistant *N. gonorrhoeae* strains is increasing. Another complication is that the symptoms of gonorrhea resemble those caused by other bacteria, such as *C. trachomatis* (see chapter 31). Because disease caused by *C. trachomatis* is now more common than disease caused by *N. gonorrhoeae*, and because people can be coinfected with both bacteria, treatment regimens are now aimed at both pathogens. Tetracyclines and macrolides such as erythromycin have been effective. As mentioned in an earlier section, cephalosporins have the advantage that they can be given in one dose to a person in a clinic. The treatment regimens for gonorrhea will continue to become more complex as the mix of efficacy and economic considerations dictates different solutions in different settings.

Despite numerous attempts to develop an effective vaccine against gonorrhea, no vaccine is in view. The

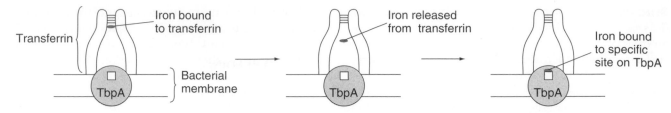

Figure 30–6 Removal of iron from transferrin by TbpA. The two parts of transferrin bind to different sites on TbpA, which causes a conformational change in transferrin that reduces the affinity for iron (Fe). The Fe migrates to an iron-binding region on TbpA, where it is captured.

hypervariability of many gonococcal surface proteins, combined with the phenomena of blocking antibodies and intracellular residence, all make vaccine development a very difficult challenge. At one time, the incidence of gonorrhea had dropped to a low enough level in some parts of the world that the possibility of eradicating the disease was discussed as a possible feat. If this is to be a viable solution to the gonorrhea problem, it will be necessary to move fast because of the increasing incidence of resistance among strains of gonococci. Countries where prostitution is legal have a better chance of controlling the disease, but in countries where prostitution is illegal, it is only possible to interrupt the chain of infection when people come to clinics for treatment. Since women are often asymptomatic carriers, this is not a very efficient solution to eliminating the disease. Condoms give some measure of protection but are not infallible in preventing the transmission of gonorrhea.

Some people think that the solution is abstinence or monogamous relationships. Certainly, if abstinence can be practiced consistently or if a relationship is truly monogamous, disease is avoided. The problem is that abstinence is not always possible; coerced sex is not unheard of. A person who is faithful in a monogamous relationship is only as safe as the behavior of the other partner allows. As we have seen with HIV, no strategy that insists on absolutely consistent human adherence to a certain code of behavior is likely to be successful.

Meningococcal Meningitis

Meningitis caused by *N. meningitidis* is treatable with penicillin and cephalosporins. Although resistance has begun to appear, making an earlier treatment with sulfonamides obsolete, there are still many antibiotics that will cure meningitis. The problem in this case is to diagnose the disease early enough for treatment to be effective. The nonspecific symptoms of meningitis in its early stages make it easy to miss. Treatment at a later stage may be effective in saving the person's life but

can leave the person with permanent neurological defects, such as vision or hearing loss. When an outbreak of meningococcal meningitis is in progress, rifampin is given prophylactically to contacts of people who develop meningitis to reduce colonization and prevent the disease from developing. How effective this has been is difficult to assess, since so few of the people colonized with *N. meningitidis* go on to develop meningitis. But rifampin prophylaxis gives the contacts of meningitis patients some measure of protection.

There is a vaccine against meningococcal meningitis. It consists of a mixture of the capsular polysaccharides of type A and type C strains. This vaccine is effective in developing countries where these two types have been common causes of meningitis. Type A in particular is often responsible for epidemics of meningitis. As a polysaccharide vaccine, it is ineffective in infants but protects children and adults, who are at highest risk for meningococcal meningitis. In the outbreaks in midwestern U.S. universities, this vaccine was offered but was probably not effective. The reason is that, in developed countries such as the United States, type B strains are responsible for about half of the cases, type C is responsible for about 20 to 25%, and types Y and W are responsible for the rest.

Why is the type B capsular polysaccharide not part of the vaccine? The reason is that type B capsular polysaccharide is a very poor antigen, probably because it consists of sialic acid residues, which are found on most human cells. Thus, it looks like "self" to the immune system. A solution to this problem is to look beyond the polysaccharide capsule for a vaccine. Surface proteins are an attractive alternative. The latest search for a vaccine against type B meningitis illustrates how vaccine development has been changed by the molecular revolution and the availability of genome sequences. The genome sequence of *N. meningitidis* type B was published in 1999. Immediately, the search began for proteins that had the characteristics of surface proteins—signal sequences and alternating hydrophobic and hydrophilic regions in the amino acid sequence. Several hundred such sequences were identified. The next goal was to weed out the ones that were likely to be hypervariable. This was done by amplifying each gene from different strains of type B *N. meningitidis* and sequencing them to find those with conserved sequences. This second criterion narrowed the search to a smaller number of genes. Proteins encoded by these genes were then overexpressed and injected into mice, which were then inoculated with the bacteria. Although *N. meningitidis* appears to be a human-specific pathogen in real life, there are strains of mice that develop a systemic disease if inoculated with the bacteria. Some proteins were identified that seemed to elicit a protective response. These proteins and the genes that encode them will now be subjected to intense scrutiny to identify those that are the most promising vaccine candidates.

It remains to be seen whether this brute force approach to finding potential vaccine components is effective, but if it works, it could completely change the way vaccines are designed in the future. Although the approach just described could shorten the initial discovery period for vaccines, there are still the years-long secondary and tertiary rounds of testing the vaccine in humans for safety and efficacy. This statement is not meant to be a criticism of the very exciting advances in vaccine development that have occurred as the result of the molecular revolution but rather as a reminder of the fact that the next frontier in vaccine research could well be finding ways to assess vaccine safety and efficacy more expeditiously.

SELECTED READINGS

Dehio, C., S. Gray-Owen, and T. Meyer. 2000. Host cell invasion by pathogenic *Neisseriae*. *Subcell. Biochem.* **33:**61–96.

Dorr, J., T. Hurek, and B. Reinhold-Hurek. 1998. Type IV pili are involved in plant-microbe and fungus-microbe interactions. *Mol. Microbiol.* **30:**7–17.

Giardina, P. C., R. Williams, D. Lubaroff, and M. A. Apicella. 1998. *Neisseria gonorrhoeae* induces focal polymerization of actin in primary human urethral epithelium. *Infect. Immun.* **66:**3416–3419.

Klee, S. R., X. Nassif, B. Kusecek, P. Merker, J. Beretti, M. Achtman, and C. Tinsley. 2000. Molecular and biological analysis of eight genetic islands that distinguish *Neisseria meningitidis* from the closely related pathogen *Neisseria gonorrhoeae*. *Infect. Immun.* **68:**2082–2095.

Nassif, X., C. Pujol, P. Morand, and E. Eugene. 1999. Interactions of pathogenic *Neisseria* with host cells. Is it possible to assemble the puzzle? *Mol. Microbiol.* **32:**1124–1132.

Schryvers, A., and I. Stojiljkovic. 1999. Iron acquisition systems in pathogenic *Neisseria*. *Mol. Microbiol.* **32:**1117–1123.

Vogel, U., and M. Frosch. 1999. Mechanisms of neisserial serum resistance. *Mol. Microbiol.* **32:**1133–1139.

SUMMARY OUTLINE

N. gonorrhoeae

Gram-negative diplococcus

Disease—gonorrhea
  Characterized by inflammation and purulent discharge
  Sexually transmitted
  Incidence declining but still a common disease
  Localized to mucosal surface
    Urethra or cervix—genital transmission
    Throat—oral transmission
    Anus—anal transmission
    Eyes—acquired during passage through infected birth canal
  Asymptomatic carriage
    Higher in females than in males
    May ascend to fallopian tubes in women unaware of being infected
  Diagnosis
    Gram stain in men (gram-negative diplococci plus PMNs)
    Must be cultivated and identified in women
    Often treated without culture-based diagnosis
  Complications
    Infertility or ectopic pregnancy due to salpingitis or pelvic inflammatory disease
    In 1% of cases (both male and female) disease becomes systemic

(continued)

SUMMARY OUTLINE (*continued*)

Arthritis most common
Heart and meninges may be affected

Virulence factors
  Difficult to study because human-specific pathogen
  Adherence and invasion
    Type 4 pili bind to CD46 on human cells
      Bundle-forming pili (glycosylated proteins)
    Outer surface porin proteins PorA and PorB—may trigger phagocytosis
      Nucleate actin
      Can enter cell membrane of eukaryotic cells
    Opa (opacity) proteins—outer membrane proteins
      Not essential for uptake
      Bind receptors on basolateral surface
      Role in progression of infection unclear
  Evading host defenses
    Hypervariability of pilin genes
      Production of PilE (pilin subunit) controlled by two-component regulatory system
        (PilA, PilB)
      Phase variation—switching between Pil⁺ and Pil⁻
        Two different processing sites on newly translated protein (P⁺ and Pˢ)
        Homologous recombination between *pilE* and *pilS* may result in large form of PilE that
          is not processed
        Slipped-strand mispairing—produces frameshift mutation in *pilC* (involved in assembly
          and maturation)
      Antigenic variation
        Changes in DNA sequence of *pilE*
        Results from recombination between different versions of *pilS* and *pilE*
        DNA may come from elsewhere on chromosome or by transformation
      Phase variation and antigenic variation occur at a frequency of 10^{-2} to 10^{-4}
    LOS—lipo-oligosaccharide
      Responsible for most symptoms of gonorrhea
      Contributes to serum resistance
      Some strains attach sialic acid to LOS
        Appear as self to immune system
        Block access of bactericidal antibodies to bacterial surface proteins
    Blocking antibodies
      Antibodies formed against Rmp, a bacterial surface protein
      Prevent binding of bactericidal antibodies to LOS and Por
    Iron acquisition
      Surface receptors bind siderophores produced by other bacteria
      TbpA—surface protein that removes iron bound to transferrin
      Remove iron from lactoferrin
      Acquire iron from heme and hemoglobin

Prevention and treatment
  Penicillin previously effective
  Multidrug resistance becoming a problem
  No vaccine for several reasons
    Hypervariability of surface proteins
    Blocking antibodies
    Intracellular residence

(*continued*)

SUMMARY OUTLINE (*continued*)

N. meningitidis

Gram-negative diplococcus

Disease—meningitis

Bacteria enter bloodstream and colonize meninges

Inflammation of meninges allows phagocytes and blood proteins to enter spinal fluid

Relatively rare in most of world

Asymptomatic carriage common

First signs are fever, stiff neck, headache, or rash

Virulence factors

Bind to and invade epithelial cells

Serum resistant

Mechanisms of iron sequestration

Polysaccharide capsule

Types A, B, C, Y, and W135 most important

Antiphagocytic

Contributes to serum resistance

Prevention and treatment

Penicillin and cephalosporins used

Resistance beginning to appear

Rifampin given prophylactically to contacts of patients

Vaccine

Consists of capsular polysaccharides of A and C

Type B capsule nonimmunogenic because it consists of sialic acid residues

QUESTIONS

Answers to the questions can be found in Appendix 2.

1. Respond to the statement: "Yes, I had sexual relations with a person who was later diagnosed as having gonorrhea, but I did not go to see a doctor because I did not develop any symptoms." To what extent does your answer depend on the sex of the person making the statement?

2. Only a fraction of babies will be born with eyes infected with *N. gonorrhoeae*, yet hospitals routinely put antiseptic drops in the eyes of all newborns. Why not simply identify the mothers with gonorrhea and treat those babies specifically?

3. Respond to the statement: "Now that we know that many cases of infertility are caused by *N. gonorrhoeae*, we can cure infertility with antibiotics."

4. Compare and contrast the diseases caused by and the virulence factors of *N. gonorrhoeae* with those of *N. meningitidis*. How can these two closely related bacteria cause such different diseases?

5. Explain how the different types of phase and antigenic variation probably work together to aid survival of *N. gonorrhoeae* in a human host.

6. Which types of variation in surface antigens would still be seen in a strain of *N. gonorrhoeae* that was deficient in the ability to carry out homologous recombination?

7. Propose an explanation, based on what is known about virulence factors of *N. gonorrhoeae*, of how nonsymptomatic infections might arise. How could a strain cause a nonsymptomatic infection in one person and yet cause symptomatic infection in a sexual contact?

8. If you had to suggest a possible vaccine formulation without any further information about *N. gonorrhoeae*, what would it contain? Explain what each component is designed to do.

9. How does sialylation of LOS impair the host response to *N. gonorrhoeae* infection? How does it interfere with vaccine development?

31

Chlamydia trachomatis

KEY FEATURES

Chlamydia trachomatis

CHARACTERISTICS

Intracellular pathogen

Gram-negative-type cell wall but no peptidoglycan

Cross-linked outer membrane proteins—stability

Two-stage life cycle—reticulate body (replicating form), elementary body (survival form)

Smaller than most bacteria

DISEASES

Women: cervical infection (usually asymptomatic); pelvic inflammatory disease (PID); infertility; ectopic pregnancy

Infants: conjunctivitis; pneumonia; trachoma (also in older children)

Men: painful urination, discharge; reactive arthritis

RESERVOIR

Infected humans

MAJOR VIRULENCE FACTORS

Intracellular lifestyle

Tough elementary body stage—infective form

Proteinaceous surface projections—penetrate through endosome membrane to host cell cytoplasm

PREVENTION AND TREATMENT

Avoid multiple sex partners

Antibiotic treatment

Most infections in females are asymptomatic—importance of new detection methods

---

The Hidden Epidemic

In an Institute of Medicine report published in 1997, the sexually transmitted bacterial diseases were called "the hidden epidemic." Cervical infection caused by *Chlamydia trachomatis* is the most common of the bacterial sexually transmitted diseases. There are at least 4 million cases a year in the United States alone. Costs of treating these infections and their consequences have been estimated to be

$2 billion a year. Yet, chlamydial disease has attracted remarkably little public notice. Lack of interest by the public and the media in an infectious disease can usually be attributed to the fact that the disease affects primarily the poor and underserved. This is certainly the case with syphilis and gonorrhea, which have their highest incidence in rural and urban poor young adults. It is not the case for chlamydial disease, however. Chlamydial disease can be found on college campuses and in rich neighborhoods as well as in inner cities.

One reason the sexually transmitted bacterial diseases get so little attention is that they are insidious in their action. Like *Neisseria gonorrhoeae* (chapter 30), *C. trachomatis* causes few symptoms in most women with an infected cervix. Men are more likely to develop urethral discharge, but infections of the male urethra can be asymptomatic, too. The fact that chlamydial infections can be asymptomatic in their early stages is misleading, however. In some women with a cervical chlamydial infection, the infection ascends to the fallopian tubes (Figure 31–1). Inflammation of the fragile fallopian tubes can result in narrowing of the tube to the point that eggs produced by the ovary are not able to reach the uterus. No one knows how many cases of chlamydia-induced infertility there are, but *C. trachomatis* is clearly a major cause of involuntary infertility.

A woman with blocked fallopian tubes may still conceive, but if the egg is fertilized in the fallopian tube and trapped there, a serious condition called ectopic pregnancy may occur. As the fetus develops, the fallopian tube is ruptured, sending the woman into shock. Ectopic pregnancy can be fatal. One small study detected *C. trachomatis* in 7 of 10 women who had experienced a case of ectopic pregnancy. So *C. trachomatis* may well be the leading cause of ectopic pregnancy. Women with an infected fallopian tube may also develop a condition called **pelvic inflammatory disease (PID),** which is painful and can result in release of bacteria into the peritoneal cavity (**peritonitis**) and bloodstream (**septicemia**).

An aspect of primary chlamydial cervical infection that has only recently been revealed is that such infections make women more likely to contract an HIV infection if they are exposed. Usually, a woman must be exposed 7 to 8 times to acquire an HIV infection. (This is an average figure; some women are infected the first time, and some are not infected until they have had many exposures.) Having a cervical infection caused by *C. trachomatis* reduces this figure significantly and increases the risk of acquiring HIV. The reason for this is not known, but it makes sense when you consider that the cells of the immune system that travel to an infected

Women

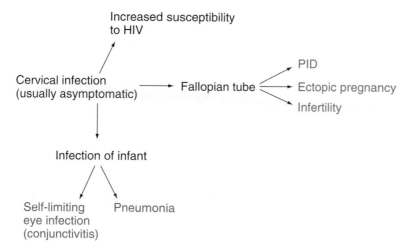

Men

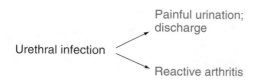

Figure 31–1 Differences between men and women in progression and outcome of disease caused by *C. trachomatis*.

area (macrophages, T cells) are also the primary targets of HIV.

As with all sexually transmitted diseases, infection of the mother has consequences for an infant that passes through an infected birth canal. In the case of *C. trachomatis,* inoculation of an infant during birth can cause conjunctivitis or pneumonia. In most cases, the conjunctivitis caused by *C. trachomatis* is self-limiting and does not do any long-term damage to the eye. This is true of the strains of *C. trachomatis* currently circulating in developed countries, but in some developing countries, such as Nepal, there are strains that cause blindness (trachoma). It is unclear whether this is due to an extraordinary genetic susceptibility of this population to chlamydiae or to the properties of the strains responsible. If the latter, it is worrisome to think of such strains being spread more widely. The neonatal pneumonia caused by *C. trachomatis* can be serious. Fortunately, if the pneumonia is diagnosed in a timely matter, treatment with antibiotics is quite effective in controlling the infection.

Although *C. trachomatis* infections have more serious ramifications for women than for men, men are not completely out of the disease picture. First, they are far more likely to experience symptoms of urethral infection, such as painful urination and a discharge. This is actually a blessing in disguise, because the symptoms drive a man to seek treatment early in the infection. A secondary consequence of urethral infection, which seems to be more common in men than in women, is a condition called **reactive arthritis** (also called **Reiter's syndrome**). Usually, *C. trachomatis* infections remain localized and do not become disseminated, but in this case, the bacteria somehow reach the joints and infect joint tissue. The result is inflammation that produces pain in the joint.

Clearly, a *C. trachomatis* infection, even one that is asymptomatic initially, can have serious consequences, especially in women. Not all scientists take chlamydial infections that seriously, however (Box 31–1).

C. trachomatis—a Lot of Pathogenic Potential in a Very Small Package

In the chapter on *Mycoplasma pneumoniae* and *Chlamydia pneumoniae* (chapter 21), the concept of a minimal genome (<1 Mbp) was introduced. The minimal genome

---

BOX 31–1 Women, How Much Is Your Future Fertility Worth?

Given the potential seriousness of an untreated *C. trachomatis* infection and the availability of a new, rapid urine test for the disease, you would think that governments would be mounting big campaigns to screen women for infection and to treat infected women. But so far, this has not happened. The excuse usually given is that such screening programs are not cost-effective. How much is a woman's fertility worth? According to some scientists from the Netherlands, less than $15,800 (van Valkengoed et al., 2001). This is the amount they estimated it would take to locate and treat each woman who would develop a "major outcome," such as PID, infertility, ectopic pregnancy, or giving birth to a neonate who would develop *C. trachomatis* pneumonia. This figure assumes that about 3% of women in the 15- to 40-year age group are infected with *C. trachomatis* and that about 480 women would have to be screened and treated to avoid one potentially serious case. In some parts of the United States, the infection rate is closer to 20%, but even at that level of infection, which would bring the cost per major outcome down to around $7,000, the thrifty authors of this study still considered the cost to be too high.

An earlier 1998 study by a U.S. group (Burstein et al., 1998) reached the opposite conclusion. They found alarming the fact that, among adolescent females who were sexually active, the incidence of infection was nearly 25%, and they recommended routine testing of sexually active adolescent females every 6 months.

Sources: G. R. Burstein, C. A. Gaydos, M. Diener-West, M. R. Howell, J. M. Zenilman, and T. C. Quinn. 1998. Incident *Chlamydia trachomatis* infections among inner-city adolescent females. *JAMA* **280:**521–526; I. G. van Valkengoed, M. J. Postma, S. A. Morre, A. J. van Den Brule, C. J. Meijer, L. M. Bouter, and A. J. Boeke. 2001. Cost effectiveness analysis of a population based screening programme for asymptomatic *Chlamydia trachomatis* infections in women by means of home obtained urine specimens. *Sex. Transm. Infect.* **77:**276–282.

is the smallest number of genes needed to encode the functions required by a free-living microbe. *C. trachomatis* also has a very small genome, but that does not stop it from having a rather complex developmental life cycle. This cycle consists of two forms: an **elementary body** (EB) (0.3 to 0.6 μm in diameter) that is designed to survive outside human cells and to infect new human cells, and a larger **reticulate body** (RB) (about 1 μm in diameter) that is the much more fragile dividing form of the bacteria (Figure 31–2). With a genome size of about 1 Mbp and many genes probably devoted to this developmental cycle, chlamydiae must economize somehow to limit the genes they need to survive. Since chlamydiae replicate inside host cells, you might think that one way to reduce genome size would be to eliminate genes encoding many of the proteins of the metabolic and biosynthetic systems found commonly in free-living bacteria and use host molecules instead. The interior of a human cell is rich in nutrients, so the RB may not have to make many amino acids and other compounds that free-living cells need to provide. This is not the case, however. Although *C. trachomatis* does lack genes for amino acid biosynthesis, its genome contains genes for several energy-generating pathways, including glycolysis, the pentose phosphate pathway, and a partial TCA cycle. For years, the dogma was that *C. trachomatis* was an ATP parasite that could not make ATP and had to acquire it from the host cell. This dogma has now been disproved, at least for *C. trachomatis*. Other species of chlamydia may be ATP parasites, judging from the genes they lack.

Although chlamydiae have gram-negative-type cytoplasmic and outer membranes, neither the EB nor the RB has detectable peptidoglycan. How, then, do the bacteria avoid lysis? The RBs may be protected to some extent by the high osmolarity of the interior of a human

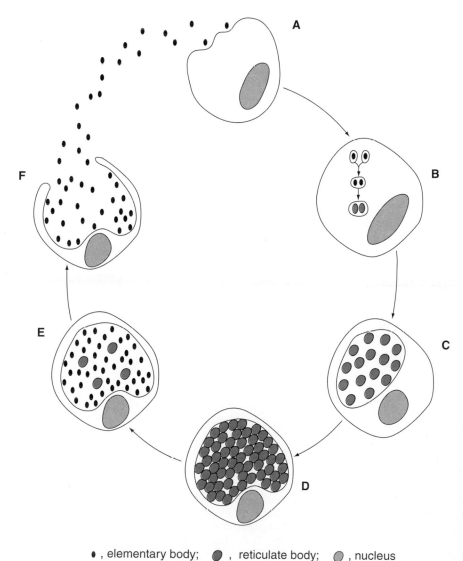

Figure 31–2 The developmental cycle of *C. trachomatis*. The elementary body is taken up into an endosome in the host cell; then endosomes fuse (**A**), and the elementary bodies differentiate into reticulate bodies (**B**). The reticulate bodies replicate (**C**) and cause the endoplasmic membrane to expand until it fills most of the cytoplasm (**D**). The reticulate bodies convert into elementary bodies (**E**). The endoplasmic membrane either ruptures and releases the elementary bodies into the host cell cytoplasm or fuses with the host cytoplasmic membrane, and the elementary bodies are released into the environment (**F**).

•, elementary body; ●, reticulate body; ●, nucleus

cell. The EBs, however, have to cope with low-osmolarity conditions outside the host cell. The answer to the question of why EBs are so resistant to lysis appears to be that the EB membranes contain proteins with multiple disulfide cross-links. These include a protein called the **major outer membrane protein (MOMP)**, a **polymorphic outer membrane protein (POMP)**, and small and large **cysteine-rich proteins (CRP)**. A model for the EB cell wall is shown in Figure 31–3.

A bigger mystery is why *C. trachomatis* is susceptible to penicillin, an antibiotic whose main mode of action is to inhibit peptidoglycan synthesis. There is still no answer to this question. Some scientists have suggested that chlamydiae may make small amounts of peptidoglycan that are not detected by standard biochemical assays. Another possibility is that secondary effects of penicillin on cellular metabolism may be responsible.

Virulence Factors

Special Problems Faced by Scientists Working on Chlamydiae

So far, no one has succeeded in growing *C. trachomatis* in cell-free medium. The bacteria must be grown in tissue culture cells. Thus, in an experiment, scientists must sort out human cellular responses from the responses of the chlamydiae themselves. Yields of *C. trachomatis* are very low. Out of 10 liters of tissue culture cells, a scientist may recover less than 200 mg of chlamydial proteins. A similar volume of medium seeded with

Escherichia coli would yield many grams of bacterial protein. Finally, there is still no method for genetic manipulation of *C. trachomatis*. Given the many frustrating limitations experienced by scientists working in this field, one has to be impressed with the progress these scientists have made.

One piece of encouraging news is that there are good animal models for chlamydial infections. Several strains of inbred mice develop genital infections and associated upper genital tract sequelae. Not all strains of mice are equally susceptible, however, and these differences may someday provide clues to the host side of the disease. There is also a murine pneumonia model that can be used to study the interactions between *C. trachomatis* and the lung.

Adherence and Invasion by EBs

The steps in the process by which EBs enter a host epithelial cell, differentiate into the replicative RB form, and exit the cell are illustrated in Figure 31–4. In contrast to *Salmonella* species and other invasive bacteria covered in earlier chapters, EBs do not mediate the kind of forced entry that involves actin rearrangements. Nonetheless, EBs have many ways of entering host cells: receptor-mediated endocytosis (in clathrin-coated pits), pinocytosis, and normal phagocytosis.

A great deal of emphasis has been placed on the characteristics of the EB entry process, because a vaccine against *C. trachomatis* would best be directed against this process. Once the bacteria are inside human cells, they are protected from antibodies and other components of the human defense systems. Human cells in-

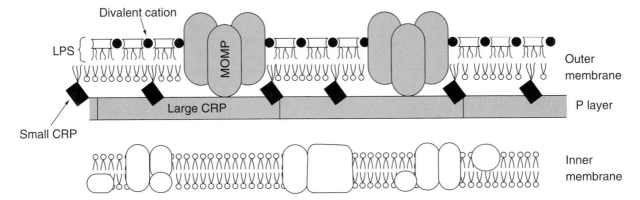

Figure 31–3 A proposed model of the structure of the elementary body membrane. The outer membrane is similar to that of other gram-negative bacteria because it has an inner leaflet and an outer membrane that contains LPS. The outer membrane is stabilized by major outer membrane proteins (MOMPs) and small and large cysteine-rich proteins (CRPs). The large CRPs form a P layer. The membrane contains no peptidoglycan. The POMPs are not shown. (Reprinted from T. P. Hatch, 1996, with permission from the publisher.)

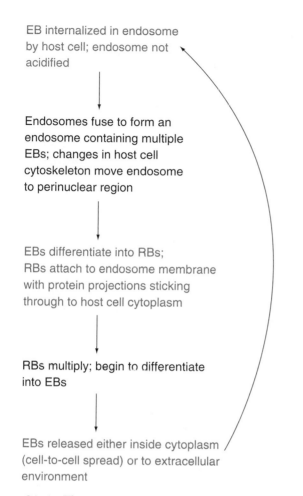

EB internalized in endosome by host cell; endosome not acidified

Endosomes fuse to form an endosome containing multiple EBs; changes in host cell cytoskeleton move endosome to perinuclear region

EBs differentiate into RBs; RBs attach to endosome membrane with protein projections sticking through to host cell cytoplasm

RBs multiply; begin to differentiate into EBs

EBs released either inside cytoplasm (cell-to-cell spread) or to extracellular environment

Figure 31–4 The steps in the life cycle of *C. trachomatis.*

fected with *C. trachomatis* do not display the antigens of the bacteria on their surfaces to any great degree, so that although T cells are attracted to the infected area, cytotoxic T cells are not very effective. Despite great interest in the process, however, little is known about EB adhesins or the host cell receptors with which they interact. What is known is that the EB enters an endosome that maintains a near-neutral pH (pH 6.6) and does not fuse with lysosomes. Endosomes containing one EB fuse with one another to produce vacuoles containing more than one EB. This is not true for other *Chlamydia* species. Scientists speculate that this may allow different strains of *C. trachomatis* to interact with one another by exchanging DNA.

During the first couple of hours after entry of the EB, the differentiating EBs seem to remodel the endosome membrane. Proteins, such as transferrin receptor, LAMP-1, and cathepsin D, that would normally be found on endosomes at this point in endosome development are not present. Phosphorylation of host cell proteins, presumably directed by the bacteria, also oc-

curs. One effect is that there are changes in the actin cytoskeleton that ultimately bring the endosome to the perinuclear region by a process that may involve dynein, a host cell protein involved in movement of organelles within the cell.

EBs are covered with nail-shaped projections (up to 30 per EB), and these are distributed randomly over the EB surface. As the EB differentiates into an RB, the RB moves to the endosomal membrane, and some of the projections penetrate the endosomal membrane to reach the host cell cytoplasm. Microscopically, these projections look like incomplete flagella that have a motor structure and a hook structure but not the shaft that is normally attached to the hook. Consistent with this hypothesis, homologs of flagellar genes have been found in the chlamydial genome sequence. These projections are not functioning as flagella, however, because both EB and RB are nonmotile. If the projections are flagellalike, they are hollow. Thus, they could function to convey nutrients from the host cell cytoplasm or to introduce bacterial proteins into the host cell cytoplasm, or both.

Once the RBs begin to replicate, they do so at a rate of about 2 to 3 h per generation, a relatively rapid multiplication rate. At first, scientists assumed that chlamydiae replicated by binary fission, but this may not be the case. The genome sequence is missing a gene called *ftsZ*, which is essential for binary fission. There is some evidence from microscopy studies that a single RB may fragment into more than two daughter cells.

As the RBs increase in number, the endosome membrane increases in surface area to accommodate the growing number of replicating bacteria. The lipids for this expansion probably come from fusion of the endosome with fragments of Golgi membranes. There are also RB proteins called Inc proteins (Inc stands for inclusion) that are inserted into the endosome membrane, so the membrane is a hybrid of host cell lipids and bacterial proteins. The RBs stay attached to the endosome membrane, but the ones that differentiate into EBs move to the internal portion of the endosome. About 40 h into the infection process, the endosomal membrane may begin to disintegrate, releasing EBs into the host cell cytoplasm. Such EBs can infect adjacent cells in contact with the infected cell. Another route of EB exit is for the endosomal membrane to fuse with the host cell cytoplasmic membrane, releasing the RBs and EBs into the extracellular space. The fragile RBs lyse rapidly, leaving the EBs to find and infect another host cell.

C. trachomatis has been called a "stealth pathogen" because multiplication of the bacteria in the endosome does little damage to the host cell, even when bacteria-filled endosomes expand to take up most of the host cell cytoplasm. It makes sense that chlamydiae would do as little damage as possible, because they depend absolutely on mammalian cells for survival and replication.

If the chlamydia-host cell interaction is so benign, how do the symptoms of cervical or urethral infections, the symptoms of reactive arthritis, or the symptoms of trachoma arise? One answer is the inflammatory response to EB proteins or other cell surface molecules. The specific defenses may also contribute to tissue damage. One indication of this is that clinical trials of a candidate trachoma vaccine consisting of EBs had to be cancelled abruptly in Nepal (a country with a high incidence of trachoma) because the vaccine appeared to be making the infection worse. This outcome could be explained by a specific host response, triggered by the vaccine, that somehow contributed to the ocular scarring that causes blindness.

Prevention and Treatment

A vaccine against *C. trachomatis* would be a highly desirable way to prevent infections and possibly to eradicate *C. trachomatis* entirely. Since *C. trachomatis* is absolutely dependent on its human host, reducing the number of infections could one day reduce the number of bacteria to a level that could not maintain the bacteria in the human population. Unfortunately, although attempts have been made to develop such a vaccine, success is a long way off.

C. trachomatis infections are treatable with antibiotics if the infection is diagnosed in time. At one time, detection was problematic because sampling was invasive. A cervical cell sample had to be obtained from women, and urethral cells had to be obtained from men (by a process called "urethral stripping," done by inserting a thin brush into the penile opening, a process which is every bit as painful as it sounds). For an initial diagnosis, a Gram stain was done. Since chlamydiae are too small to be seen with an ordinary light microscope, the result was a negative test, which can be used to rule out gonorrhea but not to prove chlamydiae are the cause. To obtain a definitive diagnosis, it was necessary to cultivate chlamydiae in the cells being tested, an expensive and time-consuming process that required the use of tissue culture cells to cultivate the bacteria.

A major breakthrough was a test based on ligase chain reaction (LCR). LCR, like PCR, is a method for amplifying specific DNA segments identified by species-specific primers (see chapter 3). PCR tests are also under development. The great thing about the gene amplification tests is that they are rapid and relatively cheap and can be done on urine samples, a noninvasive sampling method.

Chlamydia species are among the few species of bacteria that have not become resistant to antibiotics. Possibly this is due to a lifestyle that does not expose them to other bacteria, from which resistance genes could be obtained. Of course, they might be able to mutate to resistance, but so far that seems not to have happened. Although a number of antibiotics could be used to treat chlamydial infections, the antibiotics most often used are doxycycline (a tetracycline) and azithromycin (a macrolide). Patients diagnosed with gonorrhea are treated with a fourth-generation cephalosporin (β-lactam) plus either azithromycin or doxycycline. The reason for this mixed drug regimen is that people with gonorrhea are commonly coinfected with *C. trachomatis*, so it is prudent to treat for both *N. gonorrhoeae* and *C. trachomatis*.

There is another problem encountered by physicians who treat sexually transmitted bacterial diseases: patient compliance with the antibiotic regimen. Doxycycline is the cheaper drug, a feature that recommends it to cash-strapped inner city or rural clinics, but it must be taken daily for 7 days to be effective. By contrast, only one dose of azithromycin may be sufficient to cure the patient and can be given in a supervised setting. Elimination of the bacteria is more rapid than with doxycycline, a factor that can be important in the case of sex workers or sexually active teenagers who may not be willing or able to abstain from sexual intercourse for the 7-day period of doxycycline treatment. Unfortunately, azithromycin is much more expensive than doxycycline, so doxycycline is still widely used. Physicians at clinics feel that in many cases they must give the pills, not a prescription, to the patient to make it more likely that the patient will actually undergo the treatment.

Although it seems clear that chlamydiae do not have detectable amounts of peptidoglycan, if they have any at all, they are nonetheless susceptible to β-lactam antibiotics, such as members of the penicillin family. Why this should be so is yet another chlamydial mystery. One possible explanation is that the bacteria do have some penicillin-binding proteins, but they are used for a different purpose than peptidoglycan synthesis. A second possibility is that the bacteria make minute amounts of peptidoglycan. But why the bacteria would do this when they have cysteine-cross-linked membrane proteins that seem quite able to carry out the role usually played by peptidoglycan—prevention of cell lysis due to high internal osmolarity—is not clear. These observations are not particularly relevant to the treatment of chlamydial infections since β-lactam antibiotics do not penetrate mammalian cells very well and thus are not very useful for treating chlamydial infections.

Closing Observations

Chlamydia species are fascinating bacteria with a number of peculiarities that are not shared with other bacteria. In the early days of chlamydia research, scientists thought that chlamydiae might be viruses. We now know that they are bacteria, even though they are not able to live outside host cells. Certainly, however, they have the same type of multilayer interplay with host cells that characterizes the interaction between viruses and mammalian cells. The infection and replication strategies of chlamydiae are unique enough to make it virtually certain that new discoveries about mammalian cells will come out of studies of how chlamydiae cause infection. Finally, it is important to keep in mind that chlamydiae are important pathogens worldwide that can have a devastating effect (e.g., blindness, infertility) despite the fact that they often cause infections that are initially asymptomatic. More attention needs to be focused on them.

SELECTED READINGS

Buetler, A. M., A. P. Hudson, J. A. Whittum-Hudson, W. A. Salameh, H. C. Gerard, P. J. Branigan, and H. R. Schumacher. 1997. *Chlamydia trachomatis* can persist in joint tissue after antibiotic treatment in chronic Reiter's syndrome/reactive arthritis. *J. Clin. Rheumatol.* **3:**125–130.

Centers for Disease Control and Prevention. 1998. *CDC/ MMWR 1998 Guidelines for Treatment of Sexually Transmitted Diseases.* http://www.cdc.gov/mmwr/preview/mmwrhtml/00050909.

Gerard, H. C., P. J. Branigan, G. R. Balsara, C. Heath, S. S. Minassian, and A. P. Hudson. 1998. Viability of *Chlamydia trachomatis* in fallopian tubes of patients with ectopic pregnancy. *Fertil. Steril.* **70:**945–948.

Hackstadt, T. 1999. Cell biology, p. 101–138. *In* R. S. Stephens (ed.), *Chlamydia: Intracellular Biology, Pathogenesis, and Immunity.* American Society for Microbiology, Washington, D.C.

Hatch, T. P. 1996. Disulfide cross-linked envelope proteins: the functional equivalent of peptidoglycan in Chlamydiae. *J. Bacteriol.* **178:**1–5.

Iliffe-Lee, E. R., and G. McClarty. 1999. Glucose metabolism in *Chlamydia trachomatis*: the "energy parasite" hypothesis revisited. *Mol. Microbiol.* **33:**177–187.

Stephens, R. S. (ed.). 1999. *Chlamydia: Intracellular Biology, Pathogenesis, and Immunity.* American Society for Microbiology, Washington, D.C.

VanDoornum, G. J., M. Buimer, M. Prins, J. M. Henquet, R. A. Coutinho, P. K. Plier, S. Tomazic-Allen, H. Hu, and H. Lee. 1995. Detection of *Chlamydia trachomatis* infection in urine samples from men and women by ligase chain reaction. *J. Clin. Microbiol.* **33:**2024–2027.

Wyrick, P. B. 2000. Intracellular survival by *Chlamydia.* *Cell. Microbiol.* **2:**275–282.

SUMMARY OUTLINE

Characteristics of *C. trachomatis*

Very small genome (≈1 Mbp)

Complex developmental cycle
  EB—survives in external environment
  RB—intracellular replicative form

Gram-negative cytoplasmic and outer membranes

No peptidoglycan

EB membrane stability due to MOMPs, POMPs, and CRPs

Virulence factors

Difficult to study because *C. trachomatis* must be grown in tissue culture cells

Several animal models available

Adherence and invasion
  Little known about adhesins
  EBs taken up in endosomes
    Maintain near-neutral pH
    Do not fuse with lysosomes
    Endosomes containing a single EB fuse to produce vacuoles with multiple EBs

(continued)

SUMMARY OUTLINE (*continued*)

EBs begin to differentiate
  Remodel endosome membrane
  Actin cytoskeleton changes
  Endosome brought close to nucleus
Projections extend from EB surface
  Look like incomplete flagella
  During change to RB form, RB moves to endosomal membrane
  Projections penetrate endosomal membrane into host cell cytoplasm
  May convey nutrients from host to bacterium
  May introduce bacterial proteins into host cell cytoplasm
RBs replicate rapidly
  Endosome membrane expands
    Hybrid of Golgi membrane fragments and bacterial proteins
  RBs remain attached to endosomal membrane
  RBs differentiate into EBs; move to interior of endosome
EBs may be released into host cell cytoplasm; infect adjacent cells
Endosomal membrane may fuse with host cell cytoplasmic membrane
  RBs and EBs released into extracellular space
  Host cell usually not killed

Prevention and treatment

No vaccine available

Recently developed LCR test makes diagnosis rapid and reliable

Antibiotics effective
  No resistance observed yet
  Surprising that β-lactams work because no peptidoglycan

QUESTIONS

Answers to the questions can be found in Appendix 2.

1. Why might chlamydiae have a two-stage life cycle, with a nonreplicating form and a replicating form?

2. In what way does the intracellular lifestyle of chlamydiae limit possible options for prevention and treatment?

3. How do chlamydiae differ from other gram-negative bacteria that are described in this book?

4. There is currently no way to make mutants of *C. trachomatis*. Why is this such a difficult problem?

5. Do you think there should be extensive screening programs to identify and treat *C. trachomatis* infections that may not be symptomatic? What are the arguments for and against such a massive effort? What are some problems that might be encountered?

6. Suppose you learned that you had a chlamydial infection from a one-time sexual encounter caused by your imprudent use of alcohol. Your fiancé(e), with whom you are having sexual relations, does not develop disease symptoms. You are worried that telling him or her about your momentary lapse in judgment could destroy your relationship. Would you tell him or her, and what factors might influence your decision? (This is a question that we have used in an undergraduate laboratory course to get students to think about the social and psychological aspects of sexually transmitted diseases. Almost always, the women are more likely to say they would confess and the men say they would not. What is wrong with this picture?)

Overview of Bacterial Secretion Systems, Bacterial Adhesins and Their Mechanisms of Assembly, and Major Bacterial Toxins

A. Secretion Systems of Bacteria

General Secretory Pathway (Sec)

Characteristics

Pore through which proteins are secreted is composed of three proteins (heterotrimers)

A total of at least 11 proteins involved in process

Requires signal peptide on protein to be secreted (15 to 30 amino acids in length)

Mediates secretion of many bacterial proteins

Location

Cytoplasmic membrane (pore proteins embedded, others associated)

Found in both gram-positive and gram-negative bacteria

Action

Permits protein to weave itself through hydrophobic membrane

Three steps

Protein guided to proper site in membrane (ushers and chaperones involved)

Protein chain crosses lipid bilayer

Translocated protein is released (signal peptide cleaved off)

Type I Secretion System (ABC Transporters)

Characteristics

Sec independent

Composed of three proteins

Specific for certain secreted proteins

Location

Spans both inner and outer membranes

Probably forms a pore through both membranes

Found only in gram-negative bacteria

Action

Secretes proteins directly into external environment; bypasses periplasm

Example

Alpha-hemolysin of uropathogenic *Escherichia coli* (HlyA)

Type II Secretion System (Two-Step System)

Characteristics

Sec dependent

Composed of 12 to 14 proteins

Similar to system that catalyzes synthesis of type 4 (IV) pili

Location

Outer membrane proteins (secretins)

Most components located in cytoplasmic membrane

Some components may form a piluslike structure in the periplasm that guides folded proteins to other components (secretins) located in outer membrane

Found only in gram-negative bacteria

Action

Secretins form pores in outer membrane

Other components act as chaperones

Specific for certain proteins

Examples

Xcp system of *Pseudomonas aeruginosa* for export of exotoxin A as well as other proteins

Type III Secretion System (Contact-Dependent System)

Characteristics

Sec independent

Composed of more than 20 proteins

Some components similar to those of the flagellar apparatus

Location

Most of the components form a channel that spans both membranes of gram-negative bacteria

Two components fuse with eukaryotic cell membrane to form the injection pore

Found only in gram-negative bacteria

Action

Injects toxic proteins directly from bacterial cytoplasm into host cell cytoplasm

Secretion triggered by low calcium concentration

Specific for certain secreted proteins

Example

Yop proteins of *Yersinia pestis*

Type IV Secretion System (Conjugal Transfer System)

Characteristics

Sec independent

Composed of a large number of proteins

Location

Formation of piluslike structure occurs in periplasm and transits both membranes

Found only in gram-negative bacteria

Action

Can transfer monomeric proteins, multimeric proteins, or single-stranded DNA complexed to proteins (conjugation)

In most systems, protein transferred directly into host cell

In some cases, protein may be secreted into external environment

Examples

Legionella pneumophila Dot/Icm system, pertussis toxin export system of *Bordetella pertussis*

SELECTED READINGS

Christie, P. J., and J. P. Vogel. 2000. Bacterial type IV secretion: conjugation systems adapted to deliver effector molecules to host cells. *Trends Microbiol.* **8:**354–360.

Economou, A. 1999. Following the leader: bacterial protein export through the Sec pathway. *Trends Microbiol.* **7:**315–320.

Harper, J. R., and T. J. Silhavy. 2001. Germ warfare: the mechanisms of virulence factor delivery, p. 43–74. *In* E. Groisman (ed.), *Principles of Bacterial Pathogenesis.* Academic Press, Inc., San Diego, Calif.

B. Adhesins and Mechanisms of Assembly

Chaperone-Usher Pathway

Consists of a periplasmic chaperone protein and an outer membrane usher protein. The pilus subunits are secreted by the Sec system from the cytoplasm to the periplasmic side of the cytoplasmic membrane. The chaperone removes the pilus subunits from the cytoplasmic membrane and mediates their folding. The usher protein facilitates assembly of the pili on the surface of the cell. The distal (tip) end of the pilus is assembled first.

Examples:

Adhesin	Organism	Host cell type or receptor	Disease	Gene designation
P fimbriae	Uropathogenic *Escherichia coli* (UPEC)	Globobiose on uroepithelium	Pyelonephritis	*pap*
Type I pili	Enterotoxigenic *Escherichia coli* (ETEC; enteropathogenic *E. coli* (EPEC); UPEC; *Salmonella typhimurium*	Mannose residues	Diarrhea, dysentery, urinary tract infections	*fim*
S pili	Extraintestinal strains of *E. coli* (ExPEC)	Unknown	Neonatal meningitis	*sfa*
AFA-III/Dr afimbrial adhesions	UPEC	Dr determinants on erythrocytes	Pyelonephritis, urinary tract infections	*afa*
Pef pili	*S. typhimurium*	Intestinal epithelial cells	Gastroenteritis	*pef*
Long polar fimbriae	*S. typhimurium*	Peyer's patches	Gastroenteritis	*lpf*

Type II Secretion Pathway

Subunits are transported through the cytoplasmic membrane by the Sec system and then assembled in the periplasm at the surface of the inner membrane. Protein complexes at the outer membrane translocate the newly formed pilus to the external environment. This is a major difference from the chaperone-usher pathway, in which the pilus is assembled on the cell surface. The distal end of the pilus is formed first.

Examples:

Adhesin	Organism	Host cell type or receptor	Disease	Gene designation
Type 4 pili	*Neisseria gonorrhoeae*	CD46 on epithelial cells	Gonorrhea	*pil*
Tcp (type 4) pili	*Vibrio cholerae*	Unknown	Cholera	*tcp*
Bundle-forming pili	EPEC	Nonintimate binding	Infant diarrhea, traveler's diarrhea	*bfp*

Extracellular-Nucleation Pathway

Pilus subunits are secreted as soluble proteins and precipitated onto thin fibers on the surface of the bacteria. Branching of pili may occur.

Example:

Adhesin	Organism	Host cell type or receptor	Disease	Gene designation
Curli	*S. typhimurium*	Intestinal epithelial cells	Gastroenteritis	*agf*

Alternate Chaperone Pathway

Similar in action to the chaperone-usher pathway, although the components of the two pathways are unrelated. Pilus subunits are partially assembled in the periplasm. The pilus is then formed on the surface of the bacteria as the subunits move across the outer membrane.

Example:

Adhesin	Organism	Host cell or receptor	Disease	Gene designation
CFA-I	ETEC	Glycoproteins (?)	Diarrhea	*cfa*

SELECTED READINGS

Hultgren, S. J., and C. H. Jones. 1995. Utility of the immunoglobulin-like fold of chaperones in shaping organelles of attachment in pathogenic bacteria. *ASM News* **61**:457–464.

Lory, S. 1998. Secretion of proteins and assembly of bacterial surface organelles: shared pathways of extracellular protein targeting. *Curr. Opin. Microbiol.* **1**:27–35.

Soto, G. E., and S. J. Hultgren. 1999. Bacterial adhesins: common themes and variation in architecture and assembly. *J. Bacteriol.* **181**:1059–1071.

C. Major Bacterial Toxins

Toxin (disease)	Bacterial source	Host cell specificity	Mechanism of action	Role in disease
A-B (Type III) Toxins				
Diphtheria toxin (diphtheria)	*Corynebacterium diphtheriae* (gram positive)	Many cell types	B region binds HB-EGF; A region ADP-ribosylates diphthamide on host EF-2; stops protein synthesis	Formation of pseudomembrane; responsible for damage to heart, other organs
Cholera toxin (cholera)	*Vibrio cholerae* (gram negative)	Intestinal epithelial cells	B region binds G_{M1}; A region ADP-ribosylates host regulatory protein; disrupts control of cAMP	Responsible for profuse diarrhea
LT (heat-labile toxin) (infant diarrhea; traveler's diarrhea)	Enterotoxigenic *Escherichia coli* (ETEC) (gram negative)	Intestinal epithelial cells	Same as cholera toxin	Responsible for profuse diarrhea
Shiga toxin (dysentery)	Enterohemorrhagic *Escherichia coli* O157:H7 (EHEC); *Shigella dysenteriae* (both gram negative)	Many cell types	Cleaves host cell rRNA; stops protein synthesis	Uncertain; may cause hemolytic uremic syndrome (HUS)
Botulinum toxin (botulism)	*Clostridium botulinum* (gram positive)	Neurons	Proteolytic activity; nicks synaptobrevins; affects control of nerve transmission	Responsible for flaccid paralysis

(continued)

Toxin (disease)	Bacterial source	Host cell specificity	Mechanism of action	Role in disease
A-B (Type III) Toxins (*continued*)				
Tetanus toxin (tetanus)	*Clostridium tetani* (gram positive)	Neurons	Same as botulinum toxin	Responsible for spastic paralysis
Pertussis toxin (whooping cough)	*Bordetella pertussis* (gram negative)	Respiratory epithelial cells	ADP-ribosylates host regulatory protein; disrupts control of cAMP	Contributes to cough; excess mucus production
Invasive adenylate cyclase (whooping cough)	*Bordetella pertussis* (gram negative)	Respiratory epithelial cells; other cell types	Synthesizes cAMP after binding host cell calmodulin	Same as pertussis toxin
Exotoxin A (lung infections in cystic fibrosis patients)	*Pseudomonas aeruginosa* (gram negative)	Many cell types	ADP-ribosylates host cell EF-2; stops protein synthesis; synthesis regulated by iron	Causes tissue damage; inhibits phagocytes
Membrane-Disrupting (Type II) Toxins				
Alpha-toxin (gas gangrene)	*Clostridium perfringens* (gram positive)	Many cell types	Phospholipase	Kills phagocytes, causes tissue damage
Alpha-toxin (necrosis)	*Staphylococcus aureus* (gram positive)	Many cell types	Forms pores in cell membranes	Causes tissue damage; spreading
Listeriolysin O (LLO) (listeriosis)	*Listeria monocytogenes* (gram positive)	Many cell types	Forms pores in cell membranes	Allows bacteria to escape phagocytic vesicle
Pneumolysin (pneumonia)	*Streptococcus pneumoniae* (gram positive)	Alveolar and endothelial cells; ciliated cells	Binds cholesterol; forms pores in lung cells; inhibits activity of ciliated cells	Causes lung damage; activates complement; antiphagocytic; inflammatory
Streptolysin O (SLO) (rheumatic fever)	*Streptococcus pyogenes* (gram positive)	Many cell types	Binds cholesterol; forms pores in host cell membranes	May cause heart damage in rheumatic fever, rheumatic heart disease
Hemolysin A (HlyA) (urinary tract infections)	Uropathogenic *Escherichia coli* (UPEC) (gram negative)	Many cell types	Calcium-activated pore-forming cytotoxin	Kidney damage
Superantigens (Type I Toxins)				
Toxic shock syndrome toxin (TSST) (toxic shock syndrome)	*Staphylococcus aureus* (gram positive)	T cells and macrophages	Elicits cytokine production by T cells	Responsible for fever and other symptoms of toxic shock syndrome
Streptococcal pyrogenic exotoxin (Spe) (toxic shock-like syndrome; scarlet fever)	*Streptococcus pyogenes* (gram positive)	T cells and macrophages	Elicits cytokine production by T cells	Responsible for fever and other symptoms of toxic shock-like syndrome

(continued)

Toxin (disease)	Bacterial source	Host cell specificity	Mechanism of action	Role in disease
Superantigens (Type I Toxins) *(continued)*				
Staphylococcal enterotoxin (food-borne disease)	*Staphylococcus aureus* (gram positive)	Vagus nerve; T cells and macrophages	Elicits cytokine production by T cells	Stimulates vagus nerve; leads to vomiting, other symptoms
Hormone Analog				
STa (heat-stable toxin) (diarrhea)	Enterotoxigenic *Escherichia coli* (ETEC) (gram negative)	Intestinal epithelial cells	Hormone analog; binds to guanylate cyclase on host cells; stimulates overproduction of cGMP	Contributes to diarrhea

Answers to End-of-Chapter Questions

CHAPTER 1

1. Death is clearly the most serious outcome of infectious diseases, but some diseases that do not kill can have long-term serious effects. For example, some of the bacteria that cause sexually transmitted diseases can infect a woman's fallopian tubes, rendering her unable to conceive because the egg cannot reach the uterus. Surgical repair may not be possible. To a woman who wants to have children, this outcome can be a serious tragedy. Bacterial skin infections can be disfiguring, causing scars. A serious infection of an extremity may lead to amputation of that extremity. Infections also can have social and economic costs (see next question).

2. The most obvious effect on others is transmission of the disease, but there are social and economic costs that are being taken more seriously. Lost days of work due to an infection disrupt family life and may cause a reduction of income. Infections acquired in hospitals cost millions of dollars in extra days spent in the hospital and increased need for the intervention of additional medical specialists. There have now been a number of studies on the effect of antibiotic-resistant bacteria on medical costs. A patient with such an infection may cost the health care system many times what it costs to care for a person with an infection caused by a susceptible bacterium. Food-borne diseases cost the food industry millions of dollars in recalls and damage reputations of food processors. Finally, an outbreak of a serious disease in a community causes fear and even panic. Anyone who has witnessed the effect on a community of an outbreak of bacterial meningitis can attest to the destructive effects of fear and changed social behavior.

3. Intervention has the advantage that only those with disease are singled out for treatment. The disadvantage of this approach, of course, is that the person first has to suffer the effects of contracting the disease. Intervention also has a psychological advantage in the sense that patients see the services of the medical community at work and are thus more likely to be willing to pay for these services and to have a high regard for the medical personnel who deliver them. Prevention is almost always more cost-effective than intervention, however. This is not the case for some diseases that are not very serious and do not strike many members of an exposed population, but most prevention strategies (clean food and water supply, vaccination) pay for themselves many times over. Also, people do not get the disease in the first place. This is actually a disadvantage in the public relations sense, because out of sight is all too often out of mind. In the chapter on vaccination, some examples will be given of cases in which the success of a vaccine caused people to take the disease (and vaccine) less seriously.

4. Surveys of bacteria isolated before the antibiotic era often turn up bacteria that were already resistant to antibiotics that were introduced much later. No one understands how these bacteria arose, but it is clear that until antibiotic use became widespread, there was not the strong selective pressure for the resistant bacteria to become predominant. Similarly, *Escherichia coli* O157:H7 has probably been around for thousands, some say millions, of years. Only in recent times, however, has our centralized food distribution system made it possible for infections caused by this pathogen to spread so widely. Scientists also suspect that changes in the way cattle are raised, such as increased crowding or type of feed used, may have made carriage of the bacteria by cattle more common, but so far there is little experimental support for this belief.

5. Prevention once again. A clean water supply virtually eliminated cholera, a water-borne disease, from developed countries. Programs to identify people with tuberculosis and treat them have considerably reduced the incidence of tuberculosis in the developed countries. (In the chapter on tuberculosis, however, you will learn that cutbacks in these preventive programs and a general belief that tuberculosis was under control contributed to a reemergence of tuberculosis in countries such as the United States.) Opportunistic infections occurred in wounded people even before the modern era, but the incidence of these infections increased dramatically with such modern medical innovations as surgery, organ transplants, and cancer chemotherapy. Opportunistic infections can be just as deadly as the classical epidemic diseases such as cholera.

6. A relaxation of vigilance in keeping up the preventive barriers that have so effectively reduced the incidence of many infectious diseases could allow old infectious diseases to reemerge. This has already happened with tuberculosis in the United States. Many cities have aging water systems that are allowing sewage to leak into tap water lines. Another way infectious diseases could move back to a number one cause of death in developed countries is if diseases now thought not to be caused by infectious agents (e.g., heart disease and some forms of cancer) proved to be caused by bacteria or viruses. The diseases would not be new, but the attributable cause would be. Of course, if heart disease has an infectious cause, it might well be possible to develop treatments or vaccines to prevent it, thus reducing the number of deaths.

7. In a sense, humans have won the battle against bacteria. After all, we are still around despite living in a sea of bacteria, and our numbers are increasing. Instead of focusing on the relatively small number of cases in which bacteria cause disease, it is instructive to note how many cases of human-bacterium interactions there are in which

symptomatic disease does not develop. This is the reason why many scientists are advocating a change in view of the human-bacterium interaction from the war analogy to a gentler view of the interaction as a dynamic equilibrium. The dynamic equilibrium view is also desirable in our opinion because it is more consistent with a prevention-based approach to keeping the equilibrium in a state that is desirable for us.

8. The fact that new infections continue to emerge raises the question of whether there are any bacteria that cannot cause infections, given the appropriate conditions. The answer to this is almost certainly "yes." After all, a bacterium that grows optimally at 60°C is not likely to do very well in the human body. Also, one would expect that obligately photosynthetic bacteria would not do well in the interior of the human body, but there may be many more potential pathogens out there than we have realized. At first, the possibility that human pathogens could have arisen on Mars (assuming that there are microbes there) seems ridiculous. How could pathogens arise in the absence of the creatures they infect? An answer of sorts is provided by observing that some of the bacteria that are responsible for emerging infectious diseases may have developed their ability to cause disease through interaction with eukaryotic microbes such as protozoa, which have a lot of features in common with the phagocytic cells that are a key defense of the human body. Legionnaires' disease is the best-documented example of this phenomenon.

9. Bacteria and other microbes made Earth livable for humans and other animals, as noted briefly in this chapter. The bacteria that normally occupy many parts of the human body throughout life (the normal microbiota) seem to be more protective than otherwise, and some may provide us with nutrients. The concept of bacteria as dangerous germs is inaccurate. Some scientists even believe that by becoming too clean we have set ourselves up for diseases such as asthma. The idea is that in the absence of sufficient immune stimulation by interaction with microbes early in life, the defense systems of the human body—evolved to provide protection against hordes of bacteria—turn on the body itself. Eat dirt and live!

CHAPTER 2

1. We give only a superficial answer to this question here, but you might keep these three views in mind as you move through other chapters in this book. A bacterium that belongs to one of the first two categories would be expected to have humans (or humans and closely related animals) as its sole host. A pathogen that is out to get you would be expected to have a high rate of symptomatic infection, whereas one that is only using you as a food source and occasionally runs afoul of you would be expected to have a high rate of asymptomatic carriage. A bacterium in the third category should have other niches than the human

body, e.g., water or soil, and spend most of its time there, not in the human body. Two examples of diseases that fit this criterion are cholera and Legionnaires' disease.

2. For all their shortcomings, Koch's postulates remain the best way to establish cause and effect in infectious disease. They have the appeal of simplicity and logic and have a long record of establishing that a microbe causes an infectious disease. In some cases, such as heart disease (if that proves to be caused by bacteria) and periodontal disease, effective antibiotic treatment may replace Koch's third postulate for ethical reasons, but the postulates are needed to introduce a degree of rigor into infectious disease research.

3. Go back and review the criteria for selecting an animal model. Briefly, the infection in an animal may not mimic the infection in humans. Leeches may suck blood, but they do not turn you into a leech or render you immortal (or do they?). The body site affected is important. The hand is not the neck. As for advantages, what would your choice be if asked to submit either to a real live vampire or to a leech. Safety and ethical considerations often dictate the use of an animal model even if it is not a very good one.

4. Obviously, these criteria will shift depending on how serious the disease is in humans and thus how important it is to have a nonhuman animal model. Ideally, the bacteria are administered by the same route they use to enter the human body. The animal reacts to the infection the same way as humans, i.e., develops the same symptoms with the same outcome. Another consideration is cost. Primates are obviously likely to be the best animal models for human disease, but they are very expensive to maintain, and many people have ethical qualms about using them because of their close evolutionary relationship to us. Human volunteers can be used in cases in which the disease is easily treatable once symptoms begin to appear, but there are still some serious ethical barriers to overcome, especially if treatment is not 100% effective and if a chronic form of the disease can develop in some treated people.

5. Low ID_{50}, high LD_{50}. (Remember, "less is worse.") Such a disease would be highly infective but not often lethal. Flu is an example (unless, of course, the hypervirulent strains of influenza virus return). Bacteria that cause sexually transmitted diseases such as gonorrhea would be another example, even though many of the cases are asymptomatic (the person is still infected). Diseases caused by ingestion of bacterial toxins, such as botulism, would be an example of a disease with an LD_{50} but not an ID_{50} (since there is no infection). High ID_{50} but low LD_{50} should not be possible.

6. Organ cultures are very useful and increasingly popular with researchers, but they have their limitations. The main one is that the organs or tissues are maintained in a fluid and an atmosphere that are different from those encountered in the human body. We do not know how much this influences the outcome of the interaction between the bacteria and the tissue, but it may have a significant impact in some cases. Also, it is often difficult to maintain organs and tissues in vitro for long periods of time (days or weeks), and degeneration of the tissue can occur, thus further changing the connection between the organ or tissue and what it is meant to mimic.

7. Diet Koch.

CHAPTER 3

1. This question asks about the molecular version of proving cause and effect, not the molecular Koch's postulates used to show that a virulence gene causes an effect, another approach that has been called molecular Koch's postulates. The form of Koch's postulates referred to here is useful in cases in which the putative causative agent has not been cultivated or is difficult to cultivate and in cases in which scientists are looking for a lead on a possible pathogen. PCR amplification of a 16S rRNA gene replaces cultivation. So the first postulate is that the rRNA gene from a particular organism can be amplified from lesions associated with the disease. The second postulate is isolation and sequencing of the rRNA gene. The third postulate is that the loss of amplifiable rRNA genes is associated with successful antibiotic treatment that eliminates symptoms. There is, strictly speaking, no fourth postulate because the animal or human was not inoculated with the suspected pathogen. An exception arises in the case of a disease caused by a suspected pathogen, such as *Chlamydia pneumoniae* in the case of some forms of heart disease, when the organism is difficult to cultivate and PCR amplification of organism-specific sequences is more convenient. An advantage of using PCR amplification of rRNA genes is that it is only necessary to suspect that a pathogenic bacterium is there, even if one does not know its identity. If a PCR product is obtained, the DNA sequence gives a tentative identification of the causative microbe. So far, this approach, which has been wildly successful in characterization of microbes in environmental (nonpathological) settings, has not yielded much in the case of human disease. This may be due to the fact that relatively few scientists have so far tried this approach.

2. If only one strain of a species has been sequenced, one can at least look for homologs of known virulence genes. The most useful data come from comparisons of strains of the same species. For example, the genome sequence of *Escherichia coli* O157:H7 (a pathogen) was compared with the harmless lab strain *E. coli* K12. The pathogen genome sequence proved to have 1 Mbp of sequence not found in the lab strain. Of course, this could be a reflection of the fact that the K12 strain lost DNA during thousands of passages in laboratory medium, but such comparisons identify genome regions of particular interest and may help scientists to identify so-far-undiscovered virulence genes. An abiding problem is that we still cannot recognize at least one-fifth of the genes in most genome sequences,

and the identification of another 20 to 30% could well be incorrect. This hole in the databases will limit the amount and quality of information that can be extracted from genome sequences.

3. The problem with this statement was addressed in the answer to the previous question, but it is so important that it is worth repeating. Differences in genome sequences may reflect the amount of time an organism has been in culture or the different niche it normally occupies, rather than differences in virulence. Both *Escherichia coli* and *Salmonella enterica* serovar Typhimurium spend as much time outside the human body as in it. Differences in genome sequence could reflect adaptations to other environments. Also, comparisons of strains of different species may simply reflect differences in basic metabolic features. For example, the *E. coli* sequence will contain an enzyme that encodes β-galactosidase, whereas that of serovar Typhimurium will not. This does not mean that β-galactosidase is a virulence factor. The strength of the genome sequence comparison approach is that it engenders hypotheses that must be tested further.

4. We can learn from the environmental microbiologists on this one. There have been many cases in which bacteria with closely related gene sequences have proved to have very different metabolic properties. Why physiology does not always follow phylogeny remains a major mystery. We are missing something big here. Another problem is to determine how close the sequences of two 16S rRNA genes have to be to consider two organisms members of the same species. There is great disagreement on this, although agreement may be reached in the next several years. It is most prudent to use 16S rRNA gene sequence data as a hypothesis about the identity of the microbe, a hypothesis that must be confirmed with further testing.

5. There are now enough resistance gene sequences available in the databases to construct primers that would amplify various resistance genes. Of course, unlike rRNA genes, different primer sets would have to be used for different types of resistance genes. Another drawback is that getting a PCR product only tells you that the gene is in the strain. It may be unexpressed or even mutated to an inactive form. Still, experience has shown that if a gene is present, even if inactive, it can become active very quickly under selective pressure. The advantage of using PCR to assess the resistance of clinical isolates is its speed. Whereas it takes days to isolate an organism using growth-based methods and then more days to determine its resistance profile, PCR-based detection takes hours. Given this advantage, and given the importance of rapid detection of strains resistant to a particular antibiotic, why aren't the clinical labs rushing to adopt this new approach? The authors are mystified but suspect that there is a psychological reason. Clinical microbiologists we have talked to say that this approach is impossible because there are hundreds of resistance genes. (Never mind that there are hundreds of different types of media used in growth-based ap-

proaches.) What is wrong with this objection is that there are usually only a few resistance genes of interest in the case of any bacterial pathogen. Thus, if the pathogen is *Staphylococcus aureus,* only a few resistance genes are of concern. So the solution is to use the decision tree approach commonly employed in growth-based identification schemes. Do an initial round of amplification with species-specific primers to determine if the organism is *S. aureus* or some other species and then choose resistance gene primers applicable to that species. The use of microarrays that contain thousands of resistance gene sequences may render the molecular approach even easier and more powerful.

6. The choice of the restriction enzyme used affects the degree of resolution in both methods. In the case of ribotyping, the choice of the hybridization probe also affects specificity.

7. The authors have a point of view that is not shared by many scientists working in the pathogenesis area, but since we are writing the book, we will take this chance to air our view. First, the level of expression in the animal may be a factor. Also, the choice of which laboratory medium to use will affect the outcome. If a rich medium is used, bacteria grown on the laboratory medium will downregulate such genes as amino acid biosynthetic genes, so an amino acid biosynthetic gene may appear animal specific. Second, the housekeeping genes may be a lot more important than we think they are. After all, a bacterium that cannot divide in an animal is at a decided disadvantage. We think these results are telling us that the demarcation between virulence genes and housekeeping genes may be an artificial one that is impeding discovery. What do those who do not agree with us say? Keep in mind that at least one-fifth of the genes in the sequences of even the well-studied bacteria do not have a recognizable function. As many as 20% more may be mistakenly identified. So it is not too difficult to find a "novel" gene sequence. Also, there are a lot of regulatory genes in most genome sequences, so it is easy to weave a regulatory tale involving as-yet-unknown virulence genes. Ask your professor about this. Get a fresh view of this controversy. And don't believe us just because we are such wonderful and wise people.

8. Gene fusions measure the expression of one or a few genes at a time, whereas a microarray can scan the expression of thousands of genes at a time. Scientists have had more experience with gene fusions, so one might argue that these measurements are currently more accurate than scanning a microarray, but this (some would say dubious) advantage is no match for the power of a microarray. Another difference is that the microbiological world is now dividing into the chipped and the unchipped. To have a microarray that measures expression of an organism's genes, it is necessary to have a genome sequence. Those without a genome sequence are up the proverbial creek.

9. Cloning will still have a place. There are still many genes for which there is no known function or for which the function has been improperly assigned. Also, a gene that is known to have one function might well have others that are not appreciated. Thus, a genome sequence is just the basis for further studies. In experiments to find virulence genes, scientists must take the genes they identify and determine their functions. Microarrays can help by showing whether the identified genes are regulated and, if so, by what. The identity of the signal or signals that trigger gene expression can provide a clue as to function. Even this, however, is only a start. Just because a gene is expressed preferentially under low-iron conditions, for example, does not necessarily prove that the gene encodes a protein involved in iron utilization. Biochemical and genetic tests to determine the role of a gene in the physiology of the bacterial cell are just as necessary as they ever were. Some scientists have claimed that computer analysis (bioinformatics) will reveal gene function. That may be possible someday, but the databases of protein functions are currently far too incomplete to make such an approach feasible and believable.

CHAPTER 4

1. We ask this question to underscore the role of the human brain as a defense against infectious disease. One could call this a nonspecific defense, because human understanding of how a disease is caused and what measures can be used to prevent its spread can be applied to many different diseases. It is a specific defense, however, in the sense that different diseases and different microorganisms may require different prevention strategies. Some examples of the links between the human brain defense and the nonspecific and specific defenses of the body are the use of cleanliness and, in some cases, artificial skin, to restore the protective barrier provided by intact skin; compensating for the temporary loss of PMNs caused by cancer chemotherapy by developing antibiotics or proteins that stimulate the return of PMNs to the bloodstream; the use of vaccines to prevent disease; the design and use of diagnostic techniques to determine which microbe is causing a disease; and employing the appropriate therapy. We are sure that you can think of many more.

2. *Staphylococcus epidermidis* is a normal inhabitant of skin, and disease caused by this species was almost unknown before the advent of modern hospitals and intensive care wards. Such innovations as catheters and surgery, combined with increases in the numbers of somewhat immunocompromised patients, gave *S. epidermidis* the chance to become a significant cause of hospital-acquired infections. *S. epidermidis* is an opportunist because it needs breaches in the defenses of the body (in this case, skin) to cause infections.

3. One of the most effective protections of the skin is its dryness. Liquid is more likely to be found in skin folds and under bandages (seepage from the wound) and gives bacteria a better place to grow than in the dry expanses that are exposed to the air.

4. You would think that gram-negative bacteria, whose outer membrane protects them from lysozyme (a protein too large to diffuse through outer membrane porins), would predominate in areas where lysozyme is present, but that is not the case. There are probably several reasons for the predominance of gram-positive bacteria in the microbiotas of different areas of the human body. First, not all gram-positive bacteria are equally susceptible to lysozyme; some have peptidoglycan that is resistant to lysozyme, have peptidoglycan that is protected by surface proteins, or make proteases that degrade lysozyme. Second, no single defense is perfect; each one does its job but could not alone control bacterial growth. Third, there are other defenses than lysozyme, such as iron-binding proteins (e.g., lactoferrin) and defensins. Resistance to these defenses may be as important as resistance to lysozyme, and resistance to other defenses of mucosal membranes could compensate for a partial susceptibility to lysozyme.

5. It makes sense that the defenses would be different because the areas are so different. For one thing, skin is dry and mucosal surfaces are wet; skin is many layers of cells thick, and mucosal surfaces may be composed of only one layer of cells. Thus, the strategy for protecting mucosal surfaces is to have a toxic barrier (mucus, with its many toxic proteins) that keeps bacteria away from the surface, whereas the skin needs no such protection. They resemble each other in that both keep bacteria from vulnerable areas. In the case of skin, the layers of dry, keratinized dead cells protect the tissue that lies under the skin, just as mucus protects the mucosal membrane.

6. It could prevent the phagocyte from ingesting it. If ingested, it could prevent the phagosome from fusing with the lysosome (not to be confused with lysozyme). It could escape from the phagosome before fusion with lysosomes could occur. It could develop a surface that allows it to survive the harsh environment of the phagolysosome. As will be seen in later chapters, all of these methods are employed (usually only one per bacterial species) by many invasive bacterial pathogens.

7. PMNs circulate in the blood for the same reason state police officers patrol the highways rather than sitting in a wheat field; they are better able to come to the scene of a crime (infection). Also, PMNs that move into tissue also activate their killing potential (much as a policeman might remove his gun when heading for a crime scene), and keeping them in an area where activation is less likely to occur helps to protect the body from their toxic capabilities.

8. During an infection, PMNs migrating out of the bloodstream cause blood fluids to leak into tissue at higher than normal levels. This causes the redness and swelling that often accompany an infection. Pus may also be present because of the accumulation of dead PMNs. The pain is probably due to damage to nerve endings in the vicinity of the wound caused by the pressure of excess fluids or the activities of the phagocytic cells. The same signs of inflammation occur in infected inner tissues and organs; we used infections of the skin as an example because most people have seen this but have not seen, for example, an inflamed colon lining or heart.

CHAPTER 5

1. Activated complement component C5a plays a role similar to cytokines and chemokines in helping PMNs leave the bloodstream and in activating to greater killing power the PMNs moving from the bloodstream into tissue. Complement components do not have the range of regulatory activities that cytokines and chemokines do. Cytokines cannot opsonize or kill bacteria directly the way some activated complement components do.

2. Once activated, PMNs are potentially as dangerous to human tissue as they are to bacteria. The combination of cytokine and complement actions helps keep PMNs from being activated inappropriately and ensures that they are activated only as they get close to the site of infection.

3. Actually, this is a trick question. If you look at Figure 5–1, which shows complement activation, you will see what looks like three pathways. So why do we say two? The reason is that both the mannose-binding collectins and the antibody binding to the bacterial surfaces cause essentially the same set of reactions, employing C1, C2, and C4, whereas the alternative pathway goes right to C3 and Bb. Thus, they can be considered to be two pathways to activation of complement. Now to the "why." To be honest, we do not have an authoritative answer to this question, but we can make an educated guess. In an actual infection, bacteria probably first encounter the alternative pathway, which is triggered directly by bacterial surface molecules. The action of collectins soon follows. Finally, antibodies get into the act. Having more than one pathway means that the different stimuli are not competing with each other at the beginning steps and can thus pool their efforts more effectively.

4. Activated complement components are dangerous because they call in the PMNs and stimulate them to go into a feeding frenzy, an outcome that can damage tissue. As with the PMNs, complement is kept inactive until it is needed during an infection.

5. There are several contributing factors. PMNs exiting the bloodstream all over the body cause blood fluids to leak into surrounding tissue. PMNs, activated prematurely, damage the walls of blood vessels directly, causing further decrease of blood volume. Cytokines probably contribute to this process as well. So, even though the heartbeat rate increases, the heart cannot keep enough blood in the circulatory system to keep blood pressure levels normal. See the text for more details.

6. Once the process of PMN activation, complement activation, and cytokine release gets going all over the body, eliminating the bacteria no longer stops a process that is out of control. Supportive therapy that keeps the heart beating and the lungs breathing can sometimes allow the patient to survive the period between the demise of the bacteria and the return of the inflammatory process to normal, but this works only in some cases.

7. Try complements.

CHAPTER 6

1. sIgA has a special role. It binds mucin via its Fc portion and binds bacteria with its antigen-binding sites, thus stopping further progress of the bacteria toward the mucosal membrane. If the bacteria are trapped in mucin long enough, they will be shed as the mucin blebs off and is removed from the site to be replaced by new mucin. This protective process does not require complement. Furthermore, there are few phagocytic cells and very low levels of complement in mucin, so the ability to activate complement would not be nearly as useful there as it is in blood and tissue.

2. The antigen-binding sites recognize and bind to the bacterium (or other microorganism). The Fc portion interacts with phagocytes or complement (IgG, IgM) or with mucin (sIgA). So the antigen-binding sites bind the bacteria, and the Fc portion interacts with some portion of the human body. Having more than one antigen-binding site helps to increase the avidity of the antibody for its antigen and keeps the off rate down, since two or more sites must disengage simultaneously.

3. Think about this as a lock-and-key situation. The APC is the first key (MHC), which fits in the lock (T-cell receptor) of the Th cell. The Th cell in turn fits its lock with the key (MHC complex again) of the B cell. Two locks would not be able to interact with each other.

4. The reason that the immune response kicks in so rapidly (hours to days) during the second encounter with a microbe is that the memory cells can be stimulated directly without having to wait for the APC–T-cell step to occur. The APC is needed for the first reaction to an infecting microbe, of course, but during a second encounter, the APC-mediated progression of events is available as a backup in case the memory cell response flags for some reason. It also holds out the possibility for recognizing new epitopes.

5. These are listed in the text. Review them. The reason for the interactions is that the nonspecific and specific defenses need to coordinate their activities so that they are

not at cross-purposes and are tightly regulated. Remember, in connection with the latter need, that the defense responses can be harmful to the human body if they get out of control.

CHAPTER 7

1. Antibodies are useful for neutralizing toxins (or viruses), opsonizing bacteria, and activating complement. That is, the antibody response is most effective against extracellular molecules or microbes. The cell-mediated response, the cytotoxic T cells in particular, are needed for control of intracellular pathogens. Although in some diseases caused by intracellular pathogens, the antibody response is not completely useless (recall ADCC), a cytotoxic T-cell response is also important. If the vaccine triggers the antibody response at the expense of the cytotoxic T-cell response, the immune response may not be sufficient to prevent the infection.

2. This is another trick question. Not all vaccines need to be administered several times; some can be administered one or two times. The ones that need to be administered multiple times are the ones that are not self-replicating, such as dead microbes or microbial protein or carbohydrate antigens. The multiple injections mimic the continued stimulation characteristic of a real infection that seems to be needed to generate memory cells. Live vaccines replicate for a period of time and so give the necessary continued stimulation. One reason scientists are so excited about DNA vaccines is that the expression of proteins in muscle cells continues long enough to mimic the process of an actual infection with a self-replicating microbe.

3. Using recombinant techniques, the scientist can overexpress the protein antigen, thus reducing the cost of producing vaccine components. Recall that vaccines are most likely to be widely used if they are inexpensive. There is also a safety consideration. Bacteria producing a protein naturally will leak toxic molecules such as LPS or LTA. A bacterium that is producing copious amounts of a protein will yield a product with a lower LPS or LTA content than bacteria producing low levels of the same protein. Another consideration is that if the protein involved is a toxin, recombinant technology allows scientists to produce a mutant form of the toxin, thus bypassing the need to inactivate the toxin. Safety considerations include making sure that the vaccine protein is not itself toxic, does not elicit cross-reactive antibodies, and does not contain toxic levels of compounds such as LPS or LTA. Of course, these problems also arise in connection with vaccines produced without genetic engineering.

4. There is no clear-cut answer to this, but we will provide an educated guess. An obvious mechanism would be for the vaccine to trigger an autoimmune response. Another possibility is suggested by the Th1/Th2 theory. If a vaccine generated a Th2 response, when what was needed

was a Th1 response (or vice versa), deleterious activities (e.g., excess cytokine release or IgE production) could be elicited that only caused damage and did not contribute to stopping the infection.

5. Some immunocompromised people (e.g., AIDS patients) have actually been infected with live vaccine strains that are innocuous in immunocompetent people. The live polio virus vaccine is a case in point. Since this risk does not exist for otherwise healthy people, the benefit-risk ratio is still very much on the benefit side.

6. Adjuvants probably work by causing slow release of the vaccine components, thus prolonging the period of immune stimulation. Live vaccines do not need adjuvants because they are self-replicating and thus mediate their own "slow release."

7. The best example of this strategy is the rabies vaccine. Rabies is a viral disease that develops very slowly. Thus, a vaccine can have time to stimulate an immune response that kicks in before the disease has time to develop. Other slowly developing diseases, such as HIV infection and tuberculosis, might be treatable by vaccination, whereas the rapidly developing diseases that do not allow time for the immune response to be stimulated would not be treatable with a vaccine.

8. We leave this one to you. The question has been hotly debated and presents some serious moral quandaries. In the days of the smallpox eradication effort, the fear of smallpox was sufficiently great that such niceties as civil liberties were largely ignored in the push to eliminate the disease. Something to think about in this connection is the herd effect. What portion of the population would have to be vaccinated to drop the incidence of disease to near zero in small pockets of unvaccinated people? This kind of calculation may be the answer to the question of how to respect personal beliefs and yet protect the health of the population as a whole. Another consideration is whether or not vaccinating creates a kind of unintended genocide scenario.

9. The smallpox effort combined two strategies. The first was to vaccinate as many people as possible. Yet, since there were still areas where vaccination coverage had not been complete, these areas were watched for outbreaks; if one occurred, medical personnel rushed into an area and started vaccinating people in surrounding areas, trying to contain the outbreak. The problem today is that most people under the age of 40 were not vaccinated against smallpox because of the cost of continued vaccination and the risks associated with vaccination (very low, but now no longer negligible since the benefit has disappeared). Moreover, the immunity of people older than 40 is probably waning. Thus, there is once again a highly susceptible population of people in the world. And there are still smallpox virus cultures stored in freezers in several countries. Should these stores be destroyed?

CHAPTER 8

1.   For example, a bacterium that had an antiphagocytic capsule could also produce a toxin that killed or interfered with the activities of phagocytes. A bacterium could produce two toxins that target phagocytes. A bacterium could use pili to adhere to mucosal cells so that a toxin it produces can act more effectively on them. A bacterium could produce a toxin that lysed host cells and released iron-binding proteins and could also produce a protein that removed iron from these host proteins. In Part II of this book, you will see many examples of such combinations.

2.   Protozoa that live by consuming bacteria have features in common with human phagocytes. Both ingest and kill bacteria in much the same way, although the protozoan is free living, whereas the phagocyte is not. Toxins and other virulence factors that were originally developed to protect bacteria from protozoa could later be used to combat phagocytic cells such as PMNs.

3.   We do not know how many types of bacteria can infect and kill protozoa or other simple animals such as nematodes. But such bacteria might be able to adapt to mammalian cells if they had access to them. If the hypothesis mentioned in question 2 proves correct, there might be far more bacteria in nature that are capable of causing human disease than we currently assume to be the case. Also, if bacteria can develop traits that allow them to cause human disease independently of the presence of humans, this finding would support objections raised by some against bringing back samples from Mars.

4.   A vaccine that elicits production of sIgA that binds the pili and thereby prevents the bacterium from attaching in the first place would be ideal because it would prevent invasion. A vaccine that elicits production of sIgA that binds surface proteins involved in invasion should also work. These vaccine strategies have the advantage that they block infection at an early stage, reducing the likelihood of tissue damage.

5.   The idea is to opsonize the bacteria, making them targets for phagocytes and complement. This would presumably make the natural defenses of the body stronger and faster acting.

6.   This is a common misconception. The purpose of vaccines is to prevent infection in the first place and/or to make the defenses of the body more effective. The proteins that are targets of antibodies and cytotoxic T cells may be virulence factors (e.g., pili in the answer to question 4), but they need not be. The only criterion is that the antibodies or cytotoxic T cells that target them provide a protective response.

7.   Pathogenic bacteria often have other hosts or other niches beside humans. In these other locations, different virulence factors or colonization factors may be needed, and the ones needed in the human body might be superfluous. Thus, the ability of bacterial regulatory systems to sense signals associated with the human body, and to respond to them by increasing or decreasing the expression of genes, allows the bacterium to tailor its response to the human body and to avoid making unnecessary proteins.

8.   The trouble with the term "virulence factor" is that it implies that there is a clear line between pathogens and harmless bacteria. In fact, there is a continuum. Many of the so-called opportunists have some of the same characteristics that are called virulence factors of pathogens. Perhaps the best way to think of opportunists is to think of them as almost-pathogens that are missing some key virulence factor and thus have to have some help to get an infection started. Moreover, we could ask whether many bacterial pathogens should really be considered opportunists. For example, *Streptococcus pneumoniae*, the most common cause of pneumonia, is generally classified as a true pathogen, but it is more likely to cause pneumonia in a person who has had a bout of viral influenza which has impaired the defenses of the airway.

CHAPTER 9

1.   The A portion is the toxic portion. The B portion has no toxic activity; it only binds the toxin to the host cell so that the A portion can be translocated into the cell. Since preventing binding of the toxin to the cell in the first place is the ideal solution, the B portion is not only safe without having to be toxoided but is most likely to elicit the best immune response—antibodies that prevent toxin binding to host cells.

2.   Nothing. Without the B chain, diphtheria toxin cannot get into host cells and thus is harmless. Even if taken up by phagocytosis, the A chain would be unable to escape the phagosome. As explained in the answer to question 1, the binding part of the toxin is the best immunogen because it can elicit antibodies that prevent binding. Antibodies against the A chain might impair toxin activity, but if any molecules of A did not bind the antibodies, they might still enter the cell and kill it.

3.   The idea is to use genetic engineering to create a toxin that has a new B portion that binds specifically to cancer cells. The advantage is that such a toxin would kill only cancer cells, not all rapidly growing cells as the current chemotherapy drugs do. One disadvantage is that too little is known about receptors specific to tumor cells, receptors that are not found on any other cells. Another disadvantage is that such constructs (the A chain with a new B chain) frequently do not allow the A chain to translocate normally. Obviously, we need to have a better understanding of the translocation process.

4.   The toxin is the cause of the symptoms and thus can be targeted efficiently by a vaccine that elicits antibodies that bind the B portion.

5. Botulism is so rare that it is not economical to produce a vaccine for widespread use. Antibodies that bind to the toxin should neutralize the toxin, however, in case a vaccine needs to be developed (e.g., if germ warriors decide to use botulinum toxin for bioterrorist purposes). Passive immunization is also a possibility. In the case of gangrene, the antibodies would have to get into the mass of dead tissue that develops in the infected area. Since the blood supply is cut off because of tissue damage, antibodies would only reach the outer edges of the lesion. The same can be said of streptococcal fasciitis, which is also (at least at present) a fairly rare disease.

6. It is unlikely that either toxin is doing anything for the bacteria during their residence in the human body. The spores of *Clostridium botulinum* are gone before botulinum toxin gets to work. In the case of tetanus, the toxin acts far from the wounded area. If tetanus toxin were a cytotoxin rather than a neurotoxin, one might imagine that helping to create local tissue damage would make the area of the wound more anoxic, thus making it a more congenial environment for the clostridia.

7. The number of cell types affected by the toxin and their locations determine the range of symptoms. Both of these toxins affect a variety of human cells and thus affect the body in a variety of ways.

8. The hemolytic cytotoxins are either pore-forming proteins or phospholipid-degrading enzymes. They do not have B portions that are separate from the portion of the toxin that has the toxic activity.

9. These toxins may actually contribute to development of septic shock when the bacteria infect. Since only low concentrations are needed for this effect, the toxins could conceivably have such an effect at locations distant from the infected area.

CHAPTER 10

1. Antiseptics and disinfectants have multiple targets, whereas antibiotics usually have a single target. There are two exceptions to this general rule. (i) Triclosan has a single target. (ii) Scientists are now coming to realize that antibiotics have a single primary target but that some have secondary targets. Little is known about the secondary effects of antibiotics; more information about them could help scientists make antibiotics more potent.

2. Many antiseptics and disinfectants dissolve membranes. The bacterium would have to change its membrane structure to become resistant. Antiseptics and disinfectants also attack proteins nonspecifically, so modification of the target would be an impossible strategy. Bacteria do become resistant to antiseptics and disinfectants by using efflux pumps to pump them out of the cell.

3. Metronidazole could be considered an exception. Activated metronidazole causes breaks in DNA nonspecifically.

4. Scientists can make mistakes when they solve a crystal structure, so one problem could be that the crystal structure is incorrect. A more likely difficulty arises from the fact that crystal structures are snapshots of the protein or protein complex in one configuration, whereas proteins in solution have dynamic, changing structures. Finally, binding the target molecule is only part of what an antibiotic does. If the target is in the cytoplasm, the antibiotic has to get into the cell. In some cases, the antibiotic binds to and inactivates a protein but has no effect on intact bacteria because it is not transported.

5. Uptake of aminoglycosides is much slower under anaerobic conditions for some reason than under aerobic conditions. Why this is so is not clear, but the phenomenon provides yet another example of the importance of transport of antibiotics into the bacterial cell.

6. The pharmacokinetics of an antibiotic in the body is a very important factor. Different antibiotics penetrate into tissue to varying extents. Some are absorbed from the intestinal tract and some are not. Some enter human cells and some do not. Proteins in blood may inactivate an antibiotic. The antibiotic in its active form must get to the bacteria in concentrations high enough to be effective. This is probably the reason some antibiotics that work in laboratory medium fail to work in the human body. An antibiotic could be more effective in the body than expected from laboratory tests if the growth conditions in the human body were different enough from conditions in laboratory medium that the bacteria became more susceptible in the human body than in the test tube.

7. Pharmaceutical companies need to find antibiotics that are effective, have few or no side effects, and can achieve high concentrations in the appropriate portion of the body. Companies used to seek broad-spectrum antibiotics exclusively, but now narrow-spectrum antibiotics that attack only certain types of bacteria are becoming more attractive, especially if their effect on the normal microbiota is minimized. Another new criterion is that the antibiotic should not elicit resistance readily. Finally, the antibiotic production process needs to be cost-effective. Antibiotics, once the mainstay of pharmaceutical companies, are now seen as less profitable than many other pharmaceuticals, such as mood-altering drugs.

CHAPTER 11

1. Mutant porins of gram-negative bacteria slow the diffusion of antibiotic into the periplasm, making it easier for the β-lactamase to inactivate all of the antibiotic. In the case of efflux pumps, mutant porins might also help by letting in less antibiotic that will have to be pumped out.

2. Some antibiotics, like the tetracyclines, diffuse through membranes so that the bacteria cannot keep them out by not transporting them. Why antibiotics that appear to be taken up by transport proteins are not excluded by mutant uptake proteins is unclear, but this type of resistance has so far not been seen. Possibly, antibiotics use transport proteins that are essential and cannot be changed without making the bacteria a lot less fit. Or there may be multiple transport proteins that transport the antibiotic. Not much is known about the transport of antibiotics across the cytoplasmic membrane.

3. The concentration of antibiotic must reach a certain level to bind its target effectively. The efflux pump only has to keep the internal concentration of antibiotic below that threshold.

4. This question highlights another mystery. Presumably, in some cases, mutations are well tolerated by the target protein or RNA molecule, whereas in other cases either multiple mutations are needed or mutations inactivate the target molecule or both.

5. An educated guess is that if the bacteria have to become resistant by mutating an antibiotic target, and the change requires multiple mutations, it would take longer for the bacterium to become resistant to the antibiotic than if the bacterium acquired a resistance gene by horizontal gene transfer or could become resistant with only one or a few mutations.

6. The bacterium needs to get the antibiotic all the way out of the cell, not just into the periplasm, from which the antibiotic could readily reenter the cytoplasm.

7. Conjugation involves elements that carry not only genes that allow them to transfer from a donor to a recipient but also genes that allow them to replicate or integrate in the recipient. In the case of natural transformation or phage transduction, the incoming DNA must integrate by homologous recombination. Thus, the recipient must have DNA similar enough to that of the donor for homologous recombination to occur. There is a process called illegitimate recombination that allows DNA segments to integrate independently of homologous recombination, but this process—which is poorly understood—is inefficient.

8. A compound other than an antibiotic could select for maintenance of antibiotic resistance genes in a bacterial strain by selecting, in effect, for all the genes in the cluster. Thus, disinfectant use could in some cases select for bacteria that are resistant to antibiotics.

CHAPTER 12

1. Lyme disease was probably around long before it was noticed as a disease. The increase in the deer population in some locations, plus the fashion for having primary or vacation residences in wooded areas where deer and white-footed mice were found, caused humans to encounter the bacteria much more commonly than before.

2. Since the tests for Lyme disease are less than optimal and give false-positive results in some cases, one could argue that more people are diagnosed as having Lyme disease than actually have it. Also, in areas where Lyme disease has received a lot of media attention, people are far more likely to think they have the disease and visit a physician. The argument for underreporting assumes that there are cases that resolve uneventfully without treatment and that such cases are more common than previously thought. Also, not all physicians report cases of suspected Lyme disease to the CDC. So far, the jury is still out on which of these versions of Lyme disease diagnosis and reporting is correct.

3. Until recently, scientists assumed that bacteria multiplying in laboratory medium were good models for bacteria multiplying in the human body. We now know that some of the proteins displayed on the bacterial surface when the bacteria are in the human body are not produced in high levels by bacteria growing in culture. Also, passing the bacteria through laboratory medium too many times causes changes in what surface proteins are produced. The first tests developed, the ones currently being marketed, relied heavily on antigens produced by laboratory-grown bacteria.

4. Physicians are human, and they read newspapers. Lyme disease has received so much attention that it comes readily to mind if a patient reports certain symptoms. Also, many of the symptoms of Lyme disease, such as headache, are nonspecific and are experienced by people who do not have Lyme disease. Finally, the idea that a patient has a condition that can be cured with an antibiotic is very attractive both to the physician and to the patient. Patients can also be quite insistent in their belief that they have Lyme disease, especially if they have recently read news articles that detail the symptoms.

5. Loss of plasmids is one way the bacteria can change their properties in a new setting. Clearly, they do not lose these plasmids under conditions encountered in the animals they normally infect. What is not known—and is interesting to consider—is whether the bacteria might lose plasmids and thus become less virulent in the human body as a survival mechanism, at least in some cases. Since the human body and the murine body have many similarities, this seems unlikely. But it is intriguing that the bacteria do not infect deer. The reason for this trait is not known.

6. Surface proteins are prime candidates for a vaccine. Also, they can serve as candidates for proteins detected in diagnostic tests (although internal proteins can serve this

function, too). A more expanded study of the physiological traits of *Borrelia burgdorferi* is needed, however. One reason is that we can always use new antibiotics. Perhaps more important, it would help a lot to understand why chronic Lyme disease is so refractory to antibiotic treatment. Finally, there may be some new clues to the characteristics of bacteria that have an insect host and a mammalian host. *B. burgdorferi* is an excellent model for such microorganisms.

7. An important question that needs to be answered is whether the current view of the bacteria as extracellular pathogens, at least in the skin and bloodstream phase of the disease, is correct. If it is, and if phagocytic cells are indeed the ones that clear the bacteria from the bloodstream, antibodies that bind to surface antigens could help make the phagocytic defense more effective by opsonizing the bacteria. Another question that needs to be answered is where the bacteria are hiding out in people with chronic Lyme disease. If the bacteria are inside cells, and if they are displaying their antigens on the host cell surface, a vaccine component that stimulates a cell-mediated response to antigens specific to bacteria at this stage could be helpful. Most important, it is necessary to establish which antigens are being produced in the human body, so as to avoid another OspA debacle.

8. Both start with a skin phase that may be characterized by a rash. Both have a bloodstream phase, which in some people can lead to a chronic form of the disease that is characterized by debilitating symptoms, including neurological symptoms.

9. Public education and publicity about treatment opportunities would have to be a top priority, whether the population is urban or rural. Ignorance of the disease symptoms and limited access to health care are prime contributors to the spread of diseases such as syphilis. Enlisting the aid of community leaders who know the population is essential in this effort. Providing free and easily accessible treatment is also essential. Fortunately, there are simple rapid screening tests for syphilis, and a patient can be diagnosed and treated during a single visit. Follow-up visits to patients treated by a clinic to ensure that the disease was indeed cured are expensive but should be a part of any eradication effort. Readiness of government and private funding agencies to make a substantial financial investment is also important. Impressing on people that congenital syphilis can impair a child for life may help to make people realize that syphilis eradication is cheap at almost any price.

10. We will not give a detailed reply because the information on genomics will be obsolete by the time this book is in print, but students are encouraged to go to the literature for the latest analysis of these genome sequences. Genome sequences contain valuable clues about the metabolic characteristics of the bacteria and may help to sug-

gest why *Treponema pallidum* has never been cultivated successfully in laboratory medium. An important limitation is that even in the case of well-studied bacteria, such as *Escherichia coli*, scientists do not recognize a substantial fraction of the genes and are only guessing about many of their assignments of function. The function database is in need of fleshing out.

CHAPTER 13

1. For one thing, *Yersinia pestis* is injected into the bloodstream by an insect, whereas the other yersiniae enter through the intestinal mucosa. This difference is probably less important, however, than the difference between the microorganisms themselves. *Y. pestis* is an example of a bacterium that seems to have gained virulence by losing the function of adherence and invasion genes. Perhaps the products of these genes increase the likelihood that *Yersinia enterocolitica* and *Yersinia pseudotuberculosis* are cleared more rapidly from the body. Also, *Y. pestis* has two plasmids the other yersiniae do not have. The functions of the genes carried on these plasmids, especially the large one, are poorly understood and may furnish important clues.

2. As alluded to in the answer to question 1, adherence to and invasion of human cells by the bacteria might actually make it easier for phagocytes to ingest and clear these bacteria. Loss of such properties by *Y. pestis* may enable it to escape immediate killing by phagocytes encountered by bacteria still adapting to survival in a new (human) host. Both of the intestinal yersiniae can survive in macrophagelike cell lines in the laboratory but may not do so well in human PMNs and macrophages. The intestinal yersiniae appear to use the adhesion and invasion proteins as part of their strategy for invading through the intestinal mucosa.

3. These three species are very closely related to begin with, so the 70-kbp plasmid could well have been in the ancestral strain, not acquired by horizontal transfer. The two intestinal species might encounter each other in nature, but *Y. pestis* is unlikely to have much opportunity to interact with the intestinal species.

4. Both are transmitted by insects, both have a rodent reservoir, and both enter the bloodstream in the initial phase of the infection. *Y. pestis* is much more likely to cause death than *Borrelia burgdorferi*, and no chronic form of plague is known, in contrast to the chronic form of Lyme disease. Plasmids seem to play a role in the virulence of both of these pathogens. *Y. pestis* is more successful by far in avoiding or surviving phagocytosis than is *B. burgdorferi*, a trait that may explain its greater virulence. Both diseases are examples of how changing human habits have increased human exposure to the disease.

5. Phagocytes use pseudopods to engulf their bacterial prey. Changes in cytoskeletal organization are essential for pseudopod formation, so disrupting cytoskeletal organization would prevent engulfment. In the case of the F1 capsule, the antiphagocytic effect is probably due to reduction of C3b opsonization of encapsulated bacteria by the phagocytes.

6.   Rodent control is practiced in major U.S. and European cities, with varying degrees of success, but the rat population is not as out of control as it was in medieval Europe. In the United States, the bacteria are confined primarily to rodents in the western states, where populations are low and would have to move to big cities. (If you are driving through a western state and see rats or prairie dogs hitchhiking, call 911.) The best protection, however, is awareness of the disease and how it spreads. Any outbreak would be quickly contained. Fortunately, there is a cheap and effective antibiotic treatment for plague. Only in case of massive social breakdown, as in war or natural disasters, would plague have a chance to establish a foothold.

7.   The type III secretion system essentially takes antibodies out of play, because the toxic proteins move from bacterial cell cytoplasm to host cell cytoplasm. Thus, a vaccine against the F1 capsule would seem to be the best strategy. Also, some way to kill cells in which the bacteria are multiplying would help to limit the infection. There is a vaccine against plague, but it confers limited protection for a limited time period. Still, it might make a critical difference if a significant outbreak occurred.

8.   Y. pestis is a relatively fragile organism that does not survive long outside the mammalian body. Careful control of aerosols in a laboratory setting (e.g., working in a hood) is important to prevent laboratory-acquired infections. As usual, knowing what you are working with is a big protection. Antibiotic therapy as a response to any symptoms of disease solves the infection problem. Still leery? Work with cloned genes, of course. Genes expressed in Escherichia coli (a close relative of Y. pestis) or even genes expressed in other Yersinia species provide a safer bacterial model system for Y. pestis itself.

CHAPTER 14

1.   Why, indeed? Seriously, Staphylococcus aureus is a very versatile pathogen, which can colonize the skin and other parts of the body without causing symptoms but can also cause infections in many sites of the body. Thus, it is no surprise that it has many traits that can be called virulence factors. Some of these so-called virulence factors may actually be colonization factors.

2.   The simple answer is "no," but let's not jump to conclusions. The question of what signals are sensed by these regulatory proteins has still not been answered conclusively. Biofilms have become something of a fad. There may be much more to this story. The study of S. aureus virulence factors is still in its infancy, and it would be wise

to keep an open mind about what these different traits are actually designed to do.

3.   A peptide autoinducer, such as the one produced by S. aureus, probably does not diffuse through the phospholipid bilayer. Thus, the peptides may have to interact with a second sensing system, the two-component system, which transduces the signal to proteins in the cytoplasm that the concentration of autoinducer is rising.

4.   Staphylococcus epidermidis was not considered a pathogen for a long time. It is an opportunist, but if it gets into the bloodstream, it can be deadly. Thus, in retrospect, it is perhaps not surprising that S. epidermidis is not so different at base from S. aureus. Staphylococcus saprophyticus causes urinary tract infections rather than bloodstream infections or endocarditis and thus would be expected to have properties different from those of the other pathogenic staphylococci.

5.   There are two possible explanations (or a combination of the two). The most likely one is suggested by the name S. saprophyticus. Isolating a saprophyte (an organism that lives on decaying material) would in the past have been interpreted as an indication of contamination of the specimen. Since urine is one of the most frequently contaminated specimens, S. saprophyticus would be easy to overlook if one is looking for Escherichia coli. A second contributing factor is increasing sexual activity among young women, the highest risk group for this type of infection.

6.   If you are developing a vaccine, you want it to have the widest possible applicability. Since both S. aureus and S. epidermidis are increasingly resistant to antibiotics and are a common cause of infections in some hospital populations, a vaccine that protects against both is attractive. An unanswered question: would a vaccine that targets a common component of the normal skin microbiota (S. epidermidis) have any adverse effects, given the presumed protective effects of the skin microbiota?

7.   When S. aureus (or, for that matter, S. epidermidis) contaminates and forms a biofilm on a plastic implant (e.g., heart valve implant), the resulting infection is virtually impossible to control with antibiotics. Usually, the implant must be removed surgically, and a new implant must be installed. Surgeons, a little more concern about aseptic technique, please!

8.   The comment about surgeons made in the answer to question 7 might strike some as irreverent or even snide. But there is good reason to be concerned about disregard of proper aseptic procedure by surgeons. The case cited was unusual in that it was actually reported in a medical journal rather than hushed up by the hospital. The surgeon had dermatitis, which made the full surgical scrub unpleasant, even painful. He compensated for this not only

by not doing the full surgical scrub, but also by coating his hands with mineral oil prior to donning latex surgical gloves. In heart surgery, it is necessary to saw through the rib cage, creating jagged edges that have a tendency to punch holes in latex gloves. Also, mineral oil undermines latex glove material. The combination of the incomplete surgical scrub, the mineral oil, and the perforation of double-gloved hands cost a number of his patients further surgery and longer hospital stays. A word to the wise should be sufficient.

9. Even bacteria that are less susceptible to an antibiotic can be a problem. Antibiotics must be delivered to the site of infection. Achieving high concentrations of an antibiotic in an infected site may be difficult. This allows less susceptible strains a window of opportunity for evading the action of the drug if local concentrations are marginal. The discovery that some strains of *S. aureus* exhibit tolerance to vancomycin (i.e., they do not continue to divide but do not die either) was a real shock. The clinical implications of vancomycin tolerance are still under study.

CHAPTER 15

1. *Streptococcus pyogenes* has a genetic makeup that allows it to cause a variety of infections. Not every strain can cause every type of infection, and a succession of different strains could explain the fluctuations in the types of streptococcal disease that predominate at any particular time. Only recently, with the advent of genome sequencing, has it become possible to test this hypothesis and to probe more precisely the nature of the differences between strains associated with different types of disease. Patterns of antibiotic use may also affect which strains predominate at any particular time.

2. The answer to this question depends on the factors that control the strains that are predominant at a particular time. It is unlikely that fluctuations in the past were as great as they are today. The ease and frequency of international travel, the use of antibiotics, and similar innovations of the modern era would make it easier for different strains of *S. pyogenes* to make the rounds.

3. Group A streptococcal infections generally start either in the throat or in a wound. Thus, colonization of the throat and the ability to colonize skin are likely to be important early in the infection process. This colonization process presumably involves adhesins. Since "strep throat" is an inflammatory process, as is the initial infection of a wound, production of hydrolytic enzymes and shedding of LTA would be expected to play a role at this level. In the bloodstream, the PMNs and complement come into play, so antiphagocytic mechanisms (capsule, C5a peptidase) or serum resistance (Sic) should be important at this stage. Elicitation of antibodies that cross-react with heart tissue

is associated with a later stage of the disease, as are the superantigens that can cause shock.

4. As you can see from the answer to question 3, which was largely guesswork, a lot remains to be learned about the roles of difference virulence factors. This is even truer in the case of the regulation of virulence factors, which is clearly complex. Regulatory genes of *S. pyogenes* respond to a variety of signals, such as carbon dioxide levels, that may help the bacteria to recognize different environments in the body. Learning which genes are controlled by which signals is already revealing groups of genes whose products presumably act in concert. This type of information will provide valuable clues as to which genes are important at which stage in the infection.

5. Here again, as in the answer to question 1, it is likely that strains vary widely in the kinds of virulence genes they have. For example, a strain that has a limited capacity to avoid or combat phagocytic cells is likely to cause only localized infections.

6. Group B streptococci are good at colonizing the body but seem to need some help in initiating a systemic infection. They infect groups such as infants and somewhat immunocompromised adults whose defenses are not in peak condition. Thus, group B streptococci are most likely to lack those virulence factors (or express them aberrantly) that contribute to early phases of invasive infections caused by group A streptococci. Comparing genome sequences could shed light on how the group B streptococci differ from the group A streptococci. It will also be interesting to learn why they colonize different body sites.

7. The increasing number of immunocompromised people in hospitals or nursing homes is probably responsible for this phenomenon, as is lessened concern for hygienic practices (e.g., hand washing) by hospital workers.

8. A person who is colonized with a multiply antibiotic-resistant strain of *Enterococcus* spp. has a higher likelihood of developing a difficult to treat postsurgical infection. People colonized with the antibiotic-resistant strains could be considered to be ticking time bombs with respect to nosocomial infections.

9. The answer is likely to be the same as the answer to question 6—missing virulence genes or virulence genes that are not expressed optimally. Once an enterococcal strain gets into the bloodstream, serious disease develops, so most likely the missing or less effective genes are genes important for the first stages of infection. Like the group B streptococci, enterococci are very good at colonizing the intestinal tract, so they are on the scene if opportunity knocks.

10. This is a question that has puzzled scientists for some time. Since the group A streptococci can colonize the throat and skin, if only transiently, they would have abundant opportunity to acquire virulence genes from members of the normal microbiota. In fact, part of the answer to this question is based on perception. Group A streptococci have been acquiring genes for resistance to tetracycline and erythromycin, but many clinicians seem to see penicillin resistance—which has fortunately been slow to develop—as the sentinel resistance that defines the resistance status of group A streptococci. So the lag in resistance development depends on which resistance you are focusing on.

CHAPTER 16

1. The specialists mentioned in this question are introduced into the human body by insect bite, whereas the generalists colonize various parts of the human body and are poised to take advantage of breaches in the host defenses. The ability to colonize body sites is certainly a feature that distinguishes many of the generalists. There are exceptions to this rule, but it provides one way of thinking about the distinction. So, does this mean that colonization factors should be considered virulence factors?

2. Burns, wounds, and cystic fibrosis were present before the modern era. What is new is the use of antibiotics and the fact that epidemic diseases have come under control (at least in the developed countries) so that people can live long enough to suffer *Pseudomonas aeruginosa* infections. Surgery has made its contribution, as have such modern medical practices as cancer chemotherapy and immunosuppressive therapy administered to transplant patients. Contact lenses have also increased the likelihood of eye infections.

3. Pseudomonads are opportunists, so for people with none of the risk factors associated with this type of disease, pseudomonads might be considered bacteria that could outcompete pathogenic bacteria in various body sites. This is likely to work best on skin, because *P. aeruginosa* does not do well under the anoxic conditions found in the colon and vaginal tract. The main impediment to this use of pseudomonads is that there are other bacteria that colonize the skin permanently rather than transiently. And of course there is the safety issue. A person's risk status can change abruptly if, for example, the person is burned or has surgery. So *P. aeruginosa* would be too risky to use in this way. Finally, consider the fact that we are already being inoculated daily by pseudomonads in soil and water, so there would be no need for additional application of the bacteria.

4. This is a real stumper. The apparent anomaly can probably be explained, however, by the fact that in laboratory experiments scientists are administering high concentrations of a single strain, which is known to be virulent in humans. In the soil, nematodes would encounter a mixture of bacteria, some of which might actually be protective.

5. Resistance to many antibiotics by pseudomonads is certainly part of the answer to this question. The bacteria, both gram positive and gram negative, that top the list of nosocomial pathogens all have multidrug resistance in common. Also, pseudomonads are ubiquitous in the environment, including the hospital environment, and have such great metabolic flexibility that they can adapt readily to new niches, such as the water that humidifies a respirator or dilute disinfectant solutions.

6. The tremendous metabolic versatility of the pseudomonads has made them prime candidates for use in bioremediating toxic waste sites. A relative of *P. aeruginosa*, *Burkholderia cepacia*, is already being used to degrade some of the herbicides sprayed on golf courses. At first, the use of these ubiquitous soil bacteria might seem not to be a problem because they are already present. The main safety concern has been the mode of application of these agents (e.g., spraying in aerosols) and how close such applications would be to hospitals or communities where people with cystic fibrosis live.

7. The alginate probably allows *P. aeruginosa* to form biofilms that discourage ingestion by phagocytes and place the bacteria in a metabolic state that makes them even more resistant to antibiotics. The variation in LPS structure may make the bacteria more resistant to antibacterial peptides found in the lung. The functions of hydrolytic enzymes and exotoxins are easier to imagine; they probably contribute to lung damage.

8. Alginate is a polysaccharide and is thus not as good an immunogen as a protein. Also, if the function of alginate is to facilitate formation of biofilms, which are difficult for phagocytic cells to ingest and eliminate because of their size, the antibodies would not have much of a protective effect.

9. Compounds that bind autoinducer would presumably prevent the autoinducer from entering the bacterial cell and triggering gene expression. How well this works remains to be seen. An even more critical question is whether the genes controlled by the autoinducer are sufficiently important in the disease process that inhibiting their expression would interfere with the infection process. Note that there are a number of virulence genes whose expression is not controlled by the autoinducer. Finally, given the ability of pseudomonads to catabolize a variety of organic compounds, one would have to ask whether the antagonists of the autoinducer would be one of those compounds.

10. There are two ways to look at this problem. The failure to find at least some of the known virulence factors could be used as an argument that the new model systems are not very good models for human infections. Another way to look at it is to note that IVET and signature-tagged mutagenesis have also come up with different virulence factors in the same animal model (laboratory rodents) that was used for earlier studies of virulence factors. It is not surprising that different ways of screening for virulence factors will yield different candidates for such factors. The fact that the screens using lower eukaryotes as models are turning up new candidates could be considered a strength because it might unearth new classes of virulence factors. Perhaps the best way to view these new models is to use them as initial screens that provide candidate virulence factors that need to be tested in mice or some other mammalian model. If most of them prove not to be important in mammals, then perhaps the new models will be abandoned.

CHAPTER 17

1. *Bordetella pertussis* binds preferentially to ciliated cells and kills them. The binding can be explained by the adhesin Fha, although there may be still other ciliated cell-specific adhesins to discover. The "tracheal cytotoxin," which is actually a peptidoglycan fragment, explains the death of ciliated cells. The contribution of pertussis toxin and ACase to this part of the infection process is still not clear. Pertussis toxin and ACase seem to have a role in protecting the bacteria from lung monocytes and macrophages. How the observation that Fha stimulates uptake of bacteria by phagocytes squares with the strategy of killing phagocytes with toxins delivered from outside of the phagocytes is still a mystery. Much of the work on *B. pertussis* has focused on the regulation, biochemistry, and secretion of such obvious virulence factors as the toxins, rather than on the relationship of various putative virulence factors and stages of disease as it occurs in the human body. Now that so much is known about the virulence factors, however, it should be possible to make more progress toward linking virulence factors and their regulation with the progression of the disease.

2. Children are now vaccinated to prevent them from contracting the disease, thus reducing drastically their function as reservoirs of the disease. The bacteria are still around, however, and adults whose immunity is waning but who are still immune enough not to develop the severe form of the disease are an obvious reservoir. Whether adults in the pre-vaccine era were reservoirs is unclear. Perhaps, with outbreaks of infection occurring regularly in children, adults who survived the disease in childhood might well have had their immunity boosted by periodic exposure to the bacteria, whereas today such exposure would be much less common. Adults do develop symptomatic disease, the so-called "100 days cough." Since persistent cough does not seem like much of a danger sign, such adults may inadvertently expose infants and young children to disease. Health care workers who see infants and small children regularly tell us that if they are presented with a case of infant whooping cough, they can almost guarantee that there is an adult with a persistent cough in the household.

3. Pertussis toxin is externalized by a type IV secretion system, one kind of secretion system that delivers proteins from the cytoplasm of the bacteria to the cytoplasm of a host cell. Possibly, bacteria in close proximity with human cells secrete the protein to the surface of the host cell rather than to its interior, and the toxin being secreted binds the host cell and creates a bridge of sorts between the bacteria and the host cell.

4. Phagocytic cells are very dangerous to bacteria. cAMP is a signaling molecule that controls many host cell (including phagocytic cell) functions. Perhaps it takes a one-two punch to fend off the phagocytic cells. Note that the balance between the bacteria and the phagocytes is a tenuous one for the bacteria, because ultimately the host defenses win and eliminate the bacteria. Another possible aspect of this story that has not been given much attention is that these toxins could also be involved in increasing cytokine release by host cells, an outcome that could explain some of the symptoms of the infection.

5. Not a lot is known about how peptidoglycan fragments produce toxic effects, although it is clear that they can do so. An educated guess is that the peptidoglycan fragment, like LPS, stimulates inappropriate cytokine production with the result that tissue damage is done.

6. In phenotypic modulation, all of the bacteria in a culture alter expression of a gene when the bacteria are exposed to inducing conditions. Then, when the bacteria are returned to noninducing conditions, the gene expression returns to its former level. Phase variation involves only a fraction of the cells in a bacterial culture. Phenotypic modulation occurs much more rapidly in the laboratory since all cells participate, so a new trait is quickly evident. In phase variation, the change takes more time since the rare switched cell has to be selected and become the predominant cell type. This is a way of telling the two apart if you don't know much about the genes involved. If you have information about gene sequences, you can use various molecular techniques to differentiate one from the other.

7. The BvgSA two-component system is unusual in that BvgS, the sensor, has more domains that are phosphorylated in a cascade before the phosphate group is finally passed off to BvgA, the response regulator. Why this two-component system is more complex than most is anyone's guess, but the multiple phosphorylation steps might allow the bacteria to control the amount of BvgA phosphorylation more subtly, if the phosphorylation of at least some BvgS proteins is interrupted during the cascade before transferring the phosphate to BvgA.

8. Both type III and type IV secretion systems normally transfer proteins from the cytoplasm of one cell to the cytoplasm of the other. Type III systems typically inject proteins into a eukaryotic cell, whereas type IV systems are most often associated with the conjugal transfer of

DNA, which is covalently attached to a protein. The *B. pertussis* type IV system is unlike other known type IV systems in that it seems to export the protein to the outside of the bacterial cell and there is no DNA attached to the protein. Also, the transfer of the protein to the periplasm is mediated by the general secretory pathway, not by a specialized set of proteins that are specific to the type IV apparatus.

CHAPTER 18

1.   The Gram stain is obviously still an important part of the initial diagnosis of the disease, and often the clinical laboratory stops at the point when gram-positive diplococci are detected. But if it is desirable to confirm the diagnosis (as it might be if there is an outbreak of resistant strains in a hospital or nursing home), the DNA-based tests have the advantage of speed. In theory, PCR amplification of *Streptococcus pneumoniae*-specific DNA from a sputum specimen that contains gram-positive diplococci could be done in hours, whereas culturing the bacteria (which sometimes fails) can take days. Tests like the bile solubility test are not infallible, and the antibody-based tests can require the use of many different antibodies. PCR requires one set of primers that work for all strains. If further confirmation is desirable, a partial sequence of the PCR fragment would quickly provide the ultimate identification. Also, if *S. pneumoniae* is strongly suspected from the Gram stain results, PCR amplification to detect antibiotic resistance genes found in *S. pneumoniae* could also be done to provide rapid information about possible resistance to antibiotics that might be used. Microarrays containing sequences from resistance genes could also be used for this purpose. For some reason, these molecular methods have been slow to penetrate the clinical laboratory.

2.   The first challenge is the ciliated cells that defend the upper airway. *S. pneumoniae* colonizing the throat can get past this defense if the bacteria are carried in fine aerosols, but often the bacteria get some help from a prior infection with influenza virus that kills ciliated cells. Once in the lung, the next challenge faced by the bacteria is the lung macrophages. The capsule of pneumococci protects them from phagocytosis. Toxins such as pneumolysin may contribute to killing of phagocytic cells and to generalized tissue destruction. If the bacteria enter the bloodstream, they face once again an army of phagocytes, this time mainly PMNs. Here too, their capsule protects them. What role the putative adhesins play in all this is still unclear, although it is clear from animal studies that some of them are important for virulence.

3.   A protein that sticks to the Fc portion of antibodies and activates complement by the classical pathway and also acts as a pore-forming cytotoxin can have a variety of physiological effects in vitro, depending on which assay system you are using. Recall also that low concentrations of pore-forming cytotoxins, concentrations too low to be lethal to host cells, may nonetheless stimulate cytokine production or have other adverse effects. This variety of in vitro effects could extend to damage caused by the protein in vivo. If the domains of pneumolysin that mediate these different functions are separable, mutations that alter one domain and eliminate one activity but leave other domains and other activities intact could be introduced into pneumococcal genes, and the effects of these mutations could be tested in animal models.

4.   Autolysis releases LTA and peptidoglycan fragments that can be toxic because they elicit excess release of cytokines. If you doubt this, consider the effect of penicillin-induced release of these compounds on infants with meningitis (Box 18–1). Autolysis could release still other toxic components from the cell cytoplasm.

5.   Attachment of the pneumococci to the meninges, which are composed primarily of endothelial cells, has an inflammatory effect, possibly mediated by teichoic acid, lipoteichoic acid, and peptidoglycan fragments from lysing bacteria. Inflammation causes breaches in the blood-brain barrier, admitting blood proteins (e.g., complement, coagulation proteins) and phagocytes that can cause damage to the brain by raising pressure on the brain. Especially in infants, dying bacteria can be almost as dangerous as live bacteria because their components are stimulating the intense inflammatory response that causes the damage. Therefore, steroids are administered in an attempt to damp the inflammatory response elicited by successful use of antibiotics to kill the bacteria.

6.   One reason peptidoglycan fragments would not make a good vaccine is that these fragments could well be toxic. Moreover, antibodies that bind peptidoglycan would not be opsonizing because the peptidoglycan layer lies beneath the capsule, preventing contact of the Fc portion of the antibody with phagocyte receptors. Antibodies or other compounds that bind peptidoglycan fragments, however, might be useful in combating an infection in progress (passive immunization) if they prevented the peptidoglycan fragments from interacting with host cells in such a way as to cause an inflammatory response.

7.   If pneumolysin is in fact responsible for many of the symptoms of pneumonia and meningitis, it might be useful to have pneumolysin as a component of the vaccine if antibodies that bind pneumolysin neutralize it. The most likely candidates for effective vaccine components, however, are the surface proteins that would elicit antibodies capable of opsonizing the bacteria. Since these adhesin proteins are not known to be toxic, it would probably not be necessary to modify them in order to detoxify them.

8.   Pneumonia and meningitis are extremely dangerous diseases that can be caused by bacteria other than *S. pneumoniae*. Some of these other bacteria were (and still are)

more resistant to antibiotics at that time. Thus, physicians felt they should err on the side of caution by treating patients with a broad-spectrum antibiotic, since there is not much time for second guesses about therapy.

9. Nursing home patients receive some protection from the currently available pneumococcal vaccine and even more from a combination of the influenza vaccine and the pneumococcal vaccine, but coverage is not anywhere near 100%. Vaccinating staff members, who might inadvertently transmit viruses or bacteria to their patients, is more effective given their younger ages and builds an additional firewall against transmission of the disease.

10. This is speculation, but one reason is that such a procedure helps the bacteria protect themselves from hostile takeovers by phage DNA or other DNA molecules that might be hazardous to their health. By importing fragments of genes, which can then (if, for example, they are parts of mutant penicillin-binding proteins) be incorporated into the bacterium's genome, the bacterium is less likely to acquire deleterious genes. Making the DNA single stranded protects it from nucleases and restriction enzymes. Then, when the second strand is synthesized, the double-stranded form may have DNA modifications that also protect it from enzymes that might degrade it. Another possibility is that the bacteria are using DNA for food, importing it in bite-sized pieces that can then be used as sources of carbon and energy.

CHAPTER 19

1. The fact that many people were cured of TB during the period when anti-TB programs were under way meant that the number of people capable of disseminating the disease was drastically reduced in most parts of the country. Thus, the risk of acquiring TB was lower. Also, physicians were well trained to diagnose cases of TB and were on the alert for such cases. Finally, the groups that were later to act as the primary source of new cases (homeless people, AIDS patients, and substance abusers) were only beginning to appear as a public health problem. Until these groups reached critical mass, and the crowding in prisons and in some inner city areas reached its current proportions, the chance of TB acquisition and transmission remained low enough to keep the case incidence figures low. The main reason for dismantling anti-TB programs was that they were costing tax dollars when the TB problem appeared to have been more or less solved. The medical community would have had to make a strong case for continuing the programs. To be fair, it was not easy to foresee the future rise in homeless and other susceptible populations when the decision to dismantle the programs was made. The main argument against dismantling the anti-TB programs was that these programs were the main protective barrier against TB in a country which is a magnet for immigrants from all parts of the world, including many parts where TB is endemic.

Another argument against dismantling the programs was that the capacity for training people in anti-TB measures was in effect dismantled along with the programs. Thus, when the new waves of TB cases began to appear, public health officials and clinicians were caught in a state of total unpreparedness, and there was a deficit in people trained to diagnose and supervise treatment of TB.

2. A complete answer to this question would take many pages and would involve politics and personalities of the period as much as scientific considerations. No such complete answer will be attempted. The reason for raising the question here is to highlight the scientific pros and cons. The main argument for BCG administration is that, in some populations, it has been at least partially effective. It is safe and might help. The main argument against BCG administration is that it makes the TB skin test useless. Thus, in a country where it seemed possible to control TB by a combination of skin test screening, followed by aggressive treatment of new cases discovered by screening, a nationwide BCG vaccination program had less appeal than it did in Europe, where TB rates were high in many areas as a result of hardships experienced during World War II. This question would be easier to answer if a more effective vaccine were available. The range in efficacy figures found in different BCG trials gave support to the contention of some U.S. physicians and public health officials that BCG was virtually worthless, except possibly for preventing TB in small children.

3. There is an overlap between the cell-mediated (especially activated macrophage) response that confers immunity to TB and the response that gives skin test reactivity, but it is clear that these two responses are not identical. Thus, it is conceivable that an effective vaccine might not make the person PPD positive.

4. If the frequency of spontaneous resistance to a particular drug is 10^{-7}, people taking only one drug who carry 10^7 to 10^8 bacteria in their lungs have a good chance of developing a strain resistant to that drug. The frequency of spontaneous resistance to two drugs is $10^{-7} \times 10^{-7} = 10^{-14}$. A person with 10^7 to 10^8 bacteria in the lung is highly unlikely to develop a strain that is simultaneously resistant to both drugs, if they are taken in combination as prescribed. Taking one drug for awhile and then another can allow resistance to occur in steps, giving rise to strains that are resistant to more than one drug. Also, a person who acquires a strain that is already resistant to one drug in a two-drug combination has a good chance of developing a strain with spontaneous resistance to a second drug as well as the first.

5. Many of the people who are homeless are substance abusers and/or have mental problems. People in these categories are more likely to be in crowded populations in the first place (homeless shelters, prisons, and tenements) and are thus more likely to be exposed to TB. Substance abusers with depressed immune systems and people whose inability to care for themselves results in inadequate nutrition and poor sanitation are also more susceptible to TB. Finally, such people are not tied to a particular location, a factor that makes monitoring compliance with therapy difficult. They are also less likely to take prescribed drugs regularly and to have prescriptions refilled. It has become necessary for public health workers attempting to identify homeless people with TB to exercise considerable ingenuity to find ways around these numerous problems.

6. Antibodies are useless against *Mycobacterium tuberculosis* because *M. tuberculosis* grows in macrophages and is serum resistant. It has often been noted that the higher the level of *M. tuberculosis* antibodies, the more likely a person is to develop serious disease. This could be due to the fact that high antibody levels indicate that the main type of immune response being stimulated is the type of T-helper cell that stimulates B cells to produce antibodies (Th2 cells), whereas the most important response is stimulation of the T-helper cells that activate macrophages (Th1 cells) and, to a lesser extent, the cytotoxic T-cell response.

7. Since the idea of prophylactic administration is to prevent the initiation of an infection rather than eliminate well-established bacteria, a simpler therapy is sufficient.

8. *M. tuberculosis* resembles *Legionella* species in that both can enter and multiply inside macrophages, but *M. tuberculosis* can infect normal lungs. This is probably due to the fact that *M. tuberculosis* is better able to survive the killing activities of normal macrophages. A unique virulence factor of *M. tuberculosis* is its cell wall, with its high content of unusual glycolipids. These glycolipids (including mycolic acids and lipoarabinogalactan) not only provide protection against killing by phagocytes but also (at least in the case of mycolic acids) contribute to lung damage.

9. Those who advocate this change in counting deaths argue that since HIV infection makes it more likely that an *M. tuberculosis* infection could cause serious disease, HIV is the real culprit. The problem with this change in counting deaths is that governments use these numbers to determine priorities in funding research and surveillance systems. There are some who see this more as a cynical attempt to justify the enormous sums spent on HIV research to the detriment of funding for research on TB and other infectious diseases.

Bonus question: How would Hamlet have responded to injection with PPD?
Answer: TB or not TB, that is the question.

CHAPTER 20

1. There are modifications of the Gram stain procedure that improve the staining of the bacteria. Cultivation is an option, but since it takes several days for visible colonies to form and since the medium is complex (thus introducing the problem of overgrowth by other microorganisms, necessitating the inclusion of antibiotics in the medium), this is not an attractive option unless one needs pure cultures for DNA fingerprinting in the case of a suspected single-source outbreak. There are antibody tests and DNA probe tests available. The point of this question is to point out the fact that diagnosis of Legionnaires' disease can be tricky. This is a good example of a case in which laboratory technicians with a good understanding of microbiology and experience with infectious disease outbreaks can be invaluable. It may take someone who is thinking beyond the routine tests to have the suspicion that further thought and testing are required.

2. If *Legionella pneumophila* spends a good part of its time in the environment inside amoebae, it is growing in a very complex medium indeed. Water can also contain a lot of nutrients if there is rotting vegetation. Still another consideration is that the medium often used to grow *L. pneumophila* contains charcoal, a substance used to adsorb compounds that can be toxic to bacteria. Possibly, it is toxic compounds in agar or other medium components that are responsible in part for the difficulty in cultivating the bacteria, although there is no question that the bacteria have complex growth requirements.

3. In the case of opportunists such as *L. pneumophila*, the ability to cause disease is clearly somewhat marginal. Thus, the factors involved in virulence could be harder to identify than in the case of a pathogen that causes disease in otherwise healthy people. Housekeeping genes may be more important, and genes that encode functions that do not have unambiguous phenotypes in virulence assays may come into play.

4. This question is designed to remind you that a vaccine does not have to be composed of virulence proteins to be effective. If the immune response against the metalloprotease somehow helps the mammalian body to fend off the infection, it really does not matter whether the metalloprotease has a direct role in virulence. Also, keep in mind that in the case of bacteria, such as *L. pneumophila*, that do not cause disease in healthy people, phenotypes of mutants in the animal models used to assess virulence may not be clear-cut.

5. The critical question is what is or are the factors that explain why some people are more susceptible to Legionnaires' disease than others. That is, what is the nature of the immunocompromising factors? If, for example, the problem is that lung macrophages have a less than adequate oxidative burst, then normal macrophages may not provide a very good model for what is happening in the body.

6. The bacteria appear to survive and multiply in phagocytic cells. Thus, opsonizing antibodies may not help. Stimulating the activated macrophage response is obviously a desirable outcome, but this arm of the Th response also leads to antibody production. Fine-tuning the cytokine response to encourage one aspect of the Th1-type response rather than another aspect of that same response is a problem that still stymies vaccine researchers.

CHAPTER 21

1. *Mycoplasma pneumoniae* has very complex growth requirements. It relies on human cells and the nutrient-rich environment of the human body for the compounds it needs. The ability to obtain many nutrients from the human body makes it unnecessary for the bacteria to carry the genes needed to encode amino acid and other biosynthetic enzymes. It does not make peptidoglycan, and it acquires membrane sterols from the host.

2. Although many genomes of eukaryotic viruses are less than 50 kbp in size, some, such as the poxviruses, have genomes as large as 300 kbp, which approaches the size thought to be needed for free-living microbes. One could argue with the notion that *M. pneumoniae* is free living, because it is found normally in close association with eukaryotic cells, which provide it with many nutrients. *Chlamydia* spp. are also parasitic on mammalian cells, just as mammalian viruses are.

3. The number of bacterial types in which regulation of transcription has been studied is relatively small. Most of them are in the same phylogenetic group as *Escherichia coli*. Thus, it is possible that there are families of regulatory genes that have not yet been identified and characterized. A reason for believing that there might be few regulatory genes in the *M. pneumoniae* genome, however, is that the bacteria appear to be specific for humans and do not cycle through multiple hosts and environments. Thus, they would not have the need for a complex repertoire of regulatory genes.

4. The purpose of the cytadherence organelle seems to be the same as the purpose of pili—to mediate attachment to human cells. The cytadherence organelle differs from pili in that it does not have a fibrillar shape and seems to have a more complex structure.

5. The asymmetric structure of the mycoplasma membrane (outer leaflet different from the inner leaflet) is reminiscent of the structure of the gram-negative outer membrane, except that the mycoplasmas have lipoproteins in the outer layer of their cytoplasmic membrane rather than lipopolysaccharide. Two possible hypotheses about this unusual membrane architecture come to mind. One is that it might play a structural role in preventing lysis of the bacteria. The bacteria are normally found in high-osmolarity fluids (e.g., fluids bathing human cells), so the osmotic pressure from intracellular contents is closer to that exerted by the extracellular contents than it would be in the case of a bacterium in water or other fluids with

low osmolarity. Thus, the membrane of the mycoplasmas does not have to be as strong as the cell wall of bacteria that spend some of their time in dilute solutions. A second hypothesis is that this unusual membrane structure somehow aids in the interactions between the bacteria and host cells. Attachment of the bacteria to human cells has a lot of effects on the human cells, from elicitation of cytokine production to depolarization of nerve cells. Possibly the mycoplasma membrane structure is designed to help the bacteria manipulate host cell physiology.

6. We leave it up to you to answer this question. Keep in mind that it is unlikely that Koch's third postulate will ever be satisfied directly using human subjects, for ethical reasons. Most scientists would be satisfied with a demonstration that antibiotics that eliminate the bacteria from the body also cure or prevent heart disease. Nonetheless, the effect of antibiotics on the body can be complex, and some antibiotics have an anti-inflammatory effect, so there will always be skeptics who argue that the curative effect of antibiotics is not necessarily due to elimination of the bacteria from the body.

7. Both chlamydiae and mycoplasmas are small, have relatively small genomes, and are normally parasitic on human cells. Mycoplasmas, however, can be grown independently of human cells. So far, no cell-free medium has been found that supports the growth of chlamydiae outside mammalian cells. Chlamydiae have a two-stage life cycle, whereas only one form of mycoplasmas is known.

CHAPTER 22

1. Antibodies that bind to "protective antigen," which we now know is the B portion of both *Bacillus anthracis* toxins, would prevent both toxins from binding to target human cells. Also, the B portion should be nontoxic. The A portions of the two toxins would probably not be toxic either, since they need the B portion to enter the cell, but about the best that could be expected from antibodies against the A portions is that these antibodies would block internalization of the toxin. The antibodies would have to enter the cell along with the A portion to prevent toxin action inside the cell.

2. D-Amino acids are unusual in nature, so proteins composed of this type of amino acid might not be recognized well by the immune system, although this seems unlikely. Another possibility is that antibodies that bind to the capsule contribute to ingestion of the bacteria by phagocytic cells but that the bacteria can survive in these cells. These are just educated guesses, but they serve to illustrate the problems that can arise in connection with vaccine design and implementation.

3. There is insufficient information on how infectious *B. anthracis* is in humans, but its ID_{50} may be relatively high.

In cases where humans have been infected by working with infected animals or hides, the number of exposed people who become seriously ill seems not to be very high. Most develop the cutaneous form, not the much more dangerous respiratory form. Another possibility is that for some reason the spores were no longer capable of germination. This seems unlikely because spores are very tough. A third possibility is that the terrorists used the wrong strain. The vaccine strain of *B. anthracis*, which is the strain most widely available, is avirulent.

4. The most serious form of anthrax, pulmonary (or systemic) anthrax, has such a rapid onset that antibiotics generally cannot be administered early enough to be effective. Secondary transmission from human to human seems not to occur, so there will not be a secondary outbreak that could be prevented by prophylactic antibiotic therapy. The cutaneous form of anthrax is self-limiting. Thus, antibiotics have not played a major role in containing anthrax outbreaks. Nonetheless, since antibiotics may be useful in some cases to save lives, it is not wise to dismiss as unimportant a multiply resistant strain of the bacterium.

5. We do not know whether *Bacillus thuringiensis* lost the plasmids or whether the ancestor of *B. anthracis* gained them. It is not even clear whether there are important host factors missing from *B. thuringiensis* that would prevent this species from becoming virulent if it gained the plasmids. Ultimately, the question comes down to one of likelihood. Management of farm animals in the developed world has virtually eliminated *B. anthracis*, so in countries where anthrax is under control, there would be little chance for *B. thuringiensis* to come into contact with *B. anthracis*. Also, there would presumably have to be transfer of both plasmids, transfers that would likely occur as separate events. Finally, as far as we know, there is no selection for a virulent form of *B. thuringiensis*, so the very rare event in which a strain of *B. thuringiensis* acquired both virulence plasmids would not be likely to result in the virulent strain's predominating. Perhaps the best argument that we are not in immediate danger from spraying of *B. thuringiensis* by organic farmers is that this technique of insect control has been used for decades, and so far there have been no known cases of the strain's becoming virulent. There have been some reports of allergic reactions in field workers, but no cases of anthrax.

CHAPTER 23

1. Antibiotics that eliminate *Helicobacter pylori* from the stomach cure the patient's ulcers. This is considered by many to be a strong argument in favor of the hypothesis that *H. pylori* causes ulcers. Still, there is some uncertainty. Some antibiotics also act as anti-inflammatory agents. Moreover, the treatment regimen for ulcers includes a nonantibiotic compound that was used previously to treat ulcers. Finally, many people who have the bacteria in their stomachs do not develop ulcers. These might be used as arguments against *H. pylori* as the cause of ulcers.

2. Urease seems to be needed to allow the bacteria to make a run for the mucin layer, where the pH is near neutral. Thus, urease acts very early in the infection process. Once the bacteria enter the mucin layer, urease actually becomes a hindrance for the bacteria. A urease inhibitor would be a good treatment in the sense that, if given before the bacteria enter the stomach, it would prevent infection from occurring. The problem with this approach, of course, is that a person has no way of knowing when he or she would consume the bacteria. Also, many people are already infected. Thus, the urease inhibitor would have to be taken daily from youth to adulthood, not a very practical solution.

3. There may be different strains of *H. pylori* that vary greatly in the ability to cause disease. As indicated in the text, scientists are looking for traits that characterize especially virulent strains, if such strains do in fact exist. Scientists have long suspected that there is a human genetic component to susceptibility. For example, people with certain blood types are more likely to develop ulcers. Finally, it has been noted that, in countries where children are infected at a very young age, ulcers are uncommon. Possibly, early stimulation of the immune system is important. We know that some diseases, such as the viral disease measles, are worse when acquired after childhood. So there is some precedent for this latter observation.

4. The example of *Neisseria meningitidis* shows that a bacterium that causes serious disease in some people can colonize but not cause disease in many exposed people, but it does not prove that this has to be the case for *H. pylori*. There are a number of differences. Exposure to *N. meningitidis* is uncommon for most people, and the bacteria are carried only transiently. By contrast, most people are exposed to *H. pylori* and will carry the bacteria in their stomachs for the rest of their lives. Meningitis is a much more invasive disease than ulcers and is frequently fatal if untreated, whereas death caused by ulcers—although it does occur—is uncommon, even in untreated people.

5. The O antigen of the *H. pylori* LPS resembles human antigens, the Lewis x and y antigens. Thus, the LPS of *H. pylori* may function to make the bacteria look like "self" rather than "nonself." The LPS of gram-negative bacteria is usually not involved in immune mimicry but is a "signature" used by the body as a signal that bacterial invaders are present.

6. Antibodies in the bloodstream can persist for long periods of time, so finding them does not necessarily mean that the person has an active infection at the time when the test is done. Since most people who are infected carry the infection for life unless they are treated, however, there is some reason to think that a person who is producing anti-*H. pylori* antibodies probably has a current infection. This assumption is more questionable now that antibiotic therapy is used so widely to cure ulcers. People who lose *H. pylori* because of treatment may not be re-infected later. The blood test was used because it was easier and cheaper to do than endoscopic examination of the stomach or cultivation of the bacteria. The ammonia breath test could also have been used as a screening tool.

7. This is still an open question. One guess is that, just as bacteria in biofilms become more resistant to antibiotics, presumably because of their slower metabolic rate, *H. pylori* is in a metabolic state in the mucin layer that makes it somewhat resistant to antibiotics that are effective in vitro. The need for a mixture of antibiotics could also have something to do with the distribution of antibiotic in the stomach and the difficulty of achieving high enough levels of antibiotic in the mucin layer of the stomach, where the bacteria are multiplying.

8. In this chapter, the word "cure" has been used in two ways—something that is true for the literature as well. "Cure" is sometimes used to mean the healing of the ulcer, something that is achieved just as well by the non-antibiotic medications as by the antibiotic combination. In fact, the mixture of compounds administered to ulcer patients usually contains one nonantibiotic component, the job of which is to heal the existing ulcers. This type of cure is short lived, however, because the bacteria are still present. Only if the bacteria are cleared from the site is the patient cured in the sense of no longer having the disease. This second meaning of cure—elimination of symptoms and elimination of the cause of those symptoms—is the way in which most people think of a cure.

9. *H. pylori* is unusual, but probably not unique, in its ability to live in the stomach. It does this, however, not by being able to multiply in a low-pH environment but by invading the mucin layer, something other gastrointestinal pathogens do. In effect, *H. pylori* has become a paradigm model for mucin-dwelling bacteria because scientists in this field have paid attention to the mucin as an environment, whereas scientists interested in other gastrointestinal pathogens have tended to ignore the interactions between the pathogen and the mucus. Possibly the most unique thing about *H. pylori* is its strategy for surviving to reach the mucin layer. It is also possible that *H. pylori* has special virulence and survival traits. Few bacterial pathogens manage to stay in an infected site for decades.

CHAPTER 24

1. The first and second postulates are straightforward to satisfy. As usual, the third postulate is the one causing the problem. *Clostridium difficile* causes disease only under a certain condition—when a change occurs in the colonic

microbiota that makes the microbiota less able to protect the host. So, satisfying Koch's postulates is not as simple as inoculating an animal model with the bacteria; the clostridia have to have conditions that mimic the situation in the colon of a person who is taking antibiotics. There is a hamster model in which the animals are given clindamycin prior to introduction of the bacteria. Another problem that arises is that since the microbiota is obviously playing some role in the disease, it is difficult to sort out what part, if any, of the pathology is caused by the clostridia and what part is caused by the microbiota. Is the microbiota simply playing a passive role by being present in lower numbers than normal, or does it play a more active role?

2. As far as we know, the only people at risk for developing pseudomembranous colitis are those who are taking antibiotics. Health care workers are not at immediate risk but could be considered to be at risk at some point in the future if they had to take the kinds of antibiotics that are associated with the disease.

3. At first, scientists had a hard time accepting pseudomembranous colitis as a disease that is potentially transmitted from person to person. Yet, it is now clear that the bacteria can spread from person to person, probably in the form of spores because the bacteria are so sensitive to oxygen. Also, spores would be more likely to make it through the stomach than vegetative bacteria. What actually spreads, of course, is the bacterium. The disease spreads only in the sense that a condition is set up (colonization by *C. difficile*), which under certain conditions (antibiotic use) can lead to disease. It is emerging in the sense that only recently have the conditions necessary for the disease to develop been in place.

4. This is a real mystery. If prior damage to the colon lining makes it more vulnerable to action by the toxins, then this would explain why only a subset of colonized people develop the serious form of the disease. Person-to-person differences in the type of disease progression could also be due to different strains and different concentrations of the bacteria. A possibility that cannot be ruled out is that a difference in the microbiota other than *C. difficile* makes a contribution.

5. One possible explanation is that toxin B has a different receptor from toxin A, but it is also possible that these toxins differ in susceptibility to bile salts, proteases, or other conditions found in the colon.

6. The most likely explanation is a combination of differences in numbers of patients in the ward and patterns of antibiotic use. More crowding and more patients with diarrhea make it easier to transmit the bacteria to uncolonized patients. The type of antibiotics used is also an important factor, since only certain antibiotics trigger the disease. Another factor is the existence of prior cases of the disease. Studies of surfaces in hospital wards have shown that the clostridial spores can persist in the environment for long periods of time.

7. Patients who do not have the same risk factors will be unaffected by the presence of the bacteria.

8. A vaccine consisting of toxoided toxins A and B might be effective if the toxins could be neutralized. This statement is based on the assumption, however, that the two toxins are the principal virulence factors. If there are other toxins, such a vaccine might not be effective. The most cost-effective way to control pseudomembranous colitis is to prevent it by avoiding use of the antibiotics most likely to trigger it.

9. Metronidazole and vancomycin undoubtedly have effects on the patient's microbiota and could conceivably make the condition more likely if given in combination with clindamycin. Also, there is enough overuse and abuse of antibiotics in hospitals without adding to it. There is general agreement that antibiotics such as vancomycin and metronidazole, which are still effective against some multidrug-resistant pathogens, should be used as little as possible to reduce the selection of bacteria resistant to these antibiotics.

CHAPTER 25

1. Floods, typhoons, and other major disasters that affect the water supply increase the possibility that feces-contaminated water will be used for washing and drinking. The fact that non-O1 strains of *Vibrio cholerae* appear able to cause cholera makes it more difficult to assess a water source for virulent strains of the species. Many *V. cholerae* strains either do not cause disease or cause a mild form of diarrhea. Thus, isolating a member of this species from a water source does not necessarily mean that the water will spread cholera.

2. During a meal, the stomach pH rises somewhat because of the presence of food and drink. The food and drink may help to protect the bacteria transiently. Also, children are more likely than adults to develop achlorhydria (less acidic stomach contents), a condition that makes it more likely that some bacteria will get past the stomach. There is also some evidence that malnutrition can affect the acid barrier of the stomach.

3. The most likely explanation is that the vibrios either do not invade the mucosa very readily or are quickly killed by phagocytic cells in the tissue underlying the intestinal mucosa.

4. This is just a guess, but the A1 subunit may be less able to be translocated or less stable than the full A subunit in the extracellular environment. The A subunit has to enter the host cell cytoplasm in order to act.

5. Although the different strengths of the ribosome binding sites associated with the A and B subunit genes ensure that there is more B made than A, this alone probably does not ensure an exact 1:5 ratio of A to B. Excreting B subunits allows the bacteria to dump excess B subunits.

6. See the text for an explanation of these factors and the roles they play.

7. The copious diarrhea associated with cholera seems to be successful in washing the bacteria out of the site. A person who survives the dehydration will likely survive the disease, which is of limited duration because of the inability of the bacteria to stay in the site.

8. This is a trick question. To answer this question, it would be necessary to know whether the bacteria gain any benefit from producing cholera toxin in the human intestine or whether this toxin is useful in some other location. Usually, a complex set of environmental signals allows the bacteria to produce the virulence factor only in certain specific locations.

9. This is a regulatory trait that makes some of us wonder if cholera toxin is really designed to cause diarrhea in humans or if it serves some other role wherever the vibrios hang out when they are not passing through the human intestine.

10. A live vaccine strain would replicate enough to stimulate the immune system more effectively, making it more likely to produce memory cells. Moreover, whole bacteria act as an adjuvant so that providing adjuvant is less of a problem in vaccine formulation. The problem with the live vaccine strains tested to date, of course, is that so far all the effective ones cause diarrhea. People living in areas where deadly outbreaks of cholera are most likely to occur would probably be willing to overlook this side effect, but in infants (a high-risk group), diarrhea is too dangerous to induce intentionally.

11. Some *Vibrio* species can use cAMP as a carbon source. Conceivably, cholera toxin could allow the bacteria to "farm" eukaryotic cells that have the right receptor for the toxin. In the environment, *V. cholerae* has been found associated with marine invertebrates, and these might be its normal hosts.

CHAPTER 26

1. *Salmonella typhimurium* merely has to colonize the small intestine to cause symptoms. *Salmonella typhi* has to invade the body, get into the bloodstream, and move all over the body in order to cause symptoms. Not surprisingly, people who develop the systemic form of *S. typhimurium* infection also take longer to manifest symptoms of the disease.

2. Today, typhoid fever in developed countries is almost always seen in travelers who have visited countries where the disease is endemic. Typhoid fever is spread by contaminated water or food. In developing countries, typhoid fever is most commonly seen in poor areas that lack a clean water supply, but household servants can spread it to people in higher socioeconomic groups.

3. Not all strains of laboratory mice are equally susceptible to disease caused by *S. typhimurium*, so there are clearly some host genetic factors at work. Two that seem the most likely are the ability of macrophages to kill *S. typhimurium* and the susceptibility to LPS-induced sepsis. The question of why *S. typhi* does not cause disease in mice is still puzzling scientists. It seems unlikely that *S. typhi* is unable to invade, since the bacteria are thought to enter the body through M cells. Possibly, *S. typhi* is killed more effectively by murine macrophages than by human macrophages. Scientists hope that comparisons of the genome sequences of the two species of *Salmonella* will suggest clues. Also, making hybrid *S. typhimurium-S. typhi* strains could shed some light on the problem.

4. If the bacteria enter the body through M cells, a natural conduit past the mucosal layer, they may not need specialized adhesins. The greater effect of eliminating invasin genes is harder to rationalize, unless these invasin genes have multiple roles (e.g., stimulating transit through M cells, stimulating entry into macrophages in such a fashion as to prevent phagosome-lysosome fusion, escaping from a phagosome). The type III systems may be important if they help the bacteria manipulate the activities of phagocytic cells.

5. The rationale was that *Escherichia coli* K-12 and *S. typhimurium* are very similar at the DNA sequence level, so genes unique to *S. typhimurium* might be virulence genes. This type of comparison revealed not so much differences in individual genes as the existence of "islands" containing multiple genes. The advantage of this approach is that it identifies areas of the chromosome for further testing for a role in virulence. The main drawback is that there may be shared genes whose products interact with those of unshared genes to produce a virulence trait.

6. If chromosomal genes are needed for such functions as folding and secretion of proteins encoded by plasmid genes, mutations in chromosomal genes could well have an important effect on virulence, even though the chromosomal genes are actually housekeeping genes.

7. They are trying to separate steps involved in entry of the bacteria into the body through the mucosa from steps involved in spread of the bacteria in the body. If, for example, a mutant is avirulent when introduced by the oral route but is virulent when injected intraperitoneally, the mutation probably affects the initial entry of the bacteria into the body.

8. This is one of the problems that IVET and similar methods were designed to solve. Depending on where in the body a particular fusion is expressed, scientists have been trying—with some success—to determine the gene expression pattern. This information in turn may provide clues about what signals the regulatory genes are sensing and what role the regulatory genes play in helping the bacteria to adjust to different environments encountered in the body.

9. Some people have dismissed drug resistance in *S. typhimurium* (e.g., strains such as DT104) as relatively unimportant because antibiotics are generally not used to treat gastroenteritis. What this argument overlooks is the subset of infected people who go on to develop a systemic form of the disease. Without effective antibiotic therapy, many of these people will die.

CHAPTER 27

1. Presumably, the actin tail does not move as well in the viscous host cell cytoplasm as the bacterium, so the growing actin tail moves the bacterium through the host cell interior. It is worth noting, however, that the physics of this process is far from being understood.

2. ActA could have been a chaperone that helped fold the protein that actually nucleated actin or part of the secretion apparatus that placed the true nucleation protein on the cell surface. ActA could even have been a regulatory protein that controlled synthesis of the true nucleator.

3. They disrupted genes encoding these enzymes and then tested whether such mutations trapped the bacteria in endosomes and, if so, which types. Some very elegant microscopy was done in connection with this work. Also, to test the effect on cell-to-cell spread, the ability of mutants to form plaques on lawns of tissue culture cells was determined.

4. Cloning the gene responsible for this activity was the key to answering both questions. Scientists found that mutants lacking functional ActA did not have this activity and were further able to show that the gene encoded a protein that was localized to the cell surface. Some of this work is described in the references at the end of this chapter. It is still not completely clear whether some host cell protein or proteins might be involved. The availability of an in vitro system for demonstrating actin nucleation should go a long way toward answering the question of whether there is some host protein—other than actin, of course—that participates with ActA in the actin nucleation process.

5. The most likely explanation is that *Listeria monocytogenes* is better able to survive the phagocytic cell defense than *Shigella* spp. The tissue culture cell invasion and actin polymerization assay systems do not take this phase of the infection into account.

6. If *L. monocytogenes* can survive inside phagocytic cells, an opsonizing antibody response would only help the bacteria to get into host cells. Moreover, the toxic enzymes and actin nucleating protein are important inside host cells, whereas antibodies are limited to the extracellular fluid. (There have been reports of internalization of antibodies by host cells under some conditions, but the extent of internalization is almost certainly insufficient to have a significant impact on the development of the disease.) There is no question that effective containment of *L. monocytogenes* requires a cell-mediated response to the bacteria, not an antibody response.

CHAPTER 28

1. Since the virotyping scheme based on adhesins and toxins seems to be a useful way to classify *Escherichia coli* strains according to virulence properties, probes to detect adhesin and toxin genes would be a logical place to start. DNA probes to detect adhesin genes specific for the different virotypes would separate most types, including those that produce no known toxin. ETEC strains could also be identified with probes to detect genes encoding LT and ST. Both types of probe would have to be used because some strains produce LT only, whereas others produce ST only or both LT and ST. The EHEC strains could also be identified with a probe to detect Shigella toxin. If the EAggEC strains prove to produce EAST uniformly, a probe to detect this toxin would be a possible addition to the screening system.

2. Virotyping would complement rather than replace the current serotyping system. The reason it is important to be able to identify individual strains, rather than just virulence types, is that outbreaks of intestinal disease are frequently due to a single strain. Identifying this strain helps to trace the outbreak and identify its source. In the case of EHEC, in which the single strain O157:H7 seems to be causing most current outbreaks of disease associated with HUS, serotyping is particularly important. The strength of the serotyping approach is that it identifies individual strains. Serotypes are often, but not always, associated with a particular virotype. The virotype approach has the strength that it is based on virulence factors and hence is more directly tied to the pathology of the disease than serotyping based on LPS O antigen and flagellar antibodies. On the practical level, the overwhelming advantage of the serotyping approach is that it is currently in place in clinical laboratories and has been extensively tested. A typing test based on virotypes would first have to undergo extensive field testing before it could be trusted for routine use. For this reason, it is questionable whether developing a virotype test for routine clinical screening is worthwhile, given that serotyping works so well.

3. The clinicians' view as stated here (in an extreme form, which is perhaps unfair) is correct insofar as most cases of diarrhea are concerned. If therapy is needed, rehydration therapy works equally well for most types, regardless of the infectious agent that caused the disease. There are two cases in which this view could be contested (both of which are well known to most clinicians). The first case is the EHEC strains, especially O157:H7. This type of diarrhea must be detected early so that antibiotic treatment can be given to prevent HUS, a potentially fatal complication. Equally important is to identify the source of the outbreak as quickly as possible so that further cases can be prevented. A second exception to the assertion that diarrhea need not be diagnosed by identification tests is that serotyping of strains helps to trace the source of outbreaks of diarrhea caused by ETEC and other strains and to signal the appearance of especially virulent strains.

4. The question of why so few serogroups and serotypes of *E. coli* cause intestinal disease is an interesting one that has not been answered. There are two obvious possibilities. One is that there are important factors other than adhesins and toxins that contribute to colonization of the intestinal mucosa. In particular, LPS surface structure could be more important than we think in aiding colonization. This would explain why only certain serogroups cause infections. A second possibility is that differences in LPS structure reflect other differences in cell wall structure that affect productive expression of adhesins necessary to colonize the mucosal surface. Whatever the reason, the strains that are associated with diarrheal disease are a minority of all strains in nature.

5. First, EPEC strains differ from ETEC, EAggEC, and EHEC strains in that they appear not to produce toxins. They probably cause diarrhea by the attaching and effacing effect of their binding to mucosal cells, an effect that is associated with extensive actin rearrangements and triggering of a signal transduction cascade in mucosal cells which affects intracellular Ca^{2+} levels and may affect ion pumps. EPEC strains are more invasive than ETEC and EAggEC strains and cause an inflammatory response when they infect. In this respect, they resemble EHEC and EIEC strains, which also cause an inflammatory response. Compared with EIEC strains, which resemble *Shigella* spp. in their ability to invade and move within the mucosa, EPEC strains are less invasive and may not be capable of cell-to-cell spread.

6. One way is to produce a toxin that impairs the ability of the body to retain water. LT and ST are examples of this type of toxin. The second way to produce diarrhea is to affect mucosal cells so as to prevent water absorption. Failure to absorb water will appear symptomatically as diarrhea. Absorptive capacity can be reduced by direct action of the bacteria, e.g., attachment-effacement by EPEC strains, or it can be reduced indirectly by a host inflammatory response to the bacteria that damages mucosal absorptive cells.

7. This is a question that involves economic and political issues as well as microbiological issues, so only a few comments will be made here about the basis for the debate. Grinding meat introduces bacteria from the surface of the carcass (which is often contaminated by intestinal contents during slaughter) into the interior of the ground meat products. Virtually all ground meat products contain bacteria, including *E. coli*. Thus, monitoring of meat patties would have to focus on particular strains of bacteria. O157:H7 is an obvious candidate. Routine testing of ground meat for O157:H7 would be very expensive. The meat processors correctly point out that such testing would make ground meat products more expensive and that proper cooking is a more inexpensive solution. People in favor of testing argue that this solution is not working in all cases because there have been some outbreaks of O157:H7 which originated in fast-food outlets despite the fact that cooking procedures are supposed to be rigidly standardized in these facilities.

8. Antibiotics, at best, limit the duration of symptoms. At worst, as seems to be the case with *E. coli* O157:H7 and similar EHEC strains, antibiotics might actually make the disease worse. In general, rehydration therapy or other therapies that help the patient survive the acute phase of the disease are sufficient. The decision to use or not use antibiotics ultimately depends on the severity of the symptoms. Travelers, who may be exposed to diarrheagenic strains that cause a debilitating form of diarrhea because the traveler has little or no immunity, may benefit from antibiotics in that the period of illness is shortened.

CHAPTER 29

1. Ascending infections are more common than hematogenous infections in most age groups because a person is more likely to be exposed to bacteria entering the urethra than to have a bloodstream infection. Women are more likely to have urinary tract infections than men, presumably because of their shorter urethra and the proximity of the urethral opening to the bacterial population of the colon. Other predisposing factors are malformations of the urethra that allow puddles of stagnant urine to form or the presence of an indwelling urinary catheter. Having had a previous urinary tract infection could also be considered a predisposing factor because the person is more likely to be harboring a uropathogenic strain of bacteria.

2. People can have asymptomatic bacterial colonization of the bladder. This is seen most often in people with indwelling catheters. To cause symptoms, the bacterium has to elicit an inflammatory response.

3. Some virulence factors, such as the ability to elicit an inflammatory response with LPS or the ability to acquire iron, are important in most body sites. Others, such as

production of the K1 capsule or P pili, seem to be associated with infection of specific sites.

4. Presumably, differences in amino acid sequences of the pilin subunits make it necessary to have a specific secretion system for that particular serotype.

5. For simplicity, consider mutations that abolish the gene product, and assume that the mutations do not have a polar effect on genes that are downstream in the same operon. Loss of a tip protein such as PapG might not stop the formation of pili, but, if formed, the pili would not be able to adhere to their receptor. Loss of the main pilin protein (PapA) would result in no pilin production. Similarly, loss of proteins such as PapC and PapD, proteins that are responsible for secretion of pilin subunits, would lead to a buildup of pilin subunits in the periplasm but would prevent proper assembly of the pilus.

6. Ideally, the antibiotic would not only eliminate the bacteria from the urinary tract (including intracellular bacteria) but would also eliminate the strain from the colon and vaginal tract to prevent reinfection. Also, an antibiotic that is not absorbed into tissues is desirable to prevent possible side effects in areas of the body where the antibiotic is not needed.

7. Any vaccine against urinary tract infections would probably be offered mainly to people in high-risk groups.

8. The K1 antigen is part of a capsule that prevents the bacteria from being phagocytosed. K1 capsule and serum resistance are traits associated with most of the strains of *E. coli* that cause systemic infections. Adherence is not important, as it was for urinary tract infections. LPS is, however, important here too as a mediator of inflammation.

CHAPTER 30

1. Both men and women, but especially women, can acquire a *Neisseria gonorrhoeae* infection without exhibiting symptoms. Not only can such asymptomatic carriers transmit the disease to sexual contacts, but also women can pass the disease to an infant during birth. Finally, women with asymptomatic cervical infections and both women and men with asymptomatic urethral infections can still develop complications of the disease, such as arthritis or damage to the fallopian tubes (pelvic inflammatory disease and ectopic pregnancy). Thus, all people who have had sexual relations with a person who proves to have gonorrhea should seek treatment.

2. To test all women preparing to give birth in order to detect those women whose vaginal tracts contain *N. gonorrhoeae* would be very expensive. Also, since it can take several days for results of the tests to be obtained, the infant could be born and develop an eye infection before the results are available. The eye drops used are safe and very effective. It is thus much easier, cheaper, and safer in the long run to place eye drops in every baby's eyes soon after birth.

3.   This comment is true in one sense. If all cases of gonorrhea (and nongonococcal urethritis, another bacterial disease that can cause fallopian tube scarring and infertility; see chapter 31) were diagnosed and treated early, infertility rates would decrease. An important qualifying term is "early." A woman whose infection has progressed to the stage where pelvic inflammatory disease has occurred has probably sustained enough irreversible fallopian tube damage that antibiotics will not cure infertility, although antibiotics will cure the pelvic inflammatory disease.

4.   Gonorrhea starts as a localized infection of the urethra (in men) or the cervix (in women). The main symptom at this stage is a purulent discharge, though as mentioned in an earlier answer, asymptomatic infections occur commonly in women and are also seen, less commonly, in men. The bacteria can spread to the upper genital tract of women or into the bloodstream. The most common symptom of bloodstream infection is arthritis. Death is rare. By contrast, meningitis is an acute, invasive disease in which the bacteria infect the meninges and spinal fluid. The death rate is high if the infection is not treated. *N. gonorrhoeae* has a variety of virulence factors, including pili, which presumably help the bacteria adhere to the urethra or cervix, outer membrane proteins (PorA and PorB) that may have a role in actin rearrangements, LOS (inflammatory response), and variable surface antigens. The main virulence factor of *N. meningitidis* is its antiphagocytic polysaccharide capsule, but most strains are also serum resistant. The inflammation is probably induced by LOS.

5.   There are a number of bacterial strategies for evading the host's defense systems. Some bacteria try to mimic the host, some bacteria attack immune cells (via toxins), and some bacteria minimize the effectiveness of the host's defense systems (e.g., capsules, iron sequestration systems). *N. gonorrhoeae* has perfected a different strategy, to change its surface antigens often enough to foil the host's immune response. By shedding one form of an essential surface protein, which can be rendered ineffective by binding of antibodies, and substituting another form that is different enough not to be recognized by the same antibodies, the bacteria keep one step ahead of the host's antibody response. The importance of combining phase variation with antigenic variation is that phase variation allows the bacteria to get rid of the no longer useful form of the surface proteins.

6.   Such a strain would not be much affected in its ability to carry out phase variation. Only one type of pilin phase variation, in which a longer form of pilin is made, relies on homologous recombination. Conceivably, the other mechanisms of pilin phase variation could compensate for loss of this one type of variation. A strain unable to carry out homologous recombination would, however, lose the ability to carry out antigenic variation. (A word of caution is in order. This statement is based on our current understanding of mechanisms of antigenic variation. If there are other, as yet undiscovered mechanisms of antigenic variation, these might be revealed if a strain unable to carry out recombination could still undergo antigenic variation. Someone should do the experiment.) A mutant deficient in recombination should still be able to sialylate LOS and would probably be able to vary the oligosaccharide portion of LOS (to become serum resistant), since these reactions involve enzymes rather than replacements of genes by recombination.

7.   The answer provided here is an educated guess. The student is encouraged to be appropriately critical and skeptical of what follows. All that we know about *N. gonorrhoeae* virulence factors suggests that this pathogen relies heavily on changing its surface fast enough to keep one step ahead of the host response. That this strategy is not 100% effective is evident from the fact that PMNs do engulf and destroy many bacteria. Two factors probably affect the outcome of the host-bacterium interaction. One is the number of bacteria introduced into the site. Not all infected people carry and transmit the same number of bacteria. A second factor is the rapidity with which the new host's nonspecific and specific defense systems respond. A healthy person, with a healthy immune system, who is inoculated with a relatively low dose of *N. gonorrhoeae* may well be able to limit the growth of the bacteria before the concentration of bacteria reaches the level at which overt symptoms occur. In women, the ability of the resident microflora of the cervix and vagina to act as a barrier to infection may also play a critical role in the outcome of the initial interaction between the bacteria and the host.

8.   One answer will be given, but there are probably other, equally valid ones. A vaccine would have two important goals. First, since *N. gonorrhoeae* specializes in changing its surface antigens, a vaccine should contain antigens that do not change. Second, the vaccine should prevent bacterial colonization. Once the bacteria have established themselves, the host's inflammatory response does the damage, not bacterial toxins. Thus, in contrast to diphtheria, in which a vaccine targeting a late event in infection (introduction of exotoxin into the bloodstream) is successful in preventing the disease, infections caused by bacteria that cause symptoms by evoking an inflammatory response must be stopped much earlier in the infection process. There are some epitopes of pili and Opa proteins that are not varied. Assuming that these will induce a good antibody response and that they are exposed on the bacterial surface (and not buried in the interior of pili or in the outer membrane in the case of Opa proteins, so that antibodies cannot reach them), such epitopes

could elicit a response that prevents the initial colonization step because of initial binding (pili) and tighter binding (Opa). A potential complication is illustrated by the blocking antibody phenomenon. It is conceivable that binding of antibodies to one epitope of, for example, pili could be protective, whereas binding to another might not be protective (e.g., binding to the shaft, not the adhesive portion). Antibodies are relatively large molecules, and it is possible that antibodies binding to shaft pilin subunits could prevent antibodies to adhesive proteins from binding by being more abundant and by steric hindrance. The point of this question is to encourage the student to appreciate the complications that can arise when scientists try to "rationally design" vaccines. Clearly, the mixture of antibodies produced by most people who are infected with *N. gonorrhoeae* is not effective in preventing the bacteria from colonizing the area and causing symptoms. This suggests that a vaccine must elicit not the "normal" immune response but an sIgA response that targets a subset of antigens that are lost in the "normal" response to the bacteria.

9. As already mentioned in the answers to previous questions, sialylation of LOS not only makes the bacteria resistant to the MAC but also reduces the opsonizing and PMN-attracting activities of complement. The effect of this on vaccine development depends on the way in which a vaccine is designed to act. A vaccine that elicits an sIgA response that blocks adherence of bacteria to target host cells should not be affected by sialylation of LOS, unless sialylation of LOS blocks access of antibodies to bacterial surface proteins. This is more likely to be a problem with Opa proteins, which are embedded in the outer membrane, than with pili. If the goal of a vaccine is to kill bacteria by opsonizing them and amplifying complement killing via the MAC, sialylation of LOS would be a serious problem. As with question 8, the aim of this question is to illustrate how difficult it can be to rationally design vaccines for diseases such as gonorrhea.

CHAPTER 31

1. The replicating form is very fragile; it does not have peptidoglycan and is ill adapted to survival outside a host cell. For the bacteria to be transmitted from cell to cell or from person to person, the tougher elementary bodies (which have cross-linked proteins for cell wall stability) are needed.

2. Antibiotics have to be able to enter into the host cell cytoplasm and into the vesicle in which the RB form is dividing. The low metabolic activity of the EB makes it a much less attractive antibiotic target. A vaccine will have to target the EB, since the RB is inside host cells. This limits options for vaccine development.

3. Chlamydiae have an outer membrane, but they appear not to have peptidoglycan. Instead, in the EB, highly cross-linked membrane proteins (cross-linked with disulfide bonds) give the cell wall rigidity. The RBs are unusual in that they have surface projections that penetrate the membrane of the vesicle in which they are dividing.

4. The usual target of genetic engineering techniques is rapidly dividing cells. This means the RBs, which are inside host cells. It might be possible to introduce foreign DNA into EBs, but in the absence of an active metabolism, the DNA might not be retained.

5. Nongonococcal urethritis is now so widespread that screening and treatment seem more cost-effective than would be the case for gonorrhea. The question boils down to how important one thinks infertility and pelvic inflammatory disease are in the general range of health hazards. There is no vaccine in sight, so screening and treatment are the only viable options for controlling the disease. The availability of new, noninvasive urine tests makes the screening a lot cheaper and easier. If a screening program is implemented, however, it will probably be limited to high-risk populations, such as sexually active teens and young adults.

6. In formulating your answer to this question, keep in mind that most infections in women are asymptomatic in the sense that there is no discernible vaginal discharge. But such infections can nonetheless have serious consequences, such as pelvic inflammatory disease and infertility. The longer the woman delays antibiotic treatment, the more likely these consequences are to occur.

Glossary

Note: Some terms included in this glossary have meanings in fields other than bacterial pathogenesis. This glossary focuses on the way the term is used in bacterial pathogenesis.

A-B toxin   B portion of toxin responsible for binding to target cell is separate from A portion that mediates enzymatic activity

Abscess   localized collection of pus

ACase   see **invasive adenylate cyclase**

Accessory cholera enterotoxin (Ace)   enterotoxin of *Vibrio cholerae;* gene carried on CTX phage

Accessory colonization factor   a protein involved in motility of *Vibrio cholerae*

Accessory gene regulator (Agr)   regulatory system controlling production of surface adhesins and exoproteins in *Staphylococcus aureus*

ace   gene encoding Ace toxin of *Vibrio cholerae*

Ace   see **adhesin of collagen from enterococci**

Ace toxin   see **accessory cholera enterotoxin**

Acellular pertussis vaccine (aP)   subunit form of pertussis vaccine; consists of pertussis toxoid with an additional component which differs depending on manufacturer

Acellular vaccine   vaccine consisting of purified proteins, not whole cells

Acetylcholine   a neurotransmitter molecule whose release is inhibited by botulinum toxin

acf **genes**   genes encoding accessory colonization factor of *Vibrio cholerae*

Achlorhydria   decreased acidity (due to decreased levels of HCl) of the stomach

Acid-fast staining   a harsh staining procedure using the red dye fuchsin; used to stain mycobacteria

Acid tolerance response   bacteria grown at pH 6 for a generation can survive at pH 3; regulated by Fur

acpA   *Bacillus anthracis* gene encoding AcpA; controlled by AtxA

AcpA   protein controlling expression of capsule gene in *Bacillus anthracis*

acr   gene encoding α-crystallin in *Mycobacterium tuberculosis*

actA   gene encoding ActA in *Listeria monocytogenes*

ActA   a surface protein of *Listeria monocytogenes* responsible for actin nucleation

ACTH see **adrenocorticotropic hormone**

Actin a major protein component of host cell cytoskeleton

Actinomycete a member of the group of bacteria that produces many antibiotics

Activated macrophages macrophages with an increased killing capacity due to increased generation of reactive oxygen intermediates and other toxic compounds

Active immunity immunity that develops as a result of an infection or immunization

Acute short and severe illness

Acute endocarditis infection of heart valves characterized by rapid onset of symptoms; high fatality rate; can occur in people with normal heart valves; caused by virulent organisms such as *Staphylococcus aureus*, *Streptococcus pyogenes*, *Neisseria gonorrhoeae*

Acute glomerulonephritis kidney damage following strep throat or skin infections due to *Streptococcus pyogenes*

Acute-phase proteins proteins synthesized in the liver and released during acute phase response; examples are complement proteins, C-reactive protein

Acute-phase response production of a group of serum proteins in response to infection; a form of induced nonspecific immunity

Acute respiratory distress syndrome (ARDS) accumulation of fluid and PMNs in lung; leads to insufficient gas exchange and damage to lung

Acyl-carrier protein reductase enzyme of *Mycobacterium tuberculosis* that catalyzes a step in the synthesis of mycolic acid

ADCC see **antibody-dependent cell-mediated cytotoxicity**

Adenylate cyclase a protein toxin produced by *Bordetella pertussis*; catalyzes synthesis of cAMP

Adhesin of collagen from enterococci (Ace) a collagen-binding protein of *Enterococcus faecalis*

Adhesin tip proteins proteins unique to the tip of pili; mediate binding to host cells; often different from proteins making up shaft of pilus

Adhesins microbial surface components that bind to the host cell receptor

Adjuvant a substance that enhances antigenic stimulus

ADP-ribosylation transfer of ADP-ribosyl group from NAD to host cell protein by a bacterial toxin

ADP-ribosylation factors (ARFs) host proteins that activate cholera toxin in the host cell

Adrenocorticotropic hormone (ACTH) hormone produced by pituitary gland; stimulates production of glucocorticoids by adrenal gland

Aerobactin a siderophore of *Escherichia coli*

Aerobic oxygen is terminal electron acceptor

Aerosol a fine mist

Aerotolerant anaerobes that can survive in an aerobic environment

afa **genes** genes encoding afimbrial adhesins (AFA) in *Escherichia coli*

AFA-I and AFA-III afimbrial adhesins produced by some uropathogenic strains of *Escherichia coli*

Affinity strength of interaction between an antigen-binding site and an epitope

Afimbrial adhesins surface proteins of bacteria important for adhesion but not organized in piluslike structures

agf **genes** genes encoding thin aggregative fimbriae (curli) of *Salmonella* species

Agglutination clumping of cells by specific antibody

AGN acute glomerulonephritis; causes damage to glomeruli of kidney; can be associated with infections by *Streptococcus pyogenes*

agr **genes** see **accessory gene regulator**

AgrB membrane protein that secretes AgrD in *Staphylococcus aureus*

AgrC component of two-component regulatory system of *Staphylococcus aureus*

AgrD precursor of autoinducer thiolactone in *Staphylococcus aureus*

ail attachment and invasion locus; encodes an invasion protein in *Yersinia* species

alg **genes** genes encoding alginate biosynthetic enzymes and regulators of their synthesis

Algae photosynthetic eukaryotic microbes

AlgB protein required for high-level synthesis of alginate

algC gene encoding phosphomannomutase

algD gene encoding GDP mannose dehydrogenase, the first enzyme in alginate biosynthesis

Alginate polysaccharide coating of *Pseudomonas aeruginosa*

AlgP, R components of a protein complex that regulates alginate synthesis

AlgQ sensor component of two-component regulatory system that regulates alginate synthesis

algS,T genes encoding switch allowing *Pseudomonas aeruginosa* to go from mucoid to nonmucoid state

AlgU protein involved in alginate synthesis; has amino acid sequence similar to that of sigma factors

Alpha-hemolysin enzyme that lyses red blood cells

Alpha-hemolysis partial hemolysis of red blood cells in blood agar plates; characterized by greenish color in area surrounding bacterial colonies

Alpha-hemolytic streptococci a group of streptococci that are part of the normal biota of the mouth

α_1-**Proteinase inhibitor** protease inhibitor normally present in host tissue

Alpha-toxin (i) exoprotein produced by *Staphylococcus aureus* that forms pores in human cell membranes; (ii) exotoxin produced by *Clostridium perfringens* that hydrolyzes lecithin in human cell membranes

Alternative pathway nonspecific immunity in which complement components bind to receptors on the bacterial surface

Alum an aluminum salt used as an adjuvant; only adjuvant currently used in the United States

Alveolar macrophage unactivated macrophage fixed in the alveoli of the lung

Alveolus terminal saclike structure of the lung

Aminoglycosides a family of antibiotics that bind to the 30S ribosomal subunit and inhibit protein synthesis; includes kanamycin, gentamicin

Ammonia breath test test to detect ammonia produced by urease of *Helicobacter pylori* in infected patients

Anaerobic growth under conditions lacking oxygen

Anergy loss of reactivity to an antigen

Animal model a species of animal that develops a disease similar to that in humans infected with the same organism

Antibiotic a low-molecular-weight compound that can inhibit growth of or kill microorganisms

Antibiotic resistance ability of bacteria to grow in the presence of antibiotics that would normally inhibit their growth or kill them

Antibiotic-resistant bacteria bacteria that are not killed or inhibited by antibiotics

Antibiotic tolerance ability of bacteria to survive antibiotic treatment although they are unable to divide while the antibiotic is present

Antibody an immunoglobulin molecule that interacts with an antigen

Antibody-dependent cell-mediated cytotoxicity (ADCC) infected cells coated with IgG allowing phagocytes to attach; phagocytes kill infected cells by bombarding them with toxic compounds

Antigen (i) substance (protein, lipid, or carbohydrate) that can interact with the antigen-binding sites of a specific antibody; (ii) portion of a foreign object that is displayed on MHC-I or MHC-II (see **immunogen**)

Antigen-binding site portion of the Fab region of an antibody that binds to a specific antigenic determinant

Antigen 85 complex protein complex secreted by *Mycobacterium tuberculosis* that transfers mycolic acid molecules onto cell wall polysaccharides; possible drug target

Antigen-presenting cell (APC) a cell, such as a macrophage, that engulfs a microbe or its products, degrades it, and presents the resulting peptides on its surface

Antigenic determinant site on an antigen that binds to the antigen-binding site of an antibody

Antigenic variation ability of some bacteria to change the amino acid composition of their adhesins or other surface proteins

Antiseptic antimicrobial compounds applied to skin

Antiserum serum containing antibodies against a specific antigen

Antitoxin antibody specific for a toxin

aP see **acellular pertussis vaccine**

APC see **antigen-presenting cell**

Apical surface portion of an epithelial cell exposed to the lumen

Apoptosis programmed cell death; occurs normally in mammalian cells but can be induced prematurely by some microbes or prevented by others; characterized by condensation of chromatin at boundary of nucleus

Arabinogalactan-lipid complex glycolipid component of mycobacterial cell wall

Arachidonic acid precursor of leukotrienes; component of inflammatory cascade

Archaea prokaryotic microbes that are members of a domain separate from the bacteria; along with bacteria, they were the first forms of life to appear on Earth

ARDS acute respiratory distress syndrome; may occur as a result of septic shock

ARFs see **ADP-ribosylation factors**

Ascending infection urinary tract infection in which the bacteria colonize the urethra and then move up to the bladder; bacteria may continue to move up to the kidney

Aseptic free of microorganisms

Aspiration process in which fluids are introduced into or removed from body cavities

Asymptomatic carrier a person colonized by disease-causing bacteria who does not have disease symptoms

att **site** see **attachment site**

Attaching and effacing distortion of microvilli due to extensive rearrangement of host cell actin by EPEC strains

Attachment and invasion locus see *ail*

Attachment site (i) site on integrons at which integrase integrates circular DNA segments; (ii) DNA sequences involved in phage integration into chromosome

Attenuation (i) genetic regulation that involves RNA secondary structure; (ii) decrease in virulence of microorganisms used in a vaccine

AtxA, R regulatory proteins that control expression of genes for lethal toxin and edema toxin in *Bacillus anthracis*; AtxA also controls expression of *acpA*

Atypical pneumonia a type of pneumonia in which the pattern of density on radiograms of infected lungs is patchy and diffuse

Autoimmune disease disease that occurs when immune system recognizes a host molecule as foreign

Autolysins enzymes produced by bacteria which digest peptidoglycan and can cause lysis of bacteria

Autophagy   process by which components of mammalian cytoplasm or organelles are surrounded by endoplasmic reticulum and slated for destruction or recycling

Auxotroph   a microorganism that has lost the ability to synthesize an essential nutrient

Avidity   combination of affinity and valence; a measure of the strength of binding of antigen to antibody

Avr proteins   bacterial proteins recognized by plant R proteins that trigger the plant hypersensitive response

Axial filaments   internal flagella of spirochetes located between cytoplasmic membrane and outer membrane

Azithromycin   a macrolide antibiotic

B7   macrophage surface protein required for binding to receptor on T cell

B lymphocyte (B cell)   cell type that produces antibodies

BabA   surface adhesin that mediates attachment of *Helicobacter pylori* to Lewis b antigen on epithelial cells

Bacillus   rod-shaped bacterium

Bacitracin   antibiotic that inhibits cell wall synthesis by interfering with recycling of bactoprenol

Bacteremia   bacteria present in the bloodstream

Bacteria   microbes that, along with archaea, were the first forms of life on Earth

Bacterial sexually transmitted diseases   bacterial infections transmitted by sexual intercourse

Bacterial vaginosis   shift in the vaginal microbiota from a predominantly gram-positive population dominated by *Lactobacillus* species to mostly gram-negative anaerobes

Bactericidal   substance that kills bacteria

Bacteriophage   virus that infects bacteria

Bacteriostatic   substance that inhibits the growth of bacteria but does not kill them

Bacteriuria   bacteria present in the urine

Bands   immature forms of PMNs released in response to infection

Basal lamina   the basement membrane of tissues to which epithelial cells attach; made up of glycoproteins

Basal surface   portion of epithelial cells attached to basal lamina

Basolateral surface   the side and bottom portion of epithelial cells in a confluent monolayer; portions in contact with extracellular matrix

bcg   former name of *Nramp1*

BCG   bacillus Calmette-Guérin; attenuated *Mycobacterium* strain used as a vaccine to prevent tuberculosis; stimulates activated macrophage response

β-Galactosidase (LacZ)   an enzyme commonly used as a reporter group

β-Glucuronidase (GUS)   an enzyme commonly used as a reporter group

Beta-hemolytic   complete hemolysis of red blood cells in blood agar; area around bacterial colonies is clear

β-Integrins   proteins on surface of PMNs and other human cell types; bind to intercellular adhesion molecules on endothelial cells; binding stops movement of PMNs through the bloodstream

β-Lactam antibiotics   antibiotics that contain a β-lactam ring and act by inhibiting peptidoglycan synthesis; include penicillins, cephalosporins, carbapenems, and monobactams

β-Lactamase   an enzyme that cleaves the β-lactam ring of β-lactam antibiotics and thus inactivates them

β-Phage   temperate bacteriophage that carries the gene encoding diphtheria toxin

Bfp   see **bundle-forming pilus**

bfpA   gene encoding a subunit of Bfp

Bile solubility   bile activates autolysins, which digest peptidoglycan; used as test for pneumococci

Biofilm   multilayer bacterial populations embedded in a polysaccharide matrix that is attached to some surface (plastic, mucosal membrane)

Bioterrorism   use of microbes or toxins to disrupt normal societal functions

Blocking   process in which *Yersinia pestis* cells agglutinate and form a plug that prevents flea from feeding

Blocking antibodies   antibodies that are not bactericidal but bind to bacterial surface and prevent binding of antibodies (to different antigens) that are bactericidal

Blood-brain barrier   membrane covering of brain and spinal cord (meninges); prevents substances in blood from entering central nervous system

Bone marrow stem cell   precursor cells from which PMNs and macrophages descend

Botulinum toxin (botox)   neurotoxin produced by *Clostridium botulinum*; seven serotypes (A, B, C1, D, E, F, G)

Bubo   swollen lymph node resulting from an inflammatory response to *Yersinia pestis* proliferating in lymph node

Bubonic plague   the stage of plague characterized by buboes

Bullous impetigo   skin infection caused by *Staphylococcus aureus*; characterized by blisterlike lesions

Bundle-forming pilus (Bfp)   (i) ETEC adhesin (CFA/III) localized to one end of cell; (ii) a variant of a type 4 pilus formed by *Neisseria gonorrhoeae*

bvgA,S   *Bordetella* virulence genes; encode a two-component regulatory system

C3   a complement component that is cleaved proteolytically to C3a and C3b

C5   a complement component that is cleaved proteolytically to C5a and C5b

C3 convertase   C3bBb or C1C2bC4b, complexes that convert C3 to C3a and C3b

C5 convertase   C3 convertase plus C3b; a complex that converts C5 to C5a and C5b

C domain   catalytic portion of diphtheria toxin

C4-homoserine lactone (C4-HSL) an autoinducer produced by *Pseudomonas aeruginosa;* activates protein involved in glycolipid synthesis

C-reactive protein protein that appears in serum in response to inflammation

C2 toxin toxin produced by *Clostridium botulinum;* ADP-ribosylates actin

C3 toxin toxin produced by *Clostridium botulinum;* ADP-ribosylates G protein

C3a a complement component that results from the proteolytic cleavage of C3; acts as a vasodilator

C5a a complement component that results from the proteolytic cleavage of C5; acts as a chemoattractant for PMNs

C5a peptidase an enzyme produced by *Streptococcus pyogenes* that degrades C5a

Caco-2 cells human cell line derived from a colon carcinoma

caf1 gene encoding capsular antigen fraction 1

cag island pathogenicity island of *Helicobacter pylori* containing 31 genes involved in a type IV secretion system; associated with virulence

Calmodulin mammalian protein required to activate the *Bordetella pertussis* adenylate cyclase; normally involved in Ca^{2+} binding

cap genes genes encoding capsule proteins in a variety of bacteria

Capsular antigen fraction 1 protein that forms antiphagocytic fibrillar structure on surface of *Yersinia pestis*

Capsule fibrous network (usually polysaccharide) that covers the cell wall of some bacteria; often antiphagocytic

Carbapenem a class of β-lactam antibiotics

Cardiolipin lipid found in mammalian mitochondrial membranes; used as basis for Wassermann test (nonspecific test for syphilis)

Cardiotoxin toxin that targets heart cells

Carrier apparently healthy person who harbors and sheds pathogenic microorganisms

Caseous necrosis tissue necrosis that has a cheeselike consistency; occurs in tuberculosis

cat gene encoding chloramphenicol acetyltransferase (CAT); used as a reporter gene

CAT see **chloramphenicol acetyltransferase**

Cat scratch disease new-old disease caused by *Bartonella henselae*

Catalase enzyme that converts superoxide to water; also activates isoniazid, an antituberculosis drug

Catechol a class of siderophore

Catheter tube for draining fluids from or introducing them into body cavities or blood

C3b a complement component that results from the proteolytic cleavage of C3; opsonizes bacteria; part of C3 convertase

C5b complement component that results from the proteolytic cleavage of C5; binds to bacterial surface; recruits C6-C9 to form membrane attack complex

CbpA see **choline binding protein A**

CD1 molecule on surface of antigen-presenting cells that presents lipid or glycolipid antigens

CD4 surface protein of T-helper cells

CD8 surface protein of cytotoxic T cells

CD14 receptor on monocytes and macrophages that binds the LPS-LPS binding protein complex

Cdc42 G protein targeted by toxins A and B of *Clostridium difficile*

cDNA DNA made using RNA as a template; reverse transcribed from message of interest

Cell line eukaryotic cells that have been "immortalized" so that they continue to divide

Cell-mediated immunity (CMI) acquired immunity due to T cells and activated macrophages; does not involve antibodies

Cephalosporins a class of β-lactam antibiotics

Ceramide lipid a component of human cell surface glycoprotein G_{M1}; G_{M1} serves as a receptor for some bacterial toxins

CFA/I and CFA/II see **colonization factor antigens I and II**

CFA/III see **bundle-forming pilus**

CFTR see **cystic fibrosis transmembrane conductance regulation**

cGMP cyclic GMP; a signaling molecule

C3H SCID a strain of severely immunocompromised mice

Chancre primary lesion of syphilis; localized area of necrosis

Chang conjunctival epithelial cells epithelial cell line

Chaperone protein that aids in folding of secreted proteins after translation

Checkerboard hybridization DNA probe technique that permits rapid screening for many different bacterial species at once

Chelocardin an antibiotic in the tetracycline family that acts by disrupting the function of the cytoplasmic membrane

Chemokines proteins produced by many human cell types; organize activities of cells of specific and nonspecific defenses

Chemotaxis movement of bacteria toward a particular substance; movement away from a repellant

Chemotherapy treatment of disease with drugs

Chloramphenicol acetyltransferase (CAT) (i) enzyme used as a reporter group in transcriptional fusions; (ii) enzyme that inactivates chloramphenicol by adding an acetyl group

CHO cells Chinese hamster ovary cells

Cholera severe diarrheal disease caused by *Vibrio cholerae*

Cholera toxin A-B exotoxin produced by *Vibrio cholerae* which ADP-ribosylates a G protein that activates adenylate cyclase

Choline binding protein A (CbpA) surface protein of *Streptococcus pneumoniae* that attaches to choline residues on LTA

Chromogenic substrate a substrate that changes color on plates or in liquid medium if acted on by an enzyme

Cilia surface structures of eukaryotic cells that move mucus over surfaces

Ciliated cells mucosal cells that have cilia on their apical surfaces; found among the cells lining respiratory tract and fallopian tubes

Classical pathway complement pathway that is activated by antigen-antibody complexes or mannose-collectin

Classical strain the O1 strain of *Vibrio cholerae* first associated with pandemics

Clavulanic acid an inhibitor of β-lactamase; added to many modern β-lactam preparations

CMI see **cell-mediated immunity**

CMP-*N*-acetylneuraminic acid an activated form of *N*-acetylneuraminic (sialic) acid in human blood used by *Neisseria gonorrhoeae* cells to sialylate LOS; bacteria become serum resistant

CNF-1 see **cytotoxic necrotizing factor 1**

Coagulase an extracellular or cell surface enzyme of *Staphylococcus aureus* that causes plasma to clot (coagulate); also called clumping factor

Coagulase-negative staphylococci (CNS) strains of staphylococci, such as *Staphylococcus epidermidis* and *Staphylococcus saprophyticus*, that do not produce coagulase

Coagulation pathway series of steps leading to the formation of clots; some components contribute to hypotension, shock

Coccus sphere-shaped bacterium

Coiling phagocytosis a form of phagocytosis by which *Legionella* is sometimes engulfed by amoebae and human macrophages

Colitis inflammation of the colon

Collectin calcium-binding lectins that bind mannose on surface of bacteria; activate classical complement pathway

Colonization ability of a bacterium to remain at a particular site and multiply there

Colonization factor antigens I and II different types of pili produced by ETEC

Colony discrete mass of cells derived from a single cell

Columnar cells tall, thin epithelial cells

Combinatorial chemistry process in which new antibiotics are produced by adding a large variety of chemical groups to a known core compound

Competence ability of some bacteria to take up free DNA (natural transformation)

Complement see **complement system**

Complement cascade proteolytic cleavage of complement components producing activated forms of the proteins which attract phagocytes, cause lysis of gram-negative bacteria, and opsonize bacteria

Complement system group of plasma proteins that mediate the inflammatory response when activated

Complementation protein produced from a gene provided in *trans*; can be used to determine whether two different mutants with the same phenotype are due to mutations in the same gene

Congenital syphilis syphilis acquired by a fetus from its mother; bacteria transmitted transplacentally

Conjugate vaccine polysaccharide covalently linked to protein; forces polysaccharide to be processed as a protein through T-cell-dependent pathway

Conjugation transfer of DNA from one bacterium to another via a conjugation bridge; process involves a type IV secretion system

Conjugative plasmid one that carries genes encoding proteins needed for the conjugation process

Conjugative transposons transposons that can transfer themselves by conjugation from the genome of the donor to the genome of the recipient

Conjunctivitis inflammation of membranes of eyes and eyelids

Cord factor mycolic acids from cell walls of *Mycobacterium* sp.

Corticotropin-releasing factor (CRF) factor released by hypothalamus in response to stress; causes pituitary gland to produce adrenocorticotropic hormone

CovR/S two-component regulatory system in *Streptococcus pneumoniae* that controls expression of genes responsible for capsule synthesis, streptolysins, and streptokinase

cpa gene encoding collagen-binding proteins of *Streptococcus pyogenes*

CpxA, R two-component regulatory system of *Escherichia coli* that prevents buildup of improperly folded pilus proteins in periplasm

CR3 a receptor on PMNs

CRF see **corticotropin-releasing factor**

CRP see **cysteine-rich protein**

α-Crystallin a protein chaperone synthesized by *Mycobacterium tuberculosis* in stationary phase; possible persistence factor

CS see **colonization factor antigens I and II**

CTX phage filamentous phage carrying *ctx* genes of *Vibrio cholerae*

ctxA, ctxB genes encoding the two components of cholera toxin

Cuboidal cells cube-shaped mammalian epithelial cells

Culture microorganisms growing in liquid or on solid medium

Curli pili found on strains of *Escherichia coli* that infect animals; similar to GVVPQ fimbriae of EAEC; also found in *Salmonella typhimurium*

Cutaneous anthrax form of anthrax acquired through cuts in skin; characterized by lesion with black center surrounded by edema (eschar)

cya gene encoding edema factor of *Bacillus anthracis*

Cyanobacteria photosynthetic bacteria that introduced sufficient oxygen into the atmosphere to allow oxygen-consuming forms of life to evolve; sometimes produce toxins

Cyanotic having bluish discoloration of skin due to lack of O_2 in the blood

Cysteine-rich protein a type of protein found in the outer membrane of the elementary body of *Chlamydia trachomatis*; provides stability to cell wall

Cystic fibrosis disease caused by defect in chloride secretion; characterized by production of thick mucus in lungs

Cystic fibrosis transmembrane conductance regulator (CFTR) chloride channel protein to which *Pseudomonas aeruginosa* adheres; gene mutated in people with cystic fibrosis

Cystitis infection of the urinary bladder

Cytadherence attachment of *Mycoplasma pneumoniae* to ciliated respiratory cells; mediated by specialized cytadherence organelle

Cytokines signaling proteins produced by some mammalian cells in response to stimuli; mediators of inflammation, septic shock

Cytoskeleton complex array of cytoplasmic proteins that give shape to eukaryotic cells

Cytotoxic necrotizing factor 1 (CNF-1) toxin produced by some uropathogenic strains of *Escherichia coli*; role in urinary tract infections not determined

Cytotoxic T cells T cells (with CD8 antigen on their surfaces) that kill host cells displaying foreign antigens on their surfaces

Cytotoxin a toxin that kills mammalian cells

DAEC see **diffusely adhering *Escherichia coli***

Dalfopristin a streptogramin antibiotic

Dam-mediated methylation methylation of GATC sites on DNA; determines whether activators bind to DNA in *pap* gene regulation

Database search search for sequence similarity of a given gene or protein to sequences on file in databases

DbpA see **decorin-binding proteins**

Debilitation loss of health

Debride remove dead tissue

Decorin-binding proteins surface proteins of *Borrelia burgdorferi*; produced by bacteria in human body

Defensins small lysosomal peptides that kill bacteria

degP gene encoding a protease that degrades improperly folded proteins in the periplasm during synthesis of P fimbriae in uropathogenic *Escherichia coli*

Degradative enzymes lysosomal proteins, e.g., proteases and lysozyme, that destroy bacterial surface components

Dendritic cells cells that process invading bacteria, display their antigens, and activate specific defenses; covered with projections resembling the dendrites of neurons

Derivative toxin toxic portion of botulinum toxin (see **progenitor toxin**)

Dermis connective tissue below epidermis of skin

Dermonecrotic toxin (pertussis heat-labile toxin) toxin produced by *Bordetella pertussis*; causes skin lesions when injected into mice

Desmoglein-1 (Dsg-1) protein on surface of epithelial cells; maintains keratinocyte cell-cell adhesion

Desmosomes protein structures that hold epithelial cells to dermis layer

Dexamethasone anti-inflammatory steroid; administered along with β-lactam antibiotics to treat pneumococcal meningitis; reduces brain damage

Diarrhea abnormal fluidity of stool due to secretion of water (secretory diarrhea) or impaired absorption of water (cytopathic diarrhea)

DIC see **disseminated intravascular coagulation**

Diffusely adhering *Escherichia coli* (DAEC) a type of diarrheagenic *E. coli*

Diphthamide derivative of histidine found in mammalian EF-2 which is ADP-ribosylated by diphtheria toxin

Diphtheria toxin toxin produced by *Corynebacterium diphtheriae*; ADP-ribosylates mammalian EF-2

Diphtheria toxin regulation protein (DtxR) regulatory protein of *Corynebacterium diphtheriae* that mediates iron regulation of diphtheria toxin gene expression

Diplococci cocci arranged in pairs, e.g., pneumococci

Disease an infection that causes symptoms

Disinfectant antimicrobial compound applied to inanimate objects

Disseminated intravascular coagulation (DIC) formation of numerous small clots that obstruct peripheral blood vessels; a symptom of septic shock

DNA-bending protein protein that binds and causes DNA to bend

DNA sequence database resource containing sequences of bases in DNA from many sources

Dot (defect in organelle trafficking) a component of the type IV secretion system of *Legionella pneumophila*

***dot* genes** genes encoding Dot in *Legionella pneumophila*

Dr   adhesin on uropathogens that binds the Dr blood group antigen

dsbA   gene encoding disulfide-forming enzyme; important in maturation of periplasmic enzymes

Dsg-1   see **desmoglein-1**

DTP (or DTaP) vaccine   trivalent vaccine against diphtheria, tetanus, and pertussis

dtxR   gene encoding DtxR

DtxR   see **diphtheria toxin regulation protein**

Dysentery   a type of diarrhea in which stools contain blood and mucus

eae **genes**   genes encoding proteins involved in the attachment and effacement process caused by EPEC

EAggEC   see **enteroaggregative** *Escherichia coli*

EAST   see **enteroaggregative ST**

Ectopic pregnancy   fetus starts developing in blocked fallopian tube instead of uterus; can be fatal

Edema   excessive fluid in the tissues

Edema factor   A (active) portion of edema toxin of *Bacillus anthracis;* has adenylate cyclase activity; activated by calmodulin

Edema toxin   A-B protein toxin of *Bacillus anthracis* that causes edema seen in cutaneous anthrax

Edible vaccines   plants that have been genetically modified to produce a microbial vaccine protein

EF-2   see **elongation factor-2**

Efflux mechanism   cytoplasmic membrane protein pump mediates resistance to tetracycline, macrolides, and quinolones by pumping them out of the bacterial cytoplasm

Efflux pump   see **efflux mechanism**

EHEC   see **enterohemorrhagic** *Escherichia coli*

EIEC   see **enteroinvasive** *Escherichia coli*

El Tor   the O1 strain of *Vibrio cholerae* associated with some cholera pandemics

Elastase   enzyme that degrades elastin, a component of the mammalian extracellular matrix; may be important in causing lung damage during *Pseudomonas aeruginosa* infections

Elastin   protein that accounts for 30% of protein in lung tissue; also part of blood vessel walls

Electroporation   introduction of DNA or proteins into a bacterial cell by using a sudden increase in electric field to transiently increase the permeability of cells

Elementary body   metabolically inactive survival form of *Chlamydia* species; infective form

Elongation factor-2   protein that plays essential role in host cell protein synthesis; target of diphtheria toxin

Emerging infectious diseases   new diseases that appear; often due to increased human contact with microbe that has been around for years

Endemic   disease continually present at low levels in the community

Endocarditis   inflammation of heart valves

Endocytosis   engulfment of extracellular material into a vacuole (also called endosome or vesicle) by a eukaryotic cell

Endosymbiont   microbe that lives inside the cells of its symbiotic partner

Endothelium   layer of cells lining blood vessels, lymphatic vessels, and the heart

Endotoxin   see **lipopolysaccharide**

ent **genes**   genes encoding the enterotoxins of *Staphylococcus aureus*

Enteric   relating to the gastrointestinal tract

Enteroaggregative *Escherichia coli*   strain of *E. coli* that causes a persistent form of diarrhea in children; has a distinctive patchy pattern of adherence

Enteroaggregative ST   an ST-like toxin produced by EAggEC

Enterobactin   a siderophore of uropathogenic and other *Escherichia coli* strains

Enterococci   gram-positive cocci once considered members of group D streptococci; now part of genus *Enterococcus*

Enterohemorrhagic *Escherichia coli* **(E. coli O157:H7)**   strains of *E. coli* that cause dysenterylike disease but rarely invade host cells; produce Shiga toxin; may cause HUS

Enteroinvasive *Escherichia coli*   strains of *E. coli* that cause disease indistinguishable from dysentery caused by *Shigella;* invasive; do not cause HUS; invade epithelial cells

Enteropathogenic *Escherichia coli*   strains of *E. coli* that produce ultrastructural changes in small intestinal mucosal cells; cause infant diarrhea

Enterotoxigenic *Escherichia coli*   strains of *E. coli* that produce two toxins, one a choleralike toxin (LT) and the other a peptide hormone-like toxin (ST)

Enterotoxin   an exotoxin that acts specifically on the intestinal mucosa

Epa   collagen-binding protein on surface of *Streptococcus pyogenes*

EPEC   see **enteropathogenic** *Escherichia coli*

Epidemic   disease which appears sporadically and affects many individuals in a community

Epidermal growth factor (EGF)   mammalian hormone that stimulates growth and differentiation of mammalian cells

Epidermal growth factor receptor (EGFR)   host cell receptor for EGF; EGF binding to EGFR activates signal transduction cascade

Epidermis   outermost layer of skin; composed of layers of stratified squamous epithelial cells

Epinephrine   substance produced by adrenal glands; suppresses immune activities

Epithelia   layers of cells that cover the surface of the body and line body cavities

Epitope   portion of an antigen recognized by an antibody binding site; five to seven amino acids in the case of protein antigens

erm **genes**   genes conferring resistance to macrolides, streptogramins, and lincosamides

ermA,B,F,G   genes encoding an rRNA methylase that confers resistance to macrolides, streptogramins, and lincosamides

Erps   see **OspE-related proteins**

Erythema   reddening of the skin; may be rashlike

Erythema migrans   ring-shaped rash of Lyme disease that expands and moves outward from site of inoculation; common early symptom of Lyme disease

Eschar   black necrotic lesion surrounded by edema; characteristic of cutaneous anthrax

Escherichia coli **K-12**   a nonvirulent strain of *E. coli* often used in research laboratories

Escherichia coli **O157:H7**   see **enterohemorrhagic** *Escherichia coli*

ETA   exfoliative toxin of *Staphylococcus aureus* that cleaves desmoglein-1 of epidermal cells; creates a scalded or blistered appearance

ETEC   see **enterotoxigenic** *Escherichia coli*

Ethambutol   antibiotic effective against mycobacteria; probably inhibits mycolic acid synthesis

ETs   exfoliative toxins of *Staphylococcus aureus*

Eukaryotes   organisms in which DNA is enclosed in a nuclear membrane

Exfoliative toxins   dermolytic exotoxins produced by *Staphylococcus aureus*; cause symptoms of scalded skin syndrome; bullous impetigo; one type cleaves desmoglein-1, which holds keratinocytes together

Exoenzymes S, U (ExoS, ExoU)   toxins produced by *Pseudomonas aeruginosa*; introduced into host cells by type III secretion system

Exotoxin   protein toxin produced by bacteria; usually secreted into the extracellular fluid but can be intracellular or injected directly into eukaryotic cells

Exotoxin A   toxin produced by *Pseudomonas aeruginosa*; has same mechanism of action as diphtheria toxin

Exotoxin α   protein toxin produced by *Clostridium perfringens*; see **lecithinase**

ExPEC   strains of *Escherichia coli* that cause extraintestinal infections

Extracellular matrix   protein-polysaccharide material in which mammalian cells are embedded; contains collagen, hyaluronic acid, elastin, etc.

Extravasation   see **transmigration**

Exudate   fluid, cells, and debris that have oozed through tissues into a cavity or surface; usually a result of inflammation

F   component of leukocidin of *Staphylococcus aureus*; ADP-ribosylates phosphatidylinositol

F1   capsular protein of *Yersinia pestis*

F1 and F2   surface adhesin proteins produced by *Streptococcus pyogenes*; bind fibronectin

Fab   portion of an antibody that contains the two antigen-binding sites

Facet cells   see **umbrella cells**

Factor-activating ExoS (FAS)   former name of 14-3-3 zeta protein, a host protein that activates exoenzyme S of *Pseudomonas aeruginosa*

Facultative   bacteria that can use either fermentation or respiration to obtain energy, depending on whether or not oxygen is present

FAS   see **factor-activating ExoS**

Fast killing   *Pseudomonas aeruginosa* grown in high-salt medium produces phenazine; kills *Caenorhabditis elegans* in 24 h

Fc   portion of an antibody that binds complement component C1 and surface receptors of phagocytes; mediates opsonization; region of antibody bound by some streptococcal and staphylococcal surface proteins

Febrile   having a fever

Ferric uptake repressor (Fur)   repressor protein that controls iron-regulated genes in many bacteria

Ferritin   intracellular iron storage protein of mammalian cells

Fha   see **filamentous hemagglutinin**

Fibrin   protein involved in formation of blood clots

Fibronectin   protein found on surface of many host cells

Fibronectin-binding proteins (FnBP)   staphylococcal and streptococcal surface proteins that bind fibronectin

Fibronectin-binding proteins F1 and F2   surface proteins of *Streptococcus pyogenes* that bind fibronectin

Filamentous hemagglutinin (Fha)   an adhesin produced by *Bordetella pertussis*; component of acellular pertussis vaccine

Fim2, 3   types of pili produced by *Bordetella pertussis*

fim **genes**   genes encoding type 1 fimbriae of *Salmonella* species and *Escherichia coli*

Fimbriae   short, thin fibrils on surface of bacteria; pili

FimF and FimG   components of the tip of type 1 pili of UPEC

FimH   the adhesin of the type 1 pili of UPEC that binds globobiose

flaA   gene in *Helicobacter pylori* encoding FlaA; regulated by sigma factor 28

FlaA, B   protein subunits of the flagella of *Helicobacter pylori*

flaB   gene in *Helicobacter pylori* encoding FlaB; regulated by sigma factor 54

FlaEDBA   protein subunits of the flagella of *Vibrio cholerae*; controlled by different sigma factors

***flaEDBA* genes**　genes encoding FlaEDBA

Flagella　rodlike protein structures projecting from cell; responsible for motility

flgE　gene encoding the hook protein of flagella of *Helicobacter pylori*

Flora　microorganisms normally residing in a particular area of the body

Fluoroquinolone　a member of the quinolone family of antibiotics

FnBP　see **fibronectin-binding protein**

Follicles　patches of M cells and associated immune cells found in intestinal epithelium

Food-borne infection　infection acquired from ingesting food contaminated with microbes

Foodnet　surveillance program to monitor cases of *Salmonella* and *Campylobacter* food-borne infection

Freund's adjuvant　mixture of oil and other components, including mycobacterial cell walls; used to stimulate antibody response to protein antigens

fsr　gene of *Enterococcus faecalis* that encodes proteins which control other genes that encode gelatinase and a serine protease

Fuchsin　red dye used in acid-fast staining procedure

Fur　see **ferric uptake repressor**

G proteins　GTP hydrolyzing proteins that regulate many aspects of eukaryotic cell function

gacA,S　*Pseudomonas* genes encoding two-component regulatory system that may control synthesis of secondary metabolites

α-D-Gal-(1,4)-α-D-Gal　see **globobiose**

Gal β1-4 GlcNAc　receptor on human cells to which toxin A of *Clostridium difficile* binds

GalNac β1-3 Gal　*N*-acetylgalactosamine linked to galactose by β1-3 bond

GalNac β1-4 Gal　*N*-acetylgalactosamine linked to galactose by β1-4 bond

Gα, Gβ, and Gγ　components making up G proteins

GALT　see **gastrointestinal-associated lymphoid tissue**

Gamma-amino butyric acid　inhibitor of neuronal transmission; release prevented by tetanus toxin

Gamma-delta T cells　immune cells that may play a role in limiting growth of intracellular pathogens; most numerous in intestinal mucosa

Gamma interferon (IFN-γ)　cytokine that stimulates monocytes and PMNs to leave bloodstream; stimulates endothelial cells to produce selectins; helps to activate macrophages

γ-Phage　lysogenic phage closely related to β- and ω-phage of *Corynebacterium diphtheriae*; does not encode diphtheria toxin

Gangrene　death of tissue usually associated with loss of blood supply, bacterial invasion, and putrefaction

GAPDH　see **glyceraldehyde phosphate dehydrogenase**

GAS　group A streptococci (*Streptococcus pyogenes*); most are beta-hemolytic

Gastritis　inflammation of stomach lining

Gastrointestinal anthrax　rare disease characterized by pain, bleeding, fluid-filled vesicles; acquired by ingesting undercooked meat contaminated with *Bacillus anthracis* spores

Gastrointestinal-associated lymphoid tissue (GALT)　mucosal immune system characterized by M cells and production of secretory IgA; a component of MALT

GBS　group B streptococci (*Streptococcus agalactiae*); most are beta-hemolytic

GDP mannose dehydrogenase　first enzyme in the alginate biosynthesis pathway

Gelatinase　protease produced by *Enterococcus faecalis*; synthesis controlled by products of *fsr* genes; similar enzymes produced by some other bacterial species

gelE　gene encoding *Enterococcus faecalis* gelatinase

GelE　gelatinase produced by *Enterococcus faecalis*

Gene amplification　single copy of a gene is replaced by multiple copies

General secretory pathway (GSP, Sec)　pathway through which many proteins are exported from the cytoplasm to the periplasm; requires signal sequence on protein being secreted

Genome　complete set of genes of an organism; includes chromosomes and plasmids

Genome sequence　order of bases in the genome

Genotype　genetic constitution of an organism

Gentamicin　an antibiotic in the aminoglycoside family

Germination　conversion of a bacterial spore to a vegetative state

G$_i$　host cell protein ADP-ribosylated by pertussis toxin; controls adenylate cyclase activity

Giant cells　fused macrophages in vicinity of *Mycobacterium tuberculosis* cells growing in the lung

Gifsy-1, -2　lysogenic phages of *Salmonella typhimurium* that may contribute to survival during systemic phase of the disease

GISA　see **glycopeptide intermediate susceptibility** *Staphylococcus aureus*

GlcNAc β1-3 Gal　*N*-acetylglucosamine linked to galactose by β1-3 bond; found on oral epithelial cells

Globobiose　receptor recognized by P fimbriae of uropathogenic *Escherichia coli*

Glomerulonephritis　inflammation of glomeruli of the kidney leading to kidney malfunction

Glucocorticoids　hormones produced by adrenal glands; downregulate immune system

D-Glutamate　unusual amino acid component of capsule of *Bacillus anthracis*

Glyceraldehyde phosphate dehydrogenase (GAPDH)　protein on surface of *Staphylococcus aureus* that binds transferrin and removes iron; usually associated with glycolysis, not iron acquisition

Glycopeptide intermediate susceptibility *Staphylococcus aureus* (GISA) strains of *S. aureus* that are approaching the point of resistance to glycopeptides

Glycopeptides a group of antibiotics that inhibit peptidoglycan synthesis by binding to D-Ala–D-Ala of peptidoglycan peptides; include vancomycin and teichoplanin

Glycosylphosphatidylinositol (GPI) molecule in macrophage membrane to which CD14 is attached

Glycyl-glycine tetracycline tetracycline derivative designed to overcome resistance to tetracyclines

Glyoxylate cycle pathway that bypasses part of tricarboxylic cycle

G$_{M1}$ a sialic acid residue linked to a ceramide lipid on one type of ganglioside; found in intestinal mucosal cells; host cell molecule to which cholera toxin binds

GM-CSF see **granulocyte-macrophage colony-stimulating factor**

Goblet cells cells that secrete mucus

Golgi system organelle that processes proteins destined for excretion and determines what route they take to their ultimate destination

Gonococcus *Neisseria gonorrhoeae*

Gonorrhea sexually transmitted disease caused by *Neisseria gonorrhoeae*

Granulocyte-macrophage colony stimulating factor (GM-CSF) cytokine that triggers release of monocytes and PMNs from bone marrow into bloodstream

Granulocytes cells of the human nonspecific defense system that contain granules; include PMNs, basophils, and eosinophils

Granuloma lesion containing actively growing fibroblasts, macrophages, and lymphocytes

Granulomatous response cell-mediated response that produces tuberclelike lesions

Granulysin protein produced by cytotoxic host cells that enters infected host cell; lyses intracellular bacteria

Granzymes set of proteases produced by nonspecific cytotoxic cells that enter target cell and initiate apoptosis

Group A streptococci designation of *Streptococcus pyogenes* based on surface carbohydrate antigen; Lancefield grouping system

Group B streptococci designation of *Streptococcus agalactiae* and related species based on surface carbohydrate antigen; Lancefield grouping system

grvA gene encoding GrvA of *Salmonella typhimurium*

GrvA protein (Gifsy-related virulence) of *Salmonella typhimurium* that reduces virulence

G$_s$ a host cell protein that regulates production of adenylate cyclase; target of cholera toxin

Guanylate cyclase human cell enzyme that mediates formation of cGMP

Guanylin a human hormone that binds to guanylate cyclase receptor on intestinal cells; may keep mucin layer wet; *Escherichia coli* ST mimics this hormone

Gumma granuloma in tertiary stage of syphilis

GUS see **β-glucuronidase**

GVVPQ fimbriae thin filamentous adhesins of *Salmonella* and EAggEC

H antigen antigen that is part of flagella; used to identify bacterial serotypes

HACCP see **hazard analysis and critical control point**

Halides disinfectants, such as chlorine and iodine, that oxidize and inactivate bacterial proteins

has **genes** genes encoding enzymes that synthesize antiphagocytic hyaluronic acid capsule of *Streptococcus pyogenes*

Hazard analysis and critical control point (HACCP) program to identify steps in food processing stream where contamination might occur

HB-EGF heparin-binding epidermal growth factor; mammalian cell receptor to which diphtheria toxin binds

Heat-labile toxin (LT) toxin produced by ETEC; similar to cholera toxin in mechanism of action and amino acid sequence

Heat-stable toxin (ST) diarrheal toxin produced by ETEC; STa mimics guanylin, an intestinal hormone

Heavy chain one of two types of protein making up an antibody molecule

Hemagglutination clumping of erythrocytes (red blood cells)

Hemagglutinin substance that agglutinates erythrocytes (red blood cells)

Hematogenous derived from or spread by blood

Hematogenous urinary tract infection kidney infection that results from bacteria being introduced from bloodstream; usually acquired nosocomially

Hemin an iron-containing host protein

Hemin storage phenomenon in which hemin is bound tightly to surface of *Yersinia pestis* at room temperature; iron in the hemin is not nutritionally available to the bacteria

Hemoglobin molecule in the human body that binds iron

Hemolysin protein that causes lysis of erythrocytes (red blood cells)

HEp-2 cells a line of tissue culture cells derived from human epithelial cells

Heparin-binding epidermal growth factor (HB-EFG) precursor mammalian cell-bound hormone; binding site of diphtheria toxin B chain

Hepatotoxin toxin that targets liver cells

2-Heptyl-3-hydroxy-4-quinolone   an autoinducer of *Pseudomonas aeruginosa*

Herd effect   protection of unvaccinated people in a population where most people are vaccinated due to lessened risk of disease transmission

Heterogeneous resistance   in a culture of *Staphylococcus aureus* strains carrying *mecA*, only a subset expresses the gene; rapid selection for that subset occurs when culture is exposed to methicillin

Heteroresistance   another term for heterogeneous resistance; different colonies of a strain of bacteria isolated from a patient vary widely in susceptibility to a specific antibiotic

HGE   see **human granulocytic ehrlichiosis**

Hib   conjugate vaccine against *Haemophilus influenzae* type b; consists of polysaccharide capsular antigen attached covalently to a protein; processed by immune system like a protein

hilA   virulence gene of *Salmonella typhimurium*; part of virulence cascade

Histamine   vasoactive compound released by mast cells

Histonelike proteins   proteins that may function like eukaryotic histones to organize bacterial DNA in supercoiled regions

HLA-DR4   a type of MHC-II complex; associated with development of chronic arthritis due to Lyme disease and other inflammatory diseases

hLFA-1   see **human leukocyte function-associated antigen-1**

hly   gene encoding hemolysin

HlyA   alpha-hemolysin produced by EPEC

HME   see **human monocytic ehrlichiosis**

Hmu (Hms)   heme utilization system of *Yersinia pestis*

HN-S   a bacterial histonelike protein

Holins   phage proteins that form pores in bacterial membranes

Homologs   proteins with similar DNA and amino acid sequences

Hook proteins   protein structures that connect flagellar motor in cytoplasmic membrane to part of flagellum that extends from cell surface

Hospital-acquired infection   see **nosocomial infection**

Host-parasite interaction   relationship between human body (host) and invading microorganism (parasite)

hrpM   *Pseudomonas aeruginosa* gene encoding enzyme involved in synthesis of membrane-derived oligosaccharides; homolog of *mdoH* gene of *Escherichia coli*

htpG   gene encoding heat shock protein in *Vibrio cholerae*; involved in regulation of virulence genes

Human granulocytic ehrlichiosis (HGE)   potentially fatal febrile illness due to *Ehrlichia* species infecting granulocytes

Human leukocyte function-associated antigen-1 (hLFA-1)   protein displayed on the surface of T-helper cells stimulated by APCs presenting OspA peptides of *Borrelia burgdorferi* on their surface

Human monocytic ehrlichiosis (HME)   potentially fatal febrile illness due to *Ehrlichia* species infecting monocytes

Human umbilical vein endothelial cells (HUVEC)   a line of human cells used to study bacterial transit across the endothelium

Humoral immunity   antibody-mediated immunity involving IgG and other serum (humoral) antibodies

HUS   hemolytic uremic syndrome, a complication (kidney failure) of dysentery thought to be caused by Shiga toxin produced by *Shigella* spp. and a similar toxin produced by EHEC

HUVEC   see **human umbilical vein endothelial cells**

Hyaluronic acid   mucopolysaccharide component of extracellular matrix; forms ground substance of connective tissue

Hydrogen peroxide   antiseptic that acts by oxidizing proteins and damaging DNA

Hydroxamate   a class of siderophore

Hydroxyl radical   a reactive form of oxygen that can kill bacteria

Hypersensitive response   protective reaction by plants in which plant R proteins recognize bacterial avirulence proteins and create an area of dry, dead tissue, thus making the bacteria unable to cause serious infection

Hypochlorous acid   reactive form of chlorine toxic to bacteria

Hypotension   collapse of the circulatory system; drop in blood pressure; possible consequence of septic shock

Hypothalamic-adrenal cortex-pituitary axis   connection between nervous system and immune system

icaA,B,C,D   genes encoding enzymes that produce PNSG (a polysaccharide adhesin) on the surface of *Staphylococcus aureus* and *Staphylococcus epidermidis*

ICAM   see **intercellular adhesion molecule**

iC3b   proteolytic digestion product of C3b that opsonizes but does not form C3 convertase

Ice nucleation   formation of ice crystals above freezing point of water; caused by a surface protein of *Pseudomonas syringae*

icm   gene encoding Icm in *Legionella pneumophila*

Icm   part of a type IV secretion system in *Legionella pneumophila*

ID$_{50}$ see **infectious dose**

IEL   see **intestinal epithelial lymphocyte**

IFN   see **interferon**

IgA   the major class of antibody found in secretions; dimeric form in mucus secreted through mucosal membranes

IgE   serum antibody thought to play role in control of metazoal parasites and allergies; monomer

IgG the major antibody class present in the serum; monomer

IgG1 to IgG4 subtypes of human IgG; differ in ability to opsonize and to activate complement

IgM the serum antibody class produced first in response to an antigen; pentamer

IHF see **integration host factor**

IL-1 and IL-6 interleukins 1 and 6; cytokines produced by monocytes and macrophages; normally help regulate activities of cells of the defense systems; excess production may contribute to septic shock symptoms

IL-2 cytokine produced by T cells; stimulates T-cell proliferation; in high levels, causes nausea, vomiting, malaise, and fever

IL-3 cytokine that stimulates release of monocytes and PMNs from bone marrow into bloodstream

IL-8 cytokine that stimulates monocytes, PMNs, and other granulocytes to leave bloodstream and move to site of infection

Imipenem a β-lactam antibiotic

Immortalized cell lines cells that can be maintained indefinitely in culture

Immune mimicry a microorganism makes its surface look similar to surfaces of host cells; prevents the host from mounting an inflammatory response

Immune system collection of phagocytic, cytotoxic, and antibody-producing cells that protect the body from infection; usually used to mean specific defenses

Immunogen an antigen that induces an immune response

Immunogenic ability to elicit a robust antibody or T-cell response

Immunoglobulins antibodies

Immunosuppression suppression of the normal defense response against infection

Impetigo superficial infection of the skin characterized by purulent lesions; usually caused by *Staphylococcus aureus* or *Streptococcus pyogenes*

In vitro an environment outside the body (usually a test tube)

In vivo inside the body

In vivo expression technology (IVET) means of identifying bacterial genes that are expressed only when the bacteria are in the host

Indolyl-galactoside see **X-Gal**

Induced defenses host defenses that are produced only in response to exposure to specific types of bacteria or bacteria in general; include antibodies, cytotoxic T cells, and activated macrophages

Induration hardening of inflamed area due to fibrin deposition by monocytes and macrophages

Infant botulism disease resulting when botulinum toxin is produced by *Clostridium botulinum* colonizing colon of infants and absorbed across colon epithelium

Infection successful colonization of the body by a microorganism capable of causing damage to the body

Infectious capable of causing disease

Infectious dose (ID$_{50}$) number of microorganisms required to cause infection in 50% of experimentally infected animals or humans; a measure of infectivity

Inflammation response of the body to irritants; characterized by redness, swelling, pain, and heat

Inflammatory response mobilization of the nonspecific and specific defense systems; includes PMNs, complement activation, macrophages, T cells, and antibodies

InhA a mycobacterial acyl carrier protein reductase involved in mycolic acid synthesis; inhibited by isoniazid

Inhalation anthrax see **systemic anthrax**

InlA internalin of *Listeria monocytogenes*; binds E-cadherin on host intestinal cells; facilitates adhesion and invasion

inlA and *inlB* genes encoding internalins A and B

InlB internalin important in adhesion and invasion of intestinal cells by *Listeria monocytogenes*

Inoculum suspension of microorganisms introduced into tissue culture or culture medium

Insertion sequences nucleotide sequences associated with transposons that encode a protein (transposase) that allows them to insert in new areas of DNA

Integrase enzyme encoded by phage or other integrating elements; mediates insertion of element into bacterial genome

Integration host factor (IHF) bacterial protein required for bending DNA in many integration and rearrangement reactions

Integrins proteins produced on surface of host cells; allow PMNs to bind to ICAMs on endothelial cells; also function to allow other host cells to adhere to each other

Integron an integrating element that assembles non-integron genes; probably responsible for evolution of plasmids carrying multiple antibiotic resistance genes; forms an operon under control of an integron promoter

Intercellular adhesion molecule (ICAM) a protein of endothelial cells that binds to integrins on PMNs; aids PMN migration out of blood vessels; also produced by other cells

Interferon class of host proteins produced in response to infection; IFN-α and IFN-β associated mainly with control of viral infections; IFN-γ associated with the immune response to many types of infectious agents

Interleukins (IL) protein cytokines produced by monocytes and macrophages; normally function to regulate defense responses; in high levels, mediate inflammation, septic shock, and fever; see also individual ILs

Internalins membrane proteins of *Listeria monocytogenes* involved in adherence and invasion

Intestinal epithelial lymphocytes (IELs) cytotoxic T cells of the mucosal immune system; CD8 composed of γ and δ proteins (γ-δ T cells)

Intimate binding   close association between EPEC and host cells; mediated by intimin

Intimin   outer membrane protein that mediates intimate binding (close association) of EPEC to host cells

Intracellular multiplication   bacteria survive and multiply inside a host cell

inv **genes**   genes encoding outer membrane proteins of bacteria that mediate invasion of host cells

invA-H   genes encoding *Salmonella* invasins or proteins responsible for invasin localization

Invasin   bacterial surface protein that provokes endocytic uptake by host cells

Invasive   capable of penetrating the host's defenses; capable of entering host cells or passing through mucosal surfaces into the bloodstream and spreading in body

Invasive adenylate cyclase   enzyme synthesized by *Bordetella pertussis*; enters host cells and raises cAMP levels

Iron abstinence   strategy used by some bacteria, such as *Borrelia burgdorferi*, that allows them to survive without iron

IS*6110*   insertion sequence found in virtually all *Mycobacterium tuberculosis* strains; used for detecting *M. tuberculosis* in a specimen

IS elements   see **insertion sequences**

Isocitrate lyase   enzyme of the glyoxylate cycle; may play role in persistence of *Mycobacterium tuberculosis* in the lung

Isoniazid   antibiotic effective against mycobacteria; probably inhibits synthesis of mycolic acids

ity   mouse gene that codes for resistance to *Salmonella typhimurium*

IVET   see **in vivo expression technology**

J chain   protein linking IgA monomers or IgM monomers

K antigen   capsular polysaccharide antigen used for classification of *Escherichia coli*

K1 antigen   component of antiphagocytic capsule of *Escherichia coli* strains that cause septicemia and meningitis

K12 strain   a strain of *Escherichia coli* commonly used in the laboratory

Kanamycin   an antibiotic in the aminoglycoside family

katG   gene in *Mycobacterium tuberculosis* encoding catalase-peroxidase; may be responsible for isoniazid resistance

KatG   a catalase produced by *Mycobacterium tuberculosis*

Keratinocyte   stratified squamous cell constituting up to 95% of epidermis; maintains acidic environment of skin; produces keratin and cytokines; acts as antigen-presenting cell

Ketolides   new class of macrolide antibiotics

Knockout mice   mice that have disruptions in specific genes

Koch's postulates   a set of postulates that must be met to prove that a particular bacterial pathogen causes a particular disease

Kupffer cell   fixed macrophage in the liver; antigen-presenting cell of the liver

L pilin   copies of PilE of *Neisseria gonorrhoeae* that are longer than normal

Lactoferrin   host protein that binds iron with high affinity; found in mother's milk and mucin

Lactoperoxidase   a host enzyme found in mucus that produces superoxide radicals

Lactosylceramide   receptor on ciliated respiratory cells to which S2 subunit of pertussis toxin binds

lacZ   gene encoding β-galactosidase, a commonly used reporter gene

LAMP-1, -2   see **lysosomal-associated membrane proteins**

Langerhans cells   a type of antigen-presenting cell found in deep layers of the epidermis

LasA, B   *Pseudomonas aeruginosa* enzymes that act synergistically to degrade elastin

lasA,B   genes encoding LasA and LasB of *Pseudomonas aeruginosa*, which act synergistically to degrade elastin

lasI   gene encoding LasI

LasI   enzyme that produces autoinducer in *Pseudomonas aeruginosa*

LasR   transcriptional activator of genes for LasA, B

Late-stage proteins (LAMP-1, -2)   proteins in membrane of host phagosome that indicate degree of maturation of phagosome

Latency   period of inactivity of infectious agent; potential for reactivation of infection

Latent syphilis   third stage of syphilis; bacteria difficult to find; patient relatively noninfectious; can still cause serious symptoms

Lateral surface   the portion of the membrane of an epithelial cell that is in contact with adjacent epithelial cells

Lcr   regulatory proteins of *Yersinia*; part of a type III secretion system

LCR   see **ligase chain reaction**

lcr **genes**   genes encoding Lcr proteins of *Yersinia* species

LcrV   protein excreted by *Yersinia* into extracellular medium rather than being injected into a host cell by type III system; suppresses cytokine production; regulates opening of type III gated channel

LD$_{50}$ see **lethal dose**

Leader peptide   short amino acid sequences in a bacterial protein that signal the secretion system to secrete the protein; also used to denote short peptide produced during attenuation

Leader region   encodes region at 5′ end of gene that either encodes the secretion signal leader peptide or participates in regulation by attenuation

Lecithin   phospholipid component of host cell membranes

Lecithinase   toxin produced by *Clostridium perfringens*

and other bacteria that cause wound infections; cleaves lecithin and disrupts host cell membrane

lef gene encoding lethal factor of *Bacillus anthracis*

Legionnaires' disease respiratory disease acquired from inhalation of aerosols containing *Legionella pneumophila*

Lethal dose (LD$_{50}$) the number of bacteria or the amount of toxin required to kill half of the animals experimentally inoculated

Lethal factor A (active) portion of lethal toxin of *Bacillus anthracis*; causes macrophages to release cytokines

Lethal toxin A-B protein toxin of *Bacillus anthracis*; responsible for shock and death in systemic anthrax

Leucine response protein (LRP) global regulator of many *Escherichia coli* genes; other bacteria have a similar global regulator

Leukocidin extracellular toxin of *Staphylococcus aureus* that kills leukocytes; S and F components both ADP-ribosylate host cell proteins

Leukocyte white blood cell; includes PMNs, monocytes, T cells, and B cells

Leukotoxin type of protein toxin produced by some bacteria that kills leukocytes

Leukotrienes compounds in host cells that control calcium channels

Lewis antigens carbohydrates found on surfaces of epithelial cells

Lewis antigens x and y carbohydrates on surface of gastric epithelial cells; identical to moieties of LPS O antigen produced by some strains of *Helicobacter pylori*

Lewis b antigen carbohydrate antigen on surface of host cells; receptor for BabA adhesin of *Helicobacter pylori*

Le^x and Le^y see **Lewis antigens x and y**

Ligase chain reaction (LCR) an amplification procedure using one labeled and one unlabeled primer that bind immediately adjacent to each other and are linked by DNA ligase

Light chain one of two types of protein making up the basic antibody structure

Lincosamides a family of antibiotics that binds to the 50S ribosomal subunit and stops bacterial protein synthesis

Lipid A toxic portion of LPS; embedded in the outer membrane; covalently linked to O antigen which protrudes from bacterial surface

Lipid X part of unique LPS of *Bordetella pertussis*; equivalent to lipid A in function

Lipo-oligosaccharide (LOS) component of outer membrane of some gram-negative bacteria; similar to LPS in structure but with a shorter O antigen

Lipoarabinomannan mycobacterial cell wall glycolipid that suppresses T-cell activation

Lipopolysaccharide (LPS) a component of the gram-negative outer membrane; consists of lipid A (the toxic portion), a core made up of a series of sugars, and the O antigen, a long carbohydrate chain; forms the outer leaflet of the gram-negative outer membrane

Lipoteichoic acid (LTA) lipid-linked teichoic acid produced by gram-positive bacteria; lipid can be embedded in the cytoplasmic membrane

Listeriolysin O (LLO) a pore-forming cytotoxin produced by *Listeria monocytogenes*; similar to enzymes produced by streptococci (streptolysin O and pneumolysin)

Long polar fimbriae fimbriae that mediate attachment of *Salmonella typhimurium* to Peyer's patches; encoded by *lpf* genes

Longus a very long pilus of ETEC; similar in amino acid sequence to Tcp of *Vibrio cholerae*

LOS see **lipo-oligosaccharide**

Low-calcium response see *lcr*

lpf **genes** genes encoding long polar fimbriae of *Salmonella*

lps mouse chromosomal locus that determines sensitivity of the animal to LPS

LPS see **lipopolysaccharide**

LPS binding protein mammalian plasma proteins that bind LPS; LPS-LPS binding protein complex binds to CD14 receptors on monocytes and macrophages and stimulates cytokine production

lps **nonresponder** strains of mice that do not mount an inflammatory response to LPS

LPS O antigen see **O antigen**

LPXTG amino acid sequence motif of proteins cleaved by sortase of *Staphylococcus aureus* and other gram-positive bacteria

lrgA gene encoding LrgA; may play a role in protecting *Staphylococcus aureus* from penicillin killing

LrgA bacterial antiholin that may prevent formation of pores in bacteria exposed to penicillin

lrgB gene encoding LrgB; may play a role in protecting *Staphylococcus aureus* from penicillin killing

LRP see **leucine response protein**

LT see **heat-labile toxin**

LT-I and LT-II the two types of LT; LT-I has the same structure and mechanism of action as cholera toxin

LTA see **lipoteichoic acid**

Lumen cavity in an organ or blood vessel

Lyme disease systemic disease caused by *Borrelia burgdorferi*; transmitted to humans by deer ticks

LYMErix vaccine against Lyme disease; consists of OspA of *Borrelia burgdorferi*

Lymph fluid moving through lymphatic system that takes excess liquid from tissues and returns it to bloodstream; monitored by phagocytes for infection

Lymph nodes accumulation of lymphoid tissue positioned along lymphatic vessels; contain most lymphocytes (B and T cells) of peripheral blood; site where bacteria and toxins removed from circulation

Lymphocyte   leukocyte involved in immune response; includes B cells and T cells

Lymphokine   cytokine produced by lymphocytes

Lysis   disruption of membrane and release of contents of a bacterial or host cell

Lysogenic bacteriophages   bacteriophages whose genome can integrate into the bacterial genome; may carry toxin genes

Lysogeny   bacteriophage genome integrated into the bacterial genome

Lysosomal-associated membrane proteins (LAMPs)   proteins in membrane of phagosome that indicate degree of maturation of phagosome

Lysosomal granules   see **lysosome**

Lysosome   mammalian cell granule containing hydrolytic enzymes and other compounds toxic to bacteria

Lysozyme   enzyme that degrades peptidoglycan

LysR   a large family of bacterial transcriptional activators

LytA   protein responsible for autolysis in *Streptococcus pneumoniae*

lytS,R   genes encoding a two-component regulatory system that controls expression of *lrgA* and *B* genes

M (microfold) cells   cells in Peyer's patches that bring bacteria or fragments of bacteria into contact with antigen-presenting cells in the gastrointestinal mucosa (GALT)

M protein   protein fibrils on the surface of *Streptococcus pyogenes*; play antiphagocytic role

M-related proteins   surface proteins related to M proteins of *Streptococcus pyogenes*; bind Fc region of antibodies and receptors on other plasma proteins

MAC   see **membrane attack complex**

Macrolides   family of antibiotics that inhibit bacterial protein synthesis by binding to bacterial 50S ribosomal subunit

Macrophage   large tissue mononuclear cell having phagocytic and antigen-processing activity; develops from monocyte

Macrophage infectivity promoter (Mip)   *Legionella pneumophila* protein that may aid in uptake of bacteria by phagocytes; has peptidyl-prolyl isomerase activity

Major histocompatibility complex (MHC)   protein complexes on the surface of macrophages; bind foreign (e.g., bacterial) peptides and display them on the macrophage surface, where they are recognized by T cells

Major outer membrane protein (MOMP)   a protein found in the outer membrane of elementary bodies of *Chlamydia trachomatis*; provides stability to the membrane

Malaise   not feeling well

MALT   see **mucosa-associated lymphoid tissue**

Mannose-binding lectin   protein produced by liver; binds to mannose found on bacterial surfaces and activates complement; also called a collectin

Mannose-fucose-resistant hemagglutinin   type of hemagglutinin produced by *Vibrio cholerae*; binding to host cells is not inhibited by mannose or fucose

Mannose-sensitive hemagglutinin   type of hemagglutinin produced by *Vibrio cholerae*; binding to host cells is inhibited by free mannose

Margination   flattening of PMNs against blood vessel wall followed by transmigration

Mast cells   tissue cells with granules that contain histamine, heparin, and other substances that affect nerve tissue and that can attract phagocytes to the site of bacterial invasion; also can produce cytokines; important in allergic response

mdoH   *Escherichia coli* gene encoding enzyme involved in synthesis of membrane-derived oligosaccharides

mecA   gene encoding a penicillin-binding protein (PBP2a) in *Staphylococcus aureus* that is not readily inhibited by methicillin

Mechanism of pathogenesis   see **virulence factor**

Membrane attack complex (MAC)   complex consisting of complement components C5b to C9 which binds to LPS and inserts into the gram-negative cell surface and causes lysis of bacteria

Memory B cells   see **memory cells**

Memory cells   T or B cells that persist for long periods in the body; allow body to respond rapidly to second encounter with a microbe

Meninges   membranes covering brain and spinal cord; consist primarily of endothelial cells

Meningitis   inflammation of the meninges

Meningococcus   *Neisseria gonorrhoeae*

Metalloprotease   extracellular protease produced by *Legionella*; hemolytic

Methanol-insoluble ST (STb)   a type of ST peptide produced only by porcine strains of ETEC

Methanol-soluble ST (STa)   a type of ST peptide produced by ETEC that activates guanylate synthase; resembles human hormone guanylin in amino acid sequence

Methicillin-resistant *Staphylococcus aureus* (MRSA)   strains of *S. aureus* resistant to methicillin (as well as other antibiotics); many strains are susceptible only to vancomycin

Metronidazole   antibiotic that must be activated by bacterial flavodoxin; activated form makes breaks in DNA

mexA,B   genes that, along with *oprM*, encode an efflux pump in *Pseudomonas aeruginosa* that externalizes autoinducers

Mga   see **multiple gene regulator in group A streptococci**

MHC   see **major histocompatibility complex**

MHC-I   MHC type that, when bound to an epitope and displayed on the surface of a host cell, triggers activation and proliferation of cytotoxic T cells; found on most cells in body; associated with display of epitopes of intracellular pathogens

MHC-II MHC type that, when complexed with an epitope and displayed on the surface of an antigen-presenting cell, leads to activation and proliferation of T-helper cells; found on only a few cell types (e.g., APCs)

MICA and MICB protein complexes displayed on surface of infected human cells; stimulate gamma-delta T cells

Microarrays chips containing thousands of squares, each with a portion of single-stranded DNA from a particular gene; used to detect expression of genes under a variety of conditions

Microbial surface components recognizing adhesive matrix molecules (MSCRAMMs) surface adhesins of *Staphylococcus aureus* and *Streptococcus* species that bind mammalian extracellular matrix proteins

Microbiota see **resident microbiota;** synonymous with the term microflora

Microbiota shift disease a shift in the population of microbes that normally resides in a particular site, resulting in disease at that site

Microspheres resorbable inert material in which vaccine proteins are encapsulated; serve as a type of adjuvant by slowly releasing vaccine proteins over time

Microvilli fingerlike projections on the apical surface of mucosal absorptive cells; provide a greater area of absorptive surface

Miliary TB disseminated form of tuberculosis

Minicassette regions of pilin genes of *Neisseria gonorrhoeae* that vary in DNA sequence; involved in antigenic variation

Mip see **macrophage infectivity promoter**

mob **genes** genes on mobilizable plasmids that permit them to take advantage of transfer machinery of other, self-transmissible plasmids in the same cell

Mobilizable plasmid a plasmid that is not self-transmissible but can be transferred by a self-transmissible plasmid

MOMP see **major outer membrane protein**

Monobactams a class of β-lactam antibiotics

Monocyte mononuclear phagocyte circulating in blood; differentiates into macrophage when it enters tissues

Morbidity sickness

Mortality fatality

Motif patches of similarity in an amino acid sequence where certain amino acids and their spacing are shared by proteins with similar functions

mpl gene encoding a metalloprotease *of Listeria monocytogenes* that probably has an indirect effect on virulence

MR mannose resistant; refers to pili of *Escherichia coli* that bind to glycolipids on host cells that do not contain mannose; free mannose does not prevent binding

MRSA see **methicillin-resistant *Staphylococcus aureus***

MS mannose sensitive; refers to pili of *Escherichia coli* that bind to glycolipids on host cells that contain mannose; free mannose inhibits binding

MSCRAMMs see **microbial surface components recognizing adhesive matrix molecules**

mucA gene encoding inhibitor of alginate synthesis in *Pseudomonas aeruginosa*

Mucin mucus; complex, viscous, sticky mixture of proteins and carbohydrates covering mucosal membranes; produced by goblet cells

Mucinase bacterial enzyme that degrades mucin

Mucoid wet glistening appearance of colonies of bacteria that produce capsules

Mucoidy term for *Pseudomonas aeruginosa* colonies producing alginate

Mucosa-associated lymphoid tissue (MALT) specialized immune system that protects all mucosal surfaces; includes GALT

MudJ transposon that carries a selectable marker, kanamycin resistance

Multidrug efflux pumps pumps that excrete antibiotics of more than one type from a bacterial cell

Multidrug-resistant tuberculosis tuberculosis caused by bacteria that are resistant to most commonly used antibiotics

Multiple gene regulator in group A streptococci (Mga) response regulator that represses transcription of several virulence operons in group A streptococci

Multiple organ system failure failure of major organs such as the heart, kidneys, and brain; cause of fatality in septic shock

Mupirocin antibiotic effective against most MRSA strains; targets tRNA synthetases; cannot be used systemically because of rapid degradation but is used to clear nasal colonization by MRSA

Muramyl dipeptide cell wall component of *Mycobacterium;* stimulates immune system; triggers cytokine production

Mycobacterium bovis **BCG** strain used as vaccine against tuberculosis

Mycolic acid type of lipid found only in cell walls of *Mycobacterium* and *Corynebacterium* species

Myeloperoxidase lysosomal enzyme that forms hypochlorous acid, which is highly toxic to bacteria

NADPH oxidase enzyme system located in the membrane of phagosomes; produces reactive oxygen intermediates when phagosome membrane fuses with lysosome containing myeloperoxidase

Naked DNA vaccine DNA encoding a vaccine protein; injected directly into muscle cells, which synthesize protein and present it to immune system

Nalidixic acid member of the quinolone family of antibiotics; inhibits DNA gyrase

NAP see **neutrophil activation protein**

Nasal inoculation introduction of a vaccine by inhalation; stimulates the bronchial-associated lymphoid tissue (part of MALT)

Natural killer (NK) cell type of nonspecific defense cell; attacks infected host cells

Natural resistance-associated macrophage protein (Nramp1) macrophage protein once thought to be important in resistance to tuberculosis

Necrosis death of tissue in a restricted area; characterized by chromatin flocculation and disappearance of organelles

Necrotizing fasciitis destructive wound infection caused by *Streptococcus pyogenes*; also called streptococcal gangrene

Neuraminidase enzyme that removes sialic acid residues from oligosaccharide of lumen surface molecule G_{M1}; produced by *Vibrio cholerae* and *Neisseria gonorrhoeae*

Neuronal apoptosis inhibitory protein mouse protein that prevents infection by *Legionella pneumophila*

Neurotoxin toxin specific for nerve cells

Neutralization of the microbe antibodies bind to surface of microbe; prevent attachment of microbe to host cells and facilitate its ingestion and killing by phagocytic cells

Neutropenia decrease in the number of neutrophils (PMNs) in the blood

Neutrophil leukocyte in which granules do not stain with basic or acidic dyes; PMN

Neutrophil activation protein (NAP) inflammatory protein that activates neutrophils

New-new diseases diseases caused by previously unidentified bacteria that have recently entered the human population

New-old diseases diseases caused by newly recognized pathogens that have been around a long time

Nitric oxide reactive nitrogen intermediate found in phagocytes; toxic to microbes

NK cell see **natural killer cell**

NlpE an outer membrane lipoprotein of *Escherichia coli* that may participate in stimulating CpxA to phosphorylate CpxR

Nonfermenter organism that is not capable of fermentative metabolism, e.g., *Pseudomonas aeruginosa*

Nonfibrillar adhesin molecule on surface of *Streptococcus pyogenes* that mediates attachment to fibronectin on host cells

Nonintimate binding first stage in association of EPEC bacteria and host cell; mediated by bundle-forming pili

Nonpilus (nonfibrillar) adhesins adhesive cell surface components that do not form piluslike structures

Nonspecific defense system host defenses that are effective against most bacteria and are always present; include physical barriers, complement, phagocytic cells, and washing action of fluids

Norepinephrine substance produced by sympathetic neurons; suppresses immune system

Normal microbiota see **resident microbiota**

Nosocomial infection infection acquired in the hospital

Nra regulatory protein of *Streptococcus pyogenes* that regulates *mga* and genes encoding other virulence factors

Nramp1 see **natural resistance-associated macrophage protein**

NtrC an activator that controls expression of nitrogen-regulated genes of some bacteria

Nucleation of actin actin filaments form cometlike tails at end of bacteria such as *Listeria* spp.; may propel bacteria through cytoplasm

O139 a non-O1 strain of *Vibrio cholerae*; cause of most recent epidemics of cholera

O157:H7 the major serogroup of EHEC; causes bloody diarrhea and HUS

O antigen polysaccharide side chains on LPS; used as basis for determining serogroup of a bacterial strain

Obligate required

Old-new diseases diseases caused by well-known pathogens thought to have been eliminated but which have recently reappeared

Old-old diseases diseases caused by long-known bacteria which are only recently being noticed by the public

ω-Phage temperate bacteriophage that carries gene encoding diphtheria toxin

OmpA an outer membrane porin of *Escherichia coli*; may be part of a system that mediates invasion of host cells by triggering actin rearrangement

Oncogenic cancer causing

Opa proteins gonococcal outer membrane proteins that may mediate opsonin-independent uptake of the bacteria by PMNs

Opaque colony type colony made up of *Streptococcus pneumoniae* cells that do not bind tightly to oral epithelial cells

Operon unit consisting of structural genes controlled by an adjacent operator

Operon fusion see **transcriptional fusion**

Ophthalmia neonatorum gonococcal infection of eyes of infant; can cause blindness

Opportunist an organism capable of infecting only when host defenses are compromised

OprD porin through which imipenem enters periplasmic space in gram-negative bacteria

oprM one of several genes encoding an efflux pump of *Pseudomonas aeruginosa*

Opsonin antibody or complement component C3b that attaches to the bacterial surface and enhances the ability of phagocytes to ingest the bacterium

Opsonization enhancement of phagocytosis by attachment of antibody or complement component C3b to bacteria

Opsonizing antibodies   antibodies that attach to bacteria and enhance phagocytosis

Oral vaccines   vaccines administered by mouth; stimulate MALT

org   gene on SPI1 of *Salmonella typhimurium;* encodes component of type III secretory system

ORSA   see **oxacillin-resistant** *Staphylococcus aureus*

OspA-D   outer surface proteins (lipoproteins) of *Borrelia burgdorferi*

OspE-related proteins (Erps)   outer surface proteins of *Borrelia burgdorferi* produced during early infection in mammal

Otitis media   middle ear infection; common in children

Oxacillin-resistant *Staphylococcus aureus* **(ORSA)**   new name for MRSA; required because methicillin is no longer used for treatment

Oxazolidinones   a new class of antibiotics; act by binding to 50S ribosomal subunit and inhibiting bacterial protein synthesis

Oxidase test   test in which enzyme produced by bacteria converts colorless substrate (*N,N,N',N*-tetramethyl-*p*-phenylene diamine dihydrochloride) to purple color; used in identification of some bacterial species, such as *Pseudomonas* species

Oxidative (respiratory) burst   production of reactive oxygen intermediates by phagocytes

3-Oxo-decanoate (C12) homoserine lactone (3-oxo-C12-HSL)   autoinducer to which LasR responds; synthesized by LasI

p-**Aminobenzoic acid**   substrate for first enzyme in tetrahydrofolic acid pathway; inhibited by sulfonamides

P fimbriae   major adhesins of uropathogenic *Escherichia coli;* also called P pili

PAF   see **platelet-activating factor**

pag **genes**   (i) PhoPQ-activated genes in *Salmonella;* products affect survival in macrophages; (ii) genes encoding protective antigen in *Bacillus anthracis*

PAI   pathogenicity island in *Helicobacter pylori*

PAI-1   former name of 3-oxo-decanoate (C12) homoserine lactone

PAI-2   former name of C4-homoserine lactone

PaLoc   see **pathogenicity locus**

Pandemic   epidemic involving many different countries

pap **genes**   genes encoding pyelonephritis-associated fimbriae (P fimbriae) in *Escherichia coli*

PapA   major pilus subunit of P fimbriae

PapB, I   regulatory proteins involved in synthesis of P fimbriae

PapC, D, H   processing and assembly proteins involved in synthesis of P fimbriae

PapE-G   adhesin proteins at tip of P fimbriae

Parasite   an organism that lives at the expense of another

Paroxysm   severe attack of symptoms (associated with coughing in whooping cough)

Passive immunization   injecting antibodies against a particular pathogen or toxin into a nonimmunized patient

Pasteurella multocida **toxin (PMT)**   a single polypeptide toxin that interacts with a G protein (G_q), thus disrupting host cell regulatory networks; causes bone destruction and weight loss

Pasteurellosis   disease caused by *Pasteurella multocida*

Patch   a small piece of material containing many tiny prongs; can deliver vaccines via skin

Pathogen   microorganism capable of causing disease

Pathogenicity   ability of a microorganism to cause disease

Pathogenicity island   a collection of genes involved in pathogenesis located together

Pathogenicity locus   pathogenicity island of *Clostridium difficile* containing genes encoding toxins A and B and regulatory proteins

P$_{BA}$ promoter controlling transcription of *papA* and *papB* of *Escherichia coli*

PBP2' (PBP2a)   penicillin-binding protein encoded by *mec* in *Staphylococcus aureus*

PC-PLC   broad-specificity phospholipase of *Listeria monocytogenes;* important in escape from double-membrane vacuole

pCD1   70-kbp plasmid carried by all three *Yersinia* species; carries genes for type III secretion system plus other virulence genes

PCR   see **polymerase chain reaction**

PECAM   see **platelet-endothelial cell adhesion molecule**

pef **genes**   genes encoding plasmid-encoded fimbriae of *Salmonella typhimurium*

Pelvic inflammatory disease (PID)   infection of fallopian tubes

Penicillin-binding proteins   proteins (normally located on outer surface of cytoplasmic membrane) that bind penicillins; include enzymes for peptidoglycan synthesis and turnover

Penicillins   class of β-lactam antibiotics

Peptidoglycan   polysaccharide backbone with peptide cross-links that covers surface of cytoplasmic membrane and gives bacteria their shape

Peptidyl prolyl isomerase   see **macrophage infectivity promoter**

Perforin   protein found in granules of nonspecific cytotoxic cells; forms channels in target host cell membrane

Peristalsis   wave of contractions moving along intestinal tract; moves contents through intestine

Peritonitis   infection of the peritoneal cavity

Peroxidase   enzyme that converts peroxide and NADH to water and NAD

Persistence factors traits that enable *Mycobacterium tuberculosis* to survive in lung for prolonged period of time

Pertactin an adhesin on surface of *Bordetella pertussis*

Pertussis toxin (Ptx) a protein toxin of *Bordetella pertussis*; consists of subunits S1 to S5; S1 ADP-ribosylates G_i, a G factor controlling host cell adenylate cyclase activity

Petechia rash; skin lesion

Peyer's patches follicles in the small intestine that contain cells of the mucosa-associated immune system

PFGE see **pulsed-field gel electrophoresis**

Phagocyte host cell adapted specifically to engulf and destroy bacteria or other foreign particulate matter

Phagocytosis ingestion of foreign particles by a cell

Phagolysosome vacuole resulting from fusion of phagosome and lysosome

Phagosome vacuole resulting from ingestion of particulate material by phagocytes

Pharmacokinetics study of distribution of an antimicrobial or other therapeutic compound in the body

Pharyngitis inflammation of pharynx; sore throat

Phase variation on-off control for some bacterial genes

Phenazine toxin produced by *Pseudomonas aeruginosa*; kills *Caenorhabditis elegans*

Phenotype structural and metabolic characteristics of an organism

Phenotypic modulation transcriptional gene regulation

phoP/Q genes encoding PhoP/Q

PhoP/Q two-component regulatory system of *Salmonella typhimurium*; homologs found in other bacteria

Phosphatidylethanolamine phospholipid commonly found in membranes of prokaryotes and eukaryotes

Phosphatidylinositol phospholipid that acts as a second messenger molecule in eukaryotes

Phosphatidylinositol-specific phospholipase C (PI-PLC) a phospholipase produced by *Listeria monocytogenes*; hydrolyzes phosphatidylinositol; contributes to bacterial escape from primary vacuole

Phospholipase enzyme that removes charged head groups from phospholipids that constitute the lipid bilayer of host cells, thus disrupting the cell membrane

Phospholipase C (i) Plc, an alkaline protease of *Pseudomonas aeruginosa*; may degrade lung surfactant; (ii) PC-PLC, a broad-specificity phospholipase of *Listeria monocytogenes*

Phosphomannomutase enzyme in the alginate biosynthesis pathway

Phosphonomycin antibiotic that inhibits conversion of UDP-NAG to UDP-NAM, an early step in peptidoglycan synthesis

P_I promoter controlling transcription of *papI* of *Escherichia coli*

PI-PLC see **phosphatidylinositol-specific phospholipase C**

PIA see **polysaccharide intercellular adhesin**

PID see **pelvic inflammatory disease**

pil **genes** genes encoding proteins needed for pilin assembly and regulation

pilA pilin structural gene

PilA and PilB two-component regulatory system controlling transcription of *pilE* in *Neisseria gonorrhoeae*; A is activator, B is sensor component

pilB and *pilC* genes encoding proteins involved in pilus assembly

PilC protein necessary for proper assembly and maturation of pili in *Neisseria gonorrhoeae*

pilE gene encoding pilin subunit in *Neisseria gonorrhoeae*

Pili long, thick protein structures on surface of bacteria; mediate adherence by special set of proteins at tip

Pilin protein subunits packed in helical array to form the shaft of a pilus

PilR transcriptional activator that controls expression of pilin structural genes

pilS silent version (i.e., not expressed) of *pilE* (the gene encoding PilE) of *Neisseria gonorrhoeae*

Pla (plasminogen activator protease) aids systemic spread of *Yersinia pestis*

Plant hypersensitive response protective reaction by plants in which plant R proteins recognize bacterial avirulence proteins and harpins, thus triggering local tissue damage that prevents bacteria from spreading

Plaque (i) clear area formed in a monolayer of tissue culture cells when some of the cells are killed by infecting bacteria; (ii) clear area formed by lytic bacteriophage on a confluent bacterial culture; (iii) clear area formed on fibroblast monolayers by *Listeria*; (iv) biofilm on surface of teeth

Plasma noncellular portion of blood; contains elements necessary for clot formation

Plasmid autonomously replicating extrachromosomal DNA segment; most are circular, but *Borrelia* and a few other bacterial species have linear plasmids

Plasmid-encoded fimbriae (Pef) fimbriae that mediate adherence of *Salmonella typhimurium* to microvilli of enterocytes; encoded by *pef* genes

Plasmin enzyme important in dissolving fibrin clots

Platelet-activating factor (PAF) cytokine produced by macrophages; contributes to dilation of blood vessels

Platelet-endothelial cell adhesion molecule (PECAM) protein that helps PMNs move between endothelial cells into bloodstream

Plc see **phospholipase C**

plcA gene encoding PI-PLC in *Listeria monocytogenes*

plcB gene encoding PC-PLC in *Listeria monocytogenes*

PMN see **polymorphonuclear leukocyte**

PMT see *Pasteurella multocida* **toxin**

pMT1 101-kbp plasmid found in *Yersinia pestis*; carries genes (*caf*) for F1 capsule

Pneumococcal surface adhesin A (PsaA) may mediate adherence of *Streptococcus pneumoniae* to pneumocytes

Pneumococcal surface protein A (PspA) surface protein of *Streptococcus pneumoniae* of unknown function; antibodies that bind to it are protective

Pneumocyte type of cell that lines walls of lung alveoli

Pneumolysin (PLO) cytotoxic protein produced by *Streptococcus pneumoniae*; similar to SLO and listeriolysin

Pneumonic plague last stage of plague; *Yersinia pestis* growing in lung macrophages; human-to-human spread by aerosols

PNSG see: **poly-*n*-succinyl-β-1,6 glucosamine**

Polarized mammalian cells have different surface components on different faces of the cell; most mucosal cells are polarized

Poly-Ig receptor receptor on basal surface of mucosal cell to which IgA binds; a portion becomes the secretory piece of sIgA

Poly-*n*-succinyl-β-1,6 glucosamine (PNSG) polysaccharide adhesin on surface of *Staphylococcus aureus* and *Staphylococcus epidermidis*; adheres to plastic

Polymerase chain reaction a method for amplifying a specific segment of DNA in vitro; involves oligonucleotide primers complementary to nucleotide sequences flanking a target sequence with subsequent replication of the target sequence

Polymorphic outer membrane protein (POMP) a protein found in the outer membrane of *Chlamydia trachomatis*; function unknown

Polymorphonuclear leukocyte (PMN) short-lived professional phagocyte that normally circulates in the blood

Polysaccharide capsule one type of capsule that discourages binding of C3b to a bacterial surface

Polysaccharide intercellular adhesin (PIA) sulfated polysaccharide capsule of *Staphylococcus epidermidis* that contributes to biofilm formation

POMP see **polymorphic outer membrane protein**

PorA and PorB outer membrane porin proteins of *Neisseria gonorrhoeae*; cause nucleation of actin

Pore-forming cytotoxin type of toxin that destroys integrity of mammalian cell membrane by forming protein channels in the membrane

Porin protein constituent of pores in the outer membrane of gram-negative bacteria that allows diffusion of nutrients

Positive TB skin test raised, tough red area around site of PPD injection

Posttranscriptional regulation regulation of genes at the level of translation or of protein activity by posttranslational events

Posttranslational activation activation of protein by proteolytic nicking or covalent modification

pOX1 plasmid that contains genes encoding *Bacillus anthracis* toxins and regulatory proteins

pOX2 plasmid carrying genes encoding protein capsule and regulatory proteins in *Bacillus anthracis*

pPCP1 9.6-kbp plasmid found in *Yersinia pestis*; carries genes encoding plasminogen activator (Pla) and other virulence factors

PPD see **purified protein derivative**

ppGpp compound that acts as signal to activate regulatory proteins; part of stringent response system

prfA gene encoding a positive regulatory protein that activates transcription of itself and several virulence genes in *Listeria monocytogenes*

prg genes genes repressed by PhoP/Q in *Salmonella*; encode part of type III secretory system

Primary syphilis first stage of disease; characterized by lesion (chancre) localized at site of infection; curable by antibiotics

Procoagulant factor factor released by endothelial cells; activates coagulation cascade

Progenitor toxin complex containing botulinum toxin and other proteins which probably protect botulinum toxin from digestion in the stomach

Programmed cell death see **apoptosis**

Proinflammatory cytokines cytokines that aid in the process of inflammation

Promoter site on DNA where RNA polymerase binds and initiates transcription

Prophylaxis protection against disease

Prostaglandin fatty acid that stimulates contraction of smooth muscle; produced by most cell types

Protective antigen the B (binding) portion of both edema toxin and lethal toxin of *Bacillus anthracis*

Protein A surface protein of *Staphylococcus aureus* that binds the Fc portion of antibodies

Protein sequence database resource containing sequences of amino acids in specific proteins

Protozoa single-celled eukaryotes that do not have a rigid cell wall

prtF2 *Streptococcus pyogenes* gene encoding fibronectin-binding protein F2

PsaA see **pneumococcal surface adhesin A**

Pseudomembrane sheetlike layer of debris (fibrin, mucin, dead host cells) that covers a large area of the colon (pseudomembranous colitis) or the throat (diphtheria)

pSLT virulence plasmid found in *Salmonella typhimurium*; contains genes encoding adhesins and SpvB

PspA see **pneumococcal surface protein A**

ptsA,B genes required for secretion of pertussis toxin

Ptx pertussis toxin

ptx genes genes encoding pertussis toxin subunits

Pulsed-field gel electrophoresis (PFGE) large pieces of DNA subjected to alternating bursts of electrical field in different directions migrate into gel; used to compare bacterial strains in disease outbreaks

Purified protein derivative (PPD) crude extract of *Mycobacterium tuberculosis* used for skin test for tuberculosis

Purulent associated with formation of pus

Pus accumulation of fibrin, PMNs, and fragments of host cells

Pyelonephritis infection of the kidney

Pyelonephritis-associated pili see **P fimbriae**

Pyocyanin pigment produced by *Pseudomonas aeruginosa*

Pyogenic pus forming

Pyrazinamide antibiotic effective against mycobacteria; mechanism of action unknown

Pyrogenic fever inducing

pYV *Yersinia* virulence plasmids that encode genes for outer membrane proteins (Yops) and for proteins that regulate and aid secretion of Yops

QAC pumps mechanism that mediates *Staphylococcus aureus* resistance to quaternary ammonium compounds

Quaternary ammonium compounds (QACs) disinfectants that intercalate into phospholipid bilayer membranes, causing bacteria to lose essential ions and other small molecules

Quellung test anticapsular antibody test for pneumococci; antibody binding to capsular components makes capsule appear to swell

Quinolones a family of antibiotics that inhibit DNA gyrase

Quinupristin a streptogramin antibiotic

Quorum-sensing system system that recognizes bacterial signal (autoinducer), thus sensing density of bacteria in area; can control activity of either repressor or activator

R domain portion of diphtheria toxin that binds to protein receptor on host cell

R proteins plant resistance proteins that recognize bacterial proteins; part of plant defense systems

Rac G protein targeted by toxins A and B of *Clostridium difficile*

Random-primed PCR random mixture of hexamers used as primers in PCR; mixture of different-sized amplified fragments produced

RAP see **RNAIII activator peptide**

RAPID see **random-primed PCR**

Rational drug design synthesis of chemical designed to bind to and inactivate a host target molecule

rck gene encoding Rck protein

Rck (resistance to complement killing) an outer membrane protein of *Salmonella typhimurium* that prevents insertion of C9 (last step in membrane attack complex formation) and makes the bacteria serum resistant; also serves as an adhesin

Reactivation TB *Mycobacterium tuberculosis* cells which have survived for long periods in walled-off lesions break out of lesion because of immune suppression of host and cause active disease

Reactive arthritis arthritis following an infection; commonly associated with sexually transmitted diseases

Reactive nitrogen intermediates forms of nitrogen that kill bacteria; produced after phagolysosome fusion in macrophages

RegA transcriptional activator of toxin A of *Pseudomonas aeruginosa*

Regulon virulence genes located at different locations have promoter-operator regions that all recognize the same regulatory protein(s)

Reiter's syndrome see **reactive arthritis**

Reporter gene structural gene encoding easily assayable enzyme that is fused to a heterologous promoter region by cloning or other genetic means; used in transcriptional fusions or translational fusions

Resident microbiota population of normally nonvirulent bacteria found routinely in a specific site of the body of most normal adults

Respiratory burst see **oxidative burst**

Reticulate body replicating form of *Chlamydia* species found in vacuoles of infected host cells

Rhamnolipid glycolipid of *Pseudomonas aeruginosa* that solubilizes phospholipids

Rheumatic fever febrile illness that can occur several weeks after a *Streptococcus pyogenes* sore throat; can be accompanied by damage to heart valves

Rheumatic heart disease heart valve damage following rheumatic fever

rhlA,B genes encoding enzymes involved in synthesis of rhamnolipid of *Pseudomonas aeruginosa*

RhlR protein that regulates genes encoding proteins involved in synthesis of rhamnolipid in *Pseudomonas aeruginosa*

Rho mammalian G protein targeted by toxins A and B of *Clostridium difficile*

Ribosome protection bacterial cytoplasmic protein that protects ribosomes from tetracycline

Rice water stool diarrheal fluid of a cholera patient; has appearance of water in which rice has been washed

Rifampin an antibiotic that inhibits bacterial RNA polymerase; also called rifampicin

Rmp surface protein of *Neisseria gonorrhoeae* that elicits blocking antibodies

RNAIII an RNA molecule that downregulates production of MSCRAMMs and upregulates genes encoding exotoxins in *Staphylococcus aureus*; part of Agr system

RNAIII activator peptide autoinducer that activates production of RNAIII

rpoS gene encoding RpoS

RpoS a sigma factor necessary for survival of *Escherichia* *coli* and *Salmonella typhimurium* in stationary phase; many other bacteria have a similar sigma factor

rRNA methylase enzyme that methylates 23S rRNA to block binding of macrolides and lincosamides

RTX toxins pore-forming cytotoxins produced by various strains of bacteria, especially uropathogenic strains of *Escherichia coli*; contain tandem duplications of nine amino acids

Ruffling rufflelike appearance of host cell membrane after actin rearrangement stimulated by *Salmonella* invasion

S a component of leukocidin of *Staphylococcus aureus*; binds to G_{M1} gangliosides; ADP-ribosylates enzyme involved in phospholipid metabolism

S1 toxic subunit of pertussis toxin; ADP-ribosylates G_i

S pili (S fimbriae) pili found on *Escherichia coli* strains that cause neonatal meningitis

Sak see **staphylokinase**

Salmonella enterica **serovar Typhimurium** new name for *Salmonella typhimurium*

Salmonella typhi **Ty21a** attenuated strain used as an oral vaccine against typhoid fever

Salmonella typhimurium **DT104** multidrug-resistant strain responsible for outbreaks in Europe and the United States

Salpingitis inflammation of the fallopian tube; essentially the same as pelvic inflammatory disease

SALT see **skin-associated lymphoid tissue**

Sar see **staphylococcal accessory regulator**

Scalded skin syndrome disease in infants caused by exfoliative toxins of *Staphylococcus aureus*; upper layers of skin peel off

Scarlet fever febrile disease caused by *Streptococcus pyogenes*; characterized by diffuse red rash

SCID mice severe combined immunodeficient mice; lack the ability to produce functional B and T cells

SE see **staphylococcal enterotoxins**

SEA, SEB, SEC1,2,3, SED, SEE different antigenic types of staphylococcal enterotoxins produced by *Staphylococcus aureus*; SEA is the type most commonly associated with food-borne disease

Sec see **general secretory pathway**

Secondary metabolites compounds that appear to have no direct role in energy metabolism or essential biosynthetic reactions; examples are pigments, antibiotics

Secondary syphilis bacteria enter bloodstream; invade heart, musculoskeletal system, and central nervous system; symptoms include fever and rash

Secretory IgA (sIgA) dimerized IgA with two IgA molecules linked by a protein (secretory piece) found in secretions; provides local protection to mucous membranes

Secretory piece a portion of the IgA receptor of mucosal cells that becomes attached to IgA as it passes through the mucosal cells; secretory piece and IgA become sIgA

Selectins surface proteins of endothelial cells; bind to PMNs to stop movement

Self-capping process whereby flexible domains in a protein assume a configuration that discourages dimerization; example is PapD proteins of UPEC strains

Self-transmissible plasmid see **conjugative plasmid**

Sensu lato term used along with a species name to indicate a primary species plus similar species

Sensu stricto term used along with a species name to indicate a single species

Sepsis (i) condition resulting from microbes or microbial products in the blood; (ii) SIRS plus culture-documented infection

Septic shock systemic reaction caused when bacterial cell wall components (LPS, LTA, peptidoglycan fragments) trigger release of host cytokines that have a variety of effects on body temperature control and blood pressure; symptoms include fever, hypotension, DIC, acute respiratory distress, and multiple organ system failure

Septicemia systemic disease in which microorganisms multiply in the blood or are continuously seeded into the bloodstream

Septicemic plague *Yersinia pestis* in the bloodstream

Sequela abnormal condition that develops following a particular disease

Serine (serine-type) protease a family of proteolytic enzymes that contain serine in their active sites; contribute to virulence of certain pathogens

Seroconversion induction of specific antibodies in the serum in response to stimulation by an antigen

Serogroup classification of bacterial strains based on a surface antigen (e.g., O antigen of *Escherichia coli* LPS)

Serological classification (serogroup; serotype) scheme based on reactivity of bacterial surface antigens with antibodies (e.g., O antigen of LPS, H antigen of flagella, C antigen of streptococci)

Serotype classification of bacterial strains within a serogroup based on a surface antigen (e.g., H antigen of *Escherichia coli*)

Serotyping basing classification of bacteria on reactivity of surface molecules with different antibodies

Serum fluid portion of the blood without clotting factors or erythrocytes

Serum resistant bacteria that can resist killing action of serum; in gram-negative bacteria, results from alteration in O antigen so that MAC cannot nucleate around LPS

Serum sensitivity susceptibility of bacteria to killing by serum, i.e., lysis by MAC

Severe sepsis third stage of septic shock characterized by organ dysfunction and low blood pressure

Shiga-like toxin toxin produced by some species of intestinal pathogens; has an activity like that of Shiga toxin

Shiga toxin (Stx)   A-B toxin produced by *Shigella;* cleaves rRNA and stops protein synthesis in host cells; may be responsible for HUS; similar toxin produced by EHEC strains

Sialic acid   nine-carbon sugar found commonly on mammalian cell glycolipids and glycoproteins

Sialidase   see **neuraminidase**

Sic   see **streptococcal inhibitor of complement**

Siderophores   low-molecular-weight compounds produced by bacteria that chelate iron

sIgA   see **secretory IgA**

sIgA protease   enzyme that cleaves human sIgA at the hinge region

sigF   a gene encoding a putative sigma factor in *Mycobacterium tuberculosis;* related to sporulation genes of other species of spore-forming bacteria

Sigma factor (e.g., σ^{28} and σ^{54})   subunit of bacterial RNA polymerase that allows RNA polymerase to recognize a particular class of promoter

Signal transduction   stimulation of bacterial or mammalian cell surface receptor triggers a set of phosphorylation and dephosphorylation reactions that affect gene expression and metabolism

Signature-tagged mutagenesis   a form of transposon mutagenesis used to find mutants impaired in virulence; uses a transposon mixture composed of a number of sequence variants (tags)

Simple epithelium   single layer of epithelial cells covering surfaces where absorption or secretion takes place

SipA   protein of *Salmonella typhimurium* involved in ruffling response

sirA   virulence gene of *Salmonella typhimurium;* part of virulence cascade

SIRS   see **systemic inflammatory response syndrome**

Skin-associated lymphoid tissue (SALT)   specialized set of cells that confront bacterial invaders in the area immediately underlying the skin and attempt to prevent their access to the bloodstream

Slipped-strand mispairing   occurs during DNA replication in regions of highly repetitive sequence; results in frameshift; basis of phase variation of *pilC* of *Neisseria gonorrhoeae*

SLO   see **streptolysin O**

Slow killing   *Pseudomonas aeruginosa* grown in low-salt medium invade tissue of *Caenorhabditis elegans;* kill worm in 2 to 3 days

SLS   see **streptolysin S**

sod   gene on Gifsy-2 phage of *Salmonella typhimurium;* encodes superoxide dismutase

SopE   protein of *Salmonella typhimurium* involved in ruffling response

Sortase   enzyme of *Staphylococcus aureus* that covalently attaches MSCRAMMs to pentaglycine segment of peptidoglycan

spa   a gene on SPI1 plasmid of *Salmonella typhimurium;* encodes part of type III secretion system

Sparfloxacillin   fluoroquinolone active against *Mycobacterium tuberculosis* as well as other bacteria

Spe   superantigens produced by *Streptococcus pyogenes;* have various activities

SpeA   most important streptococcal superantigen; produced by strains that cause toxic shock-like syndrome

SpeB   cysteine protease produced by *Streptococcus pyogenes*

Specific defense system   host defenses produced in response to invasion by specific bacteria or other infectious agents; includes antibodies, T cells, and activated macrophages

SPI1   pathogenicity island in *Salmonella typhimurium* encoding proteins involved in early stages of infection

SPI2   pathogenicity island in *Salmonella typhimurium* encoding proteins that inhibit phagosome-lysosome fusion; important in systemic disease

SPI3   pathogenicity island in *Salmonella typhimurium* encoding proteins that aid survival of bacteria in vacuole of invaded cell

SPI4   putative pathogenicity island in *Salmonella typhimurium;* function unknown

SPI5   putative pathogenicity island in *Salmonella typhimurium;* function unknown

Spirochete   spiral-shaped organism with a cell wall consisting of two membranes with a peptidoglycan layer between them; internal flagella are also located between the two membranes; corkscrew-type motility

Spleen macrophages   fixed macrophages in the spleen

Spore   resistant form of some bacteria derived from vegetative cells

sprE   gene encoding a serine protease in *Enterococcus faecalis*

SprE   serine protease of *Enterococcus faecalis*

SpsA   see ***Streptococcus pneumoniae* surface protein A**

sptP   gene encoding a tyrosine phosphatase in *Salmonella typhimurium* which is injected into host cells by a type III secretion system

Sputum   material coughed up from an infected lung

spvABCD **and *R* genes**   *Salmonella typhimurium* genes required for virulence; carried on pSLT

Squamous cells   flattened scalelike host cells normally found on surfaces, e.g., stomach lining

ST   see **heat-stable toxin**

STa   see **methanol-soluble ST**

Staphylococcal accessory regulator (Sar)   protein required for transcription of *agr* genes in *Staphylococcus aureus*

Staphylococcal enterotoxins (SEs)   superantigens produced by *Staphylococcus aureus*

Staphylokinase (Sak)   exoprotein produced by *Staphy-*

lococcus aureus; inactivates plasminogen, leading to dissolution of clots

STb see **methanol-insoluble ST**

Stem-loop structure structure that forms in mRNA because of the presence of adjacent inverted repeats in the sequence; can be involved in regulation

Stratified epithelium multiple layers of host epithelial cells

Strep throat pharyngitis due to *Streptococcus pyogenes*

Streptococcal gangrene see **necrotizing fasciitis**

Streptococcal inhibitor of complement (Sic) compound produced by *Streptococcus pyogenes* that prevents formation of membrane attack complex

***Streptococcus pneumoniae* surface protein A (SpsA)** protein that binds the secretory component of sIgA

Streptogramins group of antibiotics that act by binding ribosome and preventing translocation of amino acids to growing peptide chain

Streptokinase clot-dissolving enzyme produced by *Streptococcus pyogenes;* activates plasminogen to plasmin

Streptolysin O (SLO) an oxygen-labile hemolysin produced by *Streptococcus pyogenes*

Streptolysin S (SLS) an oxygen-stable hemolysin produced by *Streptococcus pyogenes*

Stringent response system system that responds to starvation for amino acids or other compounds by synthesizing signals such as ppGpp to activate regulatory proteins

Stx see **Shiga toxin**

STX element conjugative transposon in *Vibrio cholerae* O139 that carries genes for resistance to sulfonamide and trimethoprim

stx **genes** genes encoding the subunits of Shiga toxin

Subunit vaccine vaccine that consists of one or a few purified components

Sulbactam an inhibitor of β-lactamase

Sulfatide sulfated glycolipid in membrane of ciliated cells; may be receptor for Fha of *Bordetella pertussis*

Sulfonamides a family of antibiotics that inhibit a bacterial enzyme in the pathway that leads to synthesis of tetrahydrofolic acid

Superantigen toxins that nonspecifically stimulate large populations of T cells to produce cytokines

Superoxide radical a reactive form of oxygen produced during phagocytosis; toxic for bacteria

Surface adhesin molecule on surface of bacteria that recognizes host cell receptor molecule

Surfactant complex mixture of phospholipids and proteins in lung that aid lung function by reducing surface tension of lung fluids; prevent collapse of alveoli

Surveillance programs programs developed to monitor appearance of new diseases, increased incidence of known diseases, and antibiotic-resistant bacteria

Sympathetic neurons part of the nervous system that produces norepinephrine in response to stress

Symptom effect of bacterial colonization that is apparent to the infected person

Synaptobrevins proteins found in synaptic vesicles of neurons; targets of tetanus and botulinum toxins

Syndrome group of symptoms that characterize a specific disease

Synercid antibiotic combination consisting of two streptogramin antibiotics

Systemic affecting the whole organism rather than a specific organ or tissue

Systemic anthrax form of anthrax in which bacteria enter the bloodstream via lungs, cause septic shock; acquired by inhalation of spores

Systemic inflammatory response syndrome (SIRS) the first stage of septic shock

T cell thymus-dependent lymphocyte; T-helper cells activate macrophages or stimulate antibody production by B cells; cytotoxic T cells kill host cells infected by specific intracellular pathogens

T-cell receptor protein complex on surface of T cells; recognizes a specific epitope presented on MHC by an antigen-presenting cell

T domain region of diphtheria toxin responsible for translocation of enzymatically active portion into the cytoplasm

T-helper cells T cells that activate macrophages or stimulate antibody production by B cells; have CD4 on their surface

T-independent antigen antigen such as a polysaccharide or lipid that interacts directly with B cells; bypasses APCs and T cells; stimulates antibody response; no memory cells produced

tag **genes (ToxT-activated genes)** genes of *Vibrio cholerae* that respond to ToxT but for which function is unknown

Tamm-Horsfall glycoprotein most abundant glycoprotein in human urine; blocks binding of some types of pili

TbpA transferrin-binding protein of *Neisseria gonorrhoeae*

tcdA,B genes encoding toxins A and B of *Clostridium difficile*

TcdC protein that inhibits expression of *Clostridium difficile* genes encoding toxins A and B

tcdC,D regulatory genes that control expression of *tcdA* and *tcdB*; located on same pathogenicity island as *tcdA,B*

TcdD protein that activates expression of *Clostridium difficile* genes encoding toxins A and B

Tcp pili toxin coregulated pili; bundle-forming pilus of *Vibrio cholerae*

tcpA gene encoding main pilin subunit of Tcp pili of *Vibrio cholerae*

tcpB gene encoding minor pilin subunit of Tcp pili of *Vibrio cholerae*

tcpC gene encoding outer membrane protein of unknown function in *Vibrio cholerae*

tcpG gene that may encode chaperone involved in pilus secretion of *Vibrio cholerae*

TcpI negative regulatory protein involved in regulation of expression of *toxT* of *Vibrio cholerae*

tcpJ gene encoding peptidase that cleaves terminal signal sequence from TcpA of *Vibrio cholerae*

TcpP, H two-component regulatory system involved in expression of *toxT* gene of *Vibrio cholerae*

Teichoic acids polymers of sugar phosphate (or sugar alcohol phosphate) found interwoven in peptidoglycan of gram-positive bacteria; stimulate cytokine release by host cells, triggering an inflammatory response

Teichoplanin a glycopeptide antibiotic

Telomere end region of eukaryotic chromosome

Temperate bacteriophages bacteriophages that can either integrate into the bacterial chromosome (lysogeny) or enter the lytic cycle and kill the bacteria; some temperate phages carry toxin genes (e.g., diphtheria toxin, SpeA)

Tertiary syphilis terminal stage of syphilis; slowly progressive inflammatory disease; symptoms include heart damage, neurological symptoms, fatigue, skin lesions

tet **genes** regulatory and structural genes responsible for tetracycline resistance

tetA-G genes encoding tetracycline efflux proteins of gram-negative bacteria

Tetanus spastic paralysis caused by tetanus toxin

Tetanus toxin an A-B neurotoxin produced by *Clostridium tetani*; acts by cleaving synaptobrevins; causes spastic paralysis

tetK, tetL genes encoding tetracycline efflux proteins of gram-positive bacteria

tetM,O, **and** *Q* genes encoding proteins involved in ribosome protection

tetR gene encoding a repressor that regulates efflux-type tetracycline resistance genes

Tetracyclines a family of antibiotics that inhibit bacterial protein synthesis by binding to the 30S ribosomal subunit and distorting the A site

Tetrahydrofolic acid an essential cofactor in bacterial pathway leading to formylmethionine and nucleic acid precursors; synthesis prevented by trimethoprim and sulfonamides

tetX gene encoding an enzyme that modifies tetracycline under aerobic conditions

Thin aggregative fimbriae see **curli**; encoded by *agf* genes of *Salmonella typhimurium*

Thiolactone cyclic peptide that acts as autoinducer of *agr* genes of *Staphylococcus aureus*

Tight junctions areas where epithelial cells are joined tightly together by proteins; prevent fluids from moving between lumen and substratum

Tissue plasminogen activator (tPA) protein that activates plasminogen, resulting in an increase in fibrinolytic activity

TLRs see **Toll-like receptors**

TNF-α see **tumor necrosis factor alpha**

Tolerance condition in which bacteria are able to survive exposure to antibiotics even though they cannot divide; bacteria begin dividing again when antibiotic is removed

Toll transmembrane receptor in *Drosophila* required for resistance to fungal infections

Toll-like receptors (TLRs) group of mammalian proteins that interact with LPS and peptidoglycan fragments; may be part of signal transduction cascade; named for Toll receptor in insects

toxA gene encoding exotoxin A of *Pseudomonas aeruginosa*

Toxic shock syndrome (TSS) disease caused by strains of *Staphylococcus aureus* that produce superantigen, toxic shock syndrome toxin (TSST); symptoms include fever, rash, exfoliation of palms and soles of feet, shock

Toxic shock syndrome toxin (TSST) toxin produced by some strains of *Staphylococcus aureus*; superantigen

Toxin A and B toxins produced by *Clostridium difficile*; responsible for symptoms of pseudomembranous colitis

Toxin coregulated pili see **Tcp pili**

Toxin neutralization binding of antibodies to toxins; prevents binding of toxin to host target cell

Toxinoses diseases in which symptoms are due entirely to action of toxins

Toxoid protein toxin that has been treated to destroy its toxicity but retain its immunogenicity

ToxRS regulatory proteins that control the expression of at least 17 genes in *Vibrio cholerae*; regulated genes include those for toxin, pili, serum resistance, and outer membrane proteins; constitute a two-component regulatory system

toxT gene encoding ToxT in *Vibrio cholerae*

ToxT activates expression of *tcp* and other genes in *Vibrio cholerae*; its synthesis is regulated by ToxRS and TcpP and H

tPA see **tissue plasminogen activator**

tra **genes** genes encoding functions necessary for bacterial conjugation

Tracheal cytotoxin peptidoglycan fragment of *Bordetella pertussis* that kills ciliated cells and stimulates release of IL-1

Tracheal rings cross-sections of rodent trachea used to study effects of *Bordetella pertussis* on host ciliated cells

Transcriptional activator   protein that facilitates binding of RNA polymerase to promoter and initiation of transcription

Transcriptional fusion   hybrid gene with promoter-operator of one gene fused to a promoterless structural gene encoding an assayable enzyme

Transcytosis   bacteria taken up in endocytic vesicle of host cell; vesicle passes through mucosal cell, and bacteria exit from vesicle on basal side of host cell

Transduction   transfer of genetic information from one bacterial cell to another by a bacteriophage

Transferrin   a blood and tissue glycoprotein synthesized by the liver; sequesters iron

Transformation   (i) process in which bacteria take up free DNA from the environment; (ii) process by which mammalian cells become tumorigenic

Transglycosylation   process by which *N*-acetylmuramic acid and *N*-acetylglucosamine residues of peptidoglycan are linked to form the polysaccharide backbone of peptidoglycan

Translocation   movement of A subunit of an A-B toxin into the cytoplasm of a host cell

Transmigration   movement of PMNs across blood vessel wall into tissues

Transparent colony type   type of colony produced by strains of pneumococci that bind tightly to GlcNAc receptors on oral epithelial cells and pneumocytes

Transpeptidation   cross-linking of peptide units on separate chains of peptidoglycan

Transposase   enzyme that catalyzes movement of transposons and insertion sequences from one DNA segment to another

Transposon   segment of DNA containing insertion sequences plus one or more genes not related to transposition

Transposon mutagenesis   creation of mutations by inserting a transposon carrying a selectable marker into a gene or its promoter

Traveler's diarrhea   adult version of ETEC diarrhea

Trench fever   systemic disease caused by *Bartonella quintana*; spread person to person by lice

Triclosan   antiseptic-disinfectant incorporated into many plastic products to prevent bacterial damage to plastic; unlike most antiseptics and disinfectants, has a specific target

Trimethoprim   an antibiotic that inhibits an enzyme in the bacterial tetrahydrofolic acid biosynthetic pathway

TSS   see **toxic shock syndrome**

TSST   see **toxic shock syndrome toxin**

tst   gene encoding TSST

Tubercle   walled-off lesion containing *Mycobacterium tuberculosis* cells and damaged tissues; encased in fibrin

Tuberculosis   granulomatous respiratory disease caused by *Mycobacterium tuberculosis*; spread by aerosols

Tumor necrosis factor alpha (TNF-α)   a cytokine produced by monocytes and macrophages in response to LPS

Two-component regulatory system   one protein senses the signal, then phosphorylates second protein to produce the form that activates transcription

Type 1 fimbriae   fimbriae found on the surface of *Salmonella typhimurium*; encoded by *fim* genes; binds mannose residues on host cells

Type 1 pili   pili commonly found on many *Escherichia coli* strains, both resident microbiota and pathogens; bind mannose residues on host cells

Type I pneumocytes   flat pneumocytes; *Streptococcus pneumoniae* does not bind well to this type of pneumocyte

Type I secretion system   specialized bacterial proteins that mediate excretion of pore-forming cytotoxins, possibly through a pore that spans outer and cytoplasmic membranes

Type I toxin   toxin that is not translocated into host cell; may or may not bind specific receptors on host cell; example is superantigens

Type II pneumocytes   cuboidal pneumocytes; *Streptococcus pneumoniae* preferentially binds this type of pneumocyte

Type II secretion system   bacterial secretion system that relies on the general secretory pathway (Sec)

Type II toxin   toxin that acts on host cell membrane; examples are phospholipase, pore-forming cytotoxins

Type III secretion system   toxic proteins are injected directly from the cytoplasm of the bacterium into the cytoplasm of the host cell

Type III toxin   classical A-B type toxin; has binding (B) region that recognizes specific receptor, translocation region, and A portion that enters host cell cytoplasm and inactivates host protein

Type IV secretion system   protein-nucleic acid complexes injected directly from cytoplasm of one cell into another; often associated with conjugal transfer of DNA from one bacterium to another; also may inject proteins that are not complexed with DNA, such as pertussis toxin from bacterium to eukaryotic cell

Type 4 (type IV) pili   pili in which pilin subunit is processed so that the first amino acid in mature protein is *N*-methylphenylalanine

uidA   gene encoding *Escherichia coli* β-glucuronidase (GUS); a reporter gene used to create transcriptional fusions

Ulcer   circumscribed area of inflammation characterized by necrosis

Umbrella cells   a layer of poorly differentiated, multinucleate cells making up the uroepithelium

Unidentified reading frame (urf)   gene whose sequence has no similarity to any gene of known function

UPEC   uropathogenic *Escherichia coli*

Urease an enzyme that hydrolyzes urea to ammonia and CO_2

Urethritis infection of the urethra

Urf see **unidentified reading frame**

Uroepithelium epithelium lining the urinary bladder

Uropathogenic strain strain that causes urinary tract infections

Uroplakins transmembrane proteins found on the surface of top uroepithelial layer; site of attachment of type 1 pili of UPEC

UTI urinary tract infection

VacA see **vacuolating cytotoxin A**

Vaccination stimulation of a specific immune response by administering a vaccine

Vaccine suspension of microorganisms (usually killed or attenuated) or their nontoxic products that elicit a protective immune response

Vacuolating cytotoxin A (VacA) cytotoxin produced by *Helicobacter pylori* that causes vacuoles to form in cultured mammalian cells

Valence number of antigen-binding sites of an antibody that are available for binding epitopes on an antigen

vanA,B **genes** genes encoding enzyme that makes D-Ala-D-lactate; mediate resistance to vancomycin

Vancomycin a glycopeptide antibiotic

Vancomycin intermediate susceptibility *Staphylococcus aureus* (VISA) strains of *S. aureus* that are approaching the point of being resistant to vancomycin

Vancomycin-resistant enterococci (VRE) strains of *Enterococcus* (usually *E. faecium*) that are resistant to vancomycin; common cause of nosocomial infections

vanH gene encoding lactate dehydrogenase; catalyzes conversion of pyruvate to lactate; part of vancomycin resistance pathway

vanX gene encoding enzyme that cleaves D-Ala from D-Ala-D-Ala; part of vancomycin resistance pathway

Variable membrane protein (Vmp) antigenically variable surface protein of *Borrelia hermsii*

Vascular containing a blood supply; such sites called vascularized

Vasoactive compounds compounds released by mast cells; dilate blood vessels

Vasodilation dilatation of blood vessels

Vector transmitter of infectious microorganisms

Verotoxin Shiga-like toxin produced by some strains of *Escherichia coli*

Vesicle (i) internal membrane-enclosed sac of eukaryotic cells involved in phagocytosis; also called endosome or (in professional phagocytes) phagosome; (ii) blister

Vi antigen *Salmonella typhi* capsule composed of N-acetylglucosamine uronic acid

Vibrio cholerae **pathogenicity island** see **VPI**

Villi projections from the mucosa of the intestine; covered by a layer consisting of differentiated absorptive cells, goblet cells, and intraepithelial lymphocytes

Virginiamycin streptogramin used as feed additive; elicits cross-resistance to streptogramins used in human treatment

Virotype variant of a particular species of bacteria that exhibits different disease strategies and different virulence factors

Virotyping classification scheme based on virulence factors; e.g., *Escherichia coli* strains

Virulence ability of an organism to cause disease

Virulence factor (virulence mechanism) bacterial product or strategy that contributes to the ability of the bacterium to cause infection

Virulence plasmid a plasmid that carries virulence genes; example is pSLT of *Salmonella typhimurium*

VISA see **vancomycin intermediate susceptibility *Staphylococcus aureus***

Vls (Vmp-like sequence) protein antigenically variable protein on the surface of *Borrelia burgdorferi*

VlsE a Vls protein found on the surface of *Borrelia burgdorferi*

vncS gene encoding one component of a two-component regulatory system involved in vancomycin tolerance in *Streptococcus pneumoniae*

VPI *Vibrio cholerae* pathogenicity island; genome of filamentous phage VPIPhi

VPIPhi filamentous phage that infects *Vibrio cholerae*; genome is *V. cholerae* pathogenicity island

VRE vancomycin-resistant enterococci

Walking pneumonia atypical pneumonia caused by *Mycoplasma pneumoniae*

Wassermann test test that detects anti-cardiolipin antibodies; nonspecific test for syphilis

Water-borne infections infections due to bacteria acquired from contaminated water

Wound botulism caused by botulinum toxin produced by *Clostridium botulinum* growing in a wound

X-Gal a chromogenic substrate for β-galactosidase

Xcp secretion system of *Pseudomonas aeruginosa*

xcp **genes** genes encoding a protein transport system in *Pseudomonas aeruginosa*

xid mouse genes required for normal rate of synthesis of IgG and IgM

YadA see *Yersinia* **adhesin A**

yadA **genes** genes encoding *Yersinia* adhesin A

Yersinia **adhesin A** adhesin-invasin protein in *Yersinia* species

Yersinia **murine toxin** protein that is probably not a toxin; appears important for *Yersinia pestis* colonization of flea gut

Yersinia **outer membrane protein (Yop)** component of the type III secretion system of *Yersinia* species

***Yersinia* secretion (Ysc)**   component of the type III secretion system of *Yersinia* species

Yersiniabactin   iron-binding siderophore of *Yersinia* species and UPEC

Yfe   part of the iron sequestration system of *Yersinia* species

Yfu   part of the iron sequestration system of *Yersinia* species

***ymt* genes**   see ***Yersinia* murine toxin**

yop   gene encoding a Yop

Yops   secreted proteins of *Yersinia;* some are part of type III secretion system; others are toxic to eukaryotic cells

ysc   gene encoding *Yersinia* secretion; part of type III secretion system

14–3-3 Zeta protein   host protein that activates ExoS injected by *Pseudomonas aeruginosa* into host cells; formerly called FAS

Zinc-requiring endopeptidases   family of enzymes that hydrolyze peptide bonds and require zinc for activity; examples are tetanus and botulinum toxins

Zn-dependent metalloprotease (Mpl)   enzyme that may have an indirect effect on virulence in *Listeria monocytogenes*

Zonula occludens   see **tight junctions**

Zoonosis   animal disease that can be transmitted to humans

zot   gene encoding Zot toxin

Zot (zonula occludens toxin)   an enterotoxin of *Vibrio cholerae* that disrupts tight junctions; part of CTX phage

Index

525